TEXTBOOK OF CYSTIC FIBROSIS

JOHN D. LLOYD-STILL

WITH CONTRIBUTIONS

John Wright • PSG Inc

Boston Bristol London

1983

Library of Congress Cataloging in Publication Data

Lloyd-Still, John D.
Textbook of cystic fibrosis.

Bibliography: p.
Includes index.
1. Cystic fibrosis. I. Title. [DNLM: 1. Cystic fibrosis. WI 820 T355]
RC858.C95L56 1983 616.3′7 82-13586
ISBN 0-7236-7026-9

Published simultaneously by:
John Wright • PSG Inc, 545 Great Road, Littleton, Massachusetts 01460, U.S.A.
John Wright & Sons Ltd, 823–825 Bath Road, Bristol BS4 5NU, England

Medicine is an ever-changing science. As new research and clinical experience broaden our knowledge, changes in treatment and drug therapy are required. The authors and the publisher of this work have made every effort to ensure that the treatment and drug dosage schedules herein are accurate and in accord with the standards accepted at the time of publication. Readers are advised, however, to check the product information sheet included in the package of each drug they plan to administer to be certain that changes have not been made in the recommended dose or in the indications and contraindications for administration. This recommendation is of particular importance in regard to new or infrequently used drugs.

Printed in Great Britain.
Bound in the United States of America.

International Standard Book Number: 0-7236-7026-9

Library of Congress Catalog Card Number: 82-13586

TO ALL PATIENTS AND FAMILIES
WITH CYSTIC FIBROSIS.

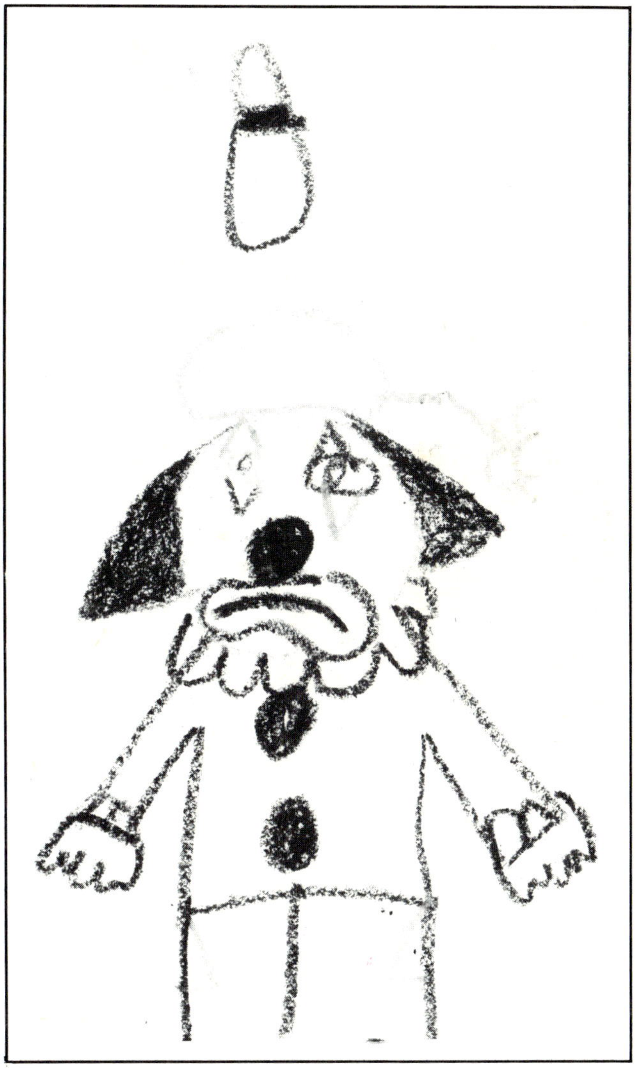

ABOUT THE AUTHOR

DR. JOHN D. LLOYD-STILL

qualified M.B.B.S. from Guys Hospital Medical School, University of London in 1960. He obtained the M.R.C.P. London in 1964. After working at Guys Hospital and the Hospital for Sick Children, Great Ormond Street, he became a senior registar in Pediatrics at St. Mary's Hospital. From 1968 to 1969 he was a Fulbright scholar on exchange at the Children's Hospital Medical Center in Boston. In 1970 Dr. Lloyd-Still returned to the United States where he was a fellow in the Nutrition Clinic at Children's Hospital Medical Center, Harvard Medical School where he worked with Dr. Harry Shwachman. From 1971 to 1972 he was a Fellow of The National Cystic Fibrosis Research Foundation before becoming Assistant Professor of Pediatrics at the Pennsylvania State College of Medicine in Hershey, Pennsylvania. At present he is Associate Professor of Pediatrics at Northwestern University, Director of the Cystic Fibrosis Center and Head of the Division of Gastroenterology at the Children's Memorial Hospital, Chicago.

Dr. Lloyd-Still is a Fellow of the American Academy of Pediatrics, and among his other memberships are included the Society for Pediatric Research, the American Gastroenterological Association, the North American Society for Pediatric Gastroenterology, and the American Association for the Study of Liver Disease. He has been a consultant in cystic fibrosis to state clinics in Massachusetts, New Hampshire, Pennsylvania, and Illinois. From 1978 to 1982 he was a member of the Center Committee of the Cystic Fibrosis Foundation, and in that capacity visited many major Cystic Fibrosis Centers throughout the United States.

Dr. Lloyd-Still has worked in many contrasting environments, including The National Health Service, the West Indies, and urban and rural areas in the United States. He was instrumental in establishing a child abuse team in rural Pennsylvania. His research interests have included various gastrointestinal disorders of children, especially protracted diarrhea of infancy, cystic fibrosis, and the effects of malnutrition on intellectual development. He has published over 50 journal articles and edited a book on malnutrition and intellectual development.

CONTRIBUTORS

David Baswell, MD
Clinical Instructor in Pediatrics
State University of New York at Buffalo
Fellow, Division of Gastroenterology and Nutrition
Children's Hospital of Buffalo
Buffalo, New York

Robert J. Beall, PhD
National Director
Cystic Fibrosis Foundation
Rockville, Maryland

Thomas F. Boat, MD
Professor and Chairman
Department of Pediatrics
University of North Carolina School of Medicine
Chapel Hill, North Carolina

Pi-Wan Cheng, PhD
Assistant Professor of Pediatrics
Case Western Reserve University
Rainbow Babies and Childrens Hospital
Cleveland, Ohio

Brian Davis, MD
Assistant Professor of Pediatrics and Medicine
Cardiovascular Research Institute
Departments of Pediatrics and Medicine
University of California San Francisco
San Francisco, California

Pamela B. Davis, MD, PhD
Assistant Professor of Medicine
Case Western Reserve University
Pulmonary Division, VAMC
Cleveland, Ohio

Philip M. Farrell, MD, PhD
Professor of Pediatrics
Department of Pediatrics and Nutritional Sciences
University of Wisconsin
Director, Cystic Fibrosis Center
Head, Division Pulmonary Medicine
Clinical Sciences Center
Madison, Wisconsin

Lewis E. Gibson, MD
Professor and Chairman
Department of Pediatrics
Loyola University
Stritch School of Medicine
Maywood, Illinois

Orville C. Green, MD
Professor of Pediatrics
Northwestern University
Head, Division of Endocrinology
Children's Memorial Hospital
Chicago, Illinois

Catharine J. Harris, MD
Fellow, Division of Genetics
Children's Memorial Hospital
Chicago, Illinois

Van S. Hubbard, MD, PhD
Senior Investigator
Pediatric Metabolism Branch
National Institutes of Arthritis, Diabetes and Digestive and Kidney Diseases
Bethesda, Maryland
Associate Professor of Child Health and Development
George Washington University

Sherry L. Keramidas, PhD
Associate Medical Director
Cystic Fibrosis Foundation
Rockville, Maryland

Franklin P. Koontz, PhD
Professor of Pathology
Director of Clinical Microbiology
University of Iowa
University of Iowa Hospitals and Clinics
Iowa City, Iowa

John V. Lavigne, PhD
Assistant Professor of Psychiatry and Pediatrics
Northwestern University
Children's Memorial Hospital
Chicago, Illinois

Emanuel Lebenthal, MD
Professor of Pediatrics
State University of New York at Buffalo
Chief, Division of Gastroenterology and Nutrition
Children's Hospital of Buffalo
Buffalo, New York

Dorothy M. Lloyd-Still, MSW, MPA
Assistant Director
Mental Health Board
City of Evanston
Evanston, Illinois

John D. Lloyd-Still, MD
Associate Professor of Pediatrics
Northwestern University
Head, Division Gastroenterology
Director, Cystic Fibrosis Center
Children's Memorial Hospital
Chicago, Illinois

Richard B. Moss, MD
Assistant Professor of Pediatrics
Stanford University
Allergy-Pulmonary Division
Children's Hospital at Stanford
Palo Alto, California

Martin G. Myers, MD
Professor of Pediatrics
University of Cincinnati
Director of Infectious Disease
Children's Hospital Medical Center
Cincinnati, Ohio

Jay A. Nadel, MD
Professor of Medicine, Physiology and Radiology
Cardiovascular Research Institute
Departments of Medicine and Physiology
University of California San Francisco
San Francisco, California

Henry L. Nadler, MD
Dean, Wayne State University
School of Medicine
Professor of Pediatrics
Wayne State University
Detroit, Michigan

Mark V. Pauly, PhD
Professor of Economics
Department of Economics
Northwestern University
Evanston, Illinois

John G. Raffensperger, MD
Professor of Surgery
Northwestern University
Head, Division of General Surgery
Children's Memorial Hospital
Chicago, Illinois

Thomas W. Riggs, MD
Assistant Professor of Pediatrics
Northwestern University
Director of Echocardiography, Division of Cardiology
Willis J. Potts Children's Heart Center
Children's Memorial Hospital
Chicago, Illinois

Harry Shwachman, MD
Emeritus Professor of Pediatrics
Harvard University
Formerly Head, Division of Clinical Nutrition
Children's Hospital Medical Center
Boston, Massachusetts

Lawrence G. Tomasi, MD, PhD
Assistant Professor of Pediatrics and Neurology
Northwestern University
Head, Division of Neurology
Children's Memorial Hospital
Chicago, Illinois

Miles Weinberger, MD
Professor of Pediatrics
Director, Division of Allergy and Pulmonary Diseases
University of Iowa
University of Iowa Hospitals and Clinics
Iowa City, Iowa

Hans U. Wessel, MD
Professor of Pediatrics and Engineering Sciences
Northwestern University
Director of Pulmonary Function and Exercise Laboratory
Division of Cardiology
Willis J. Potts Children's Heart Center
Associate Director Cystic Fibrosis Center
Children's Memorial Hospital
Chicago, Illinois

CONTENTS

SECTION TWO

CLINICAL MANIFESTATIONS

PREFACE

The term, *cystic fibrosis,* was introduced by Dorothy Andersen when she described this new pathological entity in 1938. A decade later Sidney Farber indicated the pathogenesis of the disease by renaming it, *mucoviscidosis,* a term still used in Europe, suggesting thick secretions of mucous glands.

The disease was initially thought to involve the exocrine pancreas, hence was manifested by gastrointestinal complaints and failure to thrive. However, in a very short time, the genetic and generalized nature of the disease was recognized. A significant advance in the pathophysiology was the discovery of the abnormal sweat gland secretions by Paul di Sant' Agnese in 1952. Within a few years the sweat test was developed in Boston and became the most widely accepted diagnostic procedure. It displaced the difficult and cumbersome test of pancreatic function. This led to the discovery of unrecognized cases, and helped support the concept that cystic fibrosis is a heterogeneous disease. At the same time, treatment was improved by dietary adjustments with the use of pancreatin with each meal, the administration of antibiotics, chest physical therapy, and careful periodic examinations.

These improvements are impressively reflected in mortality figures over the past 45 years. At The Children's Hospital Medical Center in Boston, as an example, most infants diagnosed in the late 1930s and in the 1940s died under two years of age. In the last five years, since 1978, and with an increasing number of patients, only two infants died under two years of age. Fifty percent of the estimated 35,000 patients with cystic fibrosis in the United States and Canada are living beyond the age of 20. The quality of life has improved immeasurably. Many adult patients have completed college and graduate education, and work in a variety of professions. Among the married patients, over 100 have had healthy children. Only three of these women have had children with cystic fibrosis.

The practitioner may harbor some common misconceptions about cystic fibrosis which will be dispelled in this volume: 1) That it is a rare disease, 2) that the patient looks too well to have cystic fibrosis, 3) that he/she needs to have some degree of pancreatic insufficiency in order to make a diagnosis, and 4) that there are few adults with cystic fibrosis. Also he may fail to recognize that the male with cystic fibrosis has abnormal wolffian duct derivatives leading to azospermia in the adult.

To date there is no method to detect the heterozygote, hence the physician is unable to provide reasonable genetic counseling, there is still no acceptable screening method of testing newborns for cystic fibrosis, and finally prenatal tests are not accepted as reliable or practical.

Dr. John Lloyd-Still presents a thorough discussion of the many problems in understanding cystic fibrosis.

HARRY SHWACHMAN, MD
Professor of Pediatrics, Emeritus
The Children's Hospital Medical Center
Boston, Massachusetts

ACKNOWLEDGMENTS

This *Textbook on Cystic Fibrosis* is the result of over two years of planning. I am deeply indebted to all the contributors to the book. These individuals, most of whom are well-known both nationally and internationally for their studies of the disease, were selected for their ability to critically evaluate their particular area of expertise in an unbiased manner. I am especially grateful to my associate, Dr. Hans Wessel, who has discussed, reviewed, criticized, and generally kept me on a level keel. Other members of our cystic fibrosis clinic team who have contributed their ideas include Ms. Alice Smith, Ms. Caroline Utech, and Ms. Sally Gorman. Special thanks are due to my colleagues, Drs. Stanford Shulman, Joel Charrow, John Lavigne, Frank Crussi, Jerry Kraut, and Sandra Fernbach who have reviewed specific chapters. I must acknowledge the unfailing courtesy, cooperation, and expertise of Ms. Leslie Goodale and the staff of the Brennemann Library. The expert illustrations and photography were done by Mr. Andrew Piper and Mr. Angelo Matas in our Audio Visual department. Very special thanks are due to my secretary, Ms. Sophie Podyma, who has been instrumental in the completion of the manuscript. From the publishers I have had the utmost cooperation and encouragement, and would like to express my gratitude to Dr. William T. Strauss, Dr. Frank N. Paparello, Ms. Bette J. Aaronson, and Mr. Steve L. Weaver.

Lastly, I would like to acknowledge my indebtedness to all my teachers, especially to Dr. Harry Shwachman who introduced me to the study of cystic fibrosis.

INTRODUCTION

Cystic fibrosis (CF) is the most common genetic disorder afflicting Caucasians. The disease is second only to asthma as a cause of chronic respiratory disease in childhood and is responsible for the majority of deaths from lung disease in this age group (especially since the dramatic improvements in the intensive care of the premature infant during the last decade). For patients and their parents, CF remains a grim sentence, usually prolonged through an unhappy adolescence to a sad, inevitable end.[1]

It cannot be stressed too strongly that cystic fibrosis is not a lung disease or a pancreatic disease, but a "generalized metabolic disorder" affecting derivatives of all three germ layers. During the last 40 years the clinicopathological features of cystic fibrosis have been clearly delineated. Thus, most new clinical observations will likely be the result of increased longevity, iatrogenic complications, and possibly an increased risk of carcinogenesis.[2,3] Since the basic gene defect is unknown, treatment is largely directed to preventing the complications of the disorder. Moreover, research is hampered by the lack of an animal model for the disease.

How does the student of cystic fibrosis approach the disease? The English and foreign language literature is vast and overwhelming. The most comprehensive approach would be to use the *Index Medicus.* This is, however, a formidable undertaking; in 1981 alone there were 243 references annotated under cystic fibrosis. The *Comprehensive Bibliography of the Medical Literature, 1813–1972,* an excellent review of the older literature, contains 5184 references to cystic fibrosis.[4] For a number of years the Cystic Fibrosis Foundation published quarterly annotated references of the literature with editorial comments, but these summaries were discontinued in 1978 with the explosion of publications. A recent publication of the Cystic Fibrosis Foundation called "Spectrum" has an updated bibliography on the disease.

"International" congresses on CF, organized by the International Cystic Fibrosis Foundation, are held at four-year intervals.

The proceedings are published in book form and usually contain the most current research to that date. The most recent international congress was held in Toronto, Canada, in 1980 and extensive references are made in the various chapters to the proceedings of that conference. The European Working Group for Cystic Fibrosis has annual meetings on recent advances in CF research; the proceedings are published in book form.[5] In the United States, the Cystic Fibrosis Club, comprising all the CF center directors and other personnel and research workers involved with the disease, organizes an annual meeting with the abstracts published by the Cystic Fibrosis Foundation.[6] Major research advances in the disease are presented at these annual meetings.

Other specific publications include the reports of the "guidance, action, projection" (GAP) conferences published by the Cystic Fibrosis Foundation and usually held once a year on a subject of topical interest. Several comprehensive reviews on CF are widely quoted in this textbook; especially useful are those on research by di Sant'Agnese and Talamo[7] and di Sant'Agnese and Davis,[8] on pulmonary disease by Wood et al,[9] and on gastrointestinal manifestations by Park and Grand.[10] Clinical descriptions of the disease are included in the major textbooks of pediatrics, medicine, metabolic disease, and genetics, but space limitations necessitate exclusion of many important manifestations of cystic fibrosis. The Cystic Fibrosis Foundation publishes a number of useful, practical booklets related to various aspects of the disease, such as genetics, diagnosis, drug therapy, teacher's guides, a guide for young adults, facts on reproduction, and vocational rehabilitation; these are discussed in Chapters 26 and 28.

The major objective in writing this textbook on cystic fibrosis was to assimilate some of this mass of data into a comprehensive reference source for a wide variety of practicing physicians, research workers, health personnel, and other students interested in the disease and/or involved in the care of these patients and their families. The book makes no pretention to include every publication on cystic fibrosis, which would have added enormously to the length, but the authors have deliberately tried to be discriminating in their selection of relevant, authoritative references. The format of the book has Chapters 1 to 11 presenting basic science aspects, and the remaining chapters presenting the clinical manifestations and complications of the disease.

Subjects covered include the genetics of cystic fibrosis, heterozygote detection, antenatal detection, and newborn screening. Despite what initially appear to be major advantages for early detection of CF, detailed examination of newborn screening programs (none of which are at present sufficiently reliable to recommend for practical use) has elicited serious problems that will have to be resolved before any program can be administered. The chapter on pathology emphasizes the classic descriptions of the disease published in the 1930s and 1940s. Since most infants with CF now survive, these histologic observations will rarely be available to current researchers. Statements regarding morphologic findings, especially those involving the mucous content of various organs such as the lungs and intestine, must be quantified by comparison with "disease" and "normal" controls.

The next five chapters (sweat abnormalities, control of secretions, glycoprotein abnormalities, cystic fibrosis factors, calcium and mucous alterations) deal with areas where many abnormal observations have been documented. Unfortunately, these changes have frequently been unreproducible, inconsistent, and difficult to interpret. The sweat abnormality is the basis for the diagnosis of the disease, but even here confusion exists in the significance of so-called "borderline" sweat values which presently account for about 5% of patients seen in large CF clinics.

The focus of current research has returned to Farber's[11] hypothesis that the primary defect may lie in the control of secretions throughout the body. The current status of this extremely difficult subject is reviewed by two authorities in this field. At present we do not know whether the abnormal gene has its primary effect on the cell membrane, in changing sodium transport or glycoprotein synthesis, whether it acts within the cell on oxygen consumption or calcium homeostasis, or whether it regulates secretion in epithelial cells.[1] The chapters on glycoproteins, cystic fibrosis factors, and calcium changes address these possibilities. While none of these come to specific conclusions, some provocative hypotheses have been suggested as possibilities for treatment in the future, including efforts to lower the calcium concentration of CF exocrine secretions, and using amiloride, an inhibitor of active sodium reabsorption, to return the excess electrical activity present in the cells in CF airways to normal.[12]

Perhaps nowhere in the care of patients with CF is there more controversy among physicians than in the therapy of their pulmonary disease. The chapter on lower respiratory infections reflects this confusion, and the authors rightly criticize us for our past failures to have addressed these problems by proper design of multicentered controlled trials of the various therapies such as prophylactic antibiotic usage, aerosol antibiotics, etc, as to their efficacy (these are currently in the planning stage by the Cystic Fibrosis Foundation). Similar considerations apply to the prophylactic use of oxygen to prevent nocturnal hypoxemia and reverse the pulmonary hypertension. This treatment is currently undergoing controlled trial.

In the past, the immunological status of patients with CF was considered to be normal, but the chapter on immunity, immunodeficiency, and hypersensitivity demonstrates the error of this statement. Numerous changes in immunological status occur in CF, and one can no longer deny the importance of the hypersensitivity disorders, such as aspergillosis, in these patients.

At one time a chapter was planned on the use of animal models for cystic fibrosis. Unfortunately, this area is still very incomplete, despite the use of such model systems as the chronically reserpinized rat[13,14] or rabbit.[15] Lebenthal and Lee[16] have reviewed animal models for pancreatic insufficiency in cystic fibrosis. An animal model for chronic *Pseudomonas* bronchitis resembling cystic fibrosis lung disease has been reported in the rat[17] and guinea pig.[18] Species differences are apparent, as for example when one uses the cat sweat gland as a model, the secretion is isotonic compared to the human sweat gland which is hypotonic.[19] Critical evaluation of all animal model systems (and indeed all claims regarding discoveries in CF) is imperative lest we repeat the mistakes of the past, such as in the selenium controversy, when a monkey supposedly succumbing from selenium deficiency was reported to show changes in the pancreas similar to cystic fibrosis. This report resulted in nationwide publicity, claiming that cystic fibrosis was not a genetic disease, but due to selenium deficiency in the mother.[20] (Chapter 23 on iatrogenic complications addresses these problems.)

Research into cystic fibrosis requires the efforts of scientists representing a broad range of basic and clinical disciplines, collaborating to approach the subject from many different perspectives. A summary of the problems presented by the disease was published by the National Institutes of Health and the Cystic Fibrosis Foundation entitled "Cystic Fibrosis: A Plea for a Future, 1978."[21] These summaries evaluated the state of the art and future directions for CF research at that time. Skillful guidance will be required in how research projects are supported. For a number of years, a major commitment went to support research into the so-called CF factor. Recently, the so-called CF factor was also found to be present in the Shwachman-Diamond syndrome, a disorder of pancreatic insufficiency in association with neutropenia.[22] Thus, it seems likely that this factor was a secondary effect of the pancreatic insufficiency, and not related to the primary gene defect.

The clinical chapters in the book are concerned with the various manifestations, complications, and treatments of the disease. The most important life-threatening effects of CF involve the lungs, and these are described in the chapters on lower respiratory tract infections, pulmonary manifestations, lung function, cor pulmonale, and the adult patient. Improvements in prognosis will require an understanding of how to prevent or delay these pulmonary complications. Each chapter approaches a problem by defining the normal pathophysiological process, and then describing the abnormalities found in patients with cystic fibrosis. Thus a complicated problem, like growth failure, is approached from a number of different perspectives including that of the endocrinologist, the pediatrician, the nutritionist, and the psychologist; alternatively, one could approach growth failure by studying the specific organ which might be involved, such as the pancreas or the liver. Correlation with the basis science chapters will be apparent when defects in the intestinal absorption of amino acids[23] and bile acids[24] secretion of bicarbonate by the pancreas,[25] or chloride/bicarbonate exchange at the apical membrane in the sweat duct[26] are demonstrated. As with many facets of CF, one ends up by asking more questions than one can answer. Several chapters are unique, such as the effects of CF on the endocrine and neurological systems. The problems of the adult with CF are referred to in numerous chapters and are integrated into a specific chapter. The two chapters on psychological problems give no easy answers. Solutions for the economic and social problems of the handicapped will not come from more and better welfare programs, but from research designed to permit development of each individual to his or her optimum.[27] The last three chapters are concerned with the administration of the Cystic Fibrosis Foundation, the organization of a CF clinic, and the economics of cystic fibrosis. Professor Pauly has written a provocative chapter that is a challenge to many of our current practices.

In a time of political change and economic uncertainty, numerous pressures are exerted in terms of where to allocate limited resources. Ultimately a compromise is usually reached between research and clinical support. Most investigators seem convinced that with increased funding and commitment, the basic gene defect in CF could be discovered. Basic understanding of this process is essential in order to devise logical treatment for the disease.

JOHN D. LLOYD-STILL

REFERENCES

1. Littlefield JW: Research on cystic fibrosis. *N Engl J Med* 1981;304:44–45.
2. Abdul-Karim FW, King TA, Dahms BB, et al: Carcinoma of extrahepatic biliary system in an adult with cystic fibrosis. *Gastroenterology* 1982;82:758–762.
3. Swender PT, Nathan EM, Sondheimer J, et al: Bowel carcinoma mimicking meconium ileus equivalent. *Cystic Fibrosis Club Abstr* 1982;23:141.
4. Holsclaw DS, Topham AL: Cystic Fibrosis: A Comprehensive Bibliography of the Medical Literature 1813–1972. DHEW Publication No. (NIH) 77-1132. Cystic Fibrosis Foundation, 6000 Executive Boulevard, Suite 309, Rockville, Maryland 20852.
5. di Sant'Agnese PA, Hubbard VS, Lowe ME: Recent developments in clinical and basic research in cystic fibrosis. *Monogr Paediatr* 1981;14:1–25.
6. Cystic Fibrosis Club Abstracts 23rd Annual Meeting, Washington, DC, May 14, 1982.
7. di Sant'Agnese PA, Talamo RC: Pathogenesis and physiopathology of cystic fibrosis of the pancreas. Fibrocystic disease of the pancreas (mucoviscidosis). *N Engl J Med* 1967; 277:1287–1295, 1343–1352, 1399–1408.
8. di Sant'Agnese PA, and Davis PB: Research in cystic fibrosis. *N Engl J Med* 1976;295: 481–485, 534–541, 597–602.
9. Wood RE, Boat TF, Doershuk CF: Cystic fibrosis. *Am Rev Respir Dis* 1976;113:833–876.
10. Park RW, Grand RJ: Gastrointestinal manifestations of cystic fibrosis : A review. *Gastroenterology* 1981;81:1143–1161.
11. Farber S: Pancreatic function and disease in early life. V. Pathological changes associated with pancreatic insufficiency in early life. *Arch Pathol* 1944;37:238–250.
12. Knowles M, Gatzy J, Boucher R: Increased bioelectric potential difference across respiratory epithelia in cystic fibrosis. *N Engl J Med* 1981;305:1489–1495.
13. Martinez JR, Martinez AM, Garrett L, et al:

Chronically reserpinized rat as a model for cystic fibrosis: Na^+ transport inhibitory effect in submaxillary saliva. *Pediatr Res* 1979;13: 1156–1159.
14. McCurdy RE, Martinez R: The chronically reserpinized rat as a model for cystic fibrosis: Alterations in pancreatic enzyme secretion and storage. *Pediatr Res* 1981;15:1308–1313.
15. Shiffman ML, Gillon MJ, Galey WR: Pancreatic function in the reserpinized rabbit—a model for cystic fibrosis. 1. Effect of secretin. *Pediatr Res* 1982;16:104–108.
16. Lebenthal E, Lee PC: Animal models for pancreatic insufficiency in cystic fibrosis. *J Pediatr Gastroenterol Nutr* 1982;1:9–11.
17. Cash HA, Woods DE, McCullough B, et al: A rat model of chronic respiratory infection with *Pseudomonas aeruginosa. Am Rev Respir Dis* 1979;119:453–459.
18. Pennington JE, Hickey WF, Blackwood LL, et al: Active immunization with lipopolysaccharide *Pseudomonas* antigen for chronic *Pseudomonas* bronchopneumonia in guinea pigs. *J Clin Invest* 1981;68:1140–1148.
19. Munger BL: Brusilow SW, Cooke RE: An electron microscopic study of exocrine sweat glands in patients with cystic fibrosis of the pancreas. *J Pediatr* 1961;59:497–511.
20. Hubbard VS, Barbero G, Chase HP: Selenium and cystic fibrosis. *J Pediatr* 1980;96: 421–422.
21. Cystic Fibrosis: A Plea for a Future. Rockville, Maryland, Cystic Fibrosis Foundation, 1978.
22. Banchini G, Harries JT, Milla PJ, et al: Short communication: Cystic fibrosis "factor(s)": Present also in sera of Shwachman's pancreatic insufficiency. *Pediatr Res* 1981; 15:1073–1075.
23. Milla PJ, Rassam UB, Kilby A, et al: Small intestinal absorption of amino acids and dipeptides in pancreatic insufficiency. In *Proceedings of the Eighth International Cystic Fibrosis Congress.* Toronto, Canadian Cystic Fibrosis Foundation, 1980, pp 177–180.
24. Fondacaro JD, Heubi JE, Kellogg FW: Intestinal bile acid malabsorption in cystic fibrosis: A primary mucosal cell defect. *Pediatr Res* 1982;16:494–498.
25. Gaskin KJ, Durie PR, Corey M, et al: Evidence for a primary defect of pancreatic HCO_3 secretion in cystic fibrosis. *Pediatr Res* 1982;16:544–557.
26. Quinton PM: Suggestion of an abnormal anion exchange mechanism in sweat glands of cystic fibrosis patients. *Pediatr Res* 1982;16:533–537.
27. Gliedman J, Roth W: *The Unexpected Minority: Handicapped Children in America.* New York, Harcourt, Brace, Jovanovich, 1980.

SECTION ONE

BASIC ASPECTS

1

Incidence, Genetics, Heterozygote, and Antenatal Detection of Cystic Fibrosis

Catharine Jean Harris

Henry L. Nadler

In the 45 years since cystic fibrosis (CF) was first recognized,[1-4] numerous investigators have attempted to elucidate the genetic and biochemical basis of the disease. Understanding the basic defect is of paramount importance if we are to understand the precise mode of inheritance, develop effective methods of heterozygote and antenatal detection, and develop effective treatment.

INCIDENCE

Cystic fibrosis is frequently stated to be the number one lethal genetic disease in the Caucasian population of the United States[5] and many Middle European countries (Table 1-1). An incidence of 1 in 2000 live births is the most widely quoted figure in the United States used to describe the homozygous live birth rate.[6] Based on this figure the carrier frequency in this group would be expected to be approximately 5%. Although the incidence varies greatly, CF has been found in all racial and ethnic groups. In the American black population the incidence of CF has been estimated to be 1 in 17,000[7] a figure

Table 1-1
Incidence Estimates of Cystic Fibrosis in Various Caucasian Populations[78]

Incidence	Country	Year	Reference
1:3,700	USA	1960	Steinberg and Brown[5]
1:2,400	USA	1962	Kramm et al[79]
1:1,900	USA	1962	Merritt et al[17]
1:8,000	Sweden	1962	Selander[14]
1:3,300	Germany	1963	Vivell et al[80]
1:2,400	Australia	1965	Danks et al[16]
1:3,000	England	1966	Carter[81]
1:2,500	USA	1966	Sultz et al[82]
1:2,900	England	1967	Pugh and Pickup[83]
1:2,600	Czechoslovakia	1967	Houstek and Vavrova[84]
1:2,400	England	1968	Hall and Simpkiss[85]
1:3,800	Hawaii	1968	Wright and Morton[8]
1:15,000	Italy	1970	Antonelli and Donfrancesco[15]
1:3,300	Czechoslovakia	1972	Brunechy[20]

eightfold less than the Caucasian population in the same area. Orientals appear to have a much lower incidence, with the homozygous frequency in this group found to be 1 in 90,000.[8] CF has also been reported in American Indians,[9] Africans,[10] Middle Easterners,[11] Malaysians,[12] Ashkenazi Jews in Israel,[13] and other European groups.[14,15]

GENETICS

Most investigators believe cystic fibrosis to be transmitted as an autosomal recessive disorder.[16] One hundred percent concordance has been found in monozygotic twin studies. Males and females appear to be affected in equal number. Second marriages of one obligate heterozygote parent produce affected offspring rarely, complying with the calculated risk of 1 in 80. In most studies the incidence of CF in siblings and other relatives approaches the expected values for an autosomal recessive disease.[16–18] Grand et al[19] reported ten women with CF who gave birth to 11 normal children, strongly supporting autosomal recessive inheritance since the theoretical risk here is only 1 in 40.

Based on the observation that the number of affected siblings in many families studied was more than the expected 25%, a number of other investigators believe their data do not support simple autosomal recessive inheritance.[20–23] However, their data did not fit a pattern of autosomal dominant inheritance either. Other investigators have argued against the method of statistical analysis and ascertainment bias in these studies.[5,24] Connealey et al[25] offer an explanation of the above data by suggesting the involvement of two or three recessive alleles at the same locus. In this model a combination of any two mutant alleles would produce the disease.

Although simple autosomal dominant inheritance appears not to fit the observed incidence, Schaap and Cohen[26] suggest that dominant alleles at two loci may be involved. Affected individuals would possess a dominant allele from each locus (*AaBb*), while one parent would carry the dominant allele from one locus (*Aabb*) and the other parent the dominant allele from the other locus (*aaBb*). Although this theory could explain the occasional reports where familial incidence of CF is higher than expected, most investigators will continue to assume a single-locus autosomal recessive pattern of inheritance until future research proves differently.

The most perplexing problem in the genetic studies of CF is the high incidence in the Caucasian population of a disease in which 98% of affected males are sterile[27] and affected females reaching childbearing age are found to have decreased fertility.[28] A gene frequency of 0.022 is thought to be too high to be explained by mutation alone. Attempts to explain the unusually high gene frequency include advocating heterozygote advantage, genetic drift, multiple loci, and genetic heterogenicity. Interestingly, in the non-Caucasian populations, the gene frequency can adequately be explained by mutation alone.

Heterozygote advantage offers an interesting explanation for the high gene frequency. A 2–2.5% advantage would be required to maintain equilibrium of the gene frequency.[5,16] Investigators have studied disease resistance among controls and heterozygotes.[29–34] However, there appears no disease now prevalent to continue to explain selection for the CF gene.

Some studies suggest sibship size in heterozygote families is larger. Danks et al[16] found there were 4.75 live born offspring to grandparents of CF cases compared to 4.129 for control families. Baumann[22] noted in a Swiss study that family size in CF families was 4.27 compared with only 2.48 children in control families. This might be explained by altered electrolyte composition of the heterozygote cervical mucus or semen, producing a more favorable environment for fertilization.[35] In reviewing these studies one must remember that there are certain built-in biases in such studies. The larger the family size in a heterozygous family, the more likely that a CF child will be born. Many families with a child born with chronic disease choose to enlarge their families over the original plan for replacement purposes.

Genetic drift may offer an answer to the high incidence of CF in isolated populations in Brittany[36] and South West Africa,[37] where there is a high incidence of inbreeding. The genetic drift theory suggests that the frequency of a gene could increase rapidly due to chance events in which a gene-containing group suddenly increases in size. It seems, however, improbable that such a mechanism could explain the difference in gene frequency found in Caucasian and non-Caucasian populations within the same area.

Genetic heterogeneity offers another explanation for the high gene frequency.[38] Many biochemical and cytogenic studies in CF families support this possibility. Patterns on polyacrylamide gel electrofocusing of plasma demonstrate an absence of an arginine esterase band.[39] The specific missing band appears to hold true in affected individuals within families but occasionally differs between families. Metachromatic staining[40–42] of cultured skin fibroblasts found CF patients in all three staining groups. Usually only one staining group is found within patients and parents in individual families. Further studies discovered a family in which fibroblasts from a mildly affected patient, his father, and some paternal relatives were ametachromatic, while fibroblasts from the mother and some maternal relatives were metachromatic-positive.[43] This individual may represent the effect of a compound with several mutant alleles. Genetic heterogeneity may then be explained by either multiple mutant alleles at a single locus or involvement of multiple CF loci. The CF gene has not yet been assigned to any specific chromosome. Affected individuals have been found to have normal karyotypes. Numerous linkage studies have failed to reveal any linkage with blood group or HLA loci.[44–47] There appear to be no strong associations between CF and any other disease.

HETEROZYGOTE DETECTION

Numerous reports have been published claiming to be able to differentiate normals, carriers, and CF patients. Some of the most recent approaches are discussed in this section. Breslow et al,[48] utilizing tissue culture techniques, claimed to be able to differentiate the three groups. In these studies they found that normal fibroblasts were killed when grown in the presence of dexamethasone but viability of CF fibroblasts was not affected. Heterozygote fibroblasts gave intermediate viability levels. A year later Kurz et al[49] published data that refuted this approach. Breslow et al[50] have recently proposed a method of carrier detection based on sodium concentration after oubain exposure of fibroblasts. Studying 13 normal fibroblast lines, 8 lines from patients, and 8 lines from obligate heterozygotes, they found decreased ^{22}Na cellular accumulation in the CF lines after drug exposure. Cells from the obligate heterozygotes have an intermediate level. However, when extended to a larger CF population, the groups could not be differentiated.[51]

Liberman et al[52] have reported the ability to detect a serum lectin-like factor by hemagglutination in 25 CF homozygotes, 70 obligate heterozygotes, and 18 of 27 CF siblings (67%). In studying 675 control sera, they found a 4.2% incidence of the CF lectin, a figure very close to the expected 5% heterozygote frequency in the general population. Although they have been unable to reproduce their studies in a blind trial, they feel this is most likely due to poorly controlled experimental collection procedures.[53] The nature of the lectin-like factor is unknown at this time.

Wilson et al[54] reported they were able to identify CF protein (CFP) in 95% of heterozygotes and homozygotes by using a technique involving isoelectric focusing on polyacrylamide gels. Although many laboratories have been able to confirm the existence of CFP in serum of patients and carriers, the separation of these two groups by the brightness of the band gave too much room for error to be useful clinically.[55,56] Manson and Brock[57] modified this technique using antiserum to CFP raised in guinea pigs in rocket immunoelectrophoresis to differentiate homozygotes and heterozygotes. Wilson[58] has also recently utilized counterimmune electrophoresis (CIE) rather than rocket immunoelectrophoresis with antisera, produced from mice. His technique is faster, requires less antisera and appears to be easier and quicker to produce antisera. He has found complete agreement between the isoelectric focusing and CIE identification of CFP in 20 controls, 10 homozygotes, and 8 obligate heterozygote sera. The heterozygote is identified by a precipitin line closer to the antigen well and fainter than the line with CF homozygote sera, indicating less CFP in the heterozygote.

Walsh Platt et al[59] have reported differences in protease activity in serum of patients with CF, heterozygotes, and controls. Although distinction of the groups is possible within families, differences between families are too great to be useful. Hopefully one of these approaches or others will provide a feasible clinical means of carrier detection. At present none can be recommended for routine clinical use.

Shapiro[69] has shown that fibroblasts from CF patients and heterozygotes utilize more O_2 than controls. When rotenone, an inhibitor of NADH dehydrogenase, was added, the inhibition of O_2 consumption was greater in CF and heterozygote fibroblasts. Further studies found the pH optimum of NADH dehydrogenase to differ between CF, carrier, and controls (pH 8.6, 8.3, 8.0, respectively).

PRENATAL DIAGNOSIS

Prenatal diagnosis for CF has been attempted in both amniotic fluid cells and cell-free amniotic fluid. Investigations have centered around such areas as metachromasis,[40,41] mucociliary inhibitors,[60–62] resistance to dexamethasone,[48,49] response to Tamm-Horsfall glycoprotein,[63–68] altered mitochondrial NADH dehydrogenase kinetics,[69] and MUGB reactive proteases.[70–73] However, at this point these approaches remain controversial at best, and presently only the latter two are being evaluated in large-scale studies.[74]

In our laboratory, studies have shown that measurement of methylumbelliferylguanidinobenzoate (MUGB) -reactive proteases in cell-free amniotic fluid appears to provide a potentially useful means for prenatal diagnosis.[70–73] The presence of MUGB-reactive proteases has been confirmed in the laboratories of Brock[75] and Blau.[76] According to our studies, gestational age, chromosomal defects, neural tube defects, and blood contamination do not appear to affect the reliability of this test during the second trimester. Presently a large number of pregnancies are being monitored from control women and women known to be at increased risk for carrying a CF fetus. MUGB reactivity is studied in amniotic fluid by quantitative analysis, polyacrylamide gel isoelectric focusing, and column filtration. Fetuses are considered affected when MUGB activity falls below the control range, benzoyl arginine ethyl ester (BAEE) stained gels are missing one of four bands in the isoelectric area 5.1–5.4, and column assay fails to reveal a 200,000-molecular-weight species. Thirty-nine pregnancies of obligate heterozygotes and 12 cases where one parent has a sibling with CF have now been monitored.[77] In all but two cases the diagnosis was accurate as confirmed by sweat test at birth. Unfortunately, confirmation of the diagnosis on abortuses is impossible. Furthermore, additional experience in approximately 100 pregnancies raises serious questions as to the usefulness of these tests as now performed. While a significant number of CF pregnancies have been identified, at least seven false negatives and three false positives have been found. Further attempts to improve these tests are in progress.

CONCLUSION

At present carrier detection and in utero diagnosis are offered only on an experimental basis. Problems exist with all the techniques described to date. Until the basic defect is defined, methods will be, at best, imprecise.

Physicians must provide families with the empiric risk of having a child with CF. In the US Caucasian population a gene frequency of 1/20 is most commonly used.[78] Some commonly encountered situations and their risks in each future pregnancy would include parents of CF child (1/4), parent of CF child in previous marriage (1/80), siblings of CF case (1/120), first cousin of CF child (1/160), and a parent with CF (1/40). It is hoped more precise methods will be forthcoming in the near future.

REFERENCES

1. Fanconi G, Uehlinger E, Knauer C: Das coeliakiesydrom bei angebeiener zystischer pankreas-fibromatose and bronchiektasien. *Wien Med Wochenschr* 1936;86:753–756.
2. Andersen DH: Cystic fibrosis of pancreas and its relation to celiac disease: Clinical and pathological study. *Am J Dis Child* 1938; 56:344–399.
3. Blackfan KD, May CD: Inspissation of secretions, dilatation of ducts and acini, atrophy and fibrosis of pancreas in infants: Clinical note. *J Pediatr* 1938;13:627–634.
4. Harper MH: Congenital steatorrhea due to pancreatic defect. *Arch Dis Child* 1938;13: 45–56.
5. Steinberg AG, Brown DC: On incidence of CF of pancreas. *Am J Hum Genet* 1960;12: 416–424.
6. di Sant'Agnese PA, Talamo RC: Pathogenesis and physiopathology of CF of the pancreas: Fibrocystic disease of the pancreas (mucoviscidosis). *N Engl J Med* 1967;277: 1287–1294.
7. Kulczycki L, Schauf V: CF in blacks in Washington DC: Incidence and characteristics. *Am J Dis Child* 1974;127:64–67.
8. Wright SW, Morton NE: Genetic studies on CF in Hawaii. *Am J Hum Genet* 1968;20: 157–169.
9. Harris RL, Riley HD: CF in the American Indian. *Pediatrics* 1968;41:733–738.
10. MacDougall LG: Fibrocystic disease of the pancreas in African children. *Lancet* 1962;2: 409–410.
11. Salem M, Idriss H: CF of the pancrease in the Middle East. *Leb Med J* 1962;15:61–74.
12. Kamdar HR: CF of the pancreas with respiratory allergy in children. *Antiseptic* 1961;58:863–870.
13. Levin S: Fibrocystic disease of the pancreas, in Goedschmidt E (ed): *Genetics of Migrant and Isolate Populations.* Baltimore, Williams and Wilkens, 1963.
14. Selander P: The frequency of CF of the pancreas in Sweden. *Acta Paediatr Scand* 1965; 51:65–67.
15. Antonelli M, Donfrancesco A: Indagine clinico-statistica sulla epidemiologia della fibrosi cistica (F.C.) in Italia nel quadriennio 1966–1969. *Fracastao (Verona)* 1970;63: 207–216.
16. Danks DM, Allan J, Anderson CM: Genetic study of fibrocystic disease of the pancreas. *Ann Human Genet* 1965;28:323–356.
17. Merritt AD, Hanna BL, Todd CW, et al: Incidence and mode of inheritance of CF, abstracted. *J Lab Clin Med* 1962;60:998–999.
18. Lave CM, May CD, Reed, SC: Fibrosis of the pancreas in infants and children: A statistical study of clinical and hereditary features. *Am J Dis Child* 1949;78:349–374.
19. Grand RJ, Talamo RC, di Sant'Agnese PA,

et al: Pregnancy in CF of pancreas. *JAMA* 1966;195:993-1000.

20. Brunechy Z: The incidence and genetics of CF. *J Med Genet* 1972;9:33-37.
21. Roberts GBS: Familial incidence of fibrocystic disease of the pancreas. *Ann Hum Genet* 1960;24:127-135.
22. Baumann T: Die mucoviscidosis als recessive und irregular dominants ebleidem: eine klinische und genetische studie. *Helv Paediatr Acta B* 1958;8(Suppl):1-79.
23. Bernhum M, Monnet P, Jeune M, et al: La maladie fibro-kystique des parenchymes glandulanes. *Pediatrie* 1961;16:17-38.
24. Bulmer MG: Fibrocystic disease of the pancreas: A comment. *Ann Hum Genet* 1961; 25:163-164.
25. Conneally PM, Merritt AD, Yu P: Cystic fibrosis: Population genetics. *Tex Rep Biol Med* 1973;31:639-650.
26. Schapp T, Cohen MM: A proposed model for the inheritance of CF, in Mangos JA, Talamo RC (eds): *Cystic Fibrosis: Projections into the Future.* New York, Stratton Intercontinental Medical Book Corp, 1976.
27. Denning CR, Sommers SC, Quigley HR: Infertility in male patients with CF. *Pediatrics* 1968;41:7-17.
28. Kopito LE, Kosasky HJ, Shwachman H: Water and electrolytes in cervical muci from patients with CF. *Fertil Steril* 1973;24: 512-516.
29. Crawford MD: A genetic study including evidence for heterosis in cystic fibrosis of the pancrease, abstracted. *Heredity* 1970;29:126.
30. Cohen FL, Daniel WL: Effects of CF sera on proteus vulgaris motility. *J Med Genet* 1974;11:253-256.
31. Sturat AB, Burdon MG: Frequency of the CF gene. *Lancet* 1974;2:1951.
32. Bauman BH, Lochhart LH, McCombs ML: Oyster ciliary inhibition by CF factor. *Science* 1969;164:325-326.
33. Edwards JH: Heterozygote advantage. *Arch Dis Child* 1977;52:343-344.
34. Super M: Cystic fibrosis in the South West African Afrikaner: An example of population drift possibly with heterozygote advantage. *S Afr Med J* 1975;49:818-820.
35. Anderson CM, Allan J, Johansen P: Comments on the possible existence and nature of a heterozygote advantage in CF. *Mod Probl Pediatr* 1967;10:381-387.
36. Bois E, Ferngold J, Demenais F, et al: Clusters of CF cases in a limited area of Brittany (France). *Clin Genet* 1978;14:73-76.
37. Super M: CF in southern Africa. *S Afr Med J* 1978;52:18-21.
38. Hirschhorn K: Genetic studies in disease, in Mangos JA, Talamo RC (eds): *Fundamental Problems in CF and Related Diseases.* New York, International Medical Book Corp, 1973.
39. Rao GJS, Nadler HL: Arginine esterase in CF of the pancreas. *Pediatr Res* 1974;8: 684-686.
40. Danes BS, Bearn AG: A genetic cell marker in CF of the pancreas. *Lancet* 1968;1: 1061-1063.
41. Danes BS, Bearn AG: CF of the pancreas, a study in cell culture. *J Exp Med* 1949;129: 775-794.
42. Danes BS, Flensberg EW: CF: Cell cultures studied on a Danish population. *Am J Hum Genet* 1971;23:297-302.
43. Danes BS, Hodson ME, Batten J: CF: Evidence for a genetic compound from a family study in cell culture. *Clin Genet* 1977;11:83-90.
44. Polynenidis A, Ludwig H, Gotz M: CF and HL-A antigens. *Lancet* 1973;2:1452.
45. Goodchild MC, Edwards JH, Glenn KP, et al: A search for linkage in CF. *J Med Genet* 1976;13:417-419.
46. Steinberg AG, Shwachman H, Allen FH, et al: Linkage studies with CF of the pancreas. *Am J Hum Genet* 1956;8:162-176.
47. Herrod HG, Ames DB, Spock A: HLA determinants in families with more than one member with CF. *J Pediatr* 1979;94:676.
48. Breslow JL, Epstein J, Fontaine JH, et al: Enhanced dexamethasone resistance in CF cells: Potential use for heterozygote detection and prenatal diagnosis. *Science* 1978;201: 180-182.
49. Kurz JB, Perkins JP, Buchwald M: Killing of fibroblast by dexamethasone a dibutynyl adenosine 3′,5′-monophosphate is not a valid test for CF. *Science* 1979;206:1317-1319.
50. Breslow JL, McPherson J, Epstein J: Distinguishing homozygous and heterozygous CF fibroblasts from normal cells by differences in sodium transport. *N Engl J Med* 1981;304:1-5.
51. Breslow L, McPherson J: Sodium transport in CF fibroblasts not different from normal. *N Engl J Med* 1981;305:98.
52. Lieberman J, Costea NV, Yahalis VJ, et at: Detection of lectin in the blood of CF homo and heterozygotes. *Trans Assoc Am Physicians* 1979;92:121.
53. Leiberman J, Kaneshiro W, Costea NV: Presence of a serum hermagglutinin (lectin-like factor) in CF homozygotes and heterozygotes. *J Lab Clin Med* 1981;97:646-653.
54. Wilson GB, Fudenberg HH, Jalon TL: Studies on CF using isoelectric focusing: I. An assay for detection of CF homozygotes and heterozygote carriers in serum. *Pediatr*

Res 1975;9:635-640.
55. Scholey J, Applegarth PA, Davidson HGF, et al: Detection of CF protein by electrofocusing. *Pediatr Res* 1978;12:800.
56. Nevin GB, Nevin NC, Redmond AO, et al: Detection of CF homozygotes and heterozygotes by serum isoelectrofocusing. *Hum Genet* 1981;56:387-389.
57. Manson J, Brock PJH: Development of a quantitative immunoassay for the CF gene. *Lancet* 1980;1:330-331.
58. Wilson GB: Monospecific antisera, hybrioduma antibodies, and immunoassays of a CF protein. *Lancet* 1980;2:313-314.
59. Walsh Platt MM, Rao GJS, Nadler HL: Protease deficiency in plasma of patients with CF: Reduced reaction of 4-methylumbelliferylguanidinobenzoate with plasma of patients with CF. *Enzyme* 1979;24:224-229.
60. Beratis NG, Conover JH, Conod EF, et al: Studies of ciliary dyskinesia factor in CF. III. Skin fibroblasts and cultured amniotic fluid cells. *Pediatr Res* 1973;7:958-964.
61. Bounan BH, Lockhart LH, Herzberg VL, et al: CF: Synthesis of ciliary inhibitor by amniotic cells. *Clin Genet* 1973;4:461-463.
62. Barnett DR, Berg K: CF: Studies with the oyster ciliary assay. *Clin Genet* 1977;12: 333-343.
63. Hosli P, Erickson RP, Vogt E: Prospects for prenatal diagnosis of CF: Induction of brochemial abnormalities in fibroblasts from patients with CF by a urinary glycoprotein. *Biochem Biophys Res Commun* 1976;73: 209-216.
64. Hosli P, Vogt E: CF: Leakage of lysosomal enzymes and of alkaline phosphatase into the extracellular space. *Biochem Biophys Res Commun* 1977;79:741-784.
65. Hosli P, Koeberg H, Vogt E: Reliable diagnosis of the major type of CF with fibroblast cultures. *Acta Pediatr Scand* 1978;67:617-620.
66. Willcox P: Secretion of β-N-acetylglucosaminidase isozymes by cultured CF fibroblasts. *Clin Chim Acta* 1979;91:81-88.
67. Butterworth J, Guy GJ: Primary amniotic fluid cells, skin fibroblasts and liver α-L-fucosidase and its relation to CF. *Clin Chim Acta* 1979;92:109-116.
68. Casola L, Dimatteo G, Romano M, et al: Glycosidases in serum of CF patients. *Clin Chim Acta* 1979;94:83-88.
69. Shapiro BL, Feigal RJ, Lam LFH: Mitochondrial NADA dehydrogenase in CF. *Proc Natl Acad Sci USA* 1979;76:2979-2983.
70. Walsh-Platt MM, Nadler HL: MUGB-reactive proteases in amniotic fluid: Possible marker for the intrauterine diagnosis of CF. *Lancet* 1979;1:622.
71. Walsh MMJ, Nadler HL: Methylumelliferylguanidinobenzoate-reactive proteases in human amniotic fluid: Promising marker for intrauterine detection of CF. *Am J Obstet Gynecol* 1980;137:978-982.
72. Nadler HL, Walsh MMJ: Intrauterine detection of CF. *Pediatrics* 1980;66:690-692.
73. Harris CJ, Mesirow K, Rembleski P, et al: Antenatal detection of cystic fibrosis, abstracted. *Pediatr Res* 1981;15:562.
74. Davis PB, di Sant'Agnese PA: A review: CF at forty—quo vadis? *Pediatr Res* 1980;14: 83-87.
75. Brouch DJH, Hayward C: Methylumbelliferylguanidinobenzoate reactive proteases and prenatal diagnosis of CF. *Lancet* 1979;1:1244.
76. Dann LG, Blau K: Arginine esterase in amniotic fluid: Possible marker for CF. *Lancet* 1979;2:907.
77. Nadler HL, Rembelski P, Mesirow K: Prenatal detection of CF, in Galjaard H (ed): *The Future of Early Diagnosis of Genetic Disease*. Edinburgh, Churchill Livingston, in press.
78. Nadler HL, Rao GJ, Taussig LM: Cystic fibrosis, in Stanbury JB, Wyngaarden JB, Fredrickson DS (eds): *The Metabolic Basis of Inherited Disease*. New York, McGraw-Hill, 1978.
79. Kramm ER, Crane MM, Sirkin MG, et al: A cystic fibrosis pilot survey in three New England states. *Am J Public Health* 1962;52:2041.
80. Vivell O, Jacobi H, Munback K: Zur mucoviscidosis im kinde salter. *Monatsschr Kinderheilkd* 1963;111:62.
81. Carter CO: Genetical aspects of cystic fibrosis of the pancreas. *Mod Probl Pediatr* 1966;10:372.
82. Sultz HA, Schlesinger AER, Mosher WE: The Erie County survey of long-term childhood illness. *Am J Public Health* 1966;56:1461.
83. Pugh RJ, Pickup JD: CF in the Leeds region. *Arch Dis Child* 1967;42:544.
84. Houstek J, Vavrova V: Notre experience á propos de la mucoviscidose. *Rev Med Liege* 1967;22:421.
85. Hall BD, Simpkiss MJ: Incidence of fibrocystic disease in Wessex. *J Med Genet* 1968; 5:262.

2

Newborn Screening Tests

John D. Lloyd-Still

Methods for the prevention of CF may be primary, aimed at preventing births of affected children, or secondary, aimed at preventing morbidity from the disease by means of presymptomatic detection (preferably neonatal screening) and treatment. The only available method of primary prevention is genetic counseling of parents known to carry the CF gene. Amniocentesis has been discussed in Chapter 1 and is still in the experimental stage. The Committee for a Study for Evaluation of Testing for CF[1] stated that screening for CF by the methods currently available can be recommended only for research purposes. Despite this negative conclusion, it is important to discuss potential approaches to screening for CF as the issues are complicated and controversial.

Genetic screening of newborns began with the development of the Guthrie test for phenylketonuria (PKU) in 1961.[2] During the 1960s additional genetic screening tests applicable to newborns became available, and by 1973 each infant born in the state of Massachusetts was being screened for over 30 genetic disorders.[3] The methodology used three filter paper specimens (cord blood, newborn peripheral blood, and urine). The most recent disease to have legislation passed for genetic screening is hypothyroidism.[4] The high incidence of CF (1 in 2000) compared with PKU (1 in 20,000) and hypothyroidism (1 in 5000) supports the rationale for attempting to devise a screening method for the disease. The subject of genetic screening was extensively reviewed and summarized by the Committee for the Study of Inborn Errors of Metabolism of the National Research Council.[5]

In the pediatric literature of the last 10 years, nearly 100 conditions have been identified as possibilities for screening programs. In order to eliminate faulty proposals, a "check-off list" has been proposed, and in Table 2-1 we have adapted a list compiled by Berwick, et al.[6]

THE DISEASE

There is no question that CF is an important cause of morbidity, mortality, and medical expense (see Chapter 28). Warwick and Pogue[7] have prepared a model based on the CF Data Registry (Figure 2-1) which suggests that there will be about 4000 adult CF patients in the next decade. They suggested that with the establishment of a newborn screening program and improved detection, the CF population will be 64,000 patients with 18,000 adults.

The question of whether early detection and treatment of CF in asymptomatic stages is advantageous is controversial. Brimblecombe and Chamberlin[8] concluded that the efficacy of prophylactic treatment in altering the natural history of the disease had not been demonstrated. Shwachman et al[9] showed that 80% of CF infants diagnosed with normal chest x-rays would survive until 18 years of age, but their study was uncontrolled. George and Norman[10] devised life tables for 128 children with CF without meconium ileus and 43 cases with meconium ileus for the five years starting in 1964. These

Table 2-1
Factors that Make Screening Advantageous

Factors	As Applicable to Cystic Fibrosis
The disease	
1. is an important cause of morbidity, mortality, or medical expense;	Yes
2. has asymptomatic stages	Yes
3. is treatable, progression is preventable during asymptomatic stages, or there is advantage to others in early detection	?
Treatment	
1. is more effective or efficient in early stages	?
2. costs are low	No
3. is acceptable to the people treated	Yes
Screening process/method	
1. is inexpensive, easy to perform, and easily transported to a central laboratory	?
2. is reliable with few false-positive or false-negative results	?
3. is possible with little trauma to the infant, is acceptable to the subject population, and has a low incidence of side effects	?
Population	
1. suffers from the disease	Yes
2. is accessible to the screening test	Yes
3. is compliant with presymptomatic treatment	?
Health care system	
1. can offer diagnostic confirmation	Yes
2. can offer therapeutic intervention	Yes
3. shows consensus about diagnostic and therapeutic policies	?

Number of cystic fibrosis (CF) patients alive and receiving care from US CF Centers at end of each calendar year. Numbers at right indicate age. Solid lines indicate observed values; dashed lines, predicted values.

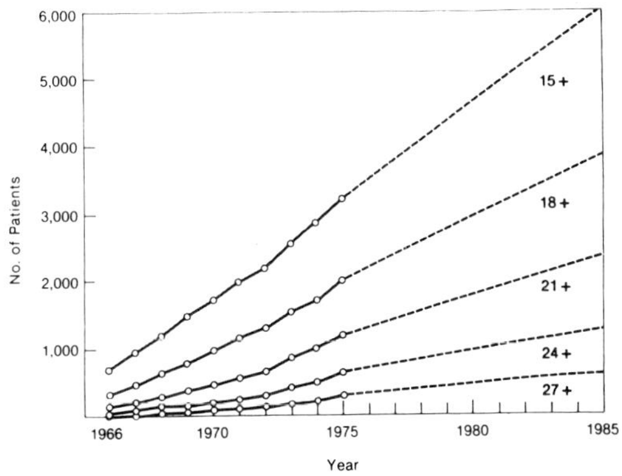

Figure 2-1. Reproduced from Warwick WJ, Pogue RE: *JAMA* 1977;238:2159 (reference 7), with permission.

were compared with similar tables constructed for the preceding 20 years and showed narrowing of the gap between the life expectancy of those entered at birth and at diagnosis and a very obvious improvement in survival rate. They suggested that this was due to early diagnosis and treatment, but their data are retrospective. Our own figures on the survival of infants treated for meconium ileus during the last 10 years show a remarkable improvement compared to published mortality rates for this disorder (see Chapter 21), but this improvement is also related to the use of a new therapeutic modality—the gastrografin enema—which can avoid the need for surgery in two thirds of these patients. Lastly, the average age of death for CF patients has increased significantly during the last decade according to the CF Data Registry, but these figures are deceptive as they fail to account for the contribution of improvements in diagnosis, especially in patients with mild disease. Thus, although the evidence for improved survival in CF as a result of therapy is suggestive, the data are still inconclusive. (See Chapter 12 for further discussion of longitudinal studies.)

TREATMENT

The same arguments can be applied when one considers whether treatment is more effective or efficient in the early stages. The cost of treatment is difficult to categorize in terms of what is considered "low." The treatment, consisting of antibiotics, vitamins, pancreatic enzyme supplements, and physical therapy, would probably be considered acceptable if screening were to become practical.

SCREENING METHODOLOGY

This is an area of considerable research activity and some of the current methodology will be summarized. In the United States today, a screening test is most conveniently and efficiently administered before a newborn baby leaves the hospital.[5] Table 2-2 lists some of the methods that have been used or advocated for the screening of newborns for CF. Measurement of the electrolyte levels of nails, saliva, and sweat (skin) have been reported, but none of these are practical. The problems with sweat testing are discussed in Chapter 4. The iontophoresis method of Gibson and Cooke[15] is the most reliable method, but it is expensive, difficult to perform accurately, and unreliable in the first few days of life, thus excluding its use as a screening tool.

Immunological, electrophoretic, and precipitation methods for the detection of albumin in meconium have been applied in screening programs.[17–23,39] The most widely used has been the Boehringer-Mannheim (B-M) test strip. This test is based on the principle that the deficiency of pancreatic enzymes secondary to CF leads to incomplete digestion of protein and a resultant increase in albumin and other proteins in the stool. The B-M test strip uses tetrabromophenolphthalein ethyl ester as the indicator and produces an intense blue color when protein is present in excess of 20 mg/g (dried weight) of meconium. Stephan et al[20] screened 69,000 meconiums by the B-M strip, and in 60 positive tests CF was confirmed later. No increased albumin was observed in four cases of CF. This test will fail to detect the 15% of CF patients with intact pancreatic function (false negatives). The incidence of false positives is 0.5–1%,

Table 2-2
Screening Tests Available for Detection of CF in Newborns

	Practicality	Expense	Specificity	Reference
Electrolytes				
Nails	Yes	High	Poor	11, 12
Saliva	No	High	Poor	13
Skin				
(Electrodes)	No		Poor	14
(Iontophoresis)	No	High	Poor	15
(Chloride plate)	Yes	Low	Poor	16
Meconium				
Albumin	Yes	Low	Fair	17–23
IgA	Yes	High	Poor	24
β-Fucosidase	No	High	Fair	25
Lactase	Yes	High	Poor	23,26
Feces				
Trypsin (colorimetric)	Yes	Low	Poor	27,28
Blood				
Trypsin (immunoreactive)	Yes	Low	Fair	29–33
CF protein	No	High	Unknown	34
Lectin	Yes	Low	Poor	35

but this is higher in conditions such as prematurity, intestinal obstruction, pancreatic achylia, etc (See Chapter 11).

The results of a collaborative study at seven CF centers in the United States and Canada[21] revealed 216 positive meconium tests in a total population of 102,159 newborns screened. Eighteen of the 216 positive tests had CF confirmed by the sweat test. An additional five patients with negative meconium tests were documented to have CF following clinical symptoms. Because of the high incidence of false negatives (21.7%) and the low incidence of the disease (1:4441) in the population studied, mass screening by this method was not recommended.

Because of the necessity to perform a sweat iontophoresis test to exclude cystic fibrosis in false-positive cases, there is the potential for parental distress. Indeed, this area has not been adequately documented in terms of whether the screening process may actually be harmful. The possibilities of inducing iatrogenic depression or even suicide in the postpartum period are real. Moreover, parents may refuse to believe their child is normal despite what appeared to be adequate genetic counseling. When choosing policies in preventative medicine, the cost–benefit ratio is used to analyze the effectiveness of a screening proposal. Thus, a false-positive test rate varying between 1%[20] and 92%[21] has considerable potential for leading to side effects for the parents of these infants. This does not seem to have been a problem in Europe, but no study has so far documented parental reaction to meconium testing. In the United States, with the legal requirements of informed consent, the potential for upset to the families is significant, especially if there is delay in the performance of the sweat test.[36] Holsclaw et al[39] documented parental apprehension, fear, nervousness, worry, and resentment in their study of 20,170 infants screened in Philadelphia. They stressed the importance of having a counselor or social worker explain the reason for the sweat test to the families and noted the expectations of parents that they would have access to physicians to discuss the reason for this test—ideals that may be very difficult to deliver in practice. When one adds to these problems the false-negative rate of 15%–21.7%, the test rates poorly for applicability to routine newborn screening.

Measurement of beta-fucosidase and lactase in meconium have been suggested for screening purposes. These are discussed in Chapter 11. Berry et al[23] compared screening meconium for CF by increased albumin levels detected by the B-M test and increased lactase activity detected by glucose production after incubation of meconium with lactose. Low-birth-weight infants accounted for more than half the positive test results with both procedures. Twelve infants with CF were identified through screening, six while testing 44,816 specimens by the lactase activity test. Three additional infants with CF were missed because meconium specimens were negative to both tests. Gibson[36] commented that these figures were not significantly different from the collaborative study.[21]

Analysis of fecal trypsin (which will be reduced in 85% of CF infants) to screen newborns for CF was reported by Robinson and Elliott,[27] but yielded a false-positive rate of 3% and a false-negative rate of 10%. A subsequent report using a different substrate, benzoylarginine-*p*-nitroaniline (BAPNAA), which is colorless and releases yellow *p*-nitroaniline after hydrolysis by trypsin, was claimed to give no false negatives for samples which were truly lacking enzymes and had a lower false-positive rate of 1.2%.[28] These data have not been confirmed, the numbers screened were small (two CF infants detected among 2500 screened), and the reason for their statements about the lack of false-negative results are inadequately documented.

Recently attention has focused on analysis of dried blood spots for CF screening.[29–33] Children with CF in the first year of life tend to have abnormally high levels of serum immunoreactive trypsin whether or not enzymatically active trypsin is measurable in the feces (Figure 2-2).[29] In older children and adults with CF the levels tend to be subnormal. This supports the hypothesis that the pancreatic duct is progressively blocked with initial "back-leakage" of acinar contents into the plasma.

Two commercial reagents (Behring and Sorin) are available, but the Sorin materials were better adapted for blood-spot analysis. Immunoreactive trypsin in blood spots rapidly decreases with specimen age but is stable in frozen serum. Values for premature infants do not differ significantly from those for full-term babies. Cystic fibrosis infants under 8 weeks of age were readily distinguished from controls,[29,32,33] but in a larger series of 185 patients with CF there was considerable overlap.[31] Further results of this test are awaited for it offers the advantages of ease (blood spots are already obtained), low cost, and detection of 15% of CF infants who have preserved some pancreatic function. A more sophisticated radioimmunoassay technique has confirmed these findings.[40]

Another approach to blood screening is by measurement of the so-called CF protein (CFP).[34] This subject is discussed in detail in Chapter 7. Lieberman et al[35] reported on a rapid screening test for the CF carrier state by detection of a serum lectin. This test failed double-blind studies and is also discussed in Chapter 7.

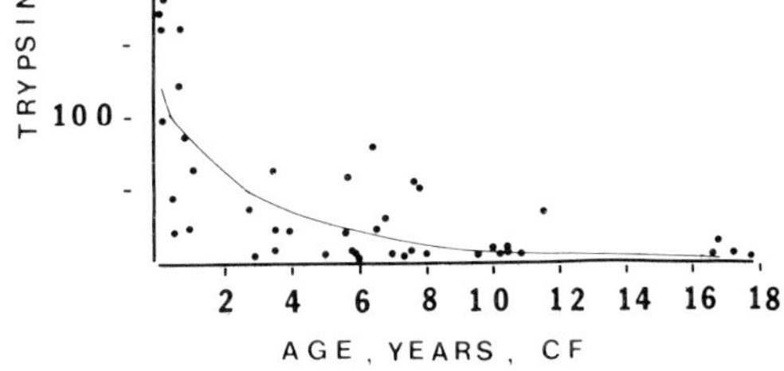

Figure 2-2 Serum immunoreactive trypsinogen levels in ng/ml plotted against age in 50 patients with cystic fibrosis. Levels in 34 control children were 10–70 ng/ml. Note the greatly elevated levels in the 14 infants (175 ± 101, range 20–400) and the decreased levels in the majority of the older children with pancreatic insufficiency (data from Lloyd-Still et al[41]).

We can conclude that at present there is no universally acceptable, practical, reliable screening test for the diagnosis of CF.[1]

POPULATION

There is no doubt that the disease is prevalent in the population and that screening in the first few days of life is theoretically possible. When discussing the population, one must consider the legal ramifications of screening. The National Academy of Sciences Committee[5] had several recommendations regarding legal requirements: (1) Participation in a genetic screening program should not be made mandatory by law but should be left to the discretion of the person tested or, if a minor, of the parents or legal guardian. (This is a surprising recommendation when in practice most states have mandated compulsory screening for PKU and hypothyroidism.) (2) Identifying information obtained through genetic screening should not be made available to anyone other than the screenee, except with the permission of the screenee or, in the case of a minor, with the permission of the parents or legal guardian. (3) Screening authorities should consult regularly with lawyers and other persons knowledgeable in ethics to avoid social consequences of screening that may be damaging. (4) For states considering legislation mandating genetic screening, it was recommended that the state create a board on hereditary disorders for advisory purposes.

These recommendations were aimed at limiting some of the side effects of other screening programs. For example, in the sickle cell screening program, numerous problems, including: (1) invasion of privacy, (2) lack of confidentiality, (3) transgression of civil rights, (4) psychological damage for being labeled or for misunderstanding about the significance of diseases and carrier states, (5) increased premiums for life insurance or health insurance, and (6) refusal for employment, were all encountered. Other stigmata found in sickle cell programs concern the marriageability of those found to be carriers. (This is certainly applicable should it ever become possible to screen for the heterozygote in CF.) During a screening program for blood diseases in Greece (where arranged marriages are common), the carriers of hemoglobinopathy were no longer considered desirable individuals for matrimony in their village.[37] Moreover, despite this deleterious effect, the frequency of the disease itself was not diminished.

Any screening program will necessitate some form of follow-up and counseling service. The organization of this service is discussed in the committee report of the National Academy of Sciences.[5] Barriers to an understanding of counseling may be related to a variety of factors, including denial, comprehension of probability, knowledge, and intelligence.

Attitudes towards further childbearing and actual reproductive performances after counseling were found to be unrelated to socioeconomic level, educational attainment, knowledge of the genetic aspects of the disease in question, general knowledge of biology, and ease in handling probabilities.[38] Thus, knowledge of genetic facts and odds, while necessary, is not all that goes into decisions made after genetic counseling.

On the other hand, enthusiasts of genetic screening programs point to the success of the Tay Sachs programs, although the thrust of these programs is carrier detection and primary prevention, not newborn screening. Tay Sachs disease is an ideal disease for screening for reproductive counseling for the following reasons: (1) It is confined to a defined population: 3–5% of Ashkenazi Jews are heterozygous. (2) There is a simple, reliable, automated, and inexpensive test for detecting the carrier state (hexosaminidase A, a lysosomal enzyme which is present in both serum and tissues), and the activity of this enzyme can be measured. (3) There is a positive reproductive alternative for couples when both are carriers, because the disorder can be diagnosed prenatally at a time when induced abortion can be carried out safely. Prescreening education is stressed and, interestingly, there is evidence that the mass media and word-of-mouth are more successful than physicians or rabbis in disseminating this information.[5] Unfortunately, few of the reasons for the success of Tay Sachs screening can be applied to CF at present (ie, higher target population, no specific test available for carrier detection, and no reproductive alternative).

HEALTH CARE SYSTEM

The health care system can offer diagnostic confirmation of CF by means of properly performed sweat tests. Therapeutic intervention is also available in the nationwide system of CF centers. The question of whether there is consensus about diagnostic and therapeutic policies is more difficult to answer and is extensively covered in this book. The natural history of the disease, lack of controlled trials of therapeutic modalities, and the genetic heterogeneity of the disease itself pose complex problems.

Methods to be employed in the screening for CF, whether for homozygotes, newborns, prenatal diagnosis, or heterozygotes, pose controversial and difficult decisions. Berwick et al[6] stated that nothing can replace the hard-learned lessons of experience in knowing whether a proposed program will succeed, but experience is not the only teacher. We could take many lessons from the authors' comprehensive analysis of alternatives for screening for cholesterol in children and its relationship to heart disease—the most important cause of mortality in developed countries. The authors have used the method of systematic cost-effective analysis to test alternative public policies. They question whether preventive medicine is a bargain compared to "curative" medicine and quote figures on single-factor intervention and screening that signify otherwise. While recognizing the importance of answering questions by basic research, studies of compliance, intervention costs, and behavioral changes have received relatively little attention and yet may have major effects on the proposed screening methodology.

SUMMARY

In the present state of knowledge, screening for CF is only recommended for research purposes. It seems doubtful that a reliable screening methodology will be available until the basic defect in the disease is identified. Even then the genetic heterogeneity of the disease may cause considerable problems in interpretation. CF screening programs that are inadequately supported in terms of confirmatory testing, genetic counseling, and public education have the potential for causing significant damage to the families involved and to those working in CF programs. These side effects of CF screening have largely been ignored by the enthusiasts of newborn screening programs. Research on the side effects of current screening programs is needed to identify and categorize these problem areas for the future.

REFERENCES

1. Report of the committee for a study for evaluation of testing for cystic fibrosis: National Academy of Sciences. Evaluation of testing for cystic fibrosis. *J Pediatr* 1976;88: 711–750.
2. Guthrie R: Blood screening for phenylketonuria. *JAMA* 1961;178:863.
3. Levy HL: Screening in the newborn, in Mangos JA, Talamo RC (eds): *Fundamental Problems of Cystic Fibrosis and Related Diseases*. New York, Intercontinental Medical Book Corporation, 1973, pp 261–268.
4. Fisher DA, Dussault JH, Foley TP: Screening for congenital hypothyroidism: Results of screening one million North American infants. *J Pediatr* 1979;94:700–705.
5. National Academy of Sciences, National Research Council, Assembly of Life Sciences, Division of Medical Sciences, Committee for the Study of Inborn Errors of Metabolism: *Genetic Screening: Programs, Principles, and Research*. Washington, DC, National Academy of Sciences, 1975.
6. Berwick DM, Cretin S, Keeler EB: *Cholesterol, Children, and Heart Disease. An Analysis of Alternatives*. New York, Oxford University Press, 1980, p 11.
7. Warwick WJ, Pogue RE: Cystic fibrosis: An expanding challenge for internal medicine. *JAMA* 1977;238:2159–2162.

8. Brimblecombe FSW, Chamberlin J: Screening for cystic fibrosis. *Lancet* 1973;2:1428-1431.
9. Shwachman H, Redmond A, Khaw KT: Studies in cystic fibrosis. A report of 130 patients diagnosed under 3 months of age over a 20-year period. *Pediatrics* 1970;46:335-340.
10. George L, Norman AP: Life tables for cystic fibrosis. *Arch Dis Child* 1971;46:139-143.
11. Kopito L, Mahmoodian A, Townley RRW, et al: Studies in cystic fibrosis. Analysis of nail clippings for sodium and potassium. *N Engl J Med* 1965;272:504-509.
12. Johnson GF, Thompson MF, Fetteroff S, et al: Neutron activation analysis technique for nail sodium concentrations in cystic fibrosis patients. *Pediatrics* 1971;47:88-92.
13. Lawson D, Westcombe P, Saggers B: Pilot trial of an infant screening programme for cystic fibrosis: Measurement of parotid salivary sodium at 4 months. *Arch Dis Child* 1969;44:715-720.
14. Kopito L, Shwachman H: Studies in cystic fibrosis: Determination of sweat electrolytes in situ with direct reading electrodes. *Pediatrics* 1969;43:794-799.
15. Gibson LE, Cooke RE: A test for concentration of electrolytes in sweat in cystic fibrosis of the pancreas utilizing pilocarpine by iontophoresis. *Pediatrics* 1959;23:545-550.
16. Shwachman H, Mahmoodian A: Reappraisal of the chloride plate test as screening test for cystic fibrosis. *Arch Dis Child* 1981;56: 137-139.
17. Green MN, Shwachman H: Presumptive tests for cystic fibrosis based on serum protein in meconium. *Pediatrics* 1968;41: 989-992.
18. Prosser R, Owen H, Bull F, et al: Screening for cystic fibrosis by examination of meconium. *Arch Dis Child* 1974;49:597-601.
19. Kollberg H, Hellsing K: Screening for cystic fibrosis by analysis of albumin in meconium. *Acta Paediatr Scand* 1975;64:477-482.
20. Stephan U, Busch EW, Kollberg H, et al: Cystic fibrosis detection by means of a test-strip. *Pediatrics* 1975;55:35-38.
21. Holsclaw AS, Berry HK, Bruns WT, et al: Meconium screening for cystic fibrosis—a collaborative study. *Cystic Fibrosis Club Abstr* 1977;17:54.
22. Shwachman H, Antonowicz I, Mahmoodian A, et al: Studies in meconium: An approach to screening tests to detect cystic fibrosis. *Am J Dis Child* 1978;132:1112-1114.
23. Berry HK, Kellogg FW, Lichstein SR, et al: Elevated meconium lactase activity. Its use as a screening test for cystic fibrosis. *Am J Dis Child* 1980;134:930-934.
24. Rule AH, Lawrence D, Hager HJ, et al: IGA: Presence in meconium obtained from patients with cystic fibrosis. *Pediatrics* 1971; 48:601-604.
25. Antonowicz I, Ishida S, Shwachman H: Studies in meconium in cystic fibrosis: The activities of alpha-D-mannosidase, beta-glucuronidase, beta-D-fucosidase, acid and alkaline phosphatase. *Biol Neonate* 1978;34: 225-230.
26. Antonowicz I, Ishida S, Shwachman H: Studies in meconium: Disaccharidase activities in meconium from cystic fibrosis patients and controls. *Pediatrics* 1975;56: 782-787.
27. Robinson PG, Elliott RB: Cystic fibrosis screening in the newborn. *Arch Dis Child* 1976;51:301-304.
28. Crossley JR, Berryman CC, Elliott RB: Cystic fibrosis screening in the newborn. *Lancet* 1977;2:1093-1095.
29. Crossley JR, Elliott RB, Smith PA: Dried-blood spot screening for cystic fibrosis in the newborn. *Lancet* 1979;1:472-474.
30. Dandona P, Hodson M, Bell J, et al: Serum immunoreactive trypsin concentrations in cystic fibrosis. *Lancet* 1979;1:1032.
31. Burlina A, Rizotti P, Tonon M, et al: Serum immunoreactive trypsin in cystic fibrosis. *Scand J Gastroenterol* 1980;15:35-43.
32. Kirby LT, Applegarth DA, Davidson AGF, et al: Use of a dried blood spot in immunoreactive trypsin assay for detection of cystic fibrosis in infants. *Clin Chem* 1981;27: 678-680.
33. Hammond KB, Hammond NB, Connor P: Immunoreactive trypsin (I.T.) in dried blood spots: An inexpensive neonatal screening test for CF. Presented at 1,000 Years of Cystic Fibrosis. University of Minnesota, May 7-9, 1981.
34. Manson JC, Brock DJH: Development of a quantitative immunoassay for the cystic fibrosis gene. *Lancet* 1980;1:330-331.
35. Lieberman J, Yakulis V, Kaneshiro W, et al: A new rapid screening test for detection of the cystic fibrosis (CF) carrier state: Detection of a serum lecitin. *Am Rev Respir Dis* 1979;119:140-148.
36. Gibson LE: Screening of newborns for cystic fibrosis. *Am J Dis Child* 1980;134:925-926.
37. Stamatoyannopoulos G: Problems of screening and counseling in the hemoglobinopathies. *Fourth International Conference on Birth Defects.* Amsterdam, Excerpta Medica Foundation, 1973, pp 14-15.
38. Leonard CO, Chase GA, Childs B: Genetic counseling: A consumer's view. *N Engl J Med* 1972;287:433-439.

39. Holsclaw DS, Keith HH, Palmer J: Meconium screening for cystic fibrosis. *Pediatr Ann* 1978;7:15–20.
40. Durie PR, Largman C, Brodrick JW, et al: Plasma immunoreactive pancreatic cationic trypsinogen in cystic fibrosis: A sensitive indicator of exocrine pancreatic dysfunction. *Pediatr Res* 1981;15:1351–1355.
41. Lloyd-Still JD, Conway JJ, Weiss SW, et al: Clinical evaluation of a serum immunoreactive trypsinogen test in cystic fibrosis. *Cystic Fibrosis Club Abstr* 1982;23:97.

3

Pathology

John D. Lloyd-Still

HISTORY

Landsteiner[1] first described the association of meconium ileus with a lesion in the pancreas. Fanconi et al[2] reported the consistent relationship between "congenital cystic pancreatic fibrosis" and bronchiectasis. Andersen, in 1938,[3] established cystic fibrosis of the pancreas as a separate entity from celiac disease. She performed the most comprehensive review of the literature to that date and reported the clinicopathological findings in a series of 49 cases (22 of these were from her personal experience, and 27 were from the literature). Farber[4] performed autopsies on 87 infants and children with pancreatic insufficiency and noted changes in the lungs, upper respiratory tract, liver, gallbladder, and upper alimentary tract which were essentially the same as those in the pancreas. A primary alteration in the character of secretions within glandular structures leading to obstruction and loss of function was suggested. He concluded that cystic fibrosis was a systemic disease with a variety of clinical appearances, the occurrence of which depended on when the obstructive changes occur and which organs are affected. Farber[5] suggested the term "mucoviscidosis" to describe the widespread defect in mucous secretions.

Other comprehensive reviews of the pathology of CF were published by Zuelzer and Newton[6] on 36 autopsied cases and by Bodian[7] who described the results of 62 autopsies in his classic monograph and coined the term "mucosis." The diagnosis of CF relied upon the demonstration of exocrine pancreatic insufficiency until di Sant'Agnese et al[8] first reported the elevated sweat electrolyte abnormalities. An extensive literature on the pathology has been published in other languages, and Nezelof and Lancret[9] reported the findings from a series of 44 autopsies in France. Oppenheimer and Esterly[10] reviewed the pathologic literature on CF and compared their own data on 146 autopsied cases. Bedrossian et al[11] performed autopsies on 82 patients with special reference to the lung and compared the prevalence of pathologic findings among different age groups. More recently, Vawter and Shwachman[12] reported their clinicopathological observations on 29 patients with CF who were 24–33 years old at death.

Other reports on the pathology can be obtained from the comprehensive bibliography published by the Cystic Fibrosis Foundation and the National Institute of Arthritis, Metabolism and Digestive Diseases publication[13] which covers the medical literature from 1813 to 1972.

DEVELOPMENT OF ORGAN SYSTEMS

During embryonic development the cells making up the germ layers—ectoderm, endoderm, and mesoderm—are undifferentiated. The ectoderm gives rise to the following structural groups and their derivatives: (1) the epidermis of the skin and its derivatives; (2) the lining of the mouth and related structures; and (3) the nervous system, brain, spinal cord, cranial and spinal nerves, and autonomic portions of the peripheral nervous system.

The endoderm develops into the epithelialized lining of the following: (1) the alimentary tract including pharynx, esophagus, stomach, intestine, liver, pancreas, and most of the cloaca; (2) the pharyngeal derivatives consisting of the larynx, trachea, lung, middle ear, eustachian tube, tonsils, thyroid, parathyroid, and thymus; and (3) miscellaneous structures including the urinary bladder.

The mesoderm differentiates into: (1) the muscles including smooth, skeletal, and cardiac; (2) the skeleton composed of cartilage, bone, and other connective tissue; (3) the excretory organs including the kidneys; (4) the reproductive organs; (5) the cardiovascular system including heart, blood vessels, spleen, and lymphatics; and (6) miscellaneous tissue, such as the dermis of the skin.

Secretory abnormalities in derivatives of all three germ layers can be deduced morphologically in CF.[12]

PRENATAL ABNORMALITIES

There is increasing evidence that the genetic defect in cystic fibrosis produces effects in utero.

1. The average birth weight of CF infants was 2.9 kg,[14,15] which is well below the national average of 3.3 kg, suggesting some degree of intrauterine growth retardation (see Chapter 19 for further discussion of this topic).

2. Anatomic defects, including ileal and jejunal stenoses and atresias, reduplications, omphalocele, congenital bands, mesenteric defects, perforation, volvulus, and intrauterine calcification are found in 50% of infants with meconium ileus.[16,17] There is also an increased incidence of inguinal hernias, hydroceles, and undescended testes compared to controls.[18]

3. Changes have been demonstrated in the male sperm transport system with an abnormal epididymus and atresia of the vas deferens.[19-21] Valman and France[21] concluded that obliteration of the mesonephric duct during the 10th–12th weeks of fetal life was responsible for this malformation.

4. Imrie et al[22] performed quantitative studies of the pancreas and showed a significant defect in the development and maturation of the exocrine pancreas in infants with CF compared to controls. This deficiency in pancreatic development could be recognized by quantitative microscopic evaluation at or before 38 weeks of gestation.

5. The elevated levels of serum immunoreactive trypsinogen in newborn infants with CF (see Chapter 2) lends support to Farber's[4] observations that the obstructive process

begins in the acini of the pancreas and that interference with the liberation or with the proper formation of pancreatic enzymes is the process of fundamental importance. Secondary obstruction of the acini and small ducts and later of the large ducts by a physically altered pancreatic secretion then takes place, to be followed in turn by atrophy of the acini and replacement fibrosis of the organ. Farber commented on the remarkable ability of the normal pancreas to regenerate following partial removal in infancy. In cystic fibrosis, regeneration does not occur, presumably reflecting the generalized nature of the disorder.

MUCOVISCIDOSIS

The literature on CF has consistently stressed the characteristic obstruction with mucus in the ducts of various tissues in the body. Andersen[23] stated that CF is a generalized familial disease that produces morphologic changes in nearly every organ of the body. The primary, most consistent, and characteristic changes are in the exocrine glands. The degree of morphological change varies greatly from case to case. The exocrine glands may be divided into three types on the basis of morphologic and chemical changes.

1. In one type the secretion precipitates or coagulates to form eosinophilic secretions in the glands and ducts, with obstruction to the outflow of secretion. Among the glands that may be affected in this way are the pancreatic acini, intestinal glands, intrahepatic bile ducts, gall bladder, prostatic glands, and sublingual salivary glands.

2. In the second type the gland appears to be hypersecreting, often with some distention of the ducts, but without the formation of solid casts. The mucous glands of the tracheobronchial tree and the upper respiratory tract belong to this group, as do the Brunners glands in the duodenum.

3. In the serous glands no morphologic changes have yet been demonstrated by the light microscope. The serous glands, however, produce an abnormal secretion high in electrolytes. The sweat glands, serous salivary glands, and lacrimal glands belong to this group.[23]

There is evidence that the physicochemical nature of mucous secretions throughout the body is abnormal in CF,[24] but more specific defects have not yet been found; this subject is discussed in detail in Chapter 6. Figure 3-1 (from Farber[4]) shows high-power photomicrographs of sections from widely differing organs including (A) duodenum, (B) sublingual gland, (C) esophagus, and (D) wall of the trachea. Distinct histologic changes, which have been interpreted as signs of mucous hypersecretion, have been reported in light microscopic studies of the large intestine in the CF patient.[7,25,26] Hypertrophic and enlarged goblet cells and crypts distended by accumulated mucus were described; these changes were considered useful in the diagnosis of CF by these authors. However, in none of these studies were quantitative morphometric methods utilized to evaluate mucosal abnormalities (Figure 3-2). Thus, whether or not a greater volume of intracellular mucus is consistently present in the large intestinal epithelium in patients with CF was not determined. When quantitative stereological methods were applied to biopsies of rectal mucosa from patients with CF, siblings, and controls,[27] the average relative volume of intracellular mucus and numbers of goblet cells were not significantly different from siblings or controls (Figures 3-3 and 3-4).

When quantitative methodology has been applied to the development of the tracheobronchial submucosal glands, infants with CF showed significant enlargement of acinar lumina compared with controls ($P < 0.005$).[28] By contrast, Oppenheimer[29] performed a retrospective study of 90 infants and young children with CF and 90 age-matched controls without CF. No histologic differences were found in the tracheobronchial mucous gland reactions with or without pulmonary infection. Reparative squamous metaplasia in the tracheobronchial tract occurred more frequently in infants with CF than in controls. She stated that the main

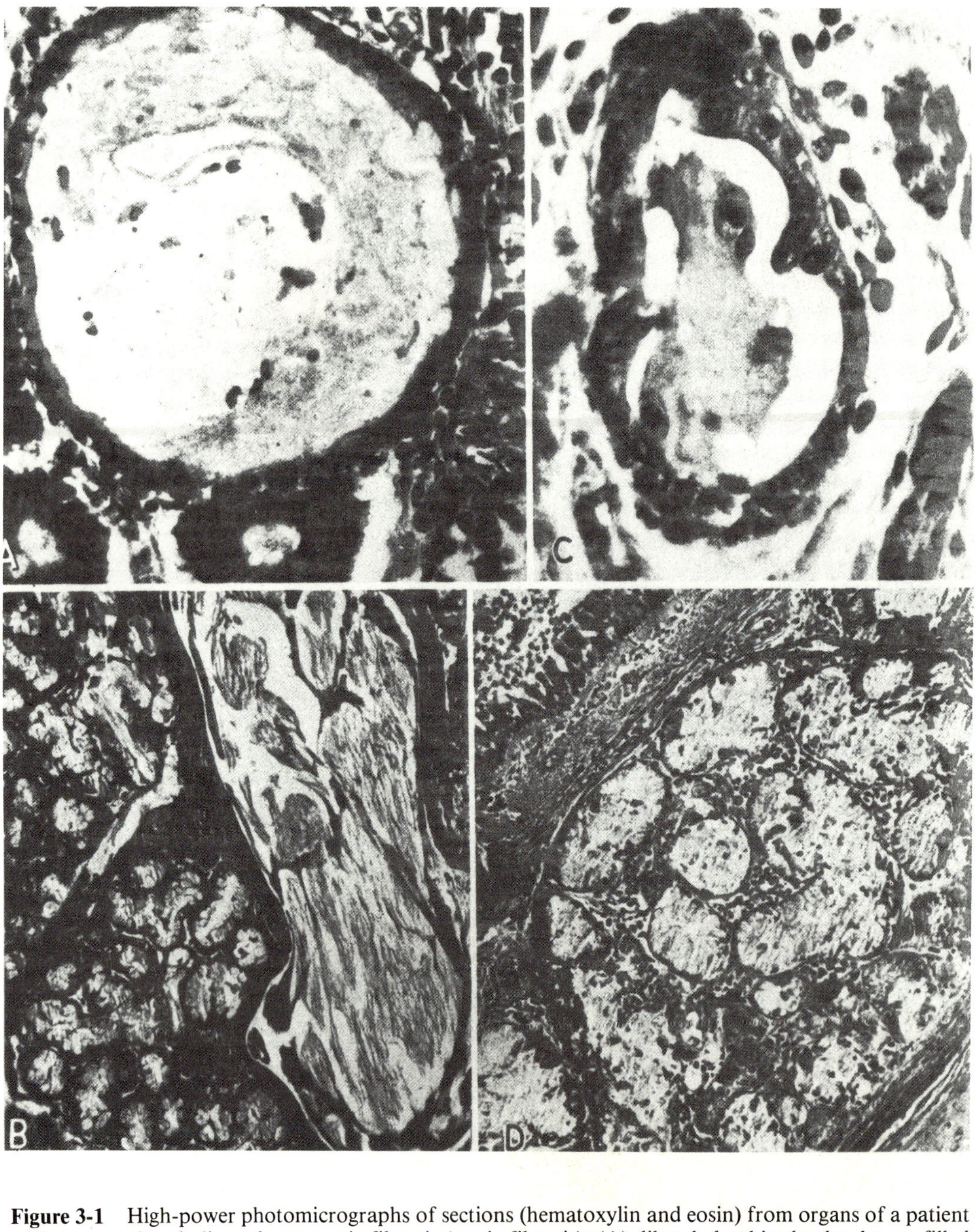

Figure 3-1 High-power photomicrographs of sections (hematoxylin and eosin) from organs of a patient with pancreatic achylia and pancreatic fibrosis (cystic fibrosis): (A) dilated gland in the duodenum filled with inspissated mucus; (B) sublingual gland, note inspissated mucus in the large duct and in the acinous cell; (C) dilated gland in the esophagus containing inspissated secretion; (D) wall of trachea, note submucosal glands distended and filled with thick mucus. Reproduced from Farber S: *Arch Pathol* 1944;37:238 (reference 4), with permission.

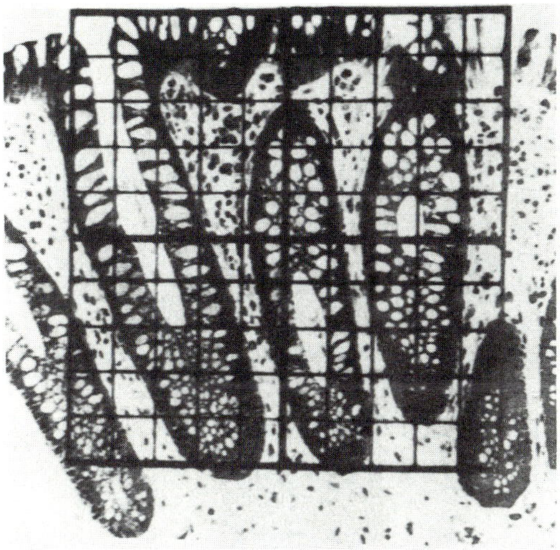

Figure 3-2 To estimate the relative volumes occupied by crypt lumina, epithelial cells, and goblet cell mucus, a 1-mm², 100-intersection ocular grid was superimposed on randomly selected mucosal areas such as this. Intersection counts from many such areas were recorded and averaged to compare quantitatively the composition of cystic fibrosis (CF) mucosa to that of sibling and adult controls. Reproduced from Neutra MR, Trier JS: *Gastroenterology* 1978;75:701 (reference 27), with permission. Copyright 1978 by The American Gastroenterological Association.

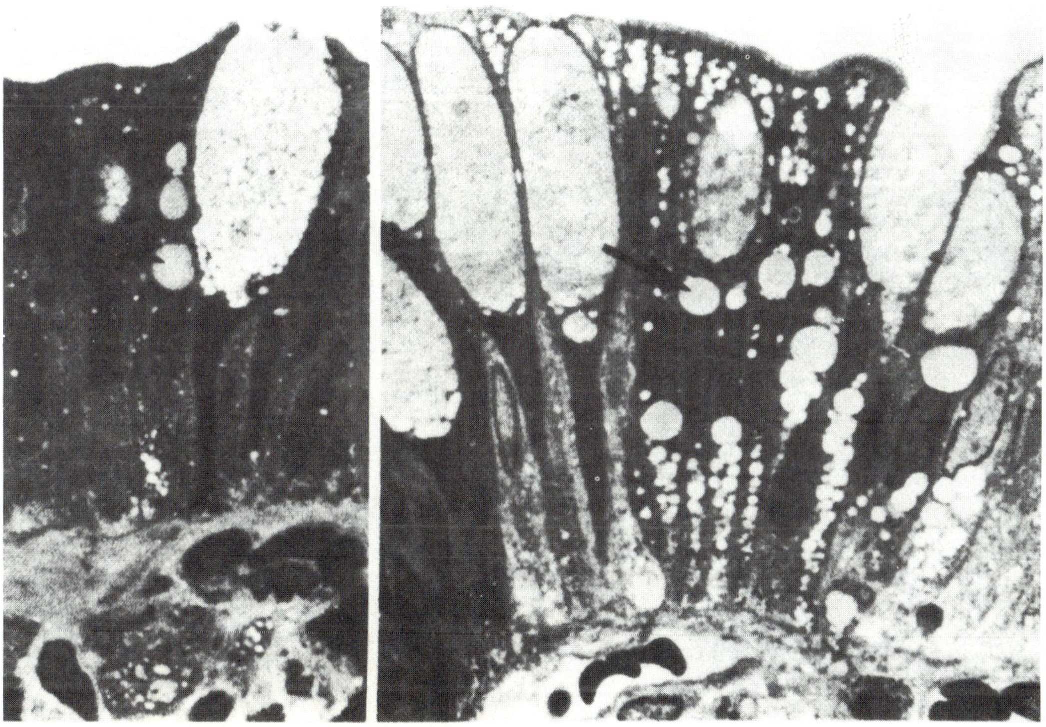

Figure 3-3 Surface epithelium of rectal biopsies (not cultured) from two cystic fibrosis patients, ages 15 and 11, respectively. Lipid-like droplets (arrows) are present in the surface absorptive cells. The number of cells affected, however, is variable (× 840). Reproduced from Neutra MR, Trier JS: *Gastroenterology* 1978;75:701 (reference 27), with permission. Copyright 1978 by The American Gastroenterological Association.

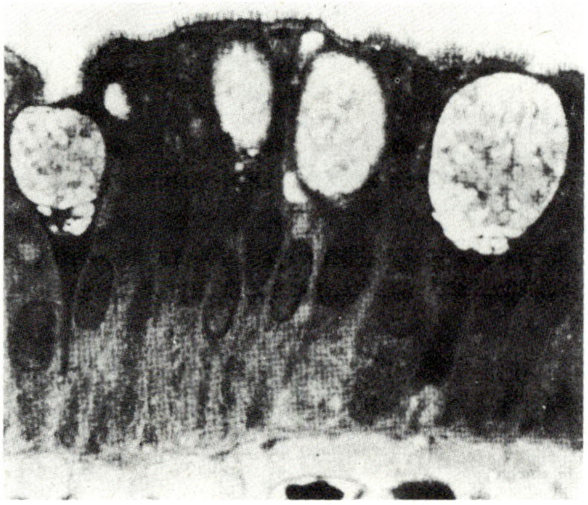

Figure 3-4 Surface epithelium of a rectal biopsy (not cultured) from a sibling control subject, age 7. No lipid-like droplets are present (×840). Reproduced from Neutra MR, Trier JS: *Gastroenterology* 1978;75:701 (reference 27), with permission. Copyright 1978 by The American Gastroenterological Association.

difference between the CF and control subjects is that in CF mucous overactivity is present throughout the body, whereas in the control patients, when mucous overactivity occurs, it is confined to the respiratory tract. Any inflammation may stimulate mucous glands to produce a preponderance of acid mucin,[30] which makes it impossible to distinguish when these changes result from CF compared to other causes of chronic lung disease. These examples demonstrate that morphologic studies in CF must be critically examined by quantitative assessment in comparison with normal and disease controls in order to prevent uncontrolled observations from becoming doctrine.

UPPER RESPIRATORY TRACT

A histologically nonspecific mucosis involves the mucosa and the accessory glands of the nose, accessory nasal sinuses, and eustachian tubes. The clinical manifestations are covered in Chapter 12 and include sinusitis and recurrent nasal polyps with or without associated atopy. Hyperplastic mucous glands, mucous cysts of various sizes, focal metaplasia of surface epithelium, and acid mucin in goblet cells were nonspecific lesions and found in both CF and non-CF nasal polyps.[31] Three differences indicated an association with CF: (1) the absence of basement membrane thickening; (2) the absence of tissue eosinophilia; and (3) the presence of predominantly acid mucin in crypts, mucous glands, and the surface mucous blanket of the polyp.

LOWER RESPIRATORY TRACT

The pulmonary findings of bronchiolitis, bronchitis, interstitial fibrosis, and progressive pneumonia leading to bronchiectasis (Figures 3-5 and 3-6) and a variety of other complications are described in Chapter 12. The associated infections and immunological alterations are described in the appropriate chapters.

HEART

The heart has never been considered a primary target organ in CF.[10] Right ventricular hypertrophy, which is the dominant adaptive change in CF, probably is directly related to the obstructive bronchial disease and pulmonary hypertension.[32] The clinical recognition of cor pulmonale, which is a late event in the natural history of CF, is covered in Chapter 14. Medial thickening of the pulmonary arteries, especially the arterioles, has been described,[33,34] and this is proportional to the degree of right ventricular hypertrophy. Deposition of mucoid material in the media of pulmonary arteries was found in seven of 35 CF cases with pulmonary hypertension.[35] Another vascular lesion reported by Oppenheimer and Esterly[10] was arterial calcification involving the internal elastic membrane and occasionally extending into the media. This calcification may involve a variety of blood vessels including iliac, mesenteric, renal, splenic, coronary, and intrarenal arteries. The cause is unknown.

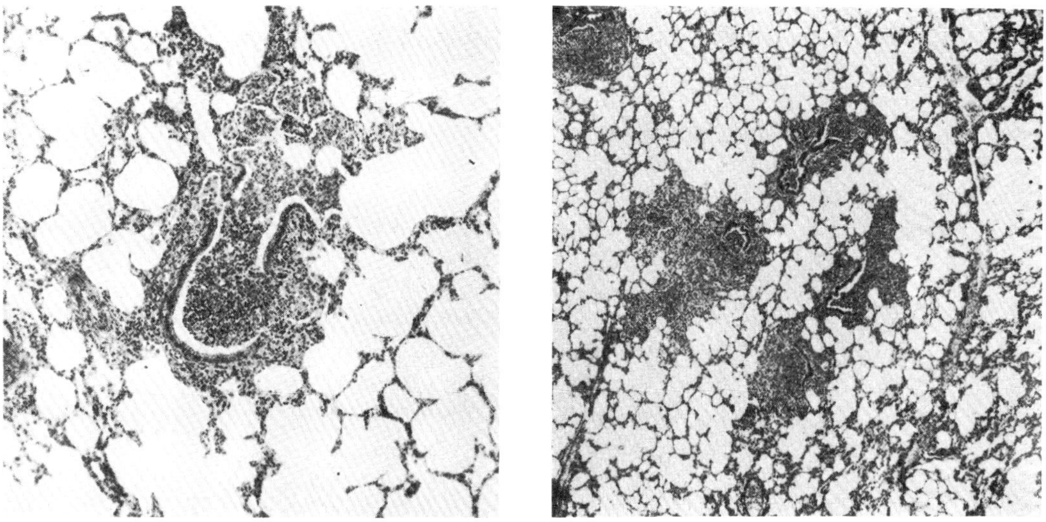

A B

Figure 3-5 Early inflammatory changes. Purulent exudate in bronchiole and few adjacent alveoli. Slight thickening and cellular infiltration of bronchial wall, × 83. (B) More marked inflammatory changes. Suppurative bronchiolitis with increase in size of pneumonic foci, × 22. Reproduced from Zuelzer WW, Newton WA: *Pediatrics* 1949;4:53 (reference 6), with permission. Copyright American Academy of Pediatrics 1949.

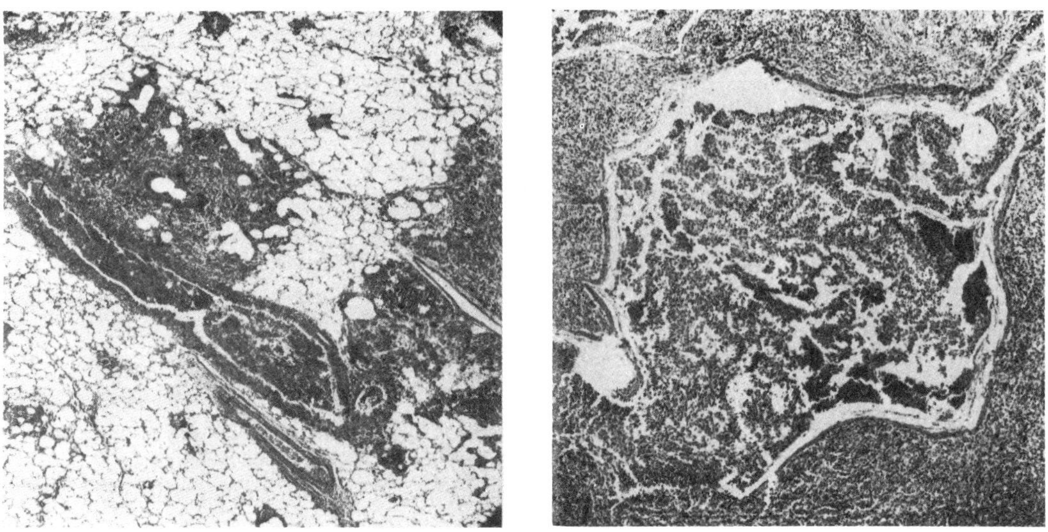

A B

Figure 3-6 (A) Further progress of inflammatory process. Marked peribronchial thickening, × 11. (B) Extreme degree of bronchial inflammatory changes. Lumen filled with purulent exudate. Lining partly ulcerated; shows extensive squamous cell metaplasia. Walls greatly thickened and densely infiltrated; marked bronchiectatic dilatation, × 27. Reproduced from Zuelzer WW, Newton WA: *Pediatrics* 1949;4:53 (reference 6), with permission. Copyright American Academy of Pediatrics 1949.

Esterly and Oppenheimer[36] stated that in no instance was myocardial disease a primary manifestation of cystic fibrosis. McGiven[37] reviewed the literature on myocardial fibrosis in CF and reported the ninth case. His patient had dilatation and hypertrophy of the heart, with patchy fibrosis of the left ventricle and endocardial fibroelastosis of the left atrium. Nezelof and Lancret[9] found such lesions in 4 of 44 autopsied cases. These children usually respond for a variable period of time to antibiotic therapy for their CF and then suddenly go into congestive cardiac failure. The myocardial lesions are thought to result from nutritional deficiency, and resemble the defects seen in the vitamin-E-deficient animal (see Chapter 22 for further discussion of these changes).

The incidence of aortic atheroma is decreased in CF,[38] with the controls having four times the incidence of the patients with cystic fibrosis. The reason for these findings are unknown and are probably not explained by simple fat malabsorption, as other children dying from malnutrition do not have this decreased incidence of atheroma. These observations could have relevance for investigators working in this area.

PANCREAS

The changes in this organ are discussed in Chapter 17, as well as in Chapter 15.

LIVER/GALLBLADDER

The histological abnormalities and complications are described in Chapter 18.

ALIMENTARY TRACT

Meconium ileus occurs in 10% of patients, and the pathology and clinical presentations are described in Chapters 11 and 21. The associated anatomical defects have been discussed and are indicative of prenatal effects on the fetus. The prognosis of meconium ileus has improved markedly in the last five years (in our experience all our patients have survived surgery during this interval), and it seems unlikely that the important findings reported in the older literature[3,4,29] will be observed again.

The light and electron microscopy of the small and large intestine are described in Chapter 15. A variety of intestinal complications, such as rectal prolapse, meconium ileus equivalent, intussusception, duodenal ulcer, and pneumatosis intestinalis are discussed. Ceroid deposits (morphologic evidence of an excessive rate of oxidation of unsaturated fatty acids) were present in the smooth muscle fibers of the gastrointestinal tract of patients with cystic fibrosis. These were first seen during the second year of life and increase with age, so that all patients over 5 years of age were affected.[39]

Similar findings were present in children dying from biliary atresia and cirrhosis of the liver. Blanc et al[39] considered extensive ceroid deposits to represent prolonged and severe Vitamin E deficiency. By contrast, involvement of striated muscle appeared to be rare and minimal in patients with cystic fibrosis. The effects of vitamin E deficiency in animals and patients with CF are detailed in Chapters 16 and 22. Lesions in the salivary glands were described by Farber,[4] and the sublingual gland shows the eosinophilic mucous plugs characteristic of the pancreatic lesions (Figure 3-1). Similar findings were found in a light and electron microscopic study of labial salivary glands.[40] Submaxillary gland enlargement was found in 2% of normal children and 92% of CF children.[41]

GENITAL TRACT

Denning et al[42] first described aspermia in male patients with cystic fibrosis. Kaplan et al[19] described the mesonephric abnormalities consisting of abnormal or absent bodies and tails of the epididymes, with the globus major usually remaining intact, abnormal atretic or absent vasa deferentia, and dilated or absent seminal vesicles (Figures 3-7 and 3-8). The testes appeared normal or diminished in size. Histologic examination of all postpubertal testes revealed decreased spermatogenesis with frequent abnormal

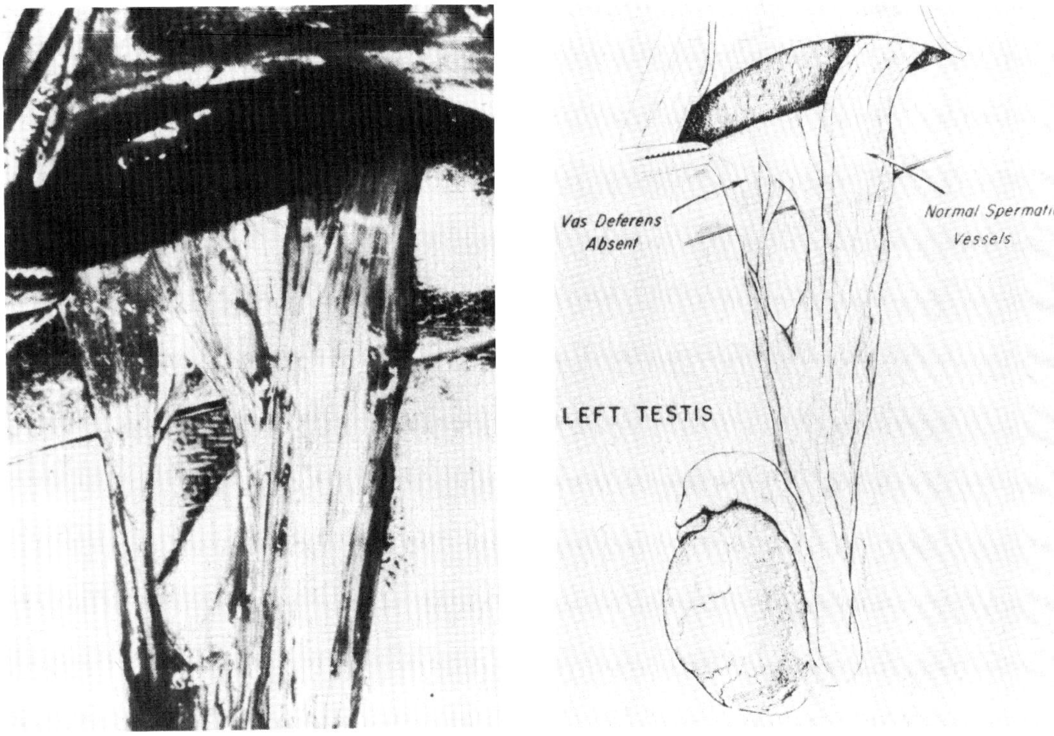

Figure 3-7 Gross specimen revealing absent vas deferens. Reproduced from Kaplan E, et al: *N Engl J Med* 1968;279:65 (reference 19), with permission.

sperm forms. The prostate gland is usually normal. Kaplan et al[19] performed semen analysis on 25 male patients with CF and noted that semen volume was reduced and more acid than that of controls. Fructose concentration was diminished. Citric acid and acid phosphatase were increased.

These findings reflect an absence of the seminal vesicles (which produce fructose) and the presence of an intact functional prostate gland (which produces citrate and acid phosphatase). Similar findings were reported in a microdissection study of 32 patients by Landing et al[20] who noted occasional normal male genital tracts. Oppenheimer and Esterly[10,43] noted normal fragments of the male genital tract to be more frequent in newborn infants than in older individuals (Figure 3-8).

There has been considerable debate whether the male genital abnormalities in patients with CF are due to a genetic developmental abnormality[19,44] or are secondary to obstruction by abnormal secretions of the mesonephros or its derivatives with consequent atresia.[10,43,45] Taussig et al[45] reported data on 117 males with CF; two were fertile and were the subject of their report; another six were believed to have fathered children, but their semen was not studied. They concluded that normal fertility occurs in 2–3% of males with cystic fibrosis.

It is of interest that all the reported fertile male patients[45,46] had mild pulmonary and gastrointestinal disease. Similar mild involvement has been reported in female patients with CF who become pregnant. Corkey et al[47] reported a total of 11 pregnancies in seven patients with cystic fibrosis. Nine of the pregnancies occurred in five mothers who had no pancreatic insufficiency. These findings add further support to the concept of mucoviscidosis of variable degree accounting for the symptoms. It is clear that the genital tract, like the pancreas, may occasionally escape involvement.[10]

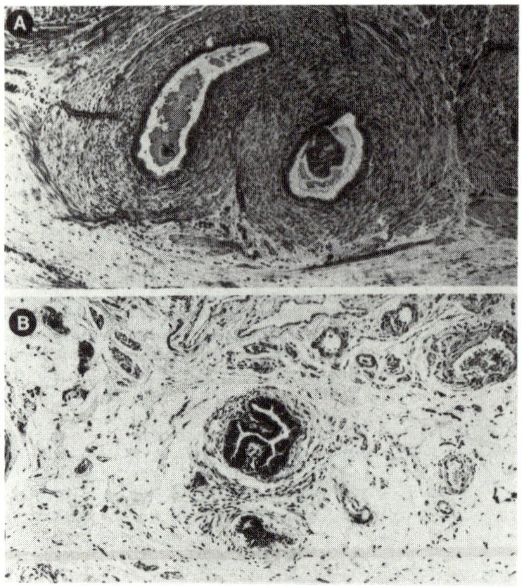

Figure 3-8 (A) In this anatomically normal vas deferens in a 3-day-old boy tenacious mucus fills the lumen. H&E, ×100. (B) The small cluster of epithelial cells represents the remains of the vas deferens in a section of spermatic cord of a 27-year-old man. H&E, ×100. Reproduced from Oppenheimer EH, et al: *Perspect Pediatr Pathol* 1975;2:241 (reference 10), with permission. Copyright 1975 by Year Book Medical Publishers, Inc., Chicago.

In contrast to men, women with CF display no major reproductive abnormalities.[48] Delayed puberty, secondary amenorrhea, acute and chronic inflammatory changes of the cervix uteri, and decreased fertility rate (20%) compared to the normal (85%) have all been encountered in increasing frequency in the female patient.[49] Oppenheimer and Esterly[50] noted mucous cell hyperplasia, obstruction of cervical glands with mucous secretions, and copious mucus in the cervical canal of 56 female patients with CF compared to 65-age-matched controls. These findings were present in all newborn infants and in over 45% of the older infants and children who had died of cystic fibrosis. Polypoid cervicitis has been reported in three adults who were receiving oral contraceptives.[51] Recently multiple small follicular cysts were described in the ovaries of female patients with CF.[52] Occasionally these cysts may replace the ovarian tissue and lead to menstrual irregularities.

Oppenheimer et al[53] suggested that there may be a biochemical abnormality in CF cervical mucus in addition to mechanical obstruction to sperm migration from increased viscosity and associated ultrastructural changes. Kopito et al[54] investigated water and electrolytes in cervical mucus from three female patients with cystic fibrosis. The cervical mucus was scanty and dehydrated containing less than 80% water. This is below the usual minimum critical level of 93–95% believed to be essential for the migration of spermatozoa. After removal of the water by desiccation, the mean concentration of sodium in the dry residue was about one third of normal during the entire cycle and about one tenth of normal during the mid-cycle period.

Further discussion of genital changes and the results of pregnancies in patients with cystic fibrosis are covered in Chapter 20.

KIDNEY

No specific abnormality has been recognized in the kidney in CF.[12] The incidence of nephrocalcinosis ranges from 5%[10] to 31%[7] and was 10% in adult patients with CF.[12] Glomerular changes thought to be associated with arterial unsaturation, with liver disease and with diabetes mellitus were found in the older patients.[12] Seven of 29 patients had interstitial nephritis which might have been the result of antibiotic therapy (see Chapter 23). Studies of renal function in patients with CF[55] suggested increased sodium reabsorption in the proximal renal tubules with decreased delivery of sodium to more distal segments of the nephron.

MISCELLANEOUS EXOCRINE GLANDS

Sweat Glands

The eccrine sweat glands (ie, exocrine sweat glands as opposed to the apocrine in which the secretions are concentrated at the free end of the cell and thrown off with that part of the cell) are under the control of the autonomic nervous system. Munger et al[56] performed an electron microscopic study of the eccrine sweat glands obtained by skin biopsies in eight patients (aged 11 months to 8 years) with cystic fibrosis; six of these were studied before and after stimulation by pilocarpine iontophoresis. Two portions of the sweat gland can be recognized in humans —a secretory segment and a duct (see Chapter 4). Eccrine sweat glands contain an acid mucopolysaccharide secretory cell (the mucoid cell) in the secretory segment. Mucoid cells in CF contain fewer secretory vacuoles than normal. Unidentified dense bodies were present in all cells of the secretory segment in large numbers in CF, but they were also present in small numbers in the normal. The eccrine duct was normal in cystic fibrosis.

Interestingly, in hypothyroidism, where elevations in the sweat electrolytes have been reported (see Chapter 4), cytologic changes are seen in the eccrine sweat glands. These changes consist of periodic acid–Schiff (PAS) -positive, diastase-resistant, granular material within the large pale cells of the secretory coil of the sweat gland. This material has never been observed in the sweat glands of normal individuals.[57] On the basis of its failure to stain with Alcian blue, the material appeared to be unrelated to the mucous substance deposited in the skin in myxedema. The exact nature of the material in the secretory cells of the sweat gland and its functional significance are unknown.

Apocrine Glands

Apocrine glands are derived from the germinal hair follicle (ectoderm) and are present at birth, but are not functional until shortly before puberty. Esterly et al[58] studied the frequency of apocrine changes in patients with CF and in unaffected infants and children, and characterized the mucin secretions of these glands. Dilatation of apocrine glands with retained secretions were found in nearly one third of autopsied patients with cystic fibrosis. The changes were most severe and frequent (8 of 13) in children over 7 years of age. Significantly less marked alterations were found in a control group. No qualitative difference in staining reactions was detected between patients with CF and controls. Apocrine gland dilatation becomes more common in normal adults after the third decade.

Breast

Ward[59] studied the histologic changes in the breast of a 20-year-old woman with cystic fibrosis. Sections showed abundant dense fibrous tissue with sparse ducts and ductules and complete lobular agenesis. Lobular agenesis is not specific for CF and may occasionally be seen in the normal young adult. Ward[59] postulated that the normal hormonal stimulation was responsible for the development of the fibrous element of the breast disk, nipples, and areolae, while the genetic defect in the epithelium modified its response and inhibited acinar development, so producing the appearance of lobular agenesis.

ENDOCRINE GLANDS

The effects of CF on the endocrine glands are discussed in a separate chapter. No primary involvement of endocrine glands has been described.[26]

SUMMARY

In summary, the autopsy diagnosis of CF is usually based on a combination of lesions rather than the changes in a single organ.[10] The spectrum of disease is broad, and tissues of each germ layer have been found involved in CF.[12] There are no histologic or histochemical features distinguishing between the mucus produced in CF and that in normal individuals. The most characteristic abnormalities in CF recognized by pathologists include focal biliary cirrhosis, distinctive obstructive lesions of the male genital tract, meconium ileus, staphylococcal and *Pseudomonas* colonization of respiratory secretions, and obstructive bronchopulmonary disease. Some form of progressive pancreatic involvement is usually present.

REFERENCES

1. Landsteiner K: Darmverschluss durch eingedicktes meconium: Pankreatitis. *Centralbl f allg Path u path Anat* 1905;16:903-907.
2. Fanconi G, Vehlinger E, Knauer C: Das coeliakiesyndrom bei angeborener zystischer pankreasfibromatose und bronchiektasien. *Wein Med Wochenschr* 1936;86:753-756.
3. Andersen DH: Cystic fibrosis of the pancreas and its relation to celiac disease. A clinical and pathological study. *Am J Dis Child* 1938;56:344-399.
4. Farber S: Pancreatic function and disease in early life. V. Pathologic changes associated with pancreatic insufficiency in early life. *Arch Pathol* 1944;37:238-250.
5. Farber S: Some organic digestive disturbances in early life. *J Mich Med Soc* 1945;44: 587-594.
6. Zuelzer WW, Newton WA: The pathogenesis of fibrocystic disease of the pancreas. A study of 36 cases with special reference to the pulmonary lesions. *Pediatrics* 1949;4:53-69.
7. Bodian M: Fibrocystic disease of the pancreas. *A Congenital Disorder of Mucus Production–Mucosis.* London, Heinemann, 1952, p 244.
8. di Sant'Agnese P, Darling R, Perera, G, et al: Abnormal electrolyte composition of sweat in cystic fibrosis of the pancreas. *Pediatrics* 1953;12:549-563.
9. Nezelof C, Lancret P: Lesions de fibrose myocardique au cours de la maladie fibrokystique du pancreas. *Arch Fr Pediatr* 1959; 16:1035-1046.
10. Oppenheimer EH, Esterly JR: Pathology of cystic fibrosis. Review of the literature and comparison with 146 autopsied cases. *Perspect Pediatr Pathol* 1975;2:241-278.
11. Bedrossian CWM, Greenberg SD, Singer DB, et al: The lung in cystic fibrosis. A quantitative study including prevalence of pathologic findings among different age groups. *Hum Pathol* 1976;7:195-204.
12. Vawter GF, Shwachman H: Cystic fibrosis in adults. An autopsy study. *Pathol Ann* 1979;14:357-382.
13. Holslaw DS, Topham AL: Cystic Fibrosis. A comprehensive bibliography of the medical literature 1813-1972. DHEW Publication No. (NIH) 77-1132. Rockville, Maryland, Cystic Fibrosis Foundation.
14. Boyer RH: Low birth weight in fibrocystic disease of the pancreas. *Pediatrics* 1955; 16:778-781.
15. Lloyd-Still JD, Hurwitz I, Wolff PH, et al: Intellectual development after severe malnutrition in infancy. *Pediatrics* 1974;54; 306-311.
16. Holsclaw DS, Eckstein HB, Nixon HH: Meconium ileus. A 20-year review of 109 cases. *Am J Dis Child* 1965;109:101-113.
17. Oppenheimer EH, Esterly JR: Cystic fibrosis of the pancreas: Morphologic findings in infants with and without diagnostic pancreatic lesions. *Arch Pathol* 1973;96:149-154.
18. Holsclaw DS, Shwachman H: Increased incidence of inguinal hernia, hydrocele, and undescended testicle in males with cystic fibrosis. *Pediatrics* 1971;48:442-445.
19. Kaplan E, Shwachman H, Perlmutter AD, et al: Reproductive failure in males with cystic fibrosis. *N Engl J Med* 1968;279:65-69.
20. Landing BH, Wells TR, Wang CI: Abnormality of the epididymis and vas deferens in cystic fibrosis. *Arch Pathol* 1969;88:569-580.
21. Valman HB, France NE: The vas deferens in cystic fibrosis. *Lancet* 1969;2:566-567.
22. Imrie JR, Fagan DG, Sturgess JM: Quantitative evaluation of the development of the exocrine pancreas in cystic fibrosis and control infants. *Am J Pathol* 1979;95:697-708.
23. Andersen DH: Pathology of cystic fibrosis. *Ann NY Acad Sci* 1962;95:500-517.
24. di Sant'Agnese PA, Davis PB: Research in cystic fibrosis. *N Engl J Med* 1976;295:481-485, 534-541, 597-602.
25. Parkins RA, Eidelman S, Rubin CE, et al: The diagnosis of cystic fibrosis by rectal suction biopsy. *Lancet* 1963;2:851-856.
26. Shwachman H, Holsclaw D: Examination of the appendix at laparotomy as a diagnostic clue in cystic fibrosis. *N Engl J Med* 1972; 386:1300-1301.
27. Neutra MR, Trier JS: Rectal mucosa in cystic fibrosis: Morphological features before and after short-term organ culture. *Gastroenterology* 1978;75:701-710.
28. Sturgess JM: Mucus secretion and clearance in the pathogenesis of cystic fibrosis. *Monogr Paediatr* 1981;14:60-74.
29. Oppenheimer EH: Similarity of the tracheobronchial mucous glands and epithelium in infants with and without cystic fibrosis. *Hum Pathol* 1981;12:36-48.
30. Lamb D, Reid L: The tracheobronchial submucosal gland in cystic fibrosis: A qualitative and quantitative histochemical study. *Br J Dis Ches* 1972;66:239-246.
31. Oppenheimer EH, Rosenstein BJ: Differential pathology of nasal polyps in cystic fibrosis and atopy. *Lab Invest* 1979;40: 445-449.

32. di Sant'Agnese PA, Talamo RC: Pathogenesis and physiopathology of cystic fibrosis of the pancreas. Fibrocystic disease of the pancreas (mucoviscidosis). *N Engl J Med* 1967;277:1287–1295, 1343–1352, 1399–1408.
33. Symchych PS: Pulmonary hypertension in cystic fibrosis. A description and morphometric analysis of the pulmonary vasculature. *Arch Pathol* 1971;92:409–414.
34. Ryland D, Reid L: The pulmonary circulation in cystic fibrosis. *Thorax* 1975;30:285–292.
35. Oppenheimer EH, Esterly JR: Medial mucoid lesions of the pulmonary artery in cystic fibrosis, pulmonary hypertension and other disorders. *Lab Invest* 1974;30:411–414.
36. Esterly JR, Oppenheimer EH: Myocardial lesions in patients with cystic fibrosis. *Johns Hopkins Med J* 1973;133:252–258.
37. McGiven AR: Myocardial fibrosis in fibrocystic disease of the pancreas. *Arch Dis Child* 1962;37:656–660.
38. Holman RL, Blanc WA, Andersen D: Decreased aortic atherosclerosis in cystic fibrosis of the pancreas. *Pediatrics* 1959; 24:34–39.
39. Blanc WA, Reid JD, Andersen DH: Avitaminosis E in cystic fibrosis of the pancreas. A morphologic study of gastrointestinal and striated muscle. *Pediatrics* 1958;22:494–506.
40. Sweney L, Warwick WJ: Involvement of the labial salivary gland in patients with cystic fibrosis. III. Ultrastructural changes. *Arch Pathol* 1968;86:413–418.
41. Barbero GJ, Sibinga MS: Enlargement of the submaxillary salivary glands in cystic fibrosis. *Pediatrics* 1962;29:788–793.
42. Denning CR, Sommers SC, Quigley HJ: Infertility in male patients with cystic fibrosis. *Pediatrics* 1968;41:7–17.
43. Oppenheimer EH, Esterly JR: Observations on cystic fibrosis of the pancreas. V. Developmental changes in the male genital system. *J Pediatr* 1969;75:806–811.
44. Holsclaw DS, Perlmutter AD, Jockin H, et al: Genital abnormalities in male patients with cystic fibrosis. *J Urol* 1971;106:568–574.
45. Taussig LM, Lobeck CC, di Sant'Agnese PA, et al: Fertility in males with cystic fibrosis. *N Engl J Med* 1972;287:586–589.
46. Feigelson J, Pecau Y, Shwachman H: A propos d'une paternite chez un malade atteint de mucoviscidose: Etudes des fonctions genitales et de la filiation. *Arch Fr Pediatr* 1969;26:937–944.
47. Corkey CWB, Newth CJL, Corey M, et al: Pregnancy in cystic fibrosis: A better prognosis in patients with pancreatic function? *Am J Obstet Gynecol* 1981;140:737–742.
48. Wood RE, Boat TF, Doerchuk CF: Cystic fibrosis. *Am Rev Respir Dis* 1976;113:833–878.
49. Denning CR: "GAP" Conference Reports, Problems in reproductive physiology and anatomy in young adults with cystic fibrosis, Atlanta, 1975. Rockville, Maryland, Cystic Fibrosis Foundation, p 2.
50. Oppenheimer EH, Esterly JR: Observations on cystic fibrosis of the pancreas. VI. The uterine cervix. *J Pediatr* 1970;77:991–995.
51. Dooley RR, Braunstein H, Osher AB: Polypoid cervicitis in cystic fibrosis patients receiving oral contraceptives. *Am J Obstet Gynecol* 1974;118:971–974.
52. Wang CI, Reid BS, Miller JH, et al: Multiple ovarian cysts in female patients with cystic fibrosis. *Cystic Fibrosis Club Abstr* 1981; 22:77.
53. Oppenheimer EH, Case AL, Esterly JR, et al: Cervical mucus in cystic fibrosis: A possible cause of infertility. *Am J Obstet Gynecol* 1970;108:673–674.
54. Kopito LE, Kosasky HJ, Shwachman H: Water and electrolytes in cervical mucus from patients with cystic fibrosis. *Fertil Steril* 1973;24:512–516.
55. Robson AM, Tateishi S, Ingelfinger JR, et al: Renal function in patients with cystic fibrosis. *J Pediatr* 1971;79:42–50.
56. Munger BL, Brusilow SW, Cooke RE: An electron microscopic study of eccrine sweat glands in patients with cystic fibrosis of the pancreas. *J Pediatr* 1961;59:497–511.
57. Means MA, Dobson RL: Cytological changes in the sweat gland in hypothyroidism. *JAMA* 1963;186:113–115.
58. Esterly NB, Oppenheimer EH, Esterly JR: Observations on cystic fibrosis of the pancreas. The apocrine gland. *Am J Dis Child* 1972;123:200–203.
59. Ward AM: The structure of the breast in mucoviscidosis. *J Clin Pathol* 1972;25:119–122.

4

The Sweat Abnormality in Cystic Fibrosis

Lewis E. Gibson

DISCOVERY

In 1948, New York City experienced a heat wave. As is usual at such times, many people were seen in metropolitan emergency rooms because of heat exhaustion. After copious sweating, they became thirsty and drank water without any added salt. This leads to hyponatremic shock. At New York Presbyterian Hospital, however, a very surprising statistic was noted. During a one-week period, ten of the cases of heat exhaustion were being followed by Dr. Dorothy Andersen for cystic fibrosis.[1] Doctor Andersen and her group were, of course, very puzzled as to why the CF patients so readily lost salt. They found that their patients' stools contained no excess sodium. The kidneys showed normal salt conservation. Dr. Paul di Sant'Agnese obtained the help of Dr. Darling, a physiologist interested in temperature control, and together they collected and analyzed sweat from CF patients.

It was found, of course, that even though the CF patients sweated at a normal rate, the concentration of sodium and chloride in their sweat greatly exceeded that of controlled subjects.[2] The cause of the heat exhaustion was obvious.

It was soon apparent that the determination of sweat sodium or chloride constituted an excellent diagnostic test for the disease.

The average concentration of either ion in CF sweat is approximately 100 mEq/liter as opposed to 20 mEq/liter in the control child. There is very little overlap between CF and control values (Figure 4-1).[3] Prior to the discovery of the sweat abnormality, the diagnosis of CF rested primarily on the chest film and on the determination of trypsin in duodenal drainage. Since the chest film is frequently normal in younger CF patients and occasionally normal in older patients, and since approximately 10% of CF patients have trypsin in their duodenal drainage, the need for a more accurate diagnostic test was quite apparent.

SWEAT PHYSIOLOGY

The discovery of this abnormality in CF sweat awakened a tremendous interest in the physiology of sweating among pediatricians interested in the disease. At the time, the mid-1950s, it was known that sweat rates were increased after acclimatization to a warm environment. The concentration of salt in sweat was known to vary with acclimatization, age, salt intake, salt-retaining steroids, and rate of sweating.[4,5] The variation with rate, although known to exist, was not well understood.

Much better data existed concerning the parotid gland.[6] The concentration of sodium in parotid saliva was known to increase with the rate of salivation and to asymptomatically approach an almost isotonic concentration (Figure 4-2). It was also known that when the sodium excretion was plotted against the rate of salivation, a straight-line relation was obtained (Figure 4-3). Mathematically it can be shown that the slope of this line repre-

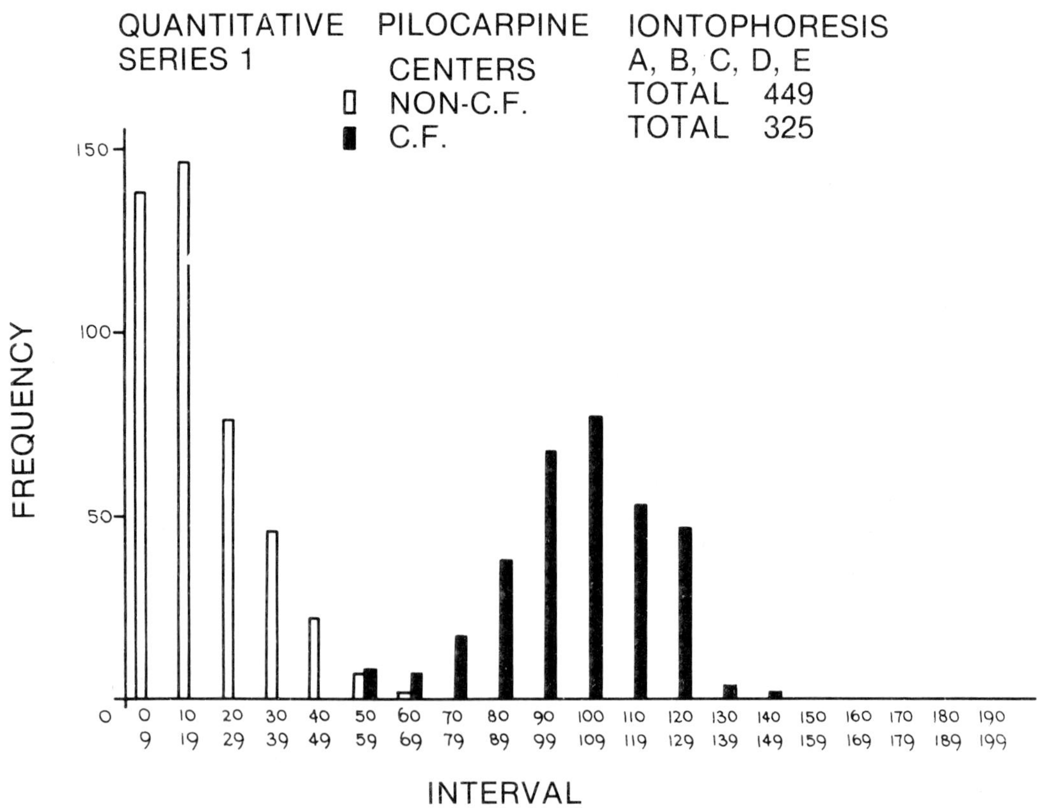

Figure 4-1 Sweat chloride determinations performed at five centers. There were 325 CF patients (solid bars) and 449 control subjects (open bars).

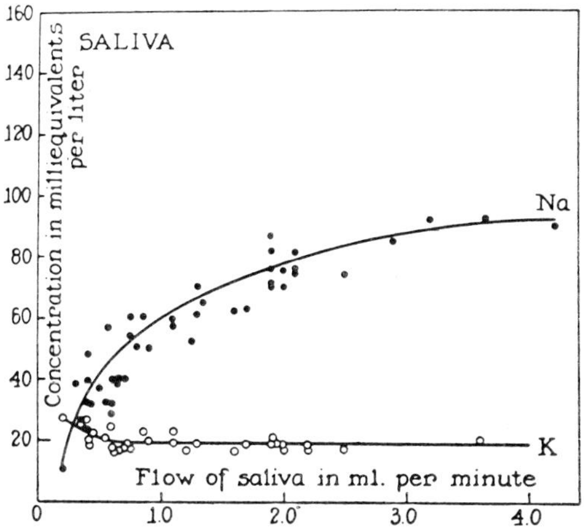

Figure 4-2 Relation between the concentration (mEq/liter) of sodium and potassium and the rate of salivary flow (ml/min). The concentration of sodium in parotid saliva increases with the rate of salivation and approaches an isotonic concentration. Reproduced from Thaysen JH et al: *Am J Physiol* 1954;178:155 (reference 6) with permission.

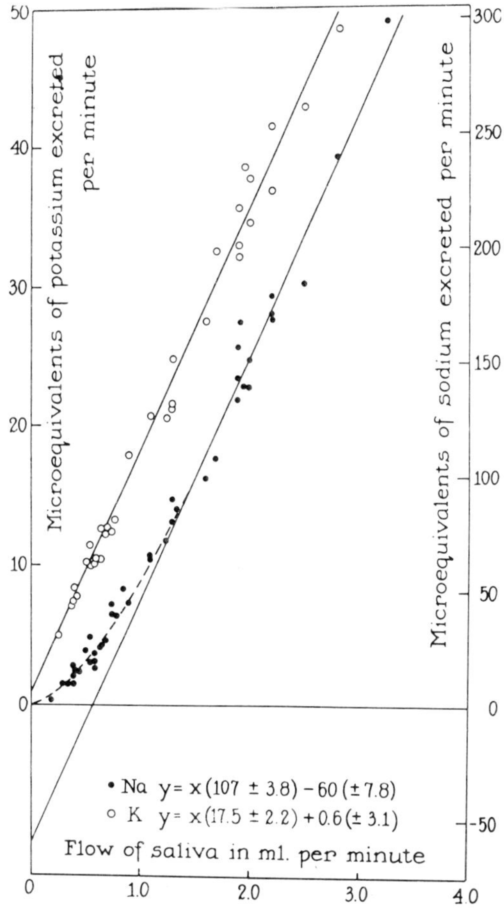

Figure 4-3 Relation between the rate of excretion (μEq/min) of sodium and potassium and the rate of salivary flow (ml/min). A straight line relation is obtained when the rate of sodium and potassium excretion is plotted against the rate of salivation. Reproduced from Thaysen JH, et al: *Am J Physiol* 1954;178:155 (reference 6) with permission.

sents the sodium concentration for a precursor solution and that an extension of the straight line to the negative intercept on the *y* axis represents the maximal rate of ductal sodium reabsorption. From data of this type it was found that the precursor solution of parotid saliva is approximately isotonic and that the ductal sodium reabsorptive system is saturated at higher rates of salivation.

Similar studies on sweat had given less clear results.[4] Concentrations of sodium in precursor solution were thought to be variable and to range from isotonic to hypotonic. Work in the author's laboratory using CF patients and control children showed that the concentration of salt in sweat definitely diminished with decreasing rates of sweating in both CF patients and control subjects.[7] We interpreted our data as showing hypotonic precursor solutions in the control subjects.

This was a mistake. The sweat precursor solution is actually slightly hypertonic in both CF patients and in controls. The mistakes in this early work were the result of inaccurate interpretation of data. It is difficult to stimulate sweating which is rapid enough to get on the straight line portion of the excretion vs rate curve.

Brusilow and Gordes[8] showed that the precursor solution in both CF patients and in normal subjects is slightly hypertonic. They did this by determining the melting points of sweat in various parts of the sweat glands of frozen biopsy specimens. This work has been confirmed by analysis of sweat obtained by micropuncture.[9]

It is now generally agreed that sweat is formed when sodium ions are pumped into the coil of the sweat gland. Chloride ions and water follow the sodium, hence the slight hypertonicity of the precursor solution. Sweat so formed then moves outwards through the sweat duct. In the sweat duct sodium is removed by a mechanism which, at high rates of sweating, becomes saturated.

SWEAT PATHOPHYSIOLOGY IN CYSTIC FIBROSIS

Although the concept of mucoviscidosis explains much of the pathophysiology of cystic fibrosis, it does not help us to understand the sweat abnormality so characteristic of the disease. Sweat glands do produce mucus, but no mucous plugs appear in the sweat ducts. The glands, in fact, appear to be entirely normal both by light and by electron microscopy.[10]

There are two conflicting theories as to the cause of the sweat abnormality in CF. At this time neither theory is entirely proven.

Mangos postulated that there is a factor in CF secretions which inhibits sodium reabsorption.[11] He collected mixed saliva from CF and control subjects and injected it in a retrograde manner into the parotid glands of rats. He then stimulated salivation and measured sodium concentrations at various rates. He found that, at equal rates, saliva from glands into which CF saliva had been introduced had higher sodium concentrations than saliva from glands with control saliva. He believed that this was due to an inhibitor of sodium reabsorption present in CF saliva. Mangos and others have attempted for some time to isolate this inhibitory factor. These efforts have been uniformly unsuccessful.

A criticism of Mangos' work is that he failed to control for the protein concentration. Cystic fibrosis saliva is well known to have a higher than normal protein concentration,[12,13] as do all CF exocrine secretions.[14] One might expect that any biological system, such as the sodium reabsorptive mechanism in the rat parotid, might be adversely affected by the injection of foreign protein.

Later, Taylor et al[15] repeated the experiment and actually measured the amount of protein injected. They found that the percentage inhibition of sodium reabsorption was extremely variable and that there was no statistically significant relationship between the amount of protein injected and the percentage inhibition. Using this data, however, we calculated the percent inhibition per milligram of protein injected. When this was done, we found no significant difference between the inhibition produced by the CF and control saliva.

Mangos also failed to control for calcium concentration, which is elevated in CF saliva. When calcium is iontophoresed into normal skin, the salt concentration of the sweat is raised. An explanation of this phenomenon is given in Chapter 8.

The present author has an entirely different view of the problem.[14] When one considers the production of human sweat, it becomes apparent that the sweat duct must be almost completely impermeable to water. Hydrostatic pressure in the duct has been measured and found to be as high as 500 mm Hg. After sodium is reabsorbed in the duct, the sweat becomes very hypotonic. Both hydrostatic and osmotic forces would tend to move water out of the sweat duct into the surrounding tissue. A permeable sweat duct would not allow fluid to reach the skin surface.

The sweat duct, then, must be fairly impermeable to water. Suppose, however, that the CF sweat duct was not quite as impermeable as the normal. The rate of sweating would be normal. Sweating is centrally mediated, and the warm subject continues to sweat until the blood flowing to the brain is cooled. Instead of diminishing the rate of sweating, a small leak in the sweat duct would lead to an increased production of precursor solution in the sweat coil. An increased amount of precursor solution could saturate the sodium reabsorptive system in the sweat duct and lead to the increased salt concentration characteristic of CF. A slightly permeable sweat duct would then explain the sweat abnormality in cystic fibrosis (Figure 4.4).

The leak theory will be discussed further in Chapter 8. Here it may be mentioned that in the normal sweat duct, sodium reabsorption occurs, to some extent, in exchange for potassium. A higher rate of sodium reabsorption would probably lead to a higher potassium concentration in sweat. The potassium concentration in CF sweat averages 15 mEq/liter while that in normal sweat averages 9 mEq/liter.[16]

PERFORMANCE OF THE SWEAT TEST

Darling and di Sant'Agnese[2] stimulated sweating by placing the patient in a hot room. This worked well, but unfortunately such rooms are prohibitively expensive to construct. Shwachman[17] stimulated sweating by placing the patient's body in a plastic bag with an elastic collar. These bags certainly made the subject sweat, although they were fairly uncomfortable. A few infants (not in Shwachman's laboratory) were inadequately watched while in sweat bags. They died of heat exhaustion.

Independently, Cooke, at Yale, and Gibson, at the National Institutes of Health, stimulated sweating by iontophoresis of a cholinergic drug. It was decided that iontophoresis was an ideal method of stimulating sweating and of performing the sweat test. The standard procedures were agreed on, the necessary data collected, and a description of the iontophoretic sweat test were published.[18]

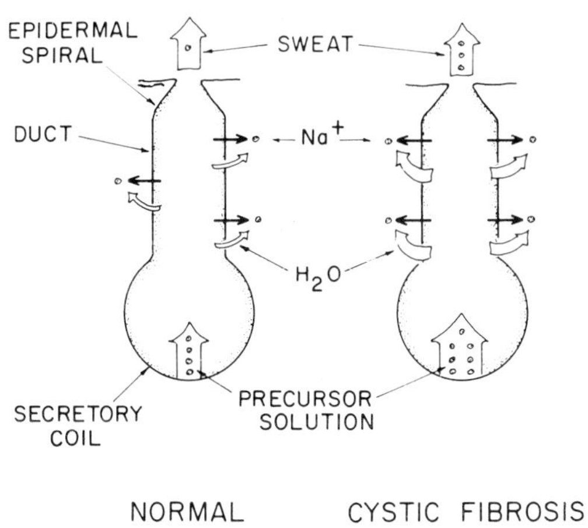

Figure 4-4 A small leak in the sweat duct will lead to increased production of precursor solution in the sweat coil, saturation of the sodium reabsorptive system in the duct, and increased salt concentration characteristic of cystic fibrosis.

Quantitative Pilocarpine Iontophoretic Test (QPIT)

Details of performing the sweat test by the QPIT method are available in the original description[18] and numerous other places. The following description is somewhat brief, but it does mention a few difficulties which should be avoided.

A 2 × 2-in. gauze square is saturated with an 0.5% pilocarpine nitrate solution and placed on the patient's forearm. This is then covered with a positive copper electrode. A saline-saturated negative electrode is placed elsewhere on the same arm. Copper electrodes seem to give fewer burns than those made of other materials, such as stainless steel. After the electrodes are secured, an electric current is started and gradually increased to 4 mamp. The 4-mamp current is continued for 5 min. This current will deliver 3.4 mg of pilocarpine nitrate which, although ineffective systematically, stimulates rapid sweating in the area covered by the electrode. A laboratory using a machine designed to do the sweat test which delivered 4 μamp of current was having difficulty getting a suffcient quantity of sweat for analysis.

If there is good contact between the skin and the entire electrode, 4 mamp will cause little discomfort and no burn. If the patient is uncomfortable, the first reaction should be to press the electrode more firmly against the skin.

After iontophoresis, the electrodes are removed and the area which was under the positive electrode is carefully washed and dried. A 2 × 2-in. collecting gauze is removed with tweezers from a weighing bottle, previously weighed, and placed over the iontophoresed area. The gauze is covered by a square sheet of plastic slightly larger than the gauze. Each edge of the plastic is carefully secured to the skin with two strips of waterproof adhesive tape. After a collection period of 30 min, the top of the plastic sheet is gently pushed down so that both the water condensing on the plastic and the sweat remaining on the skin are absorbed by the collecting gauze. The gauze is then removed from the arm with tweezers, replaced in the weighing bottle, and reweighed.

The weight of the sweat collected is obtained by subtraction. Usually between 150 and 500 mg of sweat are obtained. The sweat is eluted from the gauze and the concentration of the sodium, chloride, or both is determined by standard methods. Generally less than 100 mg of sweat is considered inadequate for determination. There is a small amount of salt in gauze squares and therefore appropriate blanks should be run. The sweat test is usually run in duplicate on both arms.

Alternative Sweat Tests

The QPIT test has the disadvantage of requiring two weighings on a chemical balance. Methods which avoid weighing have been devised but, unfortunately, they have inherent inaccuracies. Generally, the instructions say, in very small print, that they are "screening tests." The precise definition of "screening tests" is uncertain. From a practical point of view, I believe it means that the manufacturer of the equipment cannot be sued if an inaccurate diagnosis is made. When the results of "screening tests" are reported in three supposedly significant figures, their inherent inaccurracies tend to be forgotten.

The first popular screening procedure was the palm test.[19] A mixture of silver nitrate, potassium chromate, and agar were placed in a petri dish. The palm print of a CF patient was supposed to be very white while that of a control remained fairly red. The method obviously measured the amount of chloride per unit area and not chloride concentration. A sweaty control gave a false positive, while a calm and cool CF patient gave a false negative.

Methods utilizing sweat conductivity have been devised. Actually conductivity gives a fairly accurate measurement of the salt concentration in sweat.[7] The difficulty is in the method of sweat collection. A plastic cup or funnel is placed over the iontophoresed area and, after a collection period, sweat is scraped off the skin and transferred to whatever device is used to measure conductivity. During the collection the skin temperature is approximately 36°C while the cup is at room temperature. The sweat evaporates from the warm skin and condenses on the cool cup. There is then a solution with a high salt concentration on the skin and distilled water on the cup. Complete mixing is impossible. If more of the solution on the skin is analyzed, one can obtain a false positive while water from the cup can give a false negative.

A possibly less satisfactory method of performing the sweat test is by the use of a chloride-sensitive skin electrode, generally the Orion. After stimulation by pilocarpine iontophoresis, sweat is allowed to accumulate and evaporate for a variable period of time. The predictably bad results are made even worse by the fact that the instrument seems to be pressure sensitive.

Need for a Screening Test

The Cystic Fibrosis Foundation sponsored a cooperative study comparing the Medtherm conductivity test and the Orion electrode with the QPIT.[3] When the difference between two results on the same patient performed with the conductivity test were compared, it was found that the standard deviation of the difference was ± 17.4 mEq/liter. With the Orion electrode the figure was ± 26.1 mEq/liter. For the QPIT test the figure was ± 8.6 mEq/liter. Obviously the Medtherm and the Orion have some difficulties.

A good screening test for cystic fibrosis would be especially useful if it could be performed in the neonatal period. Early diagnosis would probably prolong the lives of the patients and would certainly facilitate genetic counseling. It is unlikely that sweat tests would ever be useful in the newborn period since newborns usually sweat very little. The use of a conductivity test or a skin electrode, backed up by a QPIT on all false positives, would miss a number of patients and would also be prohibitively expensive.

Another method of simplifying the sweat test which was advocated is the use of local heat.[20] As might be expected, this was ineffective since sweating is centrally mediated. Local heat will produce small amounts of sweat when the temperature is sufficient to cause local skin damage.[21]

Currently, there are no screening tests for cystic fibrosis nearly as accurate as a history and physical examination. It is unfortunate that various screening tests have been marketed since they are usually considered to be much more accurate than they actually are. Cystic fibrosis has such serious prognostic and genetic implications that mistakes in diagnosis can be catastrophic.

INTERPRETATION OF THE SWEAT TEST

Figure 4-1 shows the results of QPIT tests on a large number of CF and control children. Values between 50 and 60 mEq/liter are dubious and also infrequent. When one obtains a value in the 50–60 mEq/liter range, other diagnostic tests, such as duodenal drainage, should be considered. Although the use of salt-retaining steroids as a method of distinguishing between CF patients and normals has been considered, it should not be used. Sweat salt excretion will be lowered in both groups.[22]

Some normal adults have sweat sodium or chloride values up to 100 mEq/liter.[23] For this reason caution should be used in interpreting positive sweat tests after puberty. At one time it was suggested that obligate heterozygotes had statistically higher sweat tests. This mistake was made because obligate heterozygotes, the parents of CF children, were compared with normal children instead of normal adults.[23]

Either sodium, chloride, or both may be measured in sweat. Some authors have suggested that both ions should be measured because a large discrepancy in values will suggest laboratory error. It is the author's inclination, however, to measure one ion very carefully. The sweat test should be performed in duplicate, however.

Elevated sweat tests have been described in a number of disorders which are listed in Table 4-1. In several of these disorders (adrenal insufficiency, hypothyroidism, malnutrition, mauriac syndrome, and diabetes insipidus) the elevated sweat electrolytes will return to the normal range with treatment. These diseases should not be confused with CF. A false-negative test has occurred in a CF patient with edema.[36] It was once said that asthmatic children had slightly elevated sweat salt concentration.[37] A large series of patients did not confirm this.[38] When intradermal mecholyl is used instead of iontophoresed pilocarpine to induce sweating, sufficiently large samples for analysis can be obtained from some newborns. Using this procedure, Hardy et al[39] noted occasional false positives during the first day of life (Figure 4-5).

Values of sweat electrolytes between 50 and 60 mEq/liter are regarded as borderline values. Several of these patients have been

Table 4-1
Conditions Reported with Elevated Sweat Electrolytes

Condition	Reference
Cystic fibrosis	
Ectodermal dysplasia	24
Glycogen storage type I	25
Adrenal insufficiency	26
Familial hypoparthyroidism syndrome	27
Malnutrition	28
Fucosidosis	29
Nephrosis with edema	30
Pitressin-resistant diabetes insipidus	31
Mucopolysaccharidosis	32
Hypothyroidism	33
Mauriac syndrome	34
Familial cholestasis syndrome	35

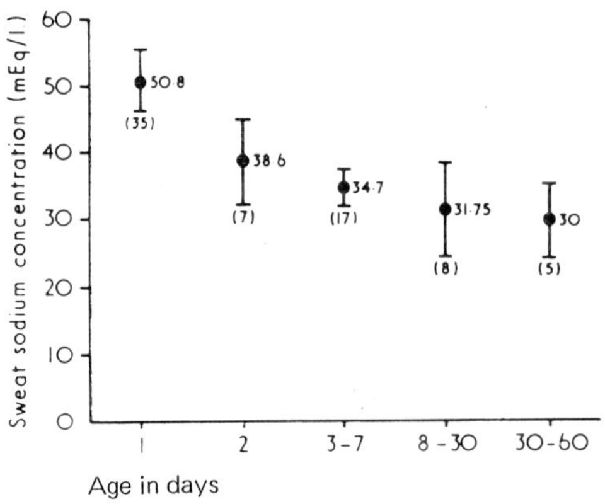

*Sweat sodium concentrations related to age. 72 tests on **64** babies. Means and standard errors of means (number of babies in parentheses).*

Figure 4-5 Details on figure. Reproduced from Hardy JD, et al: *Arch Dis Child* 1973;48:316 (reference 39) with permission.

followed for a number of years with electrolyte values varying between 40 and 70 mEq/liter. Stern et al[40] found seven patients out of a clinic population of over 700 with sweat chloride levels consistently between 40 and 60 mEq/liter, chronic staphylococcal and *Pseudomonas* bronchitis, but no overt steatorrhea. Stimulated pancreatic function tests with secretin were not performed. One of these patients died, and at autopsy the pancreas showed minor changes of fibrosis with some inspissated material. Shwachman[41] has reported similar patients. At present we are unsure whether these patients represent a cystic fibrosis variant.

There is some evidence (Figure 4-6) that the levels of sweat electrolytes in patients with CF and normal fat absorption are statistically lower than the levels in patients with CF and steatorrhea.[45]

HEAT-RELATED DIFFICULTIES IN CF PATIENTS

Human beings with and without CF develop heat-related disorders. In patients without CF, these disorders are generally divided into three syndromes: heat stroke, heat exhaustion, and heat cramps. Since all are caused by heat, however, an individual patient may have difficulties characteristic of more than one syndrome and therefore be difficult to classify.

Heat stroke occurs in unacclimatized subjects exercising in hot environments. Generally there is a cessation of sweating and a marked hyperpyrexia, with temperatures in the 106–109°F range. Brain damage frequently occurs. The cause of the cessation of sweating is not known. Both circulatory collapse and damage to sweat glands have been implicated. The only treatment is rapid cool-

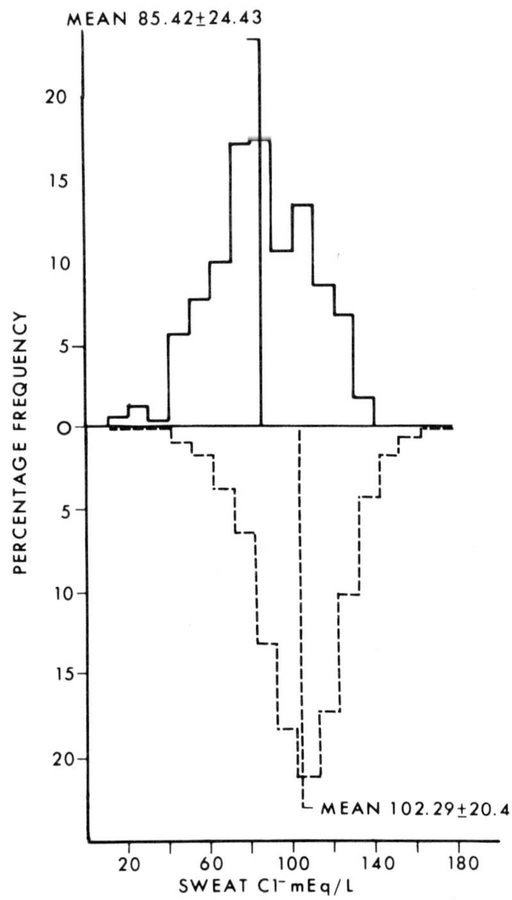

Figure 4-6 The percentage frequency of sweat chloride values: the solid line in the upper half of the figure represents the 346 sweat chloride concentrations of the group with normal fat absorption, and the broken line in the lower half, the 1367 sweat chloride concentrations of the group with steatorrhea. Mean values are indicated by the vertical lines and are significantly different ($P < 0.001$). Reproduced from Gaskin K, et al: *J Pediatr* 1982;100:857 (reference 45) with permission.

ing. The disease has a high mortality.

Heat exhaustion was mentioned earlier in the chapter. Replacing sweat loss with unsalted water leads to hyponatremia, loss of extracellular fluid volume, and shock. If neither water or salt is replaced, dehydration is more pronounced and hyponatremia less important.

Heat cramps occur in acclimated subjects doing strenuous work in hot environments. As the name implies, there is severe muscle pain. The cramps respond to oral or intravenous saline.

Cystic fibrosis patients are not prone to classic heat stroke. Even though they may become febrile after thermal stress, cessation of sweating has not been described. As mentioned, CF patients easily develop heat exhaustion. This can be prevented by increasing salt intake during hot weather. Generally, salt added to meals is sufficient, but with vigorous exercise or prolonged exposure to heat, salt tablets may be necessary. For CF patients these must be taken fairly liberally. A commonly used type of salt tablets, Thermotabs, contains 450 mg or 7.8 mEq NaCl. Since CF sweat frequently contains 120 mEq NaCl/liter, the need for liberal dosage is apparent. Oral salt is only useful to prevent heat exhaustion. Significant hyponatremia is frequently accompanied by vomiting which necessitates intravenous therapy.

There have been anecdotal reports of heat cramps in CF patients. To my knowledge these have not appeared in the literature.

Infants with CF can develop a sweat-related difficulty which is not caused by sweating in normal infants. This is hypochloremic, hypokalemic alkalosis.[42,43] These infants are fairly active and appear to sweat profusely. They have been found to have high levels of aldosterone. Presumably, the infants lose salt in their sweat, develop a chronic hyponatremia, and increase their aldosterone production.[44] The kidneys retain sodium at the expense of hydrogen and potassium ions.

We measured sodium intake and urinary output in such an infant. The child was 4 months old and weighed 4.4 kg. We found that the average daily stool and sweat sodium loss was 40 mEq. To each 8 oz of formula, 18 mEq of sodium was added as sodium chloride. The patient did well, and at age 14 months the salt supplement was stopped. During the balance study the infant appeared active and, even in the air-conditioned hospital, sweated fairly profusely. Adding salt to an infant's formula is obviously dangerous and should only be done when the blood chemistries are monitored closely.

REFERENCES

1. Kessler WR, Andersen DH: Heat prostration in fibrocystic disease of the pancreas and other conditions. *Pediatrics* 1951;8:648–656.
2. di Sant'Agnese PA, Darling RC, Perera GA, et al: Sweat electrolyte disturbances associated with childhood pancreatic disease. *Am J Med* 1953;15:777–784.
3. Denning CR, Huang NN, Cuasay LR, et al: Cooperative study comparing three methods of performing sweat tests to diagnose cystic fibrosis. *Pediatrics* 1980;66:752–757.
4. Schwartz IL, Thayson JH: Excretion of sodium and potassium in human sweat. *J Clin Invest* 1956;35:114–120.
5. Gochberg SH, Cooke RE: Physiology of the sweat gland in cystic fibrosis of the pancreas. *Pediatrics* 1956;18:701–715.
6. Thayson JH, Thorn NA, Schwartz IL: The excretion of sodium, potassium, chloride and carbon dioxide in human parotid saliva. *Am J Physiol* 1954;178:155–159.
7. Gibson LE, di Sant'Agnese PA: Studies of salt excretion in sweat. Relationship between rate, conductivity, and electrolyte composition of sweat from patients with cystic fibrosis and from control subjects. *J Pediatr* 1963;62:855–867.
8. Brusilow SW, Gordes EH: Salt and water excretion in sweat. *J Clin Invest* 1964;43: 477–484.
9. Schulz IJ: Micropuncture studies of the sweat formation in cystic fibrosis patients. *J Clin Invest* 1969;48:1470–1477.
10. Munger BL, Brusilow SW, Cooke RE: An electron microscopic study of exocrine sweat glands in patients with cystic fibrosis of the pancreas. *J Pediatr* 1961;59:497–511.
11. Mangos JA, McSherry NR: Studies on the mechanism of inhibition of sodium transport in cystic fibrosis of the pancreas. *Pediatr Res* 1968;2:378–384.
12. Chernick WS, Eighel HJ, Barbero GJ: Submaxillary salivary enzymes as a measure of

glandular activity in cystic fibrosis. *J Pediatr* 1964;65:694–700.
13. Mandel ID, Kutscher A, Denning CR, et al: Salivary studies in cystic fibrosis. *Am J Dis Child* 1967;113:431–438.
14. Gibson LE, Matthews WJ, Minihan PT, et al: Relating mucus, calcium, and sweat in a new concept of cystic fibrosis. *Pediatrics* 1971;48:695–710.
15. Taylor A, Mayo JW, Boat TF, et al: Standardized assay for the sodium reabsorption inhibitory effect and studies of its salivary gland distribution in patients with cystic fibrosis. *Pediatr Res* 1974;8:861–865.
16. di Sant'Agnese PA, Gibson LE: The exocrine sweat defect in cystic fibrosis of the pancreas (mucoviscidosis), in Montagna W, Ellis RA, Silver AF (eds): *Advances in Biology of Skin, Vol. III.* New York, Pergamon Press, 1962.
17. Shwachman H, Antonowicz C: Sweat test in cystic fibrosis. *Ann NY Acad Sci* 1961;93: 600–620.
18. Gibson LE, Cooke RE: A test for concentration of electrolytes in sweat in cystic fibrosis of the pancreas utilizing pilocarpine by iontophoresis. *Pediatrics* 1959;23:545–549.
19. Shwachman H, Gahm N: Studies in cystic fibrosis of the pancreas. A simple test for the detection of excessive chloride on the skin. *N Engl J Med* 1956;255:999–1001.
20. Warwick WJ: The silver electrode method for rapid analysis of sweat chloride. *Pediatrics* 1965;36:261–264.
21. Randall WC: Local sweat gland activity due to direct effects of radiant heat. *Am J Physiol* 1947;150:365–371.
22. Grand RJ, di Sant'Agnese PA, Talamo RC, et al: The effects of exogenous aldosterone on sweat electrolytes. I Normal subjects; II Patients with cystic fibrosis of the pancreas. *J Pediatr* 1967;70:346–356.
23. Anderson CM, Freeman M: Sweat test results in normal persons of different ages compared with families with fibrocystic disease of the pancreas. *Arch Dis Child* 1960;35:581–587.
24. Robinson GC, Miller JR, Bensimon JR: Familial ectodermal dysplasia with sensorineural deafness and other anomalies. *Pediatrics* 1962;30:797–802.
25. Harris RC, Cohen HC: Sweat electrolytes in glycogen storage disease, type I. *Pediatrics* 1963;31:1044–1046.
26. Conn JW: Electrolyte composition of sweat; clinical implications as an index of adrenal cortical function. *Arch Intern Med* 1946; 83:416–428.
27. Morse WI, Cochrane WA, Landrigan PL: Familial hypoparathyroidism with pernicious anemia, steatorrhea and adrenocortical insufficiency. *N Engl J Med* 1961;264:1021–1026.
28. Mace JW, Schanberger JE: Elevated sweat chlorides in a child with malnutrition. *Clin Pediatr* 1971;10:285–286.
29. Durand P, Borrone C, Della Cella G: Fucosidosis. *J Pediatr* 1969;75:665–674.
30. Warming-Larsen A, Wallace WM: Studies of the volume and composition of sweat during diuresis in patients with nephrosis. *J Clin Invest* 1951;30:680.
31. Lobeck CC, Barta RA, Mangos JA: Study of sweat in pitressin resistant diabetes insipidus. *J Pediatr* 1963;62:868–875.
32. Durand P, Borrone C, Della Cella G, et al: Le mucopolisaccharidose. *Recent Prog Med* 1968;44:279–300.
33. Strickland AL: Sweat electrolytes in thyroid disorders. *J Pediatr* 1973;82:284–286.
34. Rosenfeld R, Spigelblatt L, Chicione R: False positive sweat test, malnutrition, and the mauriac syndrome. *J Pediatr* 1979;94:240–242.
35. Lloyd-Still JD: Familial cholestasis with elevated sweat electrolytes. *J Pediatr* 1981; 99:580–583.
36. Goldman AS, Travis LB, Dody WF, et al: Falsely negative sweat tests in children with cystic fibrosis. *J Pediatr* 1961;59:301.
37. Hsia DY, Driscoll SG, Greenberg D, et al: Abnormal sweat electrolytes in patients with allergies. *Am J Dis Child* 1958;96:685–689.
38. Van Metre TE, Cooke RE, Gibson LE, et al: Evidence of allergy in patients with cystic fibrosis of the pancreas. *J Allergy* 1960; 31:141–150.
39. Hardy JD, Davison SHH, Higgins MU, et al: Sweat tests in the newborn period. *Arch Dis Child* 1973;48:316–318.
40. Stern RC, Boat TF, Abramowsky CR, et al: Intermediate-range sweat chloride concentration and *Pseudomonas* bronchitis. A cystic fibrosis variant with preservation of exocrine pancreatic function. *JAMA* 1978; 239:2676–2680.
41. Shwachman H: Cystic fibrosis. *Curr Probl Pediatr* 1978;8:5–72.
42. Gottlieb RP: Metabolic alkalosis in cystic fibrosis. *J Pediatr* 1971;79:930–936.
43. Beckerman RC, Taussig LM: Hypoelectrolytemia and metabolic alkalosis in infants with cystic fibrosis. *Pediatrics* 1979;63: 580–583.
44. Simopovlos AP, Lapey A, Boat TF, et al: The renin–angiotensin–aldosterone system in patients with cystic fibrosis of the pancreas. *Pediatr Res* 1971;5:626–632.
45. Gaskin K, Gurwitz D, Durie P, et al: Improved respiratory prognosis in patients with cystic fibrosis with normal fat absorption. *J Pediatr* 1982;100:857–862.

5

Control of Airway Secretions in Cystic Fibrosis

Brian Davis

Jay A. Nadel

Cystic fibrosis results from a genetically determined alteration of exocrine gland secretion.[1] In the airways, secretion from submucosal glands forms sticky respiratory tract fluid that is not cleared adequately by the mucociliary system. Narrowing of the airways by these sticky secretions leads to air trapping, atelectasis and infection. Persistent blockage and infection in the airways causes fibrosis, cystic changes, bronchitis and bronchiectasis with associated symptoms of cough, production of infected sputum and difficulty in breathing.[2] These changes cause most of the morbidity and mortality in cystic fibrosis; thus, one key to improvement in health of patients with cystic fibrosis is control of airway secretions.

Normal respiratory tract fluid is a mixture of fluids discharged from submucosal gland ducts and from goblet cells and other surface epithelial cells[3,4] (see Figure 5-1). The mixture, mainly water with small amounts of mucous glycoprotein and electrolytes,[5] forms two layers. The layer in contact with the inhaled air is an elastic gel,[6,7] the layer in contact with the epithelium is a watery sol surrounding the cilia. The cilia beat freely in the sol layer and move the gel layer with its trapped inhaled particles toward the pharynx to be swallowed. In large airways respiratory tract fluid probably originates mainly from

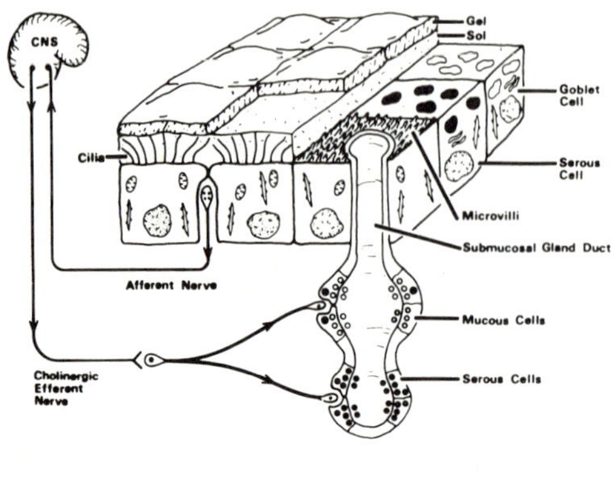

Figure 5-1 Diagram of secretory cells in airway. Serous (●) and mucous (○) secretions from the appropriate cells in the submucosal gland combine with water to form the submucosal gland secretion, which is discharged via the gland duct onto the airway luminal surface. This secretion mixes with the mucous and serous secretions from the epithelial goblet and serous cells to coat the epithelial surface with an upper gel and a lower more fluid sol in which the cilia beat and propel the gel toward the mouth. The apical surfaces of some cells are covered by microvilli whose function is unknown. Golgi apparatus (≋) of the secretory epithelial cells, and nuclei ( ), endoplasmic reticulum ( ), and mitochondria ( ) in the other surface cells are shown. Endings of afferent nerves in the lateral intercellular spaces close to the junctions between epithelial cells send impulses to the central nervous system and reflexly stimulate secretion from the serous and mucous cells of the submucosal glands via cholinergic efferent nerves. Reproduced from Nadel et al: *Ann Rev Physiol* 1979;41:369–381 with permission.

submucosal glands, since the volume of secretory cells in submucosal glands is about 40 times more than the volume of secretory cells in the surface epithelium.[8] Consequently, the consistency of respiratory tract fluid is probably determined by the secretion from submucosal glands.

SECRETION IN NORMAL AIRWAYS

Formation of mucus in submucosal glands takes place in mucous cells and serous cells.[9] Mucous glycoproteins are synthesized in the Golgi apparatus and stored in granular form in vesicles in the cells.[10] The stored granules are released by exocytosis through the apical cell membranes in response to nervous and humoral stimuli. Once released, the granular mucus rapidly takes up water to form glandular secretion which is discharged via the gland duct to become respiratory tract fluid[11] (see Figure 5-1).

Methods for studying glandular secretion have been developed recently.[12–14] Previously, the inaccessibility of submucosal glands hindered direct studies of submucosal gland regulation. New techniques using animal tracheas in vivo and in vitro allow us to visualize and measure the secretion of fluid and macromolecules from individual submucosal glands;[15] these techniques have been used to study the nervous, humoral and pharmacological control of submucosal glands.[16]

Parasympathetic Control

Tracheal submucosal glands are supplied by cholinergic nerves;[3,12,13] cholinergic nerve endings are closely associated with the secretory cells of the glands.[13] The cholinergic nerves originate in the vagi and reach the trachea via the superior laryngeal nerves and the recurrent laryngeal nerves. These nerves, when stimulated electrically, cause secretion from submucosal glands, a response that is prevented by cutting the nerve distal to the point of stimulation or by atropine, a muscarinic receptor antagonist.[3,12,13] The cholinergic nervous regulation of secretion is mediated at least in part through pulmonary reflexes. Mechanical irritation of the larynx[14,18] or stomach,[19,20] hypoxemia,[20] chemical stimulation of cough receptors[18] and of bronchial C-fibers[21] each increased glandular secretion by a reflex whose efferent pathway was in cholinergic fibers. Thus, there is conclusive evidence that the airway submucosal glands are supplied and regulated by cholinergic nerves. There is also evidence of regulation of the glands by adrenergic nerves.

Sympathetic Control

Postganglionic adrenergic nerves to the airways originate in the stellate ganglia and form a network of nerves in the periphery of the lung.[22] In cats, adrenergic nerve endings are found close to secretory cells.[17,23] Also in cats, stimulation of the stellate ganglion caused an increased output of radiolabeled macromolecules from isolated tracheal segments.[19] This increase was prevented by propranolol, suggesting that regulation of the glands was in part by a beta-adrenergic mechanism. An alpha-adrenergic agonist, phenylephrine, caused a greater increase than a beta$_2$-adrenergic agonist in the output of radiolabeled macromolecules from cat trachea in vitro.[24] Similar changes occurred in human bronchi.[25,26] In studies of ferrets in vitro, electrical stimulation of nerves in the trachea caused submucosal gland secretion that was partly prevented by phentolamine, an alpha-adrenergic antagonist.[27] Thus, alpha-adrenergic mechanisms also regulate submucosal gland secretion.

Specific Cellular Regulation

Recently, physiological and morphological evidence from the same tracheal submucosal glands showed that alpha-adrenergic agonists have a specific effect on glandular serous cells, while beta-adrenergic agonists have a proportionately greater effect on glandular mucus cells; muscarinic agonists, however, stimulate both mucus and serous cells.[28] Direct evidence that serous cells produce a different secretion from mucus cells was obtained using secretions collected from individual submucosal glands into micropipettes. Stimulation of the glands with alpha-adrenergic agonists, agents known to specifically affect serous cells, caused an increase in the volume of secretion, while total protein content remained the same; in contrast, beta-adrenergic agonists which predominantly stimulate mucus cells increased the protein concentration of the secretion with only small changes in the volume.[29] Thus, autonomic agonists have different effects on submucosal gland cells and provide one means of regulating consistency of respiratory tract fluid. Another means of modifying the consistency is by regulating the water taken up by the mucus.

Secretion and Absorption of Water

The function of the gland duct epithelium in airway submucosal glands has not been studied directly. Morphological evidence suggested that the duct cells are capable of secretion or absorption of fluid.[30] However, fluid discharged from duct openings was isotonic with respect to serum in the cat;[29,31] also, the discharged fluid did not change its tonicity when the flow rate was increased (Ueki and Nadel, unpublished observations). This evidence suggests that little or no absorption or secretion of water, electrolytes or protein occurs across the duct epithelium under normal conditions. Therefore, the airway surface epithelium remains the most likely site for modification of the primary glandular secretion by absorption or secretion of water.

Fluid discharged from gland ducts mixes with surface epithelial secretions to form a double layer of fluid. The lower watery sol layer surrounds the beating cilia. This sol, because it is watery, can be modified by absorption or secretion of water through the airway epithelium.[32]

Active transport of electrolytes is a means for movement of water across epithelia.[33] The transported electrolytes are trapped in a narrow space such as the space between adjacent lateral cell walls. There they create an osmotic force that attracts water into the space from the adjacent cells. The water, as it enters the narrow space, creates a hydrostatic pressure that moves the fluid along the space. Also, water from adjacent cells dilutes the electrolytes until isotonic fluid is discharged at the basal opening of the lateral space.

Airway epithelium has a low permeability to electrolytes and water compared to epithelia in other organs and can be classified on the basis of its spontaneous electrical potential difference and its electrical resistance as a tight epithelium.[34] Electrolytes cross the epithelium by diffusion and by transport systems that require metabolic energy. For instance, tracheal epithelium in the dog transports Cl^- toward the luminal surface and Na^+ toward the submucosal surface.[34] The transport system involves Na-K-ATPase and a neutral carrier molecule at the basolateral membrane.[35-37] In dog trachea, in vitro, active transport of electrolytes has been shown to regulate water movement across the epithelium.[32] Agents that increased Cl^- transport toward the lumen increased water movement into the lumen, and agents that increased Na^+ transport toward the submucosa caused absorption of water.[32,38] These studies indicate that active ion transport across the surface epithelium can regulate the consistency of the sol layer by changing its water and electrolyte content[32] (see Figure 5-2). The depth of the sol layer in relation to the height of the cilia may also be regulated by active ion transport.[39] Futhermore, the consistency of the upper mucus layer may depend on a balance between uptake of water from the sol and loss of water via the expired air. Each of these changes will influence the effectiveness of mucociliary clearance.

The knowledge gained from the above studies on normal control of airway secretions indicates that autonomic nerves regulate the balance of mucus glycoprotein secretion and electrolyte and water transport. However, the secretory system is complex and appears to be altered in diseases that affect the lungs, particularly cystic fibrosis (See Figure 5-3).

SECRETION IN CYSTIC FIBROSIS

Disorders of Electrolytes

Cystic fibrosis is associated with abnormal electrolyte transport across epithelial surfaces.[40,41] For instance, Na^+ reabsorption is diminished in the sweat gland duct[42,43] and salivary gland duct,[44] leading to excessive excretion of electrolytes in sweat and saliva. This loss of ductal reabsorption may depend on the presence of a "factor" in the primary secretion[45,46] (see Figure 5-2). The chemical nature and site of action of this factor have not been determined. Saliva from patients with cystic fibrosis also inhibited Na^+ absorption through channels in the apical

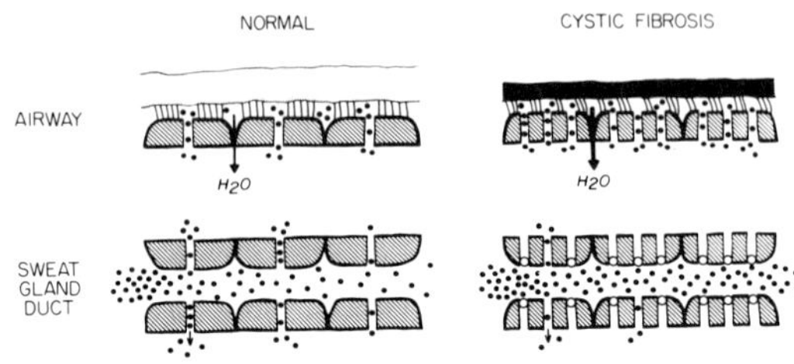

Figure 5-2 Diagram of a hypothesis explaining differences in exocrine gland secretions between normal subjects and people with cystic fibrosis. Each lower diagram shows a sweat gland duct perfused by a solution of electrolytes which is isotonic when it leaves the glandular acinus (not shown). In normals (left) electrolytes are absorbed through the duct epithelium via hypothetical channels that represent specific pathways for electrolytes, including selective ion channels, carrier molecules and metabolic ion pumps. Absorption of electrolytes from the duct results in sweat containing very little salt. In cystic fibrosis, (right) although more channels are hypothesized to be present, they are thought to be blocked by a "factor" that prevents the absorption of most of the electrolytes, leaving more salt than normal in the sweat. Each upper diagram represents airway epithelium. The luminal surfaces of the cells are coated with a watery sol containing electrolytes which supports a thick gell layer that is in contact with inhaled air. Cilia beat in the sol and move the gel to the pharynx where it is swallowed. Absorption of electrolytes through hypothetical channels creates local osmotic gradients that cause absorption of water (H_2O). In normals the absorption of water is thought to regulate the consistency of the gel and the depth of the sol so that the tips of the cilia just touch the gel during the effective part of their beat. In cystic fibrosis airways, more channels are thought to exist, but a blocking factor (o) is not present. The channels permit excessive absorption of electrolytes. In turn, this causes excessive absorption of water, reduction of the depth of the sol, impairment of ciliary movement, and dehydration of the gel layer. (This hypothesis was originally described in more detail by Ulrich Hopfer, MD, PhD, Associate Professor of Anatomy, Case Western Reserve, Cleveland, Ohio—Reference 51.)

membranes of rat colonic epithelium.[47] These channels only appear in the presence of hyperaldosteronism and are specifically blocked by the drug amiloride.[48]

The observation that some degree of hyperaldosteronism is present in many patients with CF[49] and causes hypertrophy of the adrenal zona glomerulosa[50] suggests that aldosterone might stimulate formation of amiloride sensitive Na^+ channels in the apical cell membrane of epithelia in cystic fibrosis such as airways, pancreas, intestine and biliary tract. Hopfer, Will, and Dearborn[51] have hypothesized that these channels would cause excessive reabsorption of electrolytes and water across the epithelial surfaces and account for the alterations in secretions (see Figure 5-2).

There is evidence to support this hypothesis. Human bronchi actively transport electrolytes[52–54] and are sensitive to amiloride.[52,54] Patients with cystic fibrosis have a higher electrical potential across their nasal and airway epithelium than normal subjects or patients with a wide range of diseases;[55] local application of amiloride to the epithelial surface of the nose abolished the difference in electrical potential between the two groups. In addition, amiloride inhibited ion transport in the bronchus of a patient with cystic fibrosis more than in normal human airways.[56] As a result, it has been speculated that amiloride might prove useful in the treatment of cystic fibrosis.[55] One can speculate that if amiloride was inhaled and if it inhibited Na^+ reabsorption and water reabsorption across the airway epithelium, the unabsorbed water could alter the consistency of airway secretions, the depth of the sol layer, the effectiveness of mucociliary clearance and removal of secretions by coughing.* On the other hand, the abnormal consistency of airway secretions in cystic fibrosis might also result from changes in the sensitivity of the autonomic nervous system.

*In practice it is very dangerous to inhale amiloride because it releases histamine and may cause severe bronchospasm.

Disorders of Autonomic Nerves

Patients with cystic fibrosis are abnormally sensitive to alpha-adrenergic and cholinergic agonists and abnormally insensitive to beta-adrenergic agonists.[57] Pupils of patients with cystic fibrosis were more sensitive than normal controls to dilation by phenylephrine, and to constriction by carbachol; their heart rate was less sensitive to beta adrenergic agonists than normal subjects. These findings suggested that some lesion is present in the alpha-adrenergic, beta-adrenergic and cholinergic systems at or beyond the level of the receptors. Similar pupillary responses and heart rate sensitivity have also been demonstrated in asthma,[58] suggesting that such changes in the autonomic nervous system are not specific for cystic fibrosis and could be secondary to treatment. Nevertheless, one can speculate that this imbalance of the autonomic nervous system might modify secretion of macromolecules from submucosal glands and produce a mixture of secretion from glandular serous cells and mucus cells that was thick and sticky like that in cystic fibrosis.

An alternative effect of the imbalance of the autonomic nervous system on the consistency of secretion might be mediated by changes of water movement induced by changes in ion transport across the epithelium of the airways. In animal tracheas a beta-adrenergic agonist increased Cl^- secretion,[59] and an alpha-adrenergic agonist[24] and a cholinergic agonist[60] increased Na^+ and Cl^- secretion. In normal human bronchi a cholinergic agonist increased Na^+ and Cl^- secretion, but alpha-adrenergic and beta-adrenergic agonists had no effect on ion movement.[54] Thus, the observed alteration of responsiveness to autonomic agonists in cystic fibrosis may alter the balance of water absorption across the surface epithelium and account for changes in the consistency of airway secretions. It remains to be determined whether these changes in autonomic regulation are primary or secondary effects.

The cause of these changes in autonomic regulation and in electrolyte transport across

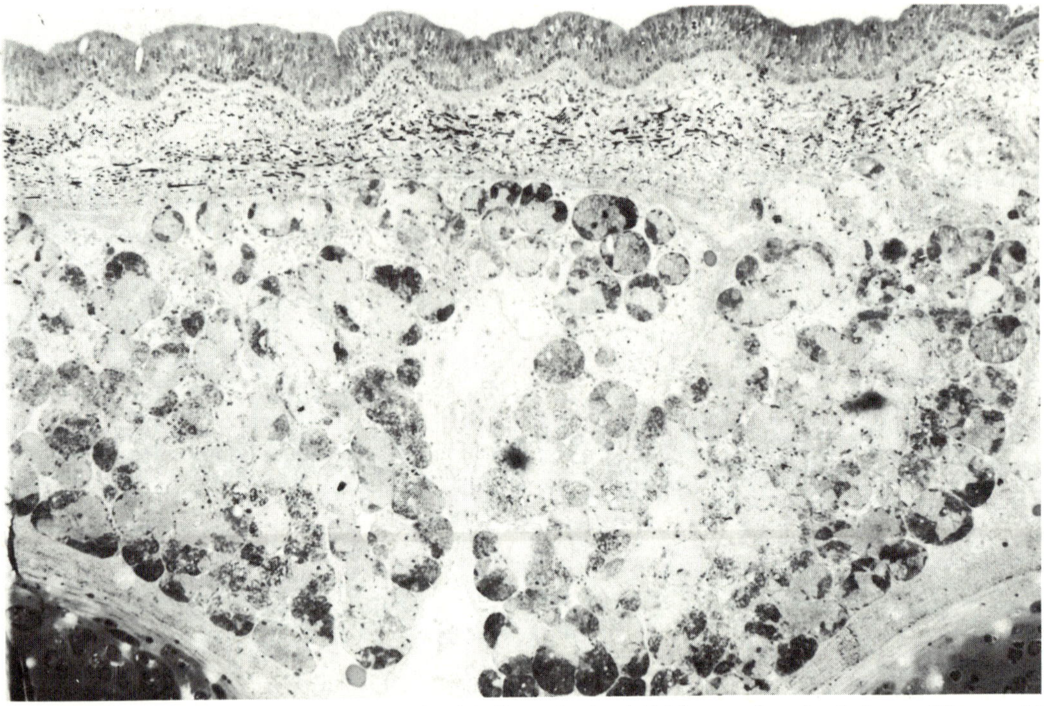

Figure 5-3 Photomicrographs of tracheal epithelium obtained 1½ hours after death from a 29-year-old male with cystic fibrosis who died of pulmonary infection. **A** Cross-section through tracheal wall shows the area occupied by tracheal glands is enlarged relative to that in normal specimens (× 100).

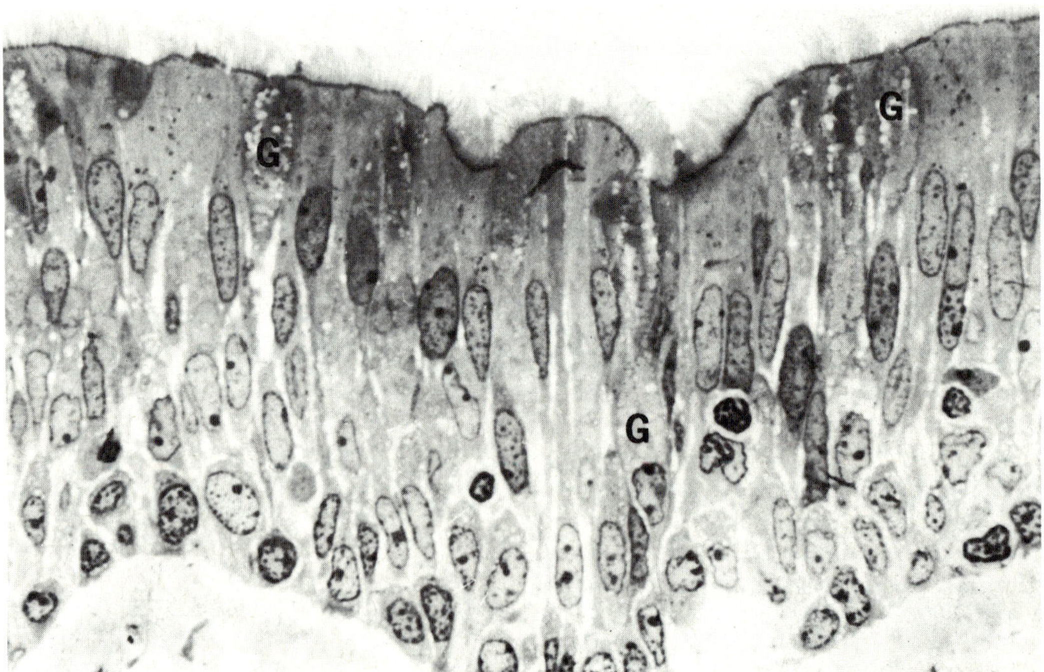

Figure 5-3B Cross-section through tracheal epithelium shows normal cilia, normal appearance and number of goblet cells (G) and somewhat enlarged lateral intercellular spaces (× 1000).

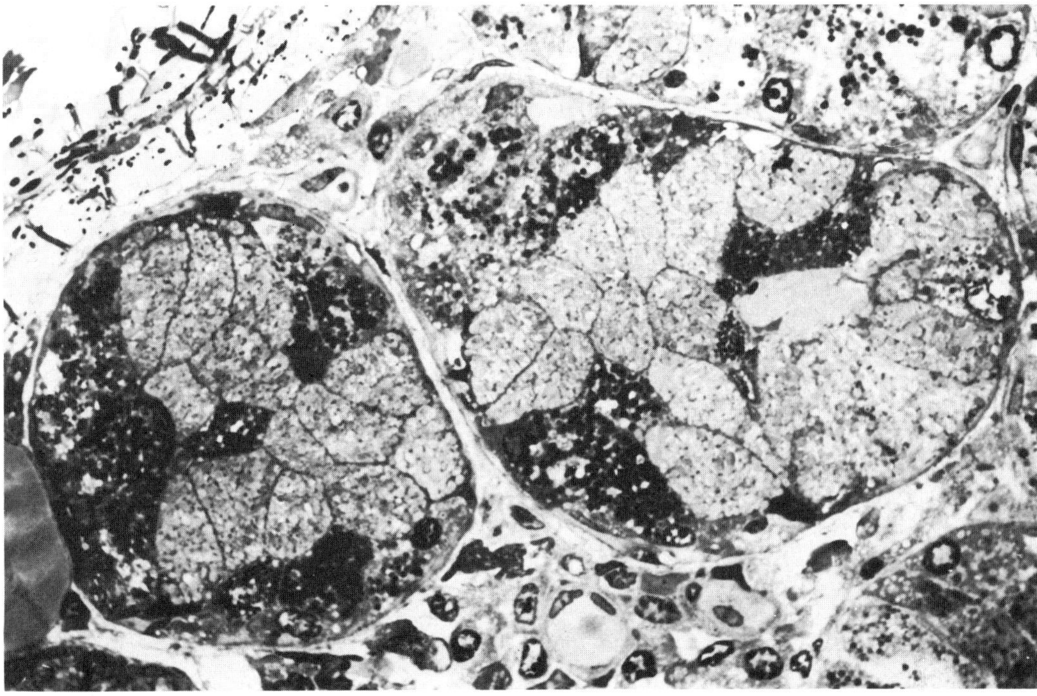

Figure 5-3C Submucosal gland acini containing mucous cells with pale staining granules and serous cells with dark staining granules. Area of each cell is enlarged relative to that in normal specimens (× 1000).

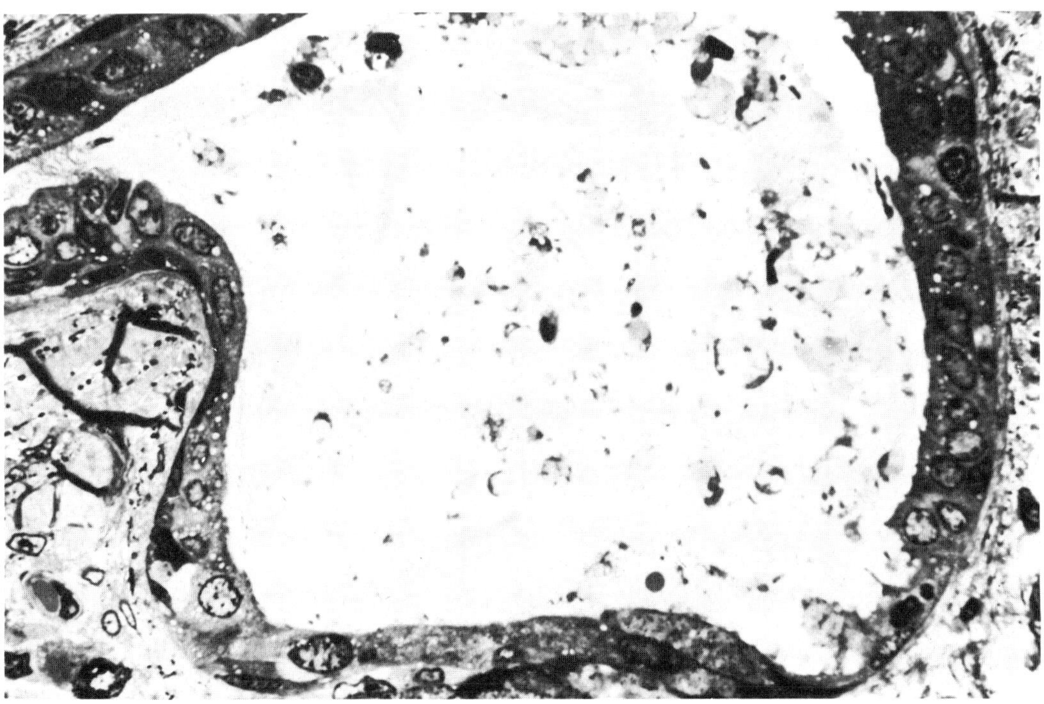

Figure 5-3D Submucosal gland duct filled with a basophilic secretion as well as clumps of granules and cell fragments (× 1000). (Photomicrographs generously provided by our colleague Carol Basbaum, PhD, Assistant Professor of Anatomy, University of California, San Francisco.)

epithelia may be less important than the effects of the changes themselves on airway secretions. If, for instance, inhalation of amiloride altered the airway secretions so that the secretion maintained a more easily cleared consistency, or if use of a drug such as atropine improved the ability of patients to clear secretions from the lung, then these changes would have important therapeutic implications.

FUTURE RESEARCH

Our knowledge of the control of airway secretions has advanced rapidly in the past decade as a result of new techniques being used to study ion transport and secretion from mucous glands in the airway. Further advances now depend on applying more sophisticated techniques for studying the functions of single cells, cellular organelles and cell membranes in animal and human tissues. Of particular importance is the isolation and culture of airway epithelial cells and submucosal gland cells, the isolation of mucous granules from secretory cells and the development of preparations of vesicles from cell membranes of airway epithelial cells. These kinds of preparations will allow us, for instance, to study the mechanisms that regulate uptake of precursors and their incorporation into mucous glycoproteins and the mechanisms in cell membranes that regulate electrolyte and water movement in cells and organelles. Also, we will be able to study how water, electrolytes and mucous glycoproteins mix to form a mucous layer with specific physicochemical properties and a regulated depth that is optimal for mucociliary clearance. In addition, we will be able to learn about the changes that occur in cell membranes during exocytosis. Finally, future clinical research will need to develop accurate methods, preferably noninvasive, to assess secretion of airway glands in patients and the effect of drugs on those secretions so that abnormal secretions in the airways of patients with cystic fibrosis can be changed back to normal and the associated chronic lung disease prevented.

ACKNOWLEDGMENTS

We thank our colleagues at the University of California, San Francisco: Carol Basbaum, PhD (Department of Anatomy) for preparing the photomicrographs; Walter Finkbeiner, MD and Martha Warnock, MD (Department of Pathology) for providing autopsy specimens; and Carol Dahlstrom for typing the manuscript. In addition we thank our colleague Ulrich Hopfer, MD, PhD (Department of Anatomy, Case Western Reserve, Cleveland, Ohio) for allowing us to reproduce his hypothesis in the form of a diagram. Supported in part by USPHS PPG HL-24136.

REFERENCES

1. Nadler HL, Rao GJS, Taussig LM: Cystic fibrosis, in Stanbury JB, Wyngaarden JB, Frederickson DS (eds): *The Metabolic Basis of Inherited Disease,* ed. 4, New York, McGraw-Hill, 1978, pp 1683–1710.
2. di Sant'Agnese P, Talamo R: Pathogenesis and physiopathology of cystic fibrosis of the pancreas. Fibrocystic disease of the pancreas (mucoviscidosis). *N Engl J Med* 1967;277 (24):1287–1294 and (25):1344–1352.
3. Kokin P: Veber die secretorischen Nerven der Kehlkopfund Luftröhrenschleimdrüsen. *Pflugers Arch ges Physiol* 1896;63:622–631.
4. Nadel JA, Davis B: Regulation of Na^+ and Cl^- transport and mucous gland secretion in airway epithelium, in Ciba Foundation Symposium 54 (new series): *Respiratory Tract Mucus.* North-Holland, Elsevier/Excerpta Medica 1978, pp 133–147.
5. Matthews LW, Spector S, Lemm J, et al: Studies on pulmonary secretions. 1. The overall chemical composition of pulmonary secretions from patients with cystic fibrosis, bronchiectasis and laryngectomy. *Am Rev Respir Dis* 1963;88:199–204.
6. Lucas MA, Douglas LC: Principles underlying ciliary activity in the respiratory tract. II. A comparison of nasal clearance in man, monkey and other mammals. *Arch Otolaryngol* 1934;20:518–541.
7. Yoneda K: Mucous blanket of rat bronchus. An ultrastructural study. *Am Rev Respir Dis* 1976;114:837–842.
8. Reid L: Chronic bronchitis and hypersecretion of mucus. *Lectures on the Scientific Basis of Medicine* 1959;8:235–254.
9. Meyrick B, Sturgess JM, Reid L: A reconstruction of the duct system and

secretory tubules of the human bronchial submucosal gland. *Thorax* 1969;24:729–736.
10. Jamieson JD, Palade GE: Condensing vacuole conversion and zymogen granule discharge in pancreatic exocrine cells: metabolic studies. *J Cell Biol* 1971;50: 135–158.
11. Nadel JA, Davis B: Autonomic regulation of mucus secretion and ion transport in airways, in Austen KF, Lichtenstein LM, (eds): *Asthma II.* New York, Academic Press, 1977, pp 197–210.
12. Gallagher JT, Kent PW, Passatore M, et al: The composition of tracheal mucus and the nervous control of its secretion in the cat. *Proc R Soc London* (Ser B) 1975;192:49–76.
13. Davis B, Marin MG, Fischer S, et al: New method for study of canine mucus gland secretion in vivo. *Am Rev Respir Dis* 1976;113: 275.
14. Ueki IF, German VF, Nadel JA: Micropipette measurement of airway submucosal gland secretion. Autonomic effects. *Am Rev Respir Dis* 1980;121:351–357.
15. Davis B, Nadel JA: New methods used to investigate the control of mucous secretion and ion transport in airways. *Environ Health Perspect* 1980;35:121–130.
16. Nadel JA, Davis B: Parasympathetic and sympathetic regulation of secretion from submucosal glands in airways. *Fed Proc* 1980;39: 3075–3079.
17. Murlas C, Nadel JA, Basbaum CB: A morphometric analysis of the autonomic inervation of cat tracheal glands. *J Auton Nerv Syst* 1980;2:23–37.
18. Phipps RJ, Richardson PS: The effects of irritation at various levels of the airway upon tracheal mucus secretion in the cat. *J Physiol* (London) 1976;261:563–581.
19. German VF, Corrales R, Ueki IF, et al: Reflex stimulation of tracheal mucus gland secretion by gastric irritation in cats. *J Appl Physiol* 1982;52:1153–1155.
20. Davis B, Chinn R, Gold J, et al: Hypoxemia reflexly increases secretion from tracheal submucosal glands in dogs. *J Appl Physiol* 1982;52:1416–1419.
21. Davis B, Roberts AM, Colleridge HM, et al: Reflex tracheal gland secretion evoked by stimulation of bronchial C-fibers in dogs. Respirat Environ Exercise Physiol 1982;53: 985–991.
22. Widdicombe JG: Regulation of tracheobronchial smooth muscle. *Physiol Rev* 1963;43: 1–37.
23. Silva D, Ross G: Ultrastructural and fluorescence histochemical studies on the innervation of the tracheabronchial muscle of normal cats and cats treated with 6-hydroxydopamine. *J Ultrastruct Res* 1974;47:310–328.
24. Phipps RJ, Nadel JA, Davis B: Effect of alpha-adrenergic stimulation on mucus secretion and ion transport in cat trachea in vitro. *Am Rev Respir Dis* 1980;121:359–365.
25. Phipps RJ, Williams IP, Richardson PS, et al: Sympathomimetic drugs stimulate the output of secretory glycoproteins from human bronchi in vitro. *Clin Sci* 1982;63: 23–28.
26. Williams IP, Phipps RJ, Wright NL, et al: Sympathomimetic agonists stimulate mucus secretion into human bronchi. *Thorax* 1981; 36:231.
27. Borson DB, Chinn RA, Davis B, et al: Adrenergic and cholinergic nerves mediate fluid secretion from tracheal glands of ferrets. *J Appl Physiol* 1980;49:1027–1031.
28. Basbaum CB, Ueki I, Brezina L, et al: Tracheal submucosal gland serous cells stimulated in vitro with adrenergic and cholinergic agonists: A morphometric study. *Cell Tiss Res* 1981;220:481–498.
29. Ueki IF, Nadel JA: Differences in total protein concentration in submucosal gland fluid: αadrenergic vs. cholinergic. *Fed Proc* 1981; 40:622.
30. Meyrick B, Reid L: Ultrastructure of cells in the human bronchial submucosal glands. *J Anat* 1970;107:281–299.
31. Quinton PM: Composition and control of secretions from tracheal bronchial submucosal glands. *Nature* 1979;279:551–552.
32. Welsh MJ, Widdicombe JH, Nadel JA: Fluid transport across the canine tracheal epithelium. *J Appl Physiol* 1980;49:905–909.
33. Diamond JM, Bossert WH: Standing-gradient osmotic flow. A mechanism for coupling of water and solute transport in epithelia. *J Gen Physiol* 1967;50:2061–2083.
34. Olver RE, Davis B, Marin MG, et al: Active transport of Na^+ and Cl^- across the canine tracheal epithelium in vitro. *Am Rev Respir Dis* 1975;112:811–815.
35. Al-Bazzaz FJ, Al-Awqati: Interaction between sodium and chloride transport in canine tracheal mucosa. *J Appl Physiol Respir Environ Exercise Physiol* 1979;46: 111–119.
36. Widdicombe JH, Ueki IF, Bruderman I, et al: The effects of sodium substitution and ouabain on ion transport by dog tracheal epithelium. *Am Rev Respir Dis* 1979;120: 385–392.
37. Widdicombe JH, Basbaum CB, Yee JW: Localization of Na pumps in the tracheal epithelium of the dog. *J Cell Biol* 1979;82: 380–390.
38. Nathanson IT, Widdicombe JH, Gashi A, et al: Effects of amphotericin B on fluid flow

across dog tracheal epithelium. *Clin Res* 1982;30:73A.

39. Davis B, Marin MG, Olver RE, et al: Active ion transport across canine tracheal epithelium: A possible control system for mucociliary transport. *Chest* 1975;67:57S.
40. Mangos JA, Bargman GJ, Martinez JR, et al: Physiology and pharmacology of secretion and cystic fibrosis. A review of past developments and projections into the future, in Mangos JA, Talamo RC (eds): *Cystic Fibrosis: Projections into the Future.* Miami, Symposia Specialists, 1976, pp 311–336.
41. Wood RE, Boat TF, Doershuk DV: State of the art. Cystic fibrosis. *Am Rev Respir Dis* 1976;113:833–878.
42. Schultz IJ: Micropuncture studies of the sweat formation in cystic fibrosis patients. *J Clin Invest* 1969;48:1470–1477.
43. Mangos JA: Microperfusion study of the sweat gland abnormality in cystic fibrosis. *Texas Rep Biol Med* 1973;31:651–663.
44. Chernick WS, Barbero GJ, Parkins FM: Studies on submaxillary saliva in cystic fibrosis. *J Pediatr* 1961;59:890–898.
45. Mangos JA, McSherry NR: Sodium transport: Inhibitory factor in sweat of patients with cystic fibrosis. *Science* 1967; 158:135–136.
46. Kaiser D, Drack E, Rossi E: Inhibition of net sodium transport in single sweat glands by sweat of patients with cystic fibrosis of the pancreas. *Pediatr Res* 1971;5:167–172.
47. Will PC, Taylor A, Lebowitz JL, et al: Saliva from patients with cystic fibrosis inhibits amiloride-sensitive sodium transport. *Pediatr Res* 1980;14:1245–1249.
48. Will PC, Lebowitz LS, Hopfer U: Induction of amiloride-sensitive sodium transport in the rat colon by mineralocorticoids. *Am J Physiol* 1980;238:F261–F268.
49. Rapaport R, Levine LS, Petrovic M, et al: The renin-aldosterone system in cystic fibrosis. *J Pediatr* 1981;98:768–771.
50. Hawkins E, Singer DB: The adrenal cortex in cystic fibrosis of the pancreas. *Am J Clin Pathol* 1976;66:710–714.
51. Hopfer U, Will PC, Dearborn DG: Cystic fibrosis: A secondary endocrine or target tissue sensitivity problem in epithelial electrolyte transport. in Sturgess JM (ed): *Perspectives in Cystic Fibrosis: Proceedings of the Eighth International Congress on Cystic Fibrosis.* Toronto, Canadian Cystic Fibrosis Foundation, 1980, p 20a.
52. Legris GJ, Will PC, Hopfer U: Human and baboon bronchial sodium absorption: Implications for airway fluid movement and the mucociliary clearance mechanism. *Chest* 1982;81(Suppl):9S–10S.
53. Knowles MR, Buntin WH, Bromberg PA, et al: In vivo measurements of tracheal and bronchial transepithelial electric potential difference (PD) in human subjects. *Am Rev Respir Dis* 1982;125(2):242.
54. Knowles MR, Murray GF, Shallal JA, et al: Ion transport in excised human bronchi and its neurohumoral control. *Chest* 1982;81 (Suppl):11S–13S.
55. Knowles MR, Gatzy JT, Boucher RC: Increased bioelectric potential difference across respiratory epithelia in cystic fibrosis. *N Engl J Med* 1981;305:1489–1495.
56. Legris GJ, Hopfer U: Electrical properties of cystic fibrosis bronchial epithelium in vitro: increased amiloride-sensitive transport. *Cystic Fibrosis Club Abstr* 1982;23:81.
57. Davis PB, Shelhamer JR, Kaliner M: Abnormal adrenergic and cholinergic sensitivity in cystic fibrosis. *N Engl J Med* 1980;302: 1453–1456.
58. Henderson WR, Shelhamer JH, Reingold DB, et al: Alpha-adrenergic hyperresponsiveness in asthma. Analysis of vascular and pupillary responses. *N Engl J Med* 1979;300:642–647.
59. Davis B, Marin MG, Yee JW, et al: Effect of terbutaline on movement of Cl^- and Na^+ across the trachea of the dog *in vitro. Am Rev Respir Dis* 1979;120:547–552.
60. Marin MG, Davis B, Nadel JA: Effect of acetylcholine on Cl^- and Na^+ fluxes across dog tracheal epithelium *in vitro. Am J Physiol* 1976;231:1546–1549.

6

Glycoproteins

Thomas F. Boat
Pi-Wan Cheng

Glycoprotein abnormalities have been implicated as a pathogenetic factor in cystic fibrosis for many years. In 1945, Farber[1] first observed that accumulation of mucous secretions in the respiratory and gastrointestinal tracts is a prominent pathological feature of this disease. Subsequently, mucous obstruction has been noted virtually wherever mucus-secreting cells are found in epithelial surfaces.[2] With recognition that mucous glycoproteins (mucins) are primary determinants of the physical properties of mucus, the question was raised, "Are these molecules altered in cystic fibrosis?" This question has generated considerable investigative interest and also considerable confusion. For example, it is now known that several categories of glycoproteins, in many respects unrelated, are synthesized by humans. Most glycoproteins are not components of mucus at all. Therefore, it is misleading to consider glycoproteins as a single category of molecules when discussing the pathophysiology of cystic fibrosis. Rather, each type of glycoprotein must be considered separately. Surprisingly, two of the three major glycoprotein types have been implicated in the pathogenesis of cystic fibrosis.

All glycoproteins are related by the fact that they are proteins to which carbohydrate is covalently attached. As reviewed by Spiro,[3] variations in the structure of this attachment have become one basis for glycoprotein categorization, namely those containing threonine- or serine-linked carbohydrate units (eg, mucous glycoproteins or mucins), those containing asparagine-linked carbohydrate units (eg, serum glycoproteins, most enzymes), and those containing hydroxylysine-linked carbohydrate units (eg, collagen, basement-membrane glycoproteins). It is now known that some glycoproteins may contain two types of carbohydrate linkage.[3] These include certain membrane glycoproteins and immunoglobulins. The biochemistry of each major glycoprotein type will be reviewed briefly before discussing the relationship of these glycoconjugates to cystic fibrosis.

PROPERTIES OF GLYCOPROTEINS

Glycoproteins with Threonine (Serine)-Linked Carbohydrate (Mucous Glycoproteins)

These glycoproteins are high-molecular-weight compounds containing a peptide core and many relatively short, sometimes branched, sugar side chains.[3,4] They contain 50–80% carbohydrate by weight. Saccharide chains are linked to threonine or serine residues of the peptide core by *O*-glycosidic bonds. This linkage is characteristically labile in dilute alkaline solutions. Mucous glycoproteins contain as many as five different sugars: fucose, sialic acid, galactose, *N*-acetylglucosamine, and *N*-acetylgalactosamine. The latter constitutes the linkage point between oligosaccharide units and the peptide moiety. Oligosaccharide chains range in complexity from a single *N*-acetylgalactosamine residue to chains containing as many as 20 sugar residues. The sugars, galactose and glucosamine, are sulfated in some mucous glycoproteins. Roussel et al[5] have demonstrated that sulfated sugars of respiratory tract mucins are present only in relatively long oligosaccharide chains, ie, those containing seven or more sugars. The sulfated sugars, along with sialic acid, provide negative charges (acidic properties) over the physiologic pH range. Repulsion of adjacent charges may be responsible, in part, for the extended (threadlike) conformation of these glycoproteins.[6] Structures of some mucin oligosaccharide chains have been worked out and are presented in Figure 6-1.

Composition of the peptide core is unique in that serine and threonine comprise 30–50% of the total amino acids. Alanine, glycine, and proline are also relatively abundant. Allen et al[7] have presented evidence that some mucins are linked by disulfide bonds to a nonglycosylated peptide which is enriched in half-cystine residues. This linkage appears to be an important determinant of the viscoelastic properties of some mucous glycoproteins.

A prominent physical property of solutions which contain mucous glycoproteins and bronchial mucins specifically is a tendency to form gels.[8] Gel formation is dependent on glycoprotein concentration, ionic composition of the fluid, and formation of intermolecular disulfide bonds.[7] Interactions of glycoproteins with divalent cations[9] and other macromolecules such as albumin[10] or lysozyme[11] also may play a role. Sugar–sugar interactions are important determinants of glycoprotein aggregation and most likely also contribute to gelation.[12] The viscoelastic properties of these gels are particularly suited for protective, lubricating, and mucociliary clearance functions of the mucous secretions. Differences in physicochemical properties have been noted as a function of organ source. For example, submaxillary saliva is a viscous solution while tracheobronchial, cervical, and gastric secretions are well-developed gels. The molecular determinants of these differences are not yet fully understood.

Following synthesis of the polypeptide core, the first sugar or sugars are added from sugar nucleotides by enzymes called glycosyltransferases in the rough or smooth endoplasmic reticulum, while completion of oligosaccharide synthesis occurs in the Golgi apparatus.[13] Sugars are added one at a time to growing oligosaccharide chains. The carbohydrate structure of mucous glycoproteins is defined by the order, specific linkages, and anomeric configuration of sugar additions. Microheterogeneity is extensive, due to incomplete synthesis of chains and/or the suitability of partially synthesized oligosaccharide chains to serve as acceptors in the different glycosyltransferase-catalyzed reactions.

Glycoproteins with Asparagine-Linked Carbohydrate

This group of glycoproteins, which includes most glycoproteins in serum, many enzymes, some membrane glycoproteins, and the Tamm-Horsfall glycoprotein in urine, is characterized by *N*-glycosidic linkages between *N*-acetylglucosamine of the oligosaccharide chains and asparagine in the peptide core which are stable under mild alkaline conditions.[14] Many glycoproteins of this type are synthesized by liver parenchymal cells, but some are produced by other cell systems, eg, the immunoglobulins which are synthesized by plasma cells in scattered submucosal tissues. Although present to a variable extent in exocrine secretions, these glycoproteins, in general, are not primary secretory products of epithelial cells and are not to be confused with the high-molecular-weight mucous glycoproteins which have very different physicochemical properties. Several serum glycoproteins such

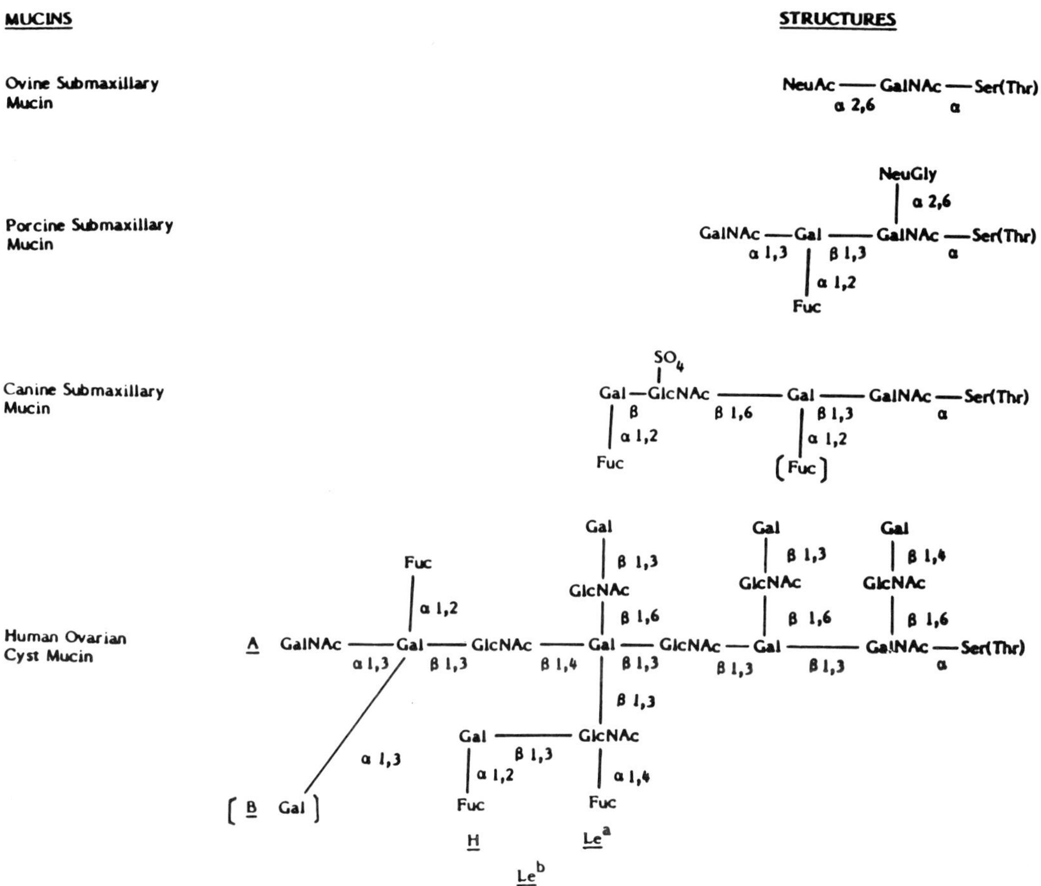

Figure 6-1 Structures of oligosaccharides found in several well-characterized mucins as discussed in Kornfeld and Kornfeld.[14] Canine submaxillary mucin is the only sulfated mucin with a defined oligosaccharide structure.[119] The structures of the highly complex oligosaccharides in human ovarian cyst mucins have not been completely elucidated. A proposed structure is shown.[120] Sugars which confer blood group A, B, H[O], Lewis[a], and Lewis[b] specificity are identified. Human tracheobronchial mucin oligosaccharides appear to resemble those of ovarian cyst mucins in complexity and blood group type and, in addition, are sulfated.

as IgG and fetuin, as well as membrane glycoproteins, are exceptional in that they contain *O*-glycosidic as well as *N*-glycosidic carbohydrate linkages. Glycoproteins with *N*-glycosidic linkages have a relatively low carbohydrate content (<40%). The most abundant sugars are *N*-acetylglucosamine and mannose. Some oligosaccharide chains contain only these sugars (simple type) while others also contain galactose, sialic acid, and fucose (complex type).

The aspargine-linked oligosaccharides are synthesized by a mechanism different from that for mucous glycoproteins.[14] The core region of the oligosaccharide chain is built by transferring sugars one at a time from sugar–nucleotide donors to a lipid carrier, dolichol phosphate. The first two sugars added, both *N*-acetylglucosamine, are followed by as many as nine mannose residues and three glucose residues. The assembled core region is then transferred intact from the lipid carrier to asparagine of the nascent peptide. Thereafter, all glucose residues and some of the mannose residues are removed to form a high-mannose-type oligosaccharide structure (Figure 6-2A). Following removal of more mannose residues and addition of sugars, such as *N*-acetylglucosamine, fucose, galactose, and sialic acid, complex type oligosaccharide chains are produced (Figure 6-2B). This biosynthetic pathway depends, for the most part, on glycosyltransferase reactions which are different from those involved in the biosynthesis of mucins. It is unlikely that the biosynthesis of these two types of glycoproteins would be disturbed by a common enzymatic deficiency. Similarly, there are few glycosidic enzymes which can degrade both glycoprotein types.

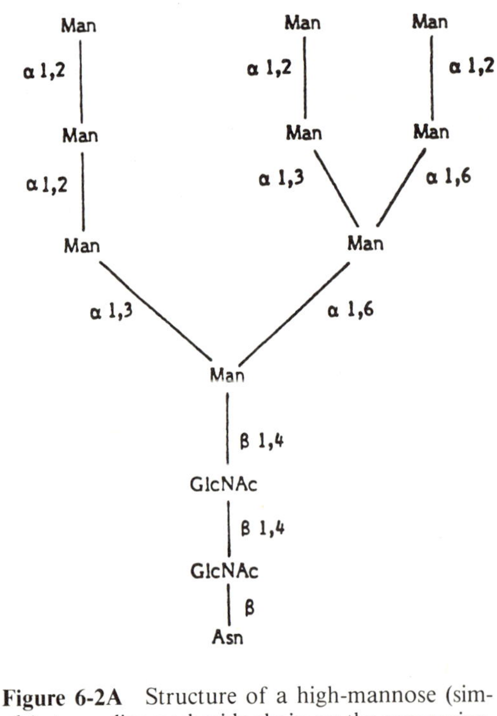

Figure 6-2A Structure of a high-mannose (simple) -type oligosaccharide chain on the asparagine-linked glycoprotein from ovary cell membranes of the Chinese hamster.[14]

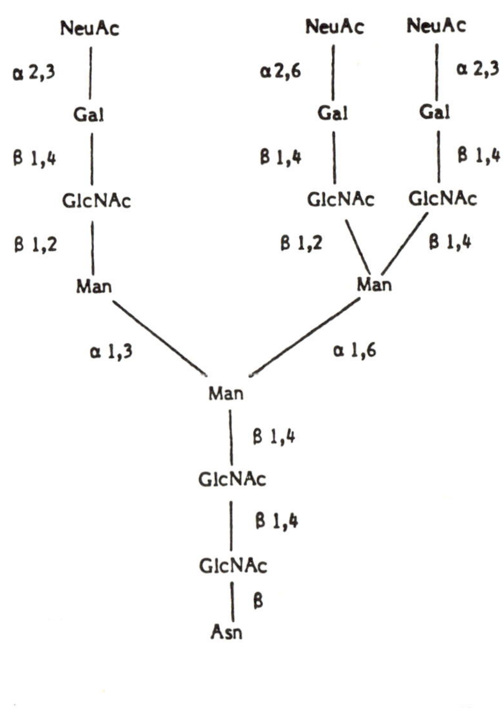

Figure 6-2B Structure of a complex-type oligosaccharide chain with asparagine linkage, found in fetuin.[121]

Glycoproteins with Hydroxylysine-Linked Carbohydrate

These glycoproteins, which include basement membrane glycoprotein and collagen, contain glucose-galactose disaccharides or single galactose residues *O*-glycosidically linked to hydroxylysine.[3] This linkage is alkaline stable. Basement membrane glycoprotein may also contain *N*-glycosidic oligosaccharide units. These glycoproteins have not been implicated in the pathology of cystic fibrosis and will not be discussed further.

MUCOUS GLYCOPROTEINS IN CYSTIC FIBROSIS

Morphologic Studies

In general, mucous glycoproteins are secreted both by goblet cells in the surface epithelium and by underlying mucous glands. Several studies of CF tissues have demonstrated increased numbers of mucus-secreting cells and increased amounts of intracellular glycoprotein in these secretory cells. For example, the goblet cells of bronchial surface epithelium are increased in number (hyperplasia) and extend peripherally into bronchioles (metaplasia)[15] where few of these cells normally reside. In addition the submucosal glands in the airways hypertrophy markedly.[16,17] In an autopsy study of 146 CF patients by Oppenheimer and Esterly,[17] hypertrophy of Brunner's glands was particularly prominent in those patients who had experienced meconium ileus. In a study using strict morphometric methods, Neutra and Trier[18] found that mucus-secreting cells of rectal mucosa from CF subjects were not unusual but that the crypt lumina were dilated. Other studies using less quantitative approaches had suggested that gastrointestinal mucus-secreting cells are enlarged and increased in number in CF subjects.[19]

Reid et al[16] have postulated that the morphologic changes of mucus-secreting elements in CF lungs are a reaction to chronic infection. This hypothesis does not account for the hyperplasia of goblet cells, gland hypertrophy, and/or dilated crypts containing excessive secretion in the esophagus,[1,17] duodenum,[20] appendix,[21] pancreatic ducts,[22] and rectum[18] where chronic infection is not a recognized feature of CF. Alternate hypotheses for morphologic changes of mucus-secreting elements include surface irritation from abnormal physicochemical properties of the secretions and long-term imbalance of autonomic or other neurohumoral influences.[23,24]

Histochemical staining reactions show increased amounts of intracellular "sulfomucin" in both the gastrointestinal and the respiratory tract[22,25] and decreased amounts of sialidase-sensitive "sialomucin"[25] in airways tissue. However, histochemical observations should be interpreted cautiously because the relationship of sulfomucin and sialomucin staining reactions to actual chemical properties of secreted mucins has not been firmly established. Nevertheless, these studies were among the first to suggest alterations of CF mucins.

Chemical Studies

Early attempts to identify abnormal mucous glycoproteins in CF were carried out with unfractionated or only partially fractionated secretions. Conflicting data resulted and apparent CF-related abnormalities were hard to interpret. Studies by di Sant'Agnese et al[26] demonstrated ethanol-benzene-precipitable substances in duodenal fluids of most patients with CF, but not in control duodenal fluids. This ethanol-benzene precipitate contained glycoprotein with a higher fucose to sialic acid ratio than glycoproteins found in soluble fractions of duodenal fluid. Additional studies by these investigators demonstrated more trichloroacetic acid (TCA) -insoluble glycoproteins in CF duodenal fluid and increased amounts of fucose relative to other sugars in TCA-soluble CF duodenal mucous glycoproteins precipitated with 50% ethanol.[27]

Dische and co-workers[27] postulated that the increased content of fucose altered the solubility, and consequently the rheologic properties, of CF mucous glycoproteins and led to the characteristic obstructive events.

Subsequent studies of CF submaxillary saliva[28] sputum,[29] and rectal mucus[30] have supported the notion that higher ratios of fucose to sialic acid are characteristic of CF mucins. More recently, Clamp and Gough[31] found more fucose and less sialic acid in glycopeptides and oligosaccharide units released from glycoproteins in CF meconium than in control meconium specimens. However, Rose (unpublished observation) has found no compositional alteration of partially purified CF meconium mucous glycoproteins, and Schacter and Dixon[32] were unable to distinguish CF and non-CF meconium by glycoprotein compositional analysis.

Other data show no alterations of fucose and/or sialic acid in CF respiratory and salivary mucous secretions.[33-36] Purified mucous glycoproteins from CF sputum[37] and nasal secretions harvested in vitro[38] do not contain increased amounts of fucose or a paucity of sialic acid relative to other sugars. Evidence for increased fucosylation of CF glycoproteins is most compelling in studies of intestinal mucus, raising the possibility that there is indeed an alteration, but that it is limited to the gastrointestinal tract.

A number of factors could alter the ratios of fucose to sialic acid and of these sugars to the other components of glycoprotein oligosaccharide chains. Glycosidic enzyme activities (sialidase, fucosidase) are present in a number of biologic fluids and may alter the carbohydrate content of mucins if the secretions are not processed promptly under conditions which inhibit these activities. Sialic acid is the most labile of the mucin sugars; for example, it can be removed with very dilute acid. Therefore, a low sialic acid content of mucins must be viewed with skepticism unless potentially degrading conditions are rigorously excluded during sample processing. To summarize, current evidence does not clearly support the contention that the monosaccharide content is altered in all CF mucous glycoproteins. Other explanations for abnormal behavior of CF mucus must be considered.

Recent evidence from several sources suggests that CF mucous glycoproteins contain increased amounts of sulfated sugars. Boat et al[38] found that cultured nasal polyp epithelium from CF subjects incorporates more $^{35}SO_4$ relative to [^{3}H]glucosamine into secreted mucous glycoproteins than does polyp tissue from allergic subjects. Fractionation of purified mucous glycoproteins from the lower respiratory tract by these investigators has demonstrated that the majority of CF mucous glycoproteins are highly sulfated; that is, they contain greater than 6% sulfate by weight.[37,39] In contrast, the bulk of the glycoproteins from respiratory tract secretions of age-matched subjects with other chronic lung diseases are sparsely sulfated.[37,39] The highly sulfated glycoproteins are more potent inhibitors of influenza B virus hemagglutination but are weaker blood group antigens than the sparsely sulfated glycoproteins. In addition, the more highly sulfated glycoproteins possess oligosaccharide units with increased average chain length.[40] These findings are supported in general by the studies of Roussel and coworkers on sputum mucins[5] and by Frates et al,[41] who have studied CF and control mucins secreted by postmortem tracheal explants.

In other respects CF respiratory tract mucous glycoproteins do not appear to be unusual. For example, carbohydrate and amino acid compositions of tracheobronchial mucins do not differ substantially from those of control glycoproteins.[37] Mucous glycoproteins in CF saliva do possess a greater-than-control capacity to interact with influenza B virus,[42] a property previously shown to be determined by sialic acid[43] and sulfate[37] content of glycoproteins. Detailed comparative analyses of oligosaccharide and peptide structure for CF and control glycoproteins have not yet been carried out. This work, although its scope is formidable, may be required to understand sulfation abnormalities at a structural level.

Currently, it is not possible to predict whether augmented sulfation of CF glycoproteins is closely related to the CF gene defect, or whether it is a response to an altered environment for the mucus-secreting epithelium. Some histochemical[22] and biochemical[6] studies of epithelial glycoproteins in other chronic respiratory tract diseases suggest that a shift to the secretion of more highly sulfated mucins in airways is not unique to CF. On the other hand, analyses of respiratory tract mucous glycoproteins from lungs of age-related subjects with chronic lung disease,[37,39] and studies of mucous glycoproteins secreted in organ culture,[44] all suggest that augmented sulfation of glycoproteins may be specific for CF.

Information concerning the relative activities and intracellular localization of glycosyltransferases in CF mucus-secreting cells would be of considerable interest. However, this information is not available at present. Studies to date of several glycosyltransferases in CF serum,[45–47] skin fibroblasts,[48,49] peripheral lung,[50] and liver[51] do not provide information about mucin biosynthesis per se. Furthermore, many of these studies have not used appropriate acceptors and/or identified the biosynthetic product. Consequently, there is very little useful information concerning the role of glycosyltransferases in CF mucin synthesis. Cheng and Bona[52] have postulated that mucous glycoprotein abnormalities in CF, namely elongated oligosaccharide chains and greater sulfation, can be explained by a preponderance of activity of those glycosyltransferases such as the galactosyltransferases and *N*-acetylglucosaminyltransferases, which act to elongate oligosaccharide chains over those glycosyltransferases, such as sialyltransferases and fucosyltransferases, which terminate chain growth. Direct evidence for this hypothesis is not yet available. However, Cheng and Bona[53] have shown that the activity of *N*-acetylgalactosaminide β1–3-galactosyltransferase in human tracheal epithelium is enhanced by spermine at a low (2.5 mM) $MnCl_2$ concentration. Similar effects of polyamines on the canine tracheal enzyme were also reported.[54] Furthermore, spermine does not affect tracheal β-*N*-acetylgalactosaminide sialyltransferase. These data suggest that spermine and other polycationic compounds may play a role in the regulation of mucin carbohydrate chain synthesis. These polycationic substances are known to be present in altered concentrations in some CF fluids and cells[55] and may play a pathogenetic role in biosynthesis of CF mucins.

Sulfotransferases required for sulfation of glycoproteins by mucus-secreting epithelia have not been studied. Factors which may influence the sulfation of mucins include cell source, nature of the stimulus for secretion, and vitamin A. Sherman et al[56] have demonstrated that cat tracheal submucosal glands secrete a more highly acidic mucin than the surface epithelium (goblet cells). This observation is supported by indirect evidence from in vivo perfusion of cat trachea and collection of radiolabeled macromolecules following cholinergic stimulation of glands and stimulation of surface cells with ammonia.[57] One possible explanation for the increased sulfation of CF tracheobronchial mucins is a disproportionate contribution from a cell source which synthesizes highly sulfated mucins.

Preliminary evidence suggests that autonomic neurotransmitters can influence the acidic properties of mucous glycoproteins released. For example, β-adrenergic stimulation with terbutaline favors the short-term release of highly sulfated glycoproteins from cat trachea.[58] Therefore an imbalance of autonomic influences could explain altered mucin properties in CF, but probably not via biosynthetic processes.

Recent studies also suggest that in the rat, vitamin A depletion not only causes squamous metaplasia of ciliated epithelium, but results in the secretion of more highly acidic, presumably sulfated mucins.[59] Vitamin A absorption in the CF intestinal tract is often hindered by a deficiency of pancreatic lipase. Even though supplemental vitamin A is prescribed, CF subjects may have lower tissue vitamin A levels than healthy subjects.[60] It is conceivable that a relative deficiency of vitamin A would also favor biosynthesis and/or secretion of highly sulfated mucins into human airways. This possibility requires additional exploration.

Degradation

Activities of α-L-fucosidase are reportedly elevated in CF fibroblasts; diminished in CF serum, lymphoblasts, and fibroblasts; or normal in serum, saliva, liver, fibroblasts, and cultured amniotic fluid cells and leukocytes.[61] In a recent article, Maler and coinvestigators[62] present evidence for decreased intracellular and extracellular specific activity of α-L-fucosidase in five CF lymphoblast lines, especially in the late log phase of growth. No α-L-fucosidase inhibitor was detected in CF cells. The K_m, pH optimum, isoelectric focusing patterns, and SDS-PAGE mobility were identical for CF and control enzyme. It is not clear that changes of α-L-fucosidase activity are more than a reflection of abnormalities in metabolism or growth of cultured CF cells. Clearly, there is as yet no link between these observations and increased fucose content reported for some CF mucous glycoproteins. Other glycosidase activities which could modify mucous glycoproteins do not seem to be altered in CF.[61]

It is conceivable that CF mucins are more highly sulfated because of diminished sulfatase activity. However, a sulfatase which degrades intact mucins has never been found. Sulfatase activities specific for the galactose-6-SO_4 and glucosamine-6-SO_4 found in glycosaminoglycans are deficient in Morquios disease and a newly described form of mucopolysaccharide storage disease, respectively.[63] Similarities between these conditions and CF are not readily discerned. Therefore, deficient sulfatase activity is, at best, only a theoretical and somewhat remote consideration for the basic defect in CF.

Regulation

Glycoprotein concentrations are increased in CF saliva[36] and, although strict quantitation is virtually impossible in vivo, excessive amounts of mucous glycoproteins appear to be secreted into the CF respiratory and gastrointestinal tracts. These observations could be explained by an increased mass of mucin-secreting cells, as noted earlier in this discussion. Increased rates of mucin secretion provide an alternative explanation. The basal rate at which radiolabeled precursors are incorporated into the secretory product of goblet cells and transported to the apical surface does not differ for CF and control explants of rectal mucosa.[64] Under baseline conditions, CF tracheal explants secrete labeled high-molecular-weight glycoproteins at a somewhat faster rate than do control explants.[44] However, when the increased secretory cell mass of CF explants is considered, the data do not support the contention that CF mucin-secreting cells are more active.

Cholinomimetic agonists stimulate mucous glycoprotein secretion in the human respiratory and gastrointestinal tracts. Increased cholinergic tone could account for mucus hypersecretion in CF. It is equally plausible that hypersecretion of mucus in CF subjects represents an exaggerated response to normal neurohumoral stimuli. CF subjects and obligate heterozygotes do display increased responsiveness to cholinergic or α-adrenergic influences.[23] This hypothesis is difficult to test in vivo for mucus hypersecretion. In vitro the response of CF tracheal explants to 30 μg/ml of methacholine did not differ from that of control explants with respect to rate of lysozyme or mucous glycoprotein release.[44] On the other hand, Sturgess and Reid[65] have suggested that cholinergic agonists disproportionately increase the rate at which radiolabeled glucose is incorporated into and transported to the apical surface by secretory cells in bronchial explants from CF and bronchitic subjects, both of whom display gland hypertrophy. These apparently contradictory data have not been resolved. In any event, there is as yet no convincing evidence for a CF-specific hypersecretory response of mucus-secreting elements.

Other mechanisms may promote mucus hypersecretion in CF. Several studies suggest that CF serum contains substances which stimulate secretion of mucus in vitro. Oyster gill epithelium appears to release increased amounts of mucus on exposure to CF sera.[66,67] A similar response may occur on incubation of rabbit tracheal epithelium with CF serum.[68] The effect was not quantitated in either study. Goblet cells in rabbit tracheal epithelium swell and then release their contents earlier in the presence of CF than control sera.[69] Increased amounts of sedimentable, sialic-acid-containing material are released from rabbit tracheal explants exposed to CF, as compared with control, sera.[70] Responses to CF and CF-heterozygote sera could not be distinguished in this system. The nature of the sedimentable material was not determined and could have been, at least in part, membranes of lysed cells, since it has been shown that respiratory epithelium is disrupted in the presence of undiluted serum within 15 min.[71] Kurlandsky et al[72] have reported greater elongation of mucous tails extruded by urn cells which are found in the coelomic cavity of the sea worm, *Sipunculus nudus,* in the presence of heat-treated CF and CF-heterozygote sera when compared with sera from controls. Release of macromolecules (presumably mucins) labeled with ^{14}C-glucosamine from isolated rat submandibular gland cells is increased on exposure to CF when compared with control sera.[73] In the latter two studies mucus-stimulating substances also were found in sera of cetain patients with other chronic diseases. Finally, studies in the authors' laboratory have demonstrated greater release of labeled mucous glycoprotein from rabbit tracheal explants in response to CF serum compared with control serum.[74]

The serum factor stimulating urn cell tail production appears to be bound noncovalently to IgG.[72] However, multiple serum fractions appear to stimulate mucin release from rabbit tracheal explants.[74] In fact, it is now evident that exoproducts of *P. aeruginosa* can stimulate the release of labeled macromolecules from tracheal epithelium in vitro. (Boat and Klinger, unpublished observation). These subtances may gain access to the circulation in individuals with chronic *Pseudomonas* lung infection and act as mucus-stimulating substances. It will be important to isolate and identify mucus-stimulating substances in CF and determine their relationship, if any, to the CF gene.

Physical Properties of Mucous Secretions in Cystic Fibrosis

Considerable attention has been directed toward turbidity of submandibular saliva, a mucous secretion, of CF subjects. Early studies by Gugler et al[75] indicated that the turbidity was due to calcium-dependent aggregation and precipitation of one or more low-molecular-weight glycoproteins. The major glycoprotein involved in development of turbidity is a phosphoglycoprotein which can be precipitated with concentrations of $CaCl_2$ in the range found in CF submandibular saliva and can be resolubilized with EDTA.[76] The calcium-precipitable glycoprotein is not a mucous glycoprotein and is not present in increased amounts in CF saliva. These studies suggest that turbidity of CF saliva is related directly to elevation of calcium levels. Small amounts of calcium-precipitable glycoprotein are present in parotid saliva, but none has been found in other exocrine secretions. Therefore, this glycoprotein does not appear to participate in the generalized obstructive processes characteristic of CF.

Early suggestions that CF mucous secretions are more viscous or "sticky" have defied definitive confirmation. Several studies of CF sputum, compared with sputum of subjects with other chronic lung diseases, have shown no evidence for increased viscosity or elasticity.[77-79] In fact, viscosity of non-purulent-looking CF sputum tends to be lower than that from subjects with other chronic lung diseases.[78] However, these secretions were not carefully characterized with respect to purulence, which would contribute additional viscosity in the form of DNA, and which might promote glycoprotein degradation by proteolytic and glycosidic enzymes released from bacteria and inflammatory cells. Rheologic comparisons of uninfected secretions from the tracheobronchial tract of CF and control subjects are obviously desirable, but very difficult to achieve because of the small amounts of secretions available and their relative inaccessibility. Duodenal mucus, but not submaxillary saliva, from patients with CF has an elevated apparent viscosity, as determined on a rotational viscometer by Lorin et al.[80] This was true whether or not the CF subjects had pancreatic insufficiency. Bettelheim et al [81] have demonstrated that a rheologic parameter representing "tackiness" is increased in submandibular secretions of some, but not all, CF patients. Cervical mucus of women with CF has been described as rubbery and highly tenacious.[82] It does not undergo the expected thinning at midcyle. Objective measures of the rheologic properties of this secretion are needed to confirm these nonquantitative observations. King[79] has noted that CF sputum is transported less well on the isolated frog palate than would be predicted from its viscoelastic properties. He postulated the presence of a ciliary inhibitor in CF sputum. Alternatively, current measurements of viscous and elastic moduli may not fully describe the properties of mucus and their constituent mucins which determine ciliary transport.

Factors which may contribute to altered properties of CF mucous secretions include water content, calcium content, and the concentrations of macromolecules which interact with mucous glycoproteins. It is clear that mucous secretions recovered at several locations from subjects with CF are deficient in water.[82-85] A relative paucity of water and inadequate hydration of mucins could explain abnormal mucus clearance properties.

Calcium can influence the viscoelastic properties of tracheal secretions,[86] and at higher calcium concentrations marked changes in mucin solubility occur.[9] Calcium interactions with cat tracheal mucins modify water adsorption to these glycoproteins.[87] Pieces of evidence such as these have prompted several investigators to postulate a pivotal role for calcium in the pathogenesis of mucus obstruction in CF. However, evidence strongly supporting this hypothesis has been elusive.

Similarly, List et al[10] have shown that albumin–mucin interactions increase the viscosity of mucin-containing solutions. This observation is particularly pertinent to the pathogenesis of intestinal obstruction with meconium (meconium ileus), in that CF meconium has a high albumin content.[88] It is not clear that albumin–mucin interactions play a more general role in initiating CF-related obstructive events, for example, in the airways. In fact, there is no evidence that albumin levels are elevated in most CF mucous secretions unless the tissue in question is highly inflamed and transudation of serum components into the secretion is enhanced.

ASPARAGINE-LINKED GLYCOPROTEINS IN CYSTIC FIBROSIS

Concentrations of many serum glycoproteins are appropriate in CF subjects.[89] A number of serum glycoproteins are acute-phase reactants, and their levels may be elevated in CF. Detailed analyses of the Tamm-Horsfall glycoprotein in CF urine have not uncovered differences of carbohydrate composition or antigenicity.[90,91] However, the carbohydrate portion of certain glycoproteins with *N*-glycosidic linkages may be altered in CF. Alhadeff and coinvestigators[92] reported altered isoenzyme patterns for the glycoprotein, α-L-fucosidase, in CF livers obtained at autopsy. Their isoelectric focusing technique showed several variations of the typical isoenzyme pattern for the CF liver enzyme. Because sialic acid is an important determinant of isoenzyme patterns for α-L-fucosidase,[93] they reasoned that altered sialic acid content of this enzyme might explain their observations. No evidence was found for altered sialidase activity in CF liver[94] or fibroblasts.[95] Decreased total activity of sialyltransferase was found in CF liver tissue, using both asialofetuin and asialo sheep submaxillary mucin as the sialic acid acceptor.[94] However, similar decreases of sialyltransferase activity were noted in other pathological livers. Isoelectric focusing revealed that the three most neutral forms of sialyltransferase were deficient or absent in CF livers.[96]

While these findings suggest that transfer of sialic acid to newly formed enzyme might be one mechanism by which α-L-fucosidase isoenzyme patterns are altered, compositional studies of α-L-fucosidase purified from CF liver have suggested a broader problem with glycosylation.[97] A reduction of mannose, *N*-acetylglucosamine, and sialic acid contents by factors of 51%, 44%, and 32%, respectively, was also noted. Decreased binding of CF liver α-L-fucosidase to concanavalin A, a lectin with mannose and glucosamine specificity, further suggested a paucity of these sugars.[98] Unfortunately, these investigators failed to report the galactose content of CF liver α-L-fucosidase. Consequently, it is difficult to predict the nature of the glycosylation abnormality suggested by their work. However, preliminary support for these observations of liver α-L-fucosidase comes from Maler et al,[62] who observed diminished activity and concanavalin A binding of α-L-fucosidase from CF lymphoblasts. On the other hand, the pH profile, Michaelis constants, subunit structure, and antigenicity of CF liver α-L-fucosidase are unremarkable.[99] Extension of this work to CF and control serum α-L-fucosidase has failed to document differences of activity,[100,101] isoenzyme patterns, thermostability, pH optimum, or K_m values.[100] Isoenzyme patterns of CF fibroblast α-L-fucosidase also do not show the alterations seen in CF liver, although they are not identical to those of control fibroblasts.[102]

These data do not clearly support a unifying hypothesis. The possibility that enzymes in CF liver obtained at autopsy reflect secondary changes is high. Genetically determined alterations of an enzyme should appear in serum or fibroblasts as well as hepatic tissue. Several recent observations, however, have rekindled curiosity concerning serum-type glycoproteins. Ben-Yoseph and coworkers[103] found decreased sialic acid content, but not total hexose content, and decreased binding to concanavalin A and wheat germ agglutinin (a lectin with sialic acid specificity) for purified CF α_2-macroglobulin. A paucity of sialic acid residues could explain the decreased affinity for wheat germ agglutinin, but not the decreased affinity for concanavalin A. In this study, the sialic acid content of α_2-macroglobulin from obligate heterozygotes for the CF gene was intermediate between CF and normal control values. Additional work from this laboratory implies that CF α_2-macroglobulin from which sialic acid has been removed is a poorer acceptor in the sialyltransferase reaction than asialo α_2-macroglobulin from control subjects,[104] suggesting a more fundamental alteration of oligosaccharide structure. On the other hand, Shapira and Menendez[105] have reported increased concanavalin A binding for CF α_2-macroglobulin, IgM, and IgG from CF plasma. Values for binding by heterozygote α_2-macroglobulin were intermediate. The discrepancy between concanavalin-A-binding results in these two studies has not been resolved.

Pearson and Lubin[106] have reported that heparin precipitates more protein from CF than control sera and that the measured carbohydrate content of precipitated CF glycoproteins reflects increased fucosylation.[107] However, recent work by Margolies et al[108] indicates that IgG is the major glycoprotein precipitated from serum by heparin and that increased amounts of precipitate merely reflect higher IgG levels in some CF sera. This finding calls into question the hypothesis forwarded by Pearson and Lubin, that glycosylation of serum proteins in general is perturbed. Systematic analytical studies are required to determine whether the carbohydrate content of IgG itself is abnormal in CF. These studies must take into consideration the possibility that IgG subclass distribution may be shifted in CF subjects.

Potential explanations for an apparent decreased sialic acid content of serum-type glycoproteins should include increased activity of circulating neuraminidase from sources such as *P. aeruginosa* in the infected lung.[109] Absence of consistent experimental results suggests that abnormal glycosylation of CF glycoproteins containing *N*-glycosidic linkages, when observed, indeed may not be a genetically controlled alteration. The most compelling evidence for this point of view comes from the study of Hunt and Summers,[110] who infected CF and control fibroblasts with vesicular stomatitis virus and analyzed newly synthesized virus envelope glycoproteins. In this situation, the virus RNA genome codes for glycoprotein polypeptide chain synthesis but fibroblast enzymes glycosylate the protein. No evidence for incomplete or aberrant oligosaccharide chain synthesis could be detected. This study provides strong evidence against a genetically determined defect in the biosynthesis of *N*-glycosidically linked oligosaccharide chains in CF.

Recent studies show that intracellular distribution of glycosidic enzymes and other glycoconjugates depends on their carbohydrate structure, including the presence of mannose-phosphate residues. These mechanisms deserve further attention with respect to putative alterations of N-linked glycoproteins in CF.

MEMBRANE GLYCOPROTEINS IN CYSTIC FIBROSIS

Abnormalities of sodium and chloride transport in sweat gland ducts have prompted investigation of membrane structure and glycoprotein content. Baig et al[111] found no qualitative or major quantitative alterations of fibroblast membrane components labeled with [^{3}H]- and [^{14}C]-amino acids and -sugars. Scanlin and Glick[112] came to a similar conclusion after labeling fibroblasts with [^{3}H]- or [^{14}C] fucose and -glucosamine. Initial attempts to compare CF with normal erythrocyte membrane proteins and glycoproteins by SDS-PAGE have yielded contradictory results.[113,114] More recently, Scanlin and Glick[102] surveyed purified membranes from fibroblast lines on 7–14% polyacrylamide gradient gel slabs and detected a 190,000-mol-wt component in six of nine CF but none of the control cell lines. This protein did not label with L-[^{3}H] fucose or by periodate oxidation followed by reduction with borotritide (indicating little or no sialic acid content). The importance of this observation remains to be established.

In yet another study, Scanlin and Glick[115] recovered glycopeptides released from CF fibroblast membranes by trypsin. Compositional analyses of these glycopeptides showed an increase of fucose relative to the amounts of sialic acid, galactose, and mannose present. The structure of these CF membrane glycopeptides has not been analyzed to ascertain whether this difference is referrable to a single or to multiple membrane components. Similar studies by Maler and Riordan[116] on lymphocyte glycopeptides released by papain (not trypsin) failed to detect an alteration of surface glycopeptide carbohydrate composition. Furthermore, they were unable to detect changes in the fucose content of CF lymphoblast plasma membranes.

Another probe for cell-surface glycoproteins is assessment of lectin (sugar-binding protein) interactions with the surface of intact cells. Cultured CF fibroblasts do not display altered binding to concanavalin A, a lectin which has primarily mannose specificity.[117] CF cell responses to concanavalin A, such as cap formation, membrane internalization, and stronger con A staining at cell contact points, do not deviate from control. While this study has not identified CF-related membrane changes, lectins with other sugar specificities should be used to survey CF cell-surface glycoproteins.

CONCLUSIONS

Isolated pieces of evidence suggest alterations of several glycoprotein types in cystic fibrosis. The most substantial evidence points to increased acidic properties (particularly sulfate content) and oligosaccharide chain length of CF mucous glycoproteins. While these alterations provide a reasonable explanation for abnormal mucus properties in CF, considerably more work is required to document that mucous glycoprotein alterations are, in fact, closely related to the gene defect in this disease. Additional studies of mucin properties and the regulation of their synthesis and secretion are also needed. Reported abnormalities of serum-type glycoproteins in CF have not been consistently confirmed, and evidence to date favors the interpretation that changes of these glycoproteins may be related to secondary effects of the disease. So little is known concerning membrane glycoproteins in CF that comment on current observations must await results of confirmatory studies and more detailed investigations.

The basic defect in cystic fibrosis, when recognized, must provide an explanation for the major pathophysiologic events, including mucous obstruction and defective electrolyte and water transport. Altered mucous glycoproteins can change the rheologic properties of secretions and may afford an explanation for mucous obstruction, but they do not relate directly to altered membrane transport of electrolytes and water. It is known that increased degree of sulfation reduces the hydration of certain complex polysaccharides such as the carrageenans.[118] On the other hand, altered electrolyte content or pH of fluids secreted by mucous epithelia may dramatically affect the hydration of CF mucus gels, thereby effecting their rheologic or clearance properties. Either mechanism could account for the relative dehydration of CF tracheobronchial mucous secretions, meconium, or cervical mucus. There is no convincing pathophysiologic corollary for the putative asparagine-linked glycoprotein abnormalities in CF. On the other hand, perturbations of membrane function secondary to an abnormality of a glycoprotein component could explain both the obstructive and electrolyte/water abnormalities characteristic of CF. In any case, glycoprotein abnormalities presently constitute only one of several promising observations related to CF pathogenesis, one of which, it is hoped, will point the way to an ultimate understanding of expression of the CF gene.

REFERENCES

1. Farber S: Pancreatic function and disease in early life. V. Pathologic changes associated with pancreatic insufficiency in early life. *Arch Pathol* 1944;37:238.
2. Boat TF: Fundamental biochemistry: Introduction, in Mangos JA, Talamo RC (eds): *Cystic Fibrosis: Projections Into The Future.* New York, Stratton Intercontinental Medical Book Corp, 1976, p 155.
3. Spiro RG: Glycoproteins. *Adv Protein Chem* 1973;27:349.
4. Pigman W: Mucus glycoproteins, in Horowitz MI, Pigman W (eds): *The Glycoconjugates.* New York, Academic Press, 1977, pp 131–256.
5. Roussel P, Lamblin G, Degand P, et al: Heterogeneity of the carbohydrate chains of sulfated bronchial glycoproteins isolated from a patient suffering from cystic fibrosis. *J Biol Chem* 1975;250:2114.
6. Lamblin G, Lhermitte M, Degand P, et al: Chemical and physical properties of human bronchial mucous glycoproteins. *Biochimie* 1979;61:23.
7. Allen A, Mantle M, Pearson JP: The structure and properties of mucus glycoproteins, in Sturgess JM (ed): *Perspectives in Cystic Fibrosis: Proceedings of the Eighth International Congress on Cystic Fibrosis.* Mississauga, Ontario, Imperial Press Ltd, 1980, pp 102–112.
8. Rose MC, Lynn WS, Kaufman B: Resolution of the major components of human lung mucosal gel and their capabilities for reaggregation and gel formation. *Biochemistry* 1979;18:4030.
9. Forstner JF, Forstner GG: Calcium binding to intestinal goblet cell mucin. *Biochim Biophys Acta* 1975;386:283.
10. List SJ, Findlay BP, Forstner GG, et al: Enhancement of the viscosity of mucin by serum albumin. *Biochem J* 1978;175:565.
11. Creeth JM, Bridge JL, Horton JP: An interaction between lysozyme and mucous glycoproteins. *Biochem J* 1979;181:717.
12. Hill HD, Reynolds JA, Hill RL: Purification, composition, molecular weight, and subunit structure of ovine submaxillary mucin. *J Biol Chem* 1977;252:3791.
13. Roseman S: The synthesis of complex carbohydrates by multiglycosyltransferase system and the potential function in intercellular adhesion. *Chem Phys Lipids* 1970;5:270.
14. Kornfeld R, Kornfeld S: The structure of glycoproteins and their oligosaccharide units, in Lennerz WJ (ed): *The Biochemistry of Glycoproteins and Proteoglycans.* New York, Plenum Press, 1980, pp 1–34.

15. Reid L, deHaller R: Lung changes in cystic fibrosis, in Hubble D (chairman): *Cystic Fibrosis: A Symposium.* London, The Chest and Heart Association, 1964, pp 21–30.
16. Reid L, deHaller R: The bronchial mucous glands—their hypertrophy and change in intracellular mucus. *Mod Probl Pediatr* 1966; 10:195.
17. Oppenheimer EH, Esterly JR: Pathology of cystic fibrosis: Review of the literature and comparison with 146 autopsied cases. *Perspect Pediatr Pathol* 1975;2:241.
18. Neutra MR, Trier JS: The rectal mucosa in cystic fibrosis: Morphological features before and after short-term organ culture. *Gastroenterology* 1978;75:701.
19. Parkins RA, Eidelman S, Rubin CE: The diagnosis of cystic fibrosis by rectal suction biopsy. *Lancet* 1963;2:851.
20. Oppenheimer EH, Esterly JR: Cystic fibrosis of the pancreas: Morphologic findings in infants with and without diagnostic pancreatic lesions. *Arch Pathol* 1973;96:149.
21. Shwachman H, Holsclaw D: Examination of the appendix at laparotomy as a diagnostic clue in cystic fibrosis. *N Engl J Med* 1972; 286:1300.
22. Spicer SS, Lev R: Histochemical comparison of human epithelial mucins in normal and in hypersecretory states including pancreatic cystic fibrosis. *Am J Pathol* 1965;46:23.
23. Davis PB, Shelhamer J, Kaliner M: Abnormal adrenergic and cholinergic sensitivity in cystic fibrosis. *N Engl J Med* 1980;302:1453.
24. Sturgess J, Reid L: The effect of isoprenaline and pilocarpine on a) bronchial mucus-secreting tissue and b) pancreas, salivary glands, heart, thymus, liver, and spleen. *Br J Exp Pathol* 1973;54:388.
25. Lamb D, Reid L: The tracheobronchial submucosa glands in cystic fibrosis: A qualitative and quantitative histochemical study. *Br J Dis Chest* 1972;66:239.
26. di Sant'Agnese PA, Dische Z, Danilczenko A: Physiochemical differences of mucoproteins in duodenal fluid of patients with cystic fibrosis of the pancreas and controls: Clinical aspects. *Pediatrics* 1957;19:252.
27. Dische Z, di Sant'Agnese P, Pallavicini C, et al: Composition of mucoprotein fractions from duodenal fluid of patients with cystic fibrosis of the pancreas and from controls. *Pediatrics* 1959;24:74.
28. Chernick WS, Barbero GJ: Studies on human tracheobronchial and submaxillary secretions in normal and pathophysiological conditions. *Ann NY Acad Sci* 1963; 106:698.
29. Johansen PG: Some observations on mucous secretions in cystic fibrosis of pancreas. *Ann NY Acad Sci* 1963;106:755.
30. Roelfs RE, Gibbs GE, Griffin GD: Composition of rectal mucus in cystic fibrosis. *Am J Dis Child* 1967;113:419.
31. Clamp JR, Gough M: Study of the oligosaccharide units from mucus glycoproteins of meconium from normal infants and from cases of cystic fibrosis with meconium ileus. *Clin Sci* 1979;57:445.
32. Schachter H, Dixon GH: A comparative study of the proteins in normal meconium and in meconium from meconium ileus patients. *Can J Biochem* 1965;43:381.
33. Potter JL, Matthews LW, Lemm J, et al: Human pulmonary secretions in health and disease. *Ann NY Acad Sci* 1963;106:692.
34. Lopez A, Vidriero MT, Das I, Reid LM: Airway secretion: Source, biochemical and rheological properties, in Brain J, Potter D, Reid L (eds): *Respiratory Defense Mechanisms.* New York, Marcel Dekker, 1977, pp 289–356.
35. Menguy R, Masters VF, Desbaillets L: Salivary mucins of patients with cystic fibrosis: Composition and susceptibility to degradation by salivary glycosidases. *Gastroenterology* 1970;59:257.
36. Mandel ID, Kutscher A, Denning CR, et al: Salivary studies in cystic fibrosis. *Am J Dis Child* 1967;113;431.
37. Boat TF, Cheng PW, Iyer R, et al: Human respiratory tract secretions: Mucous glycoproteins of nonpurulent tracheobronchial secretions and sputum of patients with bronchitis and cystic fibrosis. *Arch Biochem Biophys* 1976;177:95.
38. Boat TF, Kleinerman JI, Carlson DM, et al: Human respiratory tract secretions: Mucous glycoproteins secreted by cultured nasal polyp epithelium from subjects with allergic rhinitis and with cystic fibrosis. *Am Rev Respir Dis* 1974;110:428.
39. Boat TF, Cheng PW, Wood RE: Tracheobronchial mucus secretion in vivo and in vitro by epithelial tissues from cystic fibrosis and control subjects. *Mod Probl Paediatr* 1977; 19:141.
40. Lamblin G, Lafitte JJ, Lhermitte M, et al: Mucins from cystic fibrosis sputum. *Mod Probl Paediatr* 1977;19:153.
41. Frates RC, Kaizu T, Last JA: Glycoproteins secreted from cultured human airway tissue of cystic fibrosis and non-cystic fibrosis patients, in Sturgess JM (ed): *Perspectives in Cystic Fibrosis: Proceedings of the Eighth International Congress on Cystic Fibrosis.* Mississauga, Ontario, Imperial Press Ltd, 1980, p 14a.
42. Boat TF, Davis J, Stern RC, et al: Effect of blood group determinants on binding of human salivary mucous glycoproteins to in-

fluenza virus, in Gregory JD, Jeanloz R (eds): *Glycoconjugate Research, Vol. 1.* New York, Academic Press, 1979, pp 503–506.

43. Springer GF, Schwick HG, Fletcher MA: The relationship of the influenza virus inhibitory activity of glycoproteins to their molecular size and sialic acid content. *Biochemistry* 1969;64:634.
44. Boat TF, Cheng PW: Mucous glycoproteins, in Mangos JA, Talamo RC (eds): *Cystic Fibrosis: Projections into the Future.* Miami, Symposia Specialists, 1976, pp 165–177.
45. Kim YS, Perdomo J, Whitehead JS, et al: Glycosyltransferases in human blood. II. Study of serum galactosyltransferase and *N*-acetylgalactosaminyltransferase in patients with liver diseases. *J Clin Invest* 1972;51:2003.
46. Mookerjea S, Michaels MA, Hudgin RL, et al: The levels of nucleotide-sugar: Glycoprotein sialyl-and *N*-acetylglucosaminyltransferases in normal and pathological human sera. *Can J Biochem* 1972;50:738.
47. Singer L, Crozier O, Moscarello MA: The levels of galactosyltransferase activity in sera from normal children and patients with cystic fibrosis. *Clin Biochem* 1974;7:146.
48. Rao GLS, Spells G, Nadler HL: Enhanced UDP-galactose: glycoprotein galactosyl transferase activity in cultivated skin fibroblasts from patients with cystic fibrosis and its possible relationship to the pathogenesis of the disease. *Pediatr Res* 1977; 11:981.
49. Louisot P, Levrat C, Gilly R: A new pathogenic hypothesis for cystic fibrosis: Hyperactivity of glycosyltransferases at microsomic level. *Clin Chim Acta* 1973; 48:373.
50. Levrat C, Gilly R, Louisot P: Glycosylation des glycoconjugues dans la mucoviscidose. In *Proceedings of the VII International Cystic Fibrosis Congress,* Paris. June 1976, pp 53–59.
51. Alhadeff JA, Cimino G: Cystic fibrosis liver sialyltransferase. *Clin Genet* 1978;13:207.
52. Cheng P-W, Bona S: Mucin biosynthesis—characterization of the UDP-galactose: α-*N*-acetylgalactosaminide $\beta 1 \rightarrow 3$-galactosyltransferase from human tracheal epithelium. *J Biol Chem* 1982;257:6251.
53. Cheng P-W, Bona SJ: Properties of asialo OSM galactosyltransferase in human tracheal epithelium. *Fed Proc* 1981;40: 1674.
54. Baker AP, Hillegass LM: Enhancement of UDP-galactose: mucin galactosyltransferase activity by spermine. *Arch Biochem Biophys* 1974;165:597.
55. Lundgren DW, Farrell PM, di Sant'Agnese PA: Polyamine alterations in blood of male homozygotes and heterozygotes for cystic fibrosis. *Clin Chim Acta* 1975;62:357.
56. Sherman JM, Boat TF, Cheng PW: Analysis of mucus secreted by EDTA-separated cat tracheal glands and surface epithelium. *Am Rev Respir Dis* 1981; 124:476.
57. Kent PW: Chemical aspects of tracheal glycoproteins, in *Respiratory Tract Mucus Ciba Foundation Series* 1978;54:155–170.
58. Boat TF, Cheng PW: Regulation of tracheal mucin secretion, in Sturgess JM (ed): *Perspectives in Cystic Fibrosis: Proceedings of the Eighth International Congress on Cystic Fibrosis.* Mississauga, Ontario, Imperial Press Ltd, 1980, p 5a.
59. Clark JN, Marchok AC: The effect of vitamin A on cellular differentiation and mucous glycoprotein synthesis in long-term rat tracheal organ cultures. *Differentiation* 1979;14:175.
60. Underwood BA, Denning CR: Blood and liver concentrations of vitamins A and E in children with cystic fibrosis of the pancreas. *Pediatr Res* 1972;6:26.
61. Riordan JR, Alon N, Duthrie M, et al: Hydrolytic enzymes as markers for cystic fibrosis? in Sturgess J (ed): *Perspectives in Cystic Fibrosis: Proceedings of the Eighth International Congress on Cystic Fibrosis.* Mississauga, Ontario, Imperial Press Ltd, 1980, pp 313–321.
62. Maler T, Duthrie M, Alon N, et al: α-L-fucosidase is quantitatively reduced in cultured lymphoblasts from patients with cystic fibrosis. *J Biol Chem* 1980;256;1420.
63. DiFerrante N, Ginsberg LC, Donnelly PV, et al: Deficiencies of glucosamine-6-sulfate or galactosamine-6-sulfate sulfatases are responsible for different mucopolysaccharidases. *Science* 1978;199:79.
64. Neutra MR, Grand RJ, Trier JS: Glycoprotein synthesis, transport, and secretion by epithelial cells of human rectal mucosa: Normal and cystic fibrosis. *Lab Invest* 1977; 36:535.
65. Sturgess J, Reid L: Secretory activity of the human bronchial mucous glands in vitro. *Exp Mol Pathol* 1972;16:362.
66. Bowman BH, Lockhart LH, McCombs ML: Oyster ciliary inhibition by cystic fibrosis factor. *Science* 1969;164:325.
67. Baur PS, Brinkley BR, Bowman BH: Effects of cystic fibrosis serum ciliary inhibitor on oyster gill ultrastructure: Analysis by scanning and transmission electron microscopy. *Tex Rep Biol Med* 1976;34:1.
68. Bogart BI, Conod EJ, Conover JH: The biological activities of cystic fibrosis serum. I. The effect of cystic fibrosis sera and calcium ionophore A 23187 on rabbit tracheal explants. *Pediatr Res* 1977;11:131.
69. Czegledy-Nagy E, Sturgess JM: Cystic fibrosis: Effects of serum factors on mucus

secretion. *Lab Invest* 1976;35:588.
70. Conover JH, Conod EJ: The influence of cystic fibrosis serum and calcium on secretion in rabbit tracheal mucociliary apparatus. *Biochem Biophys Res Commun* 1978;83: 1595.
71. Bogart BI, Conod EJ, Gaerlan PF, et al: The biologic activities of cystic fibrosis serum. II. Ultrastructural aspects of the effect of cystic fibrosis sera and calcium ionophore A 23187 on rabbit tracheal explants. *Pediatr Res* 1978;12:15.
72. Kurlandsky LE, Berninger RW, Talamo RC: A quantitative in vitro model for the study of mucus-producing substances in cystic fibrosis. *Pediatr Res* 1980;14:1263.
73. Fleming N, Sturgess J: Cystic fibrosis serum stimulates glycoprotein secretion in dissociated acinar cells from rat submandibular glands. *Cystic Fibrosis Club Abstracts.* Cystic Fibrosis Foundation, Rockville, Maryland, 1979, p 40.
74. Boat TF, Polony I, Cheng PW: Mucin release from rabbit tracheal epithelium in response to sera from normal and cystic fibrosis subjects. *Pediatr Res* 1982;16:792.
75. Gugler EG, Pallavicini CJ, Swerdlow H, et al: The role of calcium in submaxillary saliva of patients with cystic fibrosis. *J Pediatr* 1967;71:585.
76. Boat TF, Wiesman UN, Pallavicini JC: Purification and properties of the calcium-precipitable protein in submaxillary saliva of normal and cystic fibrosis subjects. *Pediatr Res* 1974;8:531.
77. Sturgess J, Palfrey AJ, Reid L: Rheological properties of sputum. *Rheol Acta* 1971;10:36.
78. Charman J, Reid L: Sputum viscosity in chronic bronchitis, bronchiectasis, asthma, and cystic fibrosis. *Biorheology* 1972;9:185.
79. King M: Is cystic fibrosis mucus abnormal? *Pediatr Res* 1981;15:120.
80. Lorin MI, Denning CR, Mandel ID: Viscosity of exocrine secretions in cystic fibrosis: Sweat, duodenal fluid, and submaxillary saliva. *Biorheology* 1972;9:27.
81. Bettelheim FA, Epstein S, Gorvey JD: Rheology of submaxillary secretions of cystic fibrosis patients and normal individuals. *Biorheology* 1971;8:129.
82. Kopito LE, Kosasky HJ, Shwachman H: Water and electrolytes in cervical mucus from patients with cystic fibrosis. *Fertil Steril* 1973;24:512.
83. Matthews LW, Spector S, Lemm J, et al: Studies in pulmonary secretions. 1. The overall chemical composition of pulmonary secretions from patients with cystic fibrosis, bronchiectasis, and laryngectomy. *Am Rev Respir Dis* 1963;88:199.
84. Chernick WS, Barbero GJ: Composition of tracheobronchial secretions in cystic fibrosis of the pancreas and bronchiectasis. *Pediatrics* 1959;24:739.
85. Kopito L, Shwachman H: Mineral composition of meconium. *J Pediatr* 1966: 68:313.
86. Marriott C, Shih CK, Litt M: Changes in the gel properties of tracheal mucus induced by divalent cations. *Biorheology* 1979;16:331.
87. Boat TF, Jentoft JE, Dearborn DG, et al: Hydration of tracheal mucus: The role of calcium, abstracted. *Am Rev Respir Dis* 1980; 121:284.
88. Rule AH, Baran DT, Shwachman H: Quantitative determination of water-soluble proteins in meconium. *Pediatrics* 1970;45:847.
89. Weeke B, Flensborg EW, Jacobsen L, et al: Immunochemical quantitation of 18 proteins in sera from patients with cystic fibrosis. *Dan Med Bull* 1976;23:155.
90. Talamo RC, Raunio V, Gabriel O, et al: Immunological and biochemical comparison of urinary glycoproteins in patients with cystic fibrosis of the pancreas and normal controls. *J Pediatr* 1964;65:480.
91. Schwartz RH, Pallavicini JC: Immunologic and chemical studies of cystic fibrosis and normal urinary glycoprotein of Tamm and Horsfall. *J Lab Clin Med* 1967;70:725.
92. Alhadeff JA, Tennant L, O'Brien JS. Altered isoenzyme patterns of liver α-L-fucosidase in cystic fibrosis. *Clin Genet* 1976;10:63.
93. Alhadeff JA, Cimino G, Janowsky A: Isoenzymes of human liver α-L-fucosidase: Chemical relationships, kinetic studies, and immunochemical characterization. *Mol Cell Biochem* 1978;19:171.
94. Alhadeff JA: Lysosomal hydrolases in cystic fibrosis livers. *Clin Chim Acta* 1978; 89:469.
95. Scanlin TF, Matacic SS, Pace M, et al: Abnormal distribution of α-L-fucosidase in cystic fibrosis: Increased activity in skin fibroblasts. *Biochem Biophys Res Commun* 1977;79:869.
96. Alhadeff JA, Cimino G: Cystic fibrosis liver sialyltransferase. *Clin Genet* 1978;13: 207.
97. Alhadeff JA, Watkins P, Freeze H: Purification and characterization of altered cystic fibrosis liver α-L-fucosidase. *Clin Genet* 1978;13:417.
98. Alhadeff JA, Watkins P: Differential concanavalin A binding of cystic fibrosis and normal liver α-L-fucosidase. *Biochem Biophys Res Commun* 1979;86:787.
99. Alhadeff JA: Glycoprotein metabolism in cystic fibrosis, in Sturgess JM (ed): *Perspectives in Cystic Fibrosis: Proceedings of the Eighth International Congress on Cystic Fibrosis.* Mississauga, Ontario, Imperial Press Ltd, 1980, pp 35–43.

100. Alhadeff JA, Watkins P: Cystic fibrosis serum α-L-fucosidase: Confirmation of normal activity levels and normal kinetic and isoelectric focusing properties. *Clin Chim Acta* 1980;105(1):131–135.
101. Casola L, DiMatteo G, Romano M, et al: Glycosidases in serum of cystic fibrosis patients. *Clin Chim Acta* 1979;94:83.
102. Scanlin TF, Glick MC: Dynamic and structural aspects of cystic fibrosis fibroblast membranes, in Sturgess JM (ed): *Perspectives in Cystic Fibrosis: Proceedings of the Eighth International Congress on Cystic Fibrosis.* Mississauga, Ontario, Imperial Press Ltd, 1980, pp 44–57.
103. Ben-Yoseph Y, Defranco CL, Nadler HL: Decreased sialic acid and altered binding to lectins of purified α_2-macroglobulin from patients with cystic fibrosis. *Clin Chim Acta* 1979;99:31.
104. Ben-Yoseph J, DeFranco CL, Nadler HL: Altered carbohydrate moiety in α_2-macroglobulin purified from plasma of patients with cystic fibrosis in Sturgess JM (ed): *Perspectives in Cystic Fibrosis: Proceedings of the Eighth International Congress on Cystic Fibrosis.* Mississauga, Ontario, Imperial Press Ltd, 1980, p 4a (abstract).
105. Shapira E, Menendez R: Increased binding of concanavalin A to α_2-macroglobulin, IgM, and IgG from cystic fibrosis plasma. *Biochem Biophys Res Commun* 1980;93:50.
106. Pearson RD, Lubin AH: A simple method for estimating a heparin-binding capacity of human serum. *Health Lab Sci* 1978;15:32.
107. Pearson RD, Lubin AH: Increased heparin binding in cystic fibrosis: A reflection of altered glycoprotein biosynthesis? *Pediatr Res* 1979;13:834.
108. Margolies R: Identification of a major heparin-precipitable protein in human serum and its relationship to cystic fibrosis. *Pediatr Res* 1982;16:181.
109. Leprat R, Michel-Briand Y: Extracellular neuraminidase production by a strain of *Pseudomonas aeruginosa* isolated from cystic fibrosis. *Ann Microbiol* 1980; 131:209.
110. Hunt LA, Summers DF: Glycosylation of VSV glycoprotein is similar in cystic fibrosis, heterozygous carrier, and normal human fibroblasts. *J Supramol Struct* 1977;7:213.
111. Baig MM, Cetorelli JJ, Roberts RM: Plasma membrane components of skin fibroblasts from normal individuals and patients with cystic fibrosis. *J Pediatr* 1975;86:72.
112. Scanlin TF, Glick MC: Surface membranes from fibroblasts in cystic fibrosis. *VIIth International Cystic Fibrosis Congress Proceedings,* Paris, 1976, pp 44–52.
113. Fitzpatrick DF, Landon EJ, James V: Serum binding of calcium and the red cell membrane. *Nature (London) New Biol* 1972;235:173.
114. McEvoy FA, Davis RJ, Goodchild MC, et al: Erythrocyte membrane properties in cystic fibrosis. *Clin Chim Acta* 1974;54: 195.
115. Scanlin TF, Glick MC: Difference in monosaccharide composition of membrane glycopeptides from cystic fibrosis and control skin fibroblasts. *Pediatr Res* 1977; 11:463.
116. Maler T, Riordan JR: Altered fucose handling by cystic fibrosis lymphoblasts, in Sturgess JM (ed): *Perspectives in Cystic Fibrosis: Proceedings of the Eighth International Congress on Cystic Fibrosis.* Mississauga, Ontario, Imperial Press Ltd, 1980, pp 58–63.
117. Yokoyama M, Chang JP, Hom D, et al: An electron microscopic cytochemical study on concanavalin A binding sites and their mobility in normal and cystic fibrosis fibroblasts in vitro. *Pediatr Res* 1977;11:765.
118. Rees DA: Structure, conformation and mechanism in the formation of polysaccharide gels and networks, in *Adv Carbohydrate Chem Biochem* 1969;24:267.
119. Lombart GG, Winzler RJ: Isolation and characterization of oligosaccharides from canine submaxillary mucins. *Eur J Biochem* 1974;49:77.
120. Rovis LR, Anderson B, Kabat EA, et al: Structures of oligosaccharides produced by base-borohydride degradation of human ovarian cyst blood group H, Le^b and Le^a active glycoproteins. *Biochemistry* 1973;12: 5340.
121. Baenziger JU, Fiete D: Structure of the complex oligosaccharide of fetuin. *J Biol Chem* 1979;254:789.

7

Cystic Fibrosis Factors

Pamela B. Davis

In 1967, two laboratories reported results which profoundly affected subsequent research in cystic fibrosis (CF). Spock and co-workers[1] found a factor in the serum of patients with CF and in concentrated serum fractions from obligate heterozygotes, but not healthy controls, which caused ciliary dyskinesia. Mangos and his co-workers[2] found a factor in saliva from patients with CF which inhibited resorption of sodium along the parotid gland duct. If these factor(s) proved to be markers for the CF gene, they might be useful for heterozygote identification and prenatal diagnosis. They also might provide clues to the genetic error in CF and the pathogenesis of the clinical manifestations.[3-5]

For these reasons, enormous time, effort, and money have been invested in the so-called "CF factor(s)." Unfortunately the factors have not fulfilled our more extravagant hopes. Despite extensive and intensive efforts, critical questions about the nature, distribution, and significance of the CF factors are not yet settled. Although we should now have the technical expertise to address these questions, ambiguity remains.

Two basic classes of factors have been identified: those which appear to alter the secretion of macromolecules, and those which affect monovalent cation transport. Although the definitive experiments have not yet been done, these two categories appear to be distinct. This discussion will therefore be divided into two main sections and a third, smaller section for the miscellaneous biologic activities not clearly related to the others. The chapter will conclude with theories on the origin(s) of factor(s) and a discussion of possible future approaches to these problems.

CILIARY DYSKINESIA/MUCUS SECRETORY FACTORS

Spock and co-workers reported in 1967[1] that each of 75 sera from patients with CF contained a heat-labile, nondialyzable substance which caused ciliary dyskinesia in rabbit tracheal explants. This factor was not present in 75 sera from healthy and diseased controls. All 25 sera from CF heterozygotes had the factor, but in most, concentration of the euglobulin fraction was required to demonstrate it. Similar concentration of sera from 25 normals produced only one positive result. These observations generated much interest, and many attempts were made to demonstrate ciliary dyskinesia activity in CF serum using a variety of ciliated organisms as test systems.[6–9] However, most of these assay systems proved unsuitable, except for the oyster gill cilia assay used by Bowman and her collaborators, who had access to plentiful supplies of fresh oysters. Even they have been plagued by seasonal, water-temperature, pollution, and other variations in the oysters. For these reasons, the cilia on cultured mammalian tracheae have been the most frequently used test system.

Even the rabbit tracheal system must be rigorously standardized before acceptable assays can be performed. Maintenance of test samples in culture for several days prior to assay and selection of clean explants with vigorously beating cilia appear to be important for reproducible results.[10–12] Using such selected test systems, some investigators have been able to show that CF serum interferes with the beating of cilia to a greater extent than normal serum. However, in contrast to Spock's initial report,[1] later workers have found similar activity in the serum of patients with asthma.[13,14] The substance in sera from asthmatics which causes ciliary dyskinesia is C3a or a fragment thereof.[14] This observation highlights the lack of specificity of this bioassay: it is subject to interference from a wide variety of materials, including polyamines, bradykinin, and other naturally occurring substances. Because of this lack of specificity, the largely subjective endpoint of this assay, and the inability of some groups to replicate any of these results,[15] bioassay of whole serum for ciliary dyskinesia activity in mammalian tracheal cilia test systems will not be acceptable for identifying the CF genotype.

Bowman and co-workers,[16] using oyster gill as the test system, find ciliostasis to be quite specific for the CF genotype, although there are a number of molecules with ciliostatic activity in CF serum and urine. However, several other laboratories have been unable to confirm this result.[7,17] Thus the oyster gill bioassay apparently lacks specificity, too. In a blind trial, neither the rabbit tracheal nor the oyster gill assay system was able reliably to identify samples from persons of CF genotype.[18] Therefore, these assays are not applicable clinically. However, they are useful to test for the "CF factor" during purification and in comparative studies of biologic activities.

There is now considerable evidence that the ciliary dyskinesia or ciliotoxic factor may not act directly on cilia. CF serum has no effect on ciliary ATPase, the primary energy source for ciliary motility.[19] Ultrastructural analysis of oyster gills exposed to CF serum reveals enlarged and partially exuded goblet cells, altered mucus ultrastructure with twisted and matted cilia, and overall swelling of the gill filament.[20] In rabbit trachea, analysis of ciliary activity using high-speed cinemicrographs obtained with the use of Nomarski optics has shown that CF serum has no effect on rhythm and beat pattern of the cilia; however, it did have a cytolytic effect on tracheal epithelial cells and cell junctions.[21] Other studies with optical and scanning electron microscopy indicate that CF serum produces swelling of goblet cells, discharge of their contents, entangling of cilia, and later, some shedding of ciliated cells from rabbit tracheal epithelium.[22–24]

These observations suggest that apparent ciliary dyskinesia or ciliostasis is the result of mechanical entanglement of cilia by mucus or debris and not the result of biochemical alteration of ciliary processes per se. Using a biochemical technique, Boat and co-workers (personal communication) find that CF serum promotes release of radiolabeled mucin from rabbit tracheal explants to a greater extent than matched control serum.

If CF serum contains general secretogogue(s), it might promote secretion in other test systems besides the rabbit trachea and the oyster gill. Indeed, Conod, et al[25] reported the presence in CF serum of a "degranulation factor" which promotes the release of lysosomal enzymes from granulocytes. Kurlandsky and co-workers[26] found that CF serum promotes release of a mucus-like substance from the urn cells of a marine worm, *Sipunculus nudus*. Fleming and Sturgess[27] report increased release of radiolabeled mucins from rat submandibular cells in the presence of CF serum. Lack of specificity for the CF genotype precludes clinical use of these assays, and, like other bioassays, they are subject to interference from metabolically active, naturally occurring substances. Indeed, preliminary data indicate that substances with different properties are measured by the different assays for secretion. Nevertheless, the secretory response of a wide variety of tissues to CF serum raises the interesting possibility that the serum might contain secretogogue(s). Since a generalized derangement of mucus secretion appears to underlie the clinical syndrome of CF, participation of a mucus secretory factor in the pathogenesis of disease could easily be imagined. The multisystem clinical manifestations of CF are less easily related to a generalized abnormality of coordinated ciliary activity.

A mechanism by which a CF factor might function as a secretogogue has been suggested by Bogart et al.[28] They drew an analogy between the action of the ionophore A23187 (albeit in very high concentration) and CF serum in producing ciliary dyskinesia in tracheal explants and in morphologic effects on the tissue.[22,28] They suggested that the factor(s) might act, in part, through a calcium ionophore-like mechanism and showed that CF serum promoted uptake of ^{45}Ca by rabbit tracheal explants.[29] Banschbach and co-workers[30] found that CF serum promoted the accumulation of ^{45}Ca from the medium by leukocytes. However, Boat and co-workers (personal communication) found that the ionophore A23187 did not mimic the effects of CF serum on mucin release from rabbit tracheal explants, and other investigators, using several techniques, have been unable to demonstrate calcium ionophore-like activity in CF serum.[31]

Whatever the true biologic activities of a CF factor, an objective and specific assay is essential for research advances. Several assays have been developed to meet these needs—an assay based on inhibition of glycogen-debranching enzyme activity by the factor, isoelectric focusing to detect abnormal protein bands, and a rocket immunoelectrophoresis assay to quantitate the CF factor.

Impero et al[32] have demonstrated close correspondence between oyster gill ciliotoxic activity in CF saliva and inhibitory activity for glycogen-debranching enzyme. Presence of a salivary inhibitor of this enzyme is quite specific for the CF genotype, is unrelated to the CF donor's clinical status, and is not found in saliva from patients with diseases whose clinical manifestations resemble some of those of CF.[33] This factor is of low molecular weight, is bound to α-amylase, is a reversible noncompetitive inhibitor of glycogen-debranching enzyme, is heat-labile, is unstable to storage except under special conditions, and is labile to the extremes of pH. Although it apparently copurifies with a substance ciliotoxic for oyster gills, its low molecular weight and chemical properties make it unlikely to be identical to Bowman's ciliotoxin peptide. Detailed knowledge of the properties and instabilities of this factor may facilitate its purification and characterization.

Isoelectric focusing should offer the opportunity to purify and identify the CF factor. Indeed, the early use of this technique was in attempts to purify the oyster gill ciliotoxin.[34,35] However, the heterogeneity and complexity of protein bands from serum made it impossible to use this method as a single-step purification of a CF factor. These problems have also complicated the use of isoelectric focusing as an analytical technique.

Wilson and co-workers have championed the use of isoelectric focusing to identify a material they call cystic fibrosis protein (CFP). They have shown that fractions containing CFP invariably display ciliary dyskinesia activity.[10] CFP focuses in a band with pI 8.41–8.57, depending on the apparatus used.[36,37] It is present in serum from over 90% of CF homozygotes and heterozygotes but only in about 8% of normal sera. Wilson[38] speculates that the false negatives could result from misdiagnosis of CF or genetic heterogeneity and that the false positives are actually CF heterozygotes (thought to constitute about 5% of the general population.) However, the patient populations possessing and lacking CFP have not been described in detail, and one family study is confusing, with the heterozygous mother possessing CFP but the affected child lacking it.

Attempts of other investigators to replicate these findings have met with variable success. Some have been unable to identify a protein band unique to CF.[39,40] Others have found the band difficult to identify directly, but visible upon comparison with known positives and negatives,[41] or visible with photographic image enhancement,[42] or detectable by two-step electrofocusing/electrophoretic techniques.[43] Those who do reproduce the results of Wilson emphasize that meticulous attention to technical detail is essential for success. Therefore it seems unlikely that this assay, even if valid, will be easily applied by different laboratories as a diagnostic assay for the CF gene.

Even the best isoelectric focusing gels cannot reliably distinguish homozygotes from heterozygotes. Apparent deletions of certain protein bands in heterozygotes are not sufficiently specific to be useful,[37,44] and it is difficult to quantitate CFP on the gels. Therefore, at least two laboratories are attempting to develop immunoassays for CFP. Such assays would not depend on nuances of isoelectric focusing technique, should make CFP easier to detect unequivocally, and should be quantitative.

Manson and Brock[45] used the portion of isoelectric focusing gels containing CFP to stimulate antibody production in guinea pigs. The resulting antibodies were purified by adsorption to the same portion of gels in which CFP-negative serum had been focused. They then used this antiserum in a rocket immunoelectrophoresis assay. All sera positive, but no sera negative, for CFP by isoelectric focusing displayed a precipitin rocket. Serum from 1 of 15 normal controls, 16 of 17 patients with CF, and 8 of 9 obligate heterozygotes produced a precipitin rocket, and those of the heterozygotes were considerably smaller than those of the homozygotes. Manson and Brock[45] concluded that their antibody was specific for CFP and that, although it was comparatively weak, it could distinguish quantitatively between CF homozygotes and heterozygotes. Wilson and Middleton[46] also report raising an antibody to CFP in mice and thus should shortly have capabilities for an immunoassay. Neither of these assays is ready for clinical application yet, but both are highly promising. Such tools should facilitate evaluation of CFP as a possible marker for the abnormal CF gene.

SODIUM REABSORPTION INHIBITORY FACTOR

The discovery of a factor in CF saliva and sweat which inhibits the reabsorption of sodium along exocrine ducts[2,47] fits nicely with the clinical observations of elevated levels of sodium in the sweat and saliva of CF patients. In vitro microperfusion studies indicate that this factor in CF sweat is transducible. The CF sweat gland behaves normally when perfused with normal sweat, but both normal and CF sweat glands produce sweat containing high levels of sodium and chloride when perfused with CF sweat.[48] Thus it is likely that this transducible factor, and not an intrinsic abnormality of the CF sweat gland, accounts for the CF eccrine sweat abnormality. The factor is only effective when applied intraluminally, and recent evidence suggests that the factor in CF saliva acts upon a luminal, amiloride-sensitive transport mechanism.[49]

Although a sodium reabsorption inhibitory factor was described more than 10 years ago, and its existence has been verified by several independent groups,[2,48,50] there has been little progress on its isolation or purification. The activity appears to be quite unstable: it is heat-labile, destroyed by freezing and thawing, and adsorbed by glass. Moreover, the assays necessary to follow this activity are cumbersome and difficult. Thus, little is known of its properties and comparison with ciliary dyskinesia factor or CFP is presently not possible. However, since the sodium reabsorption inhibitory factor can be detected in deproteinized samples,[51] it is unlikely that it will be identical to the CFP of Wilson or the ciliotoxin described by Bowman. In addition, it is uncertain whether the sodium reabsorption inhibitory factor is present in serum, for this fluid cannot, for technical reasons, be directly tested in a retrograde perfusion assay.

For these reasons, simpler assays of factors altering sodium transport are highly desirable. Assays which measure some aspect of sodium-dependent glucose transport, usually in the intestine of rabbits or rats, have been tried for this purpose. Both serum and saliva have been tested in such assays. Early positive results of Brown et al[52] were followed by conflicting findings. Some laboratories confirmed the result in principle, although usually with modification of the test system.[53-56] Others could not demonstrate any specificity for CF.[57,58] One laboratory, while confirming the abnormal effects of CF serum on sugar transport in rat enterocytes, presented evidence that the changes were attributable to polyamines.[59] Other studies of sodium transport in various single cell types have also not provided a consensus.[58,60,61] Thus there is no uniformity of results in these alternate test systems, in contrast to the consistency of results in the difficult exocrine gland ductal assay for inhibition of sodium resorption.

Will and co-workers[49] have developed an assay which measures decreases in short-circuit current in the rat colon in which amiloride-sensitive sodium transport has been induced. CF saliva causes a greater decrease in short-circuit current in this system than saliva from controls. Moreover, good correlation has been demonstrated between this assay and the retrograde perfusion assay of sodium resorption in rat parotid duct. This rat colonic assay is technically easier than exocrine duct assays and, if it proves to measure the same activity and the absolute numerical differences between CF and normal samples can be amplified, it may be a useful alternative assay for following purification of the sodium resorption inhibitory activity and for elucidating its mechanism of action.

OTHER FACTORS

A number of other biologic activities of CF fluids have been reported, but have not been extensively studied. Khan and co-workers[62] found that a factor in CF saliva which copurified with the mussel gill ciliotoxin altered the colloid zeta potential of a test system of beagle tracheal mucus, but probably because the assay is so cumbersome, it has not been used by other groups. Lieberman and co-workers[63] reported an activity in CF serum which prevents the loss of protein and acid hydrolase from cultured lymphocytes and agglutinates mouse erythrocytes. The latter assay was suggested as a means of identifying a lectin-like activity in CF serum. Lieberman's assay, even in his own laboratory, is sensitive to minor methodologic and chemical source changes and has failed blind testing. Even in the same patient, the activity varies inversely with intensity of antibiotic therapy: it disappears with treatment and reappears when aggressive therapy is stopped. Thus, because of its sensitivity to technical variations and to in vivo influences, this assay is unlikely to be useful as a diagnostic, or even a research, tool.

There appear to be inherited and/or

acquired alterations in polyamine metabolism in CF,[64,65] and changes in the levels of these cations in various fluids could account for some of the biological activities attributed to the CF factors. However, because polyamine levels are altered in many biological and pathological states and vary with age and sex, they cannot be conveniently used to distinguish persons of the CF genotype. However, when bioassays are used to distinguish CF from non-CF materials, possible effects of polyamines should be considered.

ORIGINS OF FACTORS

If the CF factors are indeed small peptides which are present in biological fluids of CF homozygotes and heterozygotes, a number of possible explanations of their origins exist. They could be the product of the abnormal gene for CF or fragments thereof; they could be metabolites which accumulate due to a block at a distal metabolic point; or they could be metabolites which are overproduced by a disordered proximal enzyme system. Nonprotein factors, of course, could not be primary products of the abnormal gene, but must result from disordered metabolism.

Although Mayo and co-workers[16,66] interpret their somatic cell genetic studies to indicate that the oyster gill ciliotoxin is a direct product of the abnormal gene for CF, on balance this suggestion seems unlikely. The lack of specificity of most activities, the possibility that there are many molecules with "factor"-like activity, the probability that differences between CF and non-CF samples are quantitative and not qualitative, and the lack of consistent results in some of the assays all make this possibility remote.

Another hypothesis is that factors accumulate in CF fluids as a consequence of abnormal protease activity, due to abnormal interaction between proteases and α_2-macroglobulin. Proteases are converted to peptidases in the course of interaction with α_2-macroglobulin. In CF this conversion apparently fails to occur.[67,68] Thus peptides such as the CF factors, presumed in this model to be normal products of protein degradation, would ordinarily be further degraded by α_2-macroglobulin–protease complexes with specificity for smaller peptides, but accumulate in CF because this further degradation cannot occur. In support of this hypothesis, Wilson notes that the cell types which apparently secrete the factor(s)—fibroblasts[69,70] and monocytes[71]—are also those which manufacture α_2-macroglobulin. In Wilson's model, the primary product of the abnormal CF gene is α_2-macroglobulin. There is little chemical evidence for abnormal primary structure of α_2-macroglobulin, and in fact its amino acid composition is normal.[72] Moreover, further studies of α_2-macroglobulin in CF indicate that its function may not be disordered.[73] Thus this hypothesis may not explain the existence of small peptide factors.

FUTURE DIRECTIONS FOR RESEARCH

Real progress in the realm of the CF factors will depend on their isolation, purification, and chemical characterization. For achieving these goals, the production of antibody to a factor is a most promising development. It affords the prospect of isolation and purification. Once this is accomplished, the factor's chemical nature can be determined, its true biologic activities elucidated, and its mechanisms of action evaluated. Moreover, antibodies offer possibilities of immunoassays for the factor, with unambiguous identification and quantitation. If this goal could be achieved, the specificity of the factor for CF could be ascertained. For all these reasons, the progress of antibody production to CFP will be viewed with great interest by the CF community.

Ultimately, from the scientific point of view, it will be necessary to establish the relation of the factor(s) to the abnormal gene product in CF. Also, it will be important to evaluate what role, if any, the factor(s) play in the pathogenesis of disease. However, the lack of such knowledge may not preclude its use as a practical tool for heterozygote identification or prenatal diagnosis. Since we lack understanding of the origin and significance of factor(s), however, they should meet stringent empirical criteria in order to serve as clinical tools.

For heterozygote identification, a test should be able to distinguish CF heterozygotes from normals, but not necessarily from homozygotes, for this can be accomplished on clinical grounds and by the sweat test. Since 5% of the white population is expected to be heterozygous for CF, an "overlap" of about 5% of the "normals" into the heterozygote range is to be expected. Variation of the test parameter with age, sex, intercurrent diseases, or physiological states such as pregnancy is undesirable, but if it occurs, it should be clearly defined. Establishment of norms and variability for the test will require assays of hundreds of normal and abnormal samples. Because clinical screening is the ultimate blind sample, the test should be able to distinguish known heterozygotes from normals when the source of the samples is unknown to the investigator. In summary, the test should discriminate between CF heterozygotes and normals in blind testing and should be relatively insensitive to minor in vivo variations. For a test to be useful for mass screening, it should also be simple to perform and inexpensive. If a test is costly or difficult, it may only be reasonable to use it in high-risk situations, such as marriages including a known CF heterozygote or a sibling of a CF patient.

For prenatal diagnosis, the requirements for a suitable clinical test are slightly different. In this instance, it is critical that the homozygote be distinguishable from other genotypes; separation of heterozygotes from normals is not critical since all these subjects are phenotypically normal. Often, tests for prenatal diagnosis are developed in cultured skin fibroblasts, since a fibroblast-like cell is frequently cultured from amniotic fluid. In this case, the test in fibroblasts should be able to distinguish homozygous from other samples when they are presented in blind fashion. Even so, amniotic fluid cells may behave differently and should be tested separately.

Evaluation of a test for prenatal diagnosis is complicated by our inability to diagnose CF in an aborted fetus. It is therefore crucial to the validation of a potential prenatal diagnostic test for CF that the pregnancies tested be completed and the infants tested for CF. If a potential test gave a simple yes-or-no result (such as presence or absence of a protein), in order to be 95% confident that a test was 95% accurate the results of 60 pregnancies from the union of two obligate heterozygotes would have to be predicted accurately. Since pregnancies of parents who have previously produced a CF child are relatively unusual, nationwide cooperation would be required to accumulate such a large series expeditiously. However, many tests do not give a simple biphasic response, but rather a continuum of values with some overlap between the groups one desires to separate. A boundary is selected empirically to minimize misclassification of test subjects. The boundary may be set to minimize the error of designating an affected child as unaffected or to reduce the error of designating an unaffected child as having CF. In either case it would be important to calculate the probability of each type of misdesignation and adjust the boundary to meet the specific needs of the test populations. All such prospective evaluations, however, require that the true results of the pregnancies tested be determined, and with our present limitations, that means that the children must be delivered and sweat-tested.

These considerations are complicated by the possibility that CF is genetically heterogeneous. Thus a true marker for the abnormal gene in some families may be absent in others. However, care must be taken in interpreting the absence of a putative marker for the CF gene in some patients and parents as evidence for genetic heterogeneity. Variation in the test itself and possible secondary effects of disease (eg, malabsorption, drugs, bacterial products, etc) should be considered. Even heterozygotes may be subject to some secondary effects, such as antibody formation to the porcine pancreatic enzymes they prepare for their children.[74] Family studies may be useful in sorting out these questions and in other more practical ways. For example, if both parents demonstrate the genetic marker, then an affected child should be marker-positive. However, if neither parent has the marker, the child should not have it either. For mass screening programs, however, family studies are impractical, and if a test which identifies only one of several types of CF is used, some cases may be missed.

Since the rocket immunoelectrophoresis assay appears to distinguish CF heterozygotes from non-CF genotypes,[45] this assay might be considered for heterozygote screening. Since cultured skin fibroblasts and possibly amniotic fluid cells from persons of CF genotype reportedly produce a CF factor,[70] immunoassays for the factor might be applied for prenatal diagnosis. Other assays which do not involve the factors—such as assays for drug resistance of CF fibroblasts[75] and the protease assay[76]—have already been suggested for prenatal diagnosis. We must decide soon how to evaluate poorly understood empirical tests as clinical tools.

The checkered history of the CF factors should teach us that hasty clinical application of even very promising research findings is inappropriate and that for life-and-death decisions such as whether to conceive or to bear a child, only carefully validated assays should be used. The problems of this disease are vexing and the affected families are often eager to apply tentative laboratory conclusions to the difficult choices in their lives. However, our primary obligation as physicians and scientists is to interpret new research intelligently and cautiously for our patients. We must, however, continue to offer them hope that carefully considered and controlled research in many areas, including the factors, may someday provide not only understanding of the disease which afflicts their families, but also practical assistance with the difficult choices they face.

ACKNOWLEDGMENTS

I am grateful to Thomas F. Boat, MD, for access to data prior to publication and for his helpful comments on the manuscript, and to Mark Haacke, PhD, for statistical consultation and his reading of the paper.

REFERENCES

1. Spock A, Heick H, Cress H, et al: Abnormal serum factor in patients with cystic fibrosis of the pancreas. *Pediatr Res* 1967;1:173–177.
2. Mangos JA, McSherry NR, Benke PJ: A sodium transport inhibitory factor in the saliva of patients with cystic fibrosis of the pancreas. *Pediatr Res* 1967;1:436–442.
3. di Sant'Agnese PA, Davis PB: Research in cystic fibrosis. *N Engl J Med* 1976;295: 481–485, 534–541, 597–602.
4. Davis PB, di Sant'Agnese PA: CF at forty—quo vadis? *Pediatr Res* 1980;14:83–87.
5. Wood RE, Boat TF, Doershuk CF: Cystic fibrosis. *Am Rev Respir Dis* 1976;113: 833–876.
6. Cohen FL, Daniel WL: Effects of cystic fibrosis sera on *Proteus vulgaris* motility. *J Med Genet* 1974;11:253–256.
7. Besley GT, Patrick AD, Norman AP: Inhibition of the motility of gill cilia of *Dreissena* by plasma of cystic fibrosis patients and their parents. *J Med Genet* 1969;6:278–280.
8. Christensen J, Norrevarg A: Studies on the effect of CF serum on fresh tissue from *Dreissena* gills, oyster gills, and rabbit tracheal mucosa. In *Proceedings of the Fifth International Cystic Fibrosis Conference,* Cambridge, England, Cystic Fibrosis Research Trust, London, 1969; p 49.
9. Bowman BH, Lockhart LH, McCombs ML: Oyster ciliary inhibition by cystic fibrosis factor. *Science* 1969;164:325–326.
10. Wilson GB, Monsher MT, Fudenberg HH: Studies on cystic fibrosis using isoelectric focusing III. Correlation between cystic fibrosis protein and ciliary dyskinesia activity in serum shown by a modified rabbit tracheal bioassay. *Pediatr Res* 1977;11:143–146.
11. Conover JH, Bonforte RJ, Hathaway P, et al: Studies on ciliary dyskinesia factor in cystic fibrosis I. Bioassay and heterozygote detection in serum. *Pediatr Res* 1973;7: 220–223.
12. Gabridge MG, Bright MJ, Agee CC, et al: Development of an improved tracheal explant bioassay for the detection of the ciliary dyskinesia factor in cystic fibrosis serum. *Pediatr Res* 1979;13:31–35.
13. Conover J, Conod E, Hirschhorn K: Ciliary dyskinesia factor in immunological and pulmonary disease. *Lancet* 1973;2:1194.
14. Wilson GB, Fudenberg HH: Studies on cystic fibrosis using isoelectric focusing IV. Distinction between ciliary dyskinesia activity in cystic fibrosis and asthmatic sera and associa-

tion of cystic fibrosis protein with the activity in cystic fibrosis serum. *Pediatr Res* 1977;11: 317–324.
15. Cherry JD, Roden VJ, Rejent AJ, et al: The inhibition of ciliary activity in tracheal organ cultures by sera from children with cystic fibrosis and control subjects. *J Pediatr* 1971; 79:937–942.
16. Bowman BH, Barnett DR, Carson SD, et al: Studies of cystic fibrosis utilizing mucociliary activity in oyster gills. *Fed Proc* 1980;39: 3195–3200.
17. Posselt H, Bender S: Heterozygote testing in cystic fibrosis. *Z. Kinderheilkd* 1971;110: 93–98.
18. Wood RE, di Sant'Agnese PA: Bioassays of cystic fibrosis factor. *Lancet* 1973;2:1452–1453.
19. Farrell PM, Fox GN, Spicer SS: Biochemical assessment of ciliary activity in the presence of cystic fibrosis serum. *Pediatr Res* 1974;8: 467–474.
20. Baur PS, Brinkley BR, Bowman BH: Effects of cystic fibrosis serum and ciliary inhibitor on oyster gill ultrastructure: Analysis by scanning and transmission electron microscopy. *Tex Rep Biol Med* 1976;34:155–174.
21. Cheung ATW, Jahn TL: High-speed cinemicrographic studies on rabbit tracheal (ciliated) epithelia: Determination of the beat pattern of tracheal cilia. *Pediatr Res* 1976;10: 140–144.
22. Bogart BI, Conod EJ, Gaerlan PF, et al: Biologic activities of cystic fibrosis serum II. Ultrastructural aspects of the effect of cystic fibrosis sera and calcium ionophore A23187 on rabbit tracheal explants. *Pediatr Res* 1978; 12:15–24.
23. Kennedy JR, Allen PL: Cystic fibrosis serum effects of rabbit tracheal epithelium: An ultrastructural analysis. *Pediatr Res* 1980;14: 1173–1179.
24. Czegledy-Nagy E, Sturgess JM: Cystic fibrosis: Effects of serum factors on mucus secretion. *Lab Invest* 1976;35:588–595.
25. Conod EJ, Conover JH, Hirschhorn K: Demonstration of human leukocyte degranulation induced by sera from homozygotes and heterozygotes for cystic fibrosis. *Pediatr Res* 1975;9:724–729.
26. Kurlandsky LE, Berninger RW, Talamo RC: Mucus-stimulation activity in the sera of patients with cystic fibrosis: Demonstration and preliminary fractionation. *Pediatr Res* 1980; 14:1263–1268.
27. Fleming N, Sturgess JM: Cystic fibrosis serum stimulates glycoprotein secretion in dissociated acinar cells from rat submandibular glands. *Cystic Fibrosis Club Abstr* 1979;20:40.
28. Bogart BI, Conod EJ, Conover JH: The biologic activities of cystic fibrosis serum I. The effects of cystic fibrosis sera and calcium ionophore A23187 on rabbit tracheal explants. *Pediatr Res* 1977;11:131–134.
29. Bogart BI, Conod EJ, Gaerlan PF, et al: Biological activities of cystic fibrosis serum III. CF-serum induced uptake of 45 Ca^{++} by rabbit tracheal explants. *Biochem Biophys Res Commun* 1979;88:1398–1404.
30. Banschbach MW, Karam AG, Love PK, et al: Cystic fibrosis serum promotes [^{45}Ca] uptake by normal human leukocytes. *Biochem Biophys Res Commun* 1978;84:922–927.
31. de Salegui M, Smith H, Kattan M, et al: New approaches fail to detect in CF serum either a calcium ionophore or a gene-specific inhibitor of mucociliary function. In Sturgess JM (ed): *Perspectives in Cystic Fibrosis: Proceedings of the Eighth International Congress on Cystic Fibrosis.* Mississauga, Ontario, Imperial Press Ltd, 1980, p 12a.
32. Impero JE, Harrison GM, Nelson TE: Cystic fibrosis: Isolation and physical properties of a salivary cystic fibrosis factor. *Pediatr Res* 1978;12:108–114.
33. Impero JE, Harrison GM, Nelson TE: Specificity of an isolated salivary factor material to cystic fibrosis. *Pediatr Res* 1981;15:940–944.
34. Barnett DR, Schandfield MS, McCombs ML, et al: Isoelectric focusing and IgG allotyping of the serum fraction containing the cystic fibrosis ciliary inhibitor. *Tex Rep Biol Med* 1973;31:709–714.
35. Schmoyer IR, Brooks SP, Fischer JF: Isolation and characterization of a ciliary dyskinetic factor from cystic fibrosis heterozygous serum. *Life Sci* 1972;2:1037–1044.
36. Wilson GB, Arnaud P, Fudenberg HH: Improved method for detection of cystic fibrosis protein in serum using the LKB multiphor electrofocusing apparatus. *Pediatr Res* 1977;11:986–988.
37. Wilson GB, Fudenberg HH, Jalin TL: Studies on cystic fibrosis using isoelectric focusing I. An assay for detection of cystic fibrosis homozygotes and heterozygote carriers from serum. *Pediatr Res* 1975;9: 635–640.
38. Wilson GB: Cystic fibrosis protein, a confirmed diagnostic marker for detecting heterozygote carriers: Significance in relation to future screening and to a proposed primary defect in alpha-2-macroglobulin. *Pediatr Res* 1979;13:1079–1081.
39. Thomas JM, Merritt AD, Hodes ME: Electrophoretic analysis of serum proteins in cystic fibrosis. *Pediatr Res* 1977;11:1148–1154.
40. Smith QT, Hamilton MJ, Shapiro BL: Letter to the editor. *Pediatr Res* 1976;10:999.
41. Tully GW, Nevin, GB, Young IR, et al:

Detection of cystic fibrosis protein by isoelectric focusing of serum. *Pediatr Res* 1979;13:1078.

42. Scholey J, Applegarth DA, Davidson AGF, et al: Detection of cystic fibrosis protein by electrofocusing. *Pediatr Res* 1978;12:800.
43. Altland K, Schmidt SR, Kaiser, G, et al: Demonstration of a factor in the serum of homozygotes and heterozygotes for cystic fibrosis by a nonbiological technique. *Humangenetik* 1975;28:209.
44. Forstner G, Koheil, A, Forstner J: Isoelectric focusing of serum in cystic fibrosis: Failure to distinguish between homozygote and heterozygote sera. *Clin Chim Acta* 1976;70:459–462.
45. Manson JC, Brock DJH: Development of a quantitative immunoassay for the cystic fibrosis gene. *Lancet* 1980;1:330–331.
46. Wilson GB, Middleton S: Development of monospecific antisera, hybridoma antibodies, and immunoassays for cystic fibrosis protein, a specific marker for the gene defect. *Clin Res* 1980;28:632A.
47. Mangos JA: Microperfusion study of the sweat gland abnormality in cystic fibrosis. *Tex Rep Biol Med* 1973;31:651–663.
48. Kaiser D, Drack E, Rossi E: Inhibition of net sodium transport in single sweat glands by sweat of patients with cystic fibrosis of the pancreas. *Pediatr Res* 1971;5:167–172.
49. Will PC, Taylor A, Lebowitz JL, et al: Saliva from patients with cystic fibrosis inhibits amiloride-sensitive sodium transport. *Pediatr Res* 1980;14:1245–1249.
50. Taylor A, Mayo J, Boat T, et al: Standardized assay for the sodium reabsorption inhibitory effect and studies of its salivary gland distribution in patients with cystic fibrosis. *Pediatr Res* 1974;8:861–865.
51. Dearborn DG, Will PC, Gerken TA, et al: Partial purification of an inhibitor of sodium transport from cystic fibrosis saliva. in Sturgess JM (ed): *Perspectives in Cystic Fibrosis: Proceedings of the Eighth International Congress on Cystic Fibrosis.* Mississauga, Ontario, Imperial Press Ltd, 1980, p 11a.
52. Brown GA, Oshin A, Goodchild MC, et al: Inhibition of sugar transport by plasma from cystic fibrosis patients. *Lancet* 1971;2:639–640.
53. Araki H, Field M, Shwachman H: A new assay for cystic fibrosis factor: Effects of serum from patients with cystic fibrosis on the in vitro electrical properties of rat jejunum. *Pediatr Res* 1975;9:932–934.
54. Gilmore JP, Davis M, Gibbs GE: Influence of cystic fibrotic and heterozygous serum on rat jejunum. *Proc Soc Exp Biol Med* 1978;157:70–74.
55. Morin CL, Desjeux JF, Authier L: Effect of saliva and serum from patients with cystic fibrosis on intestinal uptake of amino acids in rat. *Biomedicine* 1973;19:133–137.
56. Tucker RD, Gibbs GE, Christensen MB: Cystic fibrosis serum effect on the short circuit current of rat jejunum. *Pediatr Res* 1979;13:1371–1374.
57. Will PC, Boat TF, Hopfer U: Evidence against a specific effect of serum from patients with cystic fibrosis on a sodium-dependent glucose transport in the rat jejunum. *Pediatr Res* 1979;13:1129–1133.
58. Taussig LM, Gardner JD: Effects of saliva and plasma from cystic fibrosis patients on membrane transport. *Lancet* 1972;1:1367–1369.
59. Arvanitakis SN, Mangos JA, McSherry NR, et al: Role of polyamines in cystic fibrosis. *Pediatr Res* 1975;9:336.
60. Araki H, Nakamura K: Effect of sera from cystic fibrosis homozygotes and heterozygotes on glucose metabolism in Vero cells. *Lancet* 1978;1:793–795.
61. Grinwald PM, Segal MB: Effect of saliva from cystic fibrosis patients and from normal subjects on red blood cell sodium transport. *Pediatr Res* 1978;12:1–3.
62. Khan MA, Litt M, Kwart H, et al: Measurement of colloid zeta potential as a test for cystic fibrosis secretion factor. *Tex Rep Biol Med* 1973;31:665–683.
63. Lieberman J, Kaneshiro W, Costea NV: Presence of a serum hemagglutinin (lectinlike factor) in cystic fibrosis homozygotes and heterozygotes. *J Lab Clin Med* 1981;97:646–656.
64. Lundgren DW, Farrell PM, di Sant'Agnese PA: Polyamine alterations in blood of male homozygotes and heterozygotes for cystic fibrosis. *Clin Chim Acta* 1975;62:357–362.
65. Baylin SB, Rosenstein BJ, Marton LJ, et al: Age-related abnormalities of circulating polyamines and diamine oxidase activity in cystic fibrosis heterozygotes and homozygotes. *Pediatr Res* 1980;14:921–925.
66. Mayo BJ, Klebe RJ, Lankford BJ, et al: Somatic cell genetic studies of cystic fibrosis. *Tex Rep Biol Med* 1976;34:107–111.
67. Wilson GB, Fudenberg HH: Studies on cystic fibrosis using isoelectric focusing II. Demonstration of deficient proteolytic cleavage of alpha 2-macroglobulin in cystic fibrosis plasma. *Pediatr Res* 1976;10:87–96.
68. Shapira E, Martin CL, Nadler HL: Comparison between purified alpha 2-macroglobulin preparations from normal controls and patients with cystic fibrosis. *J Biol Chem* 1977;252:7923–7929.
69. Bowman B, Barnett D, Matalon R, et al:

Cystic fibrosis: Fractionation of fibroblast media demonstrating ciliary inhibition. *Proc Natl Acad Sci USA* 1973;70:548–551.

70. Beratis NG, Conover JH, Conod EJ: Studies on ciliary dyskinesia factor in cystic fibrosis: III. Skin fibroblasts and cultured amniotic fluid cells. *Pediatr Res* 1973;7:958–964.

71. Wilson GB, Bahm VJ: Synthesis and secretion of cystic fibrosis ciliary dyskinesia substances by purified subpopulations of leukocytes. *J Clin Invest* 1980;66:1010–1019.

72. Roberts RC, Nelles LP, Hall P, et al: Comparison of cystic fibrosis and normal alpha-2-macroglobulin physicochemical and primary structure studies. *Cystic Fibrosis Club Abstr* 1979;20:8.

73. Choy H, Applegarth DA, Davidson AGF, et al: Antiplasmin (alpha-2-macroglobulin) activity of plasma of cystic fibrosis patients. *Biochem Biophys Res Commun* 1978;82: 1325–1332.

74. Romeo G, Parsons M, Bossen A, et al: Trypsin-binding IgG in cystic fibrosis. *Nature* 1978;274:909–910.

75. Breslow JL, Epstein J, Fontaine JH, et al: Enhanced dexamethasone resistance in cystic fibrosis cells: Potential use for heterozygote detection and prenatal diagnosis. *Science* 1978;201:180–182.

76. Nadler HL, Walsh MMJ: Intrauterine detection of cystic fibrosis. *Pediatrics* 1980;66: 690–692.

8

Calcium and Mucus in Cystic Fibrosis

Lewis E. Gibson

MUCOVISCIDOSIS

Farber's old idea of mucoviscidosis has stood the test of time.[1] It is the only theory which explains the ubiquitous dilation of mucous glands, the transformation of pancreatic acini into cysts, and the failure of the mucociliary ladder to effectively remove bacteria. This concept of recurrent pulmonary infections having a purely mechanical cause has been given negative support by the repeated failures of attempts to find abnormalities in the CF patient's immune system. (See Chapter 10 for another point of view.)

There are, however, two difficulties with the concept of mucoviscidosis. First, it does not explain the sweat abnormality. Like all exocrine glands, sweat glands produce mucus and their ducts are mucus-lined. There is, however, no plugging. CF sweat glands appear normal both by light and by electron microscopy.[2] Secondly, no chemical abnormality has been found to explain the viscidity of exocrine secretions. At one time it was thought that the fucose-to-sialic acid ratio was abnormally high in CF mucus.[3] The evidence is contradictory.[4] If the ratio is actually increased, it may well be secondary to an abnormality in autonomic stimulation.[5]

Since mucoproteins are highly antigenic, a number of investigators have attempted to find immunological differences between CF and normal mucus. Here the evidence is not contradictory. Many antibodies can be produced to human mucoproteins, but no difference between CF and normal antigens could be found.[6–8]

Although no chemical difference between normal and CF mucus has been found, there is one important difference in the composition of CF exocrine secretions. The CF secretions contain higher concentrations of total proteins and specific enzymes (Table 8-1).[4,9–11] Even pancreatic juice, taken from CF patients without malabsorption, has a higher than normal trypsin concentration.

This is an important observation. Even though viscosity is a complex property depending upon many molecular interactions, one can still observe that, generally, when water is added to a protein-containing solution, the solution becomes less viscid. It seems probable that the cause of the viscidity of CF secretions is simply that they contain an abnormally low concentration of water.

So far, one enigma has been explained only to be replaced with another. The mucoproteins in CF may be entirely normal and the viscidity of the exocrine secretions explained by a lack of water. The new puzzle is, of course, the cause of the low concentration of water. To approach this, we must first examine the physiological functions of mucus. It will help us with the water problem.

FUNCTIONS OF MUCUS

Considering the wide distribution of mucus which is produced by all exocrine glands, those of its biological functions which we understand seem few. Mucus does give mechanical defense against bacterial infections. Mucus acts as a lubricant. This is important in the vagina and probably in the intestine.

Mucus is frequently described as having a protective function. Descriptions of this function are generally vague. Victor Negus, however, performed experiments which clarified the protective effect.[12] He used eels, which can generally live in either salt or fresh water, and wiped off their mucus coating with a bicarbonate solution. After this pro-

Table 8-1
Summary of Protein and Enzyme Abnormalities Found in CF Exocrine Secretions by Various Authors*

Data	Parotid Saliva (%)	Submaxillary Saliva (%)	Pancreatic Juice (%)	Bronchial Secretions (%)
Protein		+ 36[†]		+457[¶]A +173[¶]B
Amylase	+51[†]	+484[‡] +129[†]	+140[§]	
Lysozyme	−22[†]	+ 84[†]		
Acid ribonuclease		+192[‡]		
Alkaline ribonuclease		+110[‡]		
Trypsin			+134[§]	
Carboxypeptidase			+210[§]	
Lipase			+100[§]	
Chymotrypsin			+366[§]	

*CF protein concentration and CF enzyme activities per unit volume are given as percents of normal. The high enzyme concentrations listed for CF pancreatic juice were found in patients without symptoms of malabsorption. Generally CF patients have widespread destruction of pancreatic acini and low or absent pancreatic enzymes. Proteins are obviously highly concentrated in CF exocrine secretions.
[†]Mandel et al (1967).[29]
[‡]Chernick et al (1964).[9]
[§]Hadorn et al (1968).[10]
[¶]A = Sputum from CF patients compared to bronchial secretions of laryngectomized patients without lung disease. B = The same CF patients as A compared to patients with bronchiectasis. Matthews et al (1963).[11]

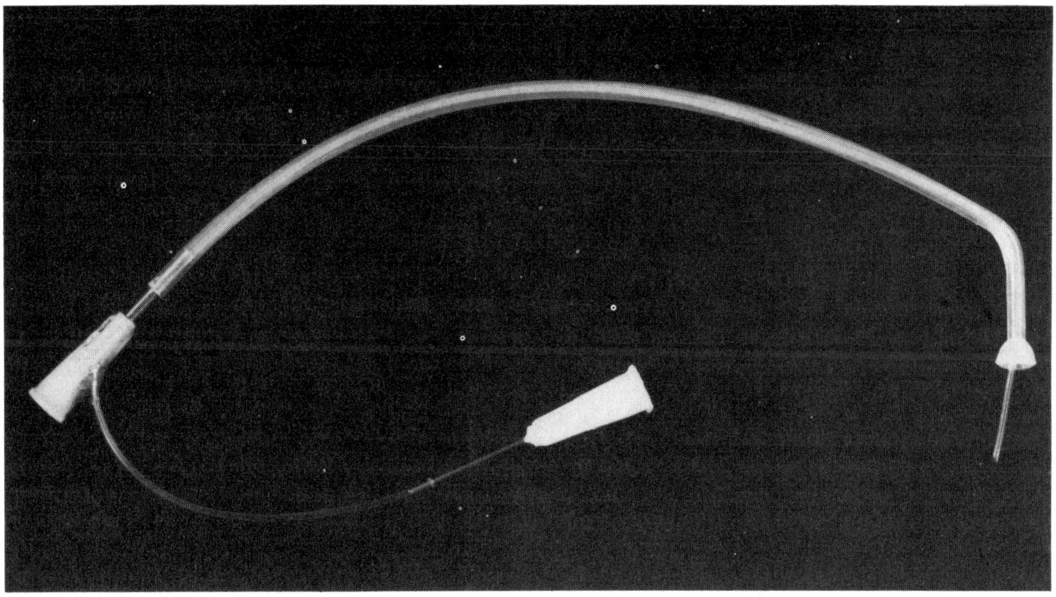

Figure 8-1 The cannulation device used to infuse isotonic saline into the human parotid gland. The small tube shown on the right is inserted into the parotid duct until the flared portion of the outer tube rests on the papilla. Suction is then applied through the outer tube so that the papilla forms a seal.

cedure, the eels were found to lose weight in sea water and gain weight in fresh water. Negus stated simply that "They seemed to have lost their raincoats." Negus also removed mucus from sections of rat intestine and placed hypertonic saline in these sections, as well as in others with a normal mucus coating. He then measured an increased osmotic flow of fluid into the segment lacking mucus. This experiment was repeated and confirmed in our laboratory.[13]

Negus demonstrated that a function of mucus is to inhibit the passive flow of water across biological membranes. This is interesting since all exocrine gland ducts are lined with mucus. Hydrostatic and, in some cases such as the sweat gland, osmotic pressures tend to push water out of the ducts. If exocrine gland ducts leak, more water than protein would be lost, and the viscid secretions characteristic of CF would be formed.

HYPERPERMEABILITY

In Chapter 4 it was shown that leakage of water from sweat gland ducts would result in an overproduction of isotonic precursor solution in the coil of the gland, saturation of the sodium reabsorption system in the duct, and the high sweat salt concentrations characteristic of the disease. Hyperpermeable mucus could then explain both the viscid secretions and the salty sweat of CF patients. The next problem was to measure the permeability of mucus.

This was done in our laboratory by forming films of the nondialyzable material in submaxillary saliva and measuring the rate at which isotonic saliva passed through the mucous film when pulled by an osmotic gradient.[13] It was found that the material from the CF patients was considerably more permeable than that from control subjects. In a more direct experiment,[14] isotonic saline was pushed at a constant rate into the parotid glands of CF patients and control subjects using an apparatus designed for this purpose (Figure 8-1). The ducts of both groups were permeable since, at the low flow rates, no swelling or discomfort occurred. Pressures were recorded during this procedure, and it was found that the pressure per unit area of parotid lumen was lower in the CF patients. The ductal luminal area was estimated by taking it as being proportional to the patient's surface area or to his height squared, or to his weight to the two-thirds power. In each case, the pressures recorded in the CF patients were significantly lower.

It seems that CF exocrine secretions are viscid because they lack water and that they lack water because the gland ducts are coated with abnormally permeable mucus. The next question is why the mucus is abnormally permeable.

CALCIUM IN CF EXOCRINE SECRETIONS

Although CF mucus is probably normal chemically and certainly normal immunologically, there is one definite abnormality in CF mucus. This is motility of the mucoproteins in submaxillary saliva in an electric field.[15] Here there is a definite quantitative, although not qualitative, difference. The difference in motility, however, is entirely due to the increased calcium content of CF submaxillary saliva. Table 8-2 shows this averages 6.1 mEq/liter in CF patients while in normal children the value is 3.7 mEq/liter.[4,16] When calcium is added to normal submaxillary saliva, its motility is like that of CF saliva. When calcium is removed from CF saliva with EDTA, its motility is normal.

In 1971, we stated that the calcium concentration was elevated in all CF exocrine secretions.[13] At that time the evidence for this statement was slightly weak, since the calcium content of the most abnormal CF secretion, sweat, was incompletely studied. Since then, one group of investigators found that the calcium concentration in the sweat of a group of CF patients averaged greater than in a group of control children.[17] The difference, however, was not statistically significant. The authors did not control for rate of sweating, and the calcium concentration in sweat varies markedly with rate. Later another group carefully controlled for rate of sweating and found a highly significant increase in the calcium content of CF sweat.[18] Since our initial statement, a definite

Table 8-2
Calcium in CF Exocrine Secretions

Secretion	Calcium (mEq/liter)		Reference
	Normals	*CF (%)*	
Sweat	0.88	+7	Paunier et al[17] A*
	0.84	+29	Hanggeli[18] B
Tears	1.40	+93	Botelho et al[19]
Parotid saliva	2.39	+16	Marmar et al[28]
	2.50	+4	Mandel et al[29]
	1.70	+53	Chauncy et al[30]
Submaxillary saliva	3.60	+69	Mandel et al[4]
	3.74	+66	Chernick et al[16]
Pancreatic juice		↑↑↑	Kopito et al[31] C
Bronchial secretions	5.9	+100	Chernick et al[32] D
	6.2	+18	Matthews et al[11] E
	9.3	−22	Matthews et al[11] F
Meconium		+53	Kopito et al[33] G
		−23	Kopito et al[33] H

* A = Not controlled for rate. Not significant.
B = Controlled for rate. Significant.
C = CF patients with malabsorption, Ca "many times higher."
D = Patients with bronchiectasis provide control sputum. Specimens obtained by bronchoscopy.
E = CF patients compared to laryngectomized controls without lung disease.
F = Same CF patients as E compared to controls with bronchiectasis. All sputum simply expectorated and pressed between gauze squares to remove saliva.
G & H = Measured as a fraction of dry weight. G patients had meconium ileus while H patients did not.

elevation in the calcium concentration of CF tears has also been demonstrated.[19] Calcium concentrations in various exocrine secretions are listed in Table 8-2.

Since the only known abnormality in CF mucus, its motility in an electric field, was secondary to an increased calcium concentration present in all CF exocrine secretions, we wondered if the hyperpermeability of CF mucus, which we had demonstrated, could be due to an increased calcium concentration.

First, calcium was added to normal submaxillary saliva so that the concentration was at the CF level. Mucous films formed with this material were more permeable than films made with unaltered saliva.[13] Calcium was then iontophoresed into normal skin prior to pilocarpine iontophoresis. This was found to decrease the rate of sweating and increase the salt concentration in the sweat.[13] This is, of course, the expected result of a permeable sweat duct. Finally, segments of rat intestine were exposed to calcium prior to instilling hypertonic saline. We recorded an increased osmotic flow into the segments which had been exposed to calcium.[13] It was noted in Chapter 4 that the effect of iontophoresed calcium into normal skin might explain the sodium reabsorption inhibitory factor described by Mangos.[20] Mixed saliva from CF patients would obviously contain more calcium than that from controls.

Calcium, then, seems to cause hyperpermeability, and hyperpermeability will explain both the viscidity of CF exocrine secretions and the high salt concentration in CF sweat. The next question is obviously why the calcium is elevated. Evidence for two possible causes for this elevation has recently been found.

INTRACELLULAR CALCIUM IN CF

The first cause could be the CF serum factor. Although the serum factor has never been isolated, and its existence may even be doubted, it has been postulated to have a number of actions. The action of importance here is that of increasing cellular uptake of calcium. Bogart et al[21] showed that serum from CF patients and, to a lesser extent, serum from heterozygotes increased the uptake of $^{45}Ca^{2+}$ in rabbit tracheal explants. This effect was inhibited by the calcium channel blocker methoxyverapamil. Bogart et al[22] also showed that K^+ efflux from rat submandibular gland slices was calcium-dependent and could be induced by CF and heterozygote serum and blocked by methoxyverapamil. Banschback et al[23] noted increased uptake of $^{45}Ca^{2+}$ in leukocytes from normal individuals when exposed to CF serum. CF leukocytes exposed to normal serum also had an increased uptake of $^{45}Ca^{2+}$.

The second cause may be an innate property of CF cells to have increased intracellular calcium. This may not be secondary to any serum factor, since it has been observed by Shapiro et al[24] in fibroblasts grown in tissue culture as well as in circulating lymphocytes. Shapiro et al[24] considered that this increased calcium was caused by an abnormally large mitochrondrial uptake secondary to altered kinetics of mitochrondrial NADH dehydrogenase. Another cause of increased intracellular calcium might be the decreased activity of Mg^{2+}-dependent Ca^{2+}-ATPase activity observed by Katz in CF erythrocyte membranes[25] and in tissue fibroblasts.[26] The increased resistance of CF fibroblasts to ouabain toxicity observed by Epstein and Breslow[27] might well be secondary to increased intracellular calcium.

CF exocrine secretions contain an abnormally high concentration of calcium. This may be caused by a serum factor which increases cellular uptake and, later, release of calcium or by an innate property of CF cells. If our ideas on mucus hyperpermeability are correct, the great problem in treating CF is to learn how to lower the calcium in the patient's exocrine secretions.

REFERENCES

1. Farber S: Pancreatic function and disease in early life. V. Pathological changes associated with pancreatic insufficiency in early life. *Arch Pathol* 1944;37:238–250.
2. Munger BL, Brusilow SW, Cooke RE: An

electron microscopic study of exocrine sweat glands in patients with cystic fibrosis of the pancreas. *J Pediatr* 1961;59:497-511.

3. Dische Z, Pallavicini JC, Smirnow N, et al: Abnormalities in composition of urinary nondialyzable glycoproteins in cystic fibrosis of the pancreas (CFP). *Am J Dis Child* 1961; 102:733-734.
4. Mandel ED, Kutscher A, Denning CR, et al: Salivary studies in cystic fibrosis. *Am J Dis Child* 1967;113:431-438.
5. Dische Z, Pallavicini JC, Cizek LJ, et al: Changes in the control of the secretion of mucous glycoproteins as possible pathogenic factor in cystic fibrosis of the pancreas. *Ann NY Acad Sci* 1962;93:526-540.
6. Talamo RC, Raunio V, Gabriel O, et al: Immunological and biochemical comparison of urinary glycoproteins in patients with cystic fibrosis of the pancreas and normal controls. *J Pediatr* 1964;65:480-494.
7. Schwartz RH, Pallavicini JC: Immunological and chemical studies of cystic fibrosis and normal urinary glycoprotein of Tamm and Horsfall. *J Lab Clin Med* 1967;70:725-735.
8. Gugler E, Pallavicini JC, Swerdlow H, et al: Immunological studies of submaxillary saliva from patients with cystic fibrosis and from normal children. *J Pediatr* 1968;73:548-559.
9. Chernick WS, Eighel HJ, Barbero GJ: Submaxillary salivary enzymes as a measure of glandular activity in cystic fibrosis. *J Pediatr* 1964;65:694-700.
10. Hadorn B, Johansen PG, Anderson CM: Pancreozymin secretin test of exocrine pancreatic function in cystic fibrosis and the significance of the result for the pathogenesis of the disease. *Can Med Assoc J* 1968;98: 377-385.
11. Matthews LW, Spector S, Lemm J, et al: Studies on pulmonary secretions. I. The overall chemical composition of pulmonary secretions from patients with cystic fibrosis, bronchiectasis and laryngectomy. *Am Rev Respir Dis* 1963;88:(2):199-204.
12. Negus V: The function of mucus: A hypothesis. *Proc R Soc Med* 1967;60:75-77.
13. Gibson LE, Matthews WJ, Minihan PT, et al: Relating mucus, calcium, and sweat in a new concept of cystic fibrosis. *Pediatrics* 1971;48:695-710.
14. Gibson LE, Duda FJ: Exocrine gland duct hyperpermeability demonstrated in cystic fibrosis patients and induced in an animal model. *J Pediatr* 1975;86:979.
15. Gugler E, Pallavicini JC, Swerdlow H, et al: Role of calcium in submaxillary saliva of patients with cystic fibrosis. *J Pediatr* 1967;71: 585-588.
16. Chernick WS, Barbero GJ, Parkins FM: Studies on submaxillary saliva in cystic fibrosis. *J Pediatr* 1961;59:890-898.
17. Paunier L, Girardin E, Sizonenko PC, et al: Calcium and magnesium concentration in sweat of normal children and patients with cystic fibrosis. *Pediatrics* 1973;52:446-448.
18. Hanggeli CA: Die kalziumkonzentration im schweiss bei patienten mit zystischer pandreasfibrose und bei gesunden kindern. *Helv Paediatr Acta* 1973;28:611-615.
19. Botelho SY, Goldstein AM, Rosenlund ML: Tear sodium, potassium, chloride, and calcium at various flow rates. Children with cystic fibrosis and unaffected siblings with and without corneal staining. *J Pediatr* 1973;83:601-606.
20. Mangos JA, McSherry NR: Studies on the mechanism of inhibition of sodium transport in cystic fibrosis of the pancreas. *Pediatr Res* 1968;2:378-384.
21. Bogart BI, Conod EJ, Gaerlan PL, et al: Biological activities of cystic fibrosis serum. III. CF serum uptake of $^{45}Ca^{++}$ by rabbit tracheal explants. *Biochem Biophys Res Commun* 1979;88:1398-1404.
22. Bogart BI, Picarelli J, Gaerlan PF, et al: CF serum induced K^+ efflux from rats submandibular gland tissue slices a calcium dependent parameter. In *Proceedings of 8th International CF Congress,* Toronto, Canada, May 26-30, 1980, pp 29-34.
23. Banschback MW, Karam AG, Love PK, et al: Cystic fibrosis serum promotes ^{45}Ca uptake by normal human leucocytes. *Biochem Biophys Res Commun* 1978;84:922-927.
24. Shapiro BL, Fiegal RJ, Lam LFH: Intracellular calcium and cystic fibrosis. In *Proceedings of the 8th International CF Congress,* Toronto, Canada, May 26-30, 1980, pp 15-28.
25. Katz S: Calcium and sodium transport processes in patients with cystic fibrosis. I. A specific decrease in Mg^{2+}-dependent, Ca^{2+}-adenosine triphosphatase activity in erythrocyte membranes from cystic fibrosis patients. *Pediatr Res* 1978;12:1033-1038.
26. Katz S: Calcium and sodium transport processes in patients with cystic fibrosis. *Res Commun Chem Pathol Pharmacol* 1978;19: 491-503.
27. Epstein J, Breslow JL: Increased resistance of cystic fibrosis fibroblasts to ouabain toxicity. *Proc Natl Acad Sci USA* 1977;74:1676-1679.
28. Marmar J, Barbero GJ, Sibinga MS: The pattern of parotid gland secretion in cystic fibrosis of the pancreas. *Gastroenterology* 1966;50:551-556.
29. Mandel ID, Thompson RH, Wotman S, et al: Parotid saliva in cystic fibrosis. II. Elec-

trolytes and protein bound carbohydrates. *Am J Dis Child* 1965;110:646–651.

30. Chauncy HH, Levine DM, Kass G, et al: Composition of human saliva; parotid gland secretory rate and electrolyte concentration in children with cystic fibrosis. *Arch Oral Biol* 1962;7:707–713.
31. Kopito L, Shwachman H: Spectroscopic analysis of tissues from patients with cystic fibrosis and controls. *Nature (London)* 1964;202:501–502.
32. Chernick WS, Barbero GJ: Composition of tracheobronchial secretions in cystic fibrosis of the pancreas and bronchiectasis. *Pediatrics* 1959;24:739–745.
33. Kopito L, Shwachman H: Mineral composition of meconium. *J Pediatr* 1966;68: 313–314.

9

Lower Respiratory Infections in Patients with Cystic Fibrosis

Martin G. Myers

Franklin P. Koontz

Miles Weinberger

EVALUATION OF MICROBIOLOGY OF THE LOWER RESPIRATORY TRACT

Extraordinary progress has been made in increasing the longevity of patients with cystic fibrosis, primarily as a consequence of improved nutritional support and aggressive management of acute pulmonary infections. As a result, chronic bacterial lower respiratory infection, the major cause of the progressive lung disease, causes the ultimate demise of most patients with cystic fibrosis. The pulmonary pathophysiology consists of defective mucociliary transport which causes chronic bronchiolar obstruction with consequent infection and, ultimately, bronchiectasis. Indeed, outside the neonatal period, bronchiectasis is a nearly universal finding in patients with cystic fibrosis.[1]

Advances in understanding the complex ecology of the lower respiratory tract in patients with cystic fibrosis have been hampered by a lack of suitable culture methodology and the frequent, chronic, and often injudicious use of antimicrobial agents. The predominant organisms recovered from the sputum have changed over the past four decades, with a decrease in the prevalence of *Staphylococcus aureus,* and an increase in rates of colonization with *Pseudomonas aeruginosa.*[1,2] Thus, prior to the advent of antibiotics, *S. aureus* was the organism most frequently isolated from patients with cystic fibrosis, but since that time *Ps. aeruginosa,* which was rarely recovered from these patients in the preantibiotic era, has become the predominant infectious agent reported. In addition, almost all authors report multiple isolates of normal oropharyngeal commensal flora, and mixed flora are found when cultures are obtained both through the bronchoscope[3] and at postmortem examination.[4]

Characterizing the lower respiratory tract flora of any patient poses a logistic problem, especially in children. For example, potential pathogens recovered from sputum or bronchial secretions obtained at bronchoscopy may include organisms present in the oropharyngeal flora, which, therefore, cannot be distinguished as commensals of oral flora or as potential lower respiratory pathogens. Although bypassing the problem of orapharyngeal contamination, transtracheal aspiration and lung aspiration may not accurately sample bronchiolar secretions. For example, three patients demonstrated significant improvement in pulmonary function tests while undergoing antimicrobial therapy for acute lower respiratory exacerbation, although no organisms were recovered by transthoracic lung aspiration (unpublished observations).

The respiratory bacterial flora of patients with cystic fibrosis has often been evaluated by nasopharyngeal culture, oropharyngeal culture, or qualitative culture of sputum performed by streaking a portion of the sputum upon an agar plate. These culture techniques may give misleading information because of the contamination of sputum by oral secretions,[5,6] the irregular distribution of bacteria in sputum,[7] and the overgrowth of slow-growing, fastidious organisms by faster-growing organisms. On examination, the tenacious sputum consists of microfoci of polymorphonuclear cells and clumps of bacteria (Figure 9-1). Because of this uneven distribution of organisms, the identification of all aerobic bacteria qualitatively may require as many as five cultures of a single sample.[7] To minimize the sampling problems associated with multiple microfoci of organisms, quantitative culture of homogenized sputum samples may be adaptable to the study of the lower respiratory flora of patients with cystic fibrosis. For example, quantitative cultures of sputum, employing homogenization and dilution, are helpful in the diagnosis of acute pneumonia,[8] and serial sputum quantitation has been utilized as an in vivo correlate of the efficacy of antimicrobial therapy.[9,10] Because surface colony counts give results which are equivalent to the pour plate method,[11] quantitative culture by serial dilution of homogenized sputum also allows the use of a variety of selective or enriched media such as chocolate agar.

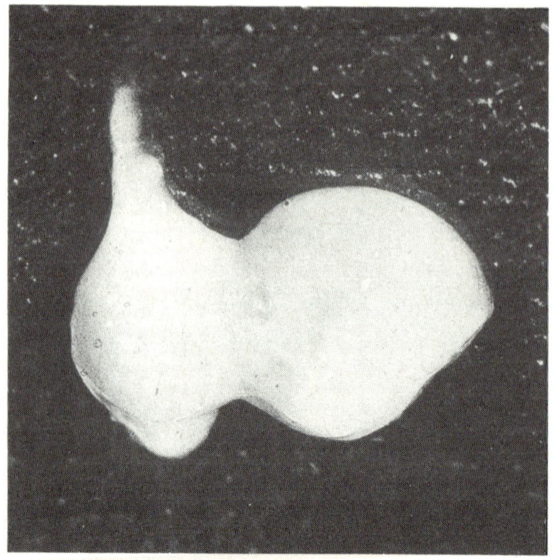

Figure 9-1 Cystic fibrosis sputum. **A** Gross examination of tenacious mucoid sputum from a child with cystic fibrosis.

The technology of quantitative cultures of homogenized sputum has been available for almost 30 years[7–10,12,13] and has been utilized as a diagnostic aid in the management of patients with pneumonia, including those with cystic fibrosis. A variety of mucolytic agents have been employed for homogenization of sputum, including *N*-acetylcysteine (NAC),

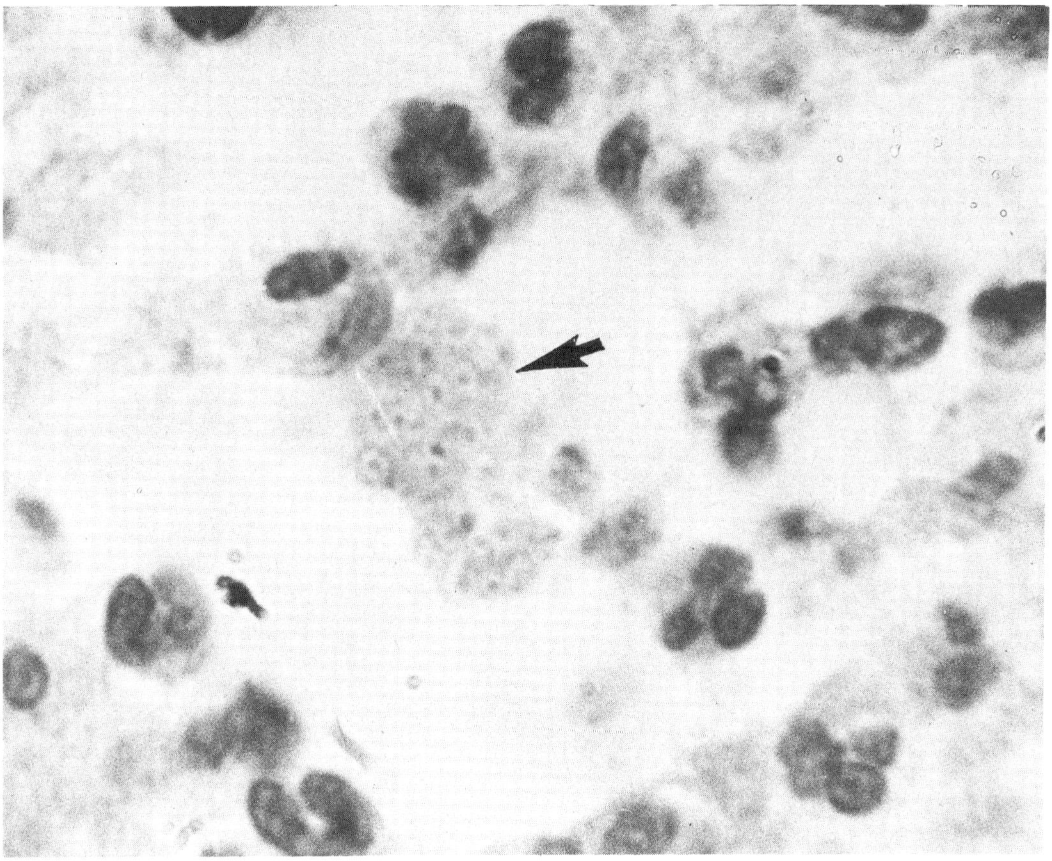

Figure 9-1B A tissue Gram stain of a section of the formalin-fixed sputum illustrating a microfocus (arrow) of organisms.

EDTA, sonication, and others. We have utilized 2% NAC because of its apparent lack of toxicity for the pathogens expected to be found in sputum from patients with cystic fibrosis. For example, to assess the possible toxicity of NAC upon sputum organisms, isolated colonies of *Hemophilus parainfluenza, H. influenzae, Ps. aeruginosa,* and *S. aureus* were selected from direct (nonhomogenized) sputum cultures from cystic fibrosis patients. Single colonies were diluted in 0.01 M, pH 7.2, phosphate-buffered saline (PBS) or PBS containing 2% NAC and were incubated for 30 min at 4°C. Little effect was seen on viability of these organisms (Table 9-1).

To limit oropharyngeal contamination of sputum specimens, we evaluated the effects of mouth-washing with water on the concentration of organisms in saliva and sputum. Before and immediately following rinsing the mouth with water, saliva was collected by syringe and then quantitatively cultured (Table 9-2). Saliva from patients with cystic fibrosis often contains organisms associated with lower respiratory illness and oropharyngeal commensals. However, these are present in saliva in concentrations $<10^4$ CFU/ml after rinsing the mouth with water. Directly washing sputum samples may be equally effective as a means to minimize oropharyngeal contamination.[14]

For quantitative culture, specimens are obtained by having patients expectorate into a sterile collection container after rinsing the mouth with water. Containers of sputum are transported on ice to the laboratory for culture within 10–20 min. If cultures are not refrigerated or rapidly transported, erroneous results may be obtained because of loss of fastidious organisms and rapid growth of faster-growing organisms. In the laboratory, equal volumes of sputum and 2% NAC in PBS are mixed in thick-walled sterile tubes containing sterile, acid-cleaned glass beads. The specimen is homogenized by vigorous mixing until liquefied. Serial 10-fold dilutions in PBS are prepared, and both selective and nonselective media may be plated with various sputum dilutions.[15] For adaptation to the clinical microbiology laboratory, a single dilution step may be utilized employing a 0.001-ml platinum loop. By employing a solid medium and a homogenized specimen, the problem of overgrowth by more rapidly growing organisms is obviated. Species present at $\geq 10^6$ CFU/ml are enumerated and speciated by usual microbiologic means[16] and then may be tested for antimicrobial susceptibility.[17]

Rinsing the mouth with water reduced the level of aerobic organisms in saliva to $< 10^4$ CFU/ml (Table 9-2). However, organisms initially present in saliva were often present at an equivalent or greater concentration in the sputum (Table 9-3). Using this methodology, the flora present in saliva are not attributed to sputum, and the sputum flora is highly stable and reproducible in the same patient over a 6-month period (Table 9-4).

In a comparison of qualitative (nonhomogenized) and quantitative sputum cultures (Table 9-5), we found that the qualitative culture may underestimate the importance of commensal oropharyngeal organisms, especially species of *Hemophilus.*[18] From one to eight (mean four) aerobic bacterial species at a concentration exceeding 10^6 CFU/ml were recovered from 97 sputum samples obtained from 45 patients. (Table 9-6). Because organisms present at a concentration exceeding 10^6 CFU/ml sputum appeared to be unaffected by previous mouth-washing with water, this concentration has been utilized in our laboratory as defining colonization. Species often considered normal oropharyngeal

Table 9-1
N-Acetyl-L-Cysteine Effect upon Viability of Organisms Recovered from Sputum of Patients with Cystic Fibrosis

	Colony-forming Units (per ml)	
	*PBS**	*PBS-NAC**
Ps. aeruginosa	5.0×10^5	4.5×10^5
	7.4×10^7	6.6×10^7
S. aureus	3.8×10^5	3.0×10^5
	4.2×10^6	3.2×10^6
H. influenzae	3.3×10^5	3.0×10^5
	3.6×10^5	2.8×10^5
	2.9×10^7	2.7×10^7
H. parainfluenza	4.7×10^7	3.7×10^7

*PBS: 0.01 M, pH 7.2, phosphate-buffered saline; PBS-NAC: 2% *N*-acetylcysteine in PBS.

Table 9-2
Effect of Mouth Rinsing with Water on Aerobic Saliva Flora of Patients with Cystic Fibrosis

	Concentration					
	Patient 1		*Patient 2*		*Patient 3*	
	Pre	Post	Pre	Post	Pre	Post
S. aureus	6.0*	-†	-	-	-	-
S. epidermidis	-	-	-	-	7.3	-
Ps. aeruginosa	-	-	4.3	-	-	-
H. influenzae	7.8	-	6.2	-	-	-
Streptococcus						
α-Hemolytic	6.7	-	6.9	-	7.0	-
Nonhemolytic	-	-	6.0	-	5.5	-
Neisseria sp.	-	-	7.3	-	-	-

*Log_{10} CFU/ml.
†$< 10^4$ CFU/ml.

Table 9-3
Effect of Mouth Rinsing with Water on Homogenized Sputum Flora of Patients with Cystic Fibrosis

	Concentration					
	Patient 1		*Patient 2*		*Patient 3*	
	Pre	Post	Pre	Post	Pre	Post
S. aureus	7.3*	†	-	-	7.5	8.0
S. epidermidis	-	-	-	-	7.5	-
Ps. aeruginosa	-	-	5.2	5.0	-	-
H. influenzae	7.8	7.8	7.5	8.0	-	-
Streptococcus						
α-Hemolytic	6.7	-	7.0	7.0	7.5	6.0
Nonhemolytic	-	-	7.5	7.3	6.0	-
Neisseria sp.	-	-	7.3	7.3	-	-

*Log_{10} CFU/ml.
†$< 10^4$ CFU/ml.

Table 9-4
Persistence of Bacterial Flora in Homogenized Sputum

	Frequency of Recovery		
	*Patient 1**	*Patient 2*	*Patient 3*
S. aureus	6/6†	0/6	6/6
S. epidermidis	0/6	1/6	1/6
Ps. aeruginosa	0/6	6/6	0/6
H. influenzae	6/6	6/6	2/6
Streptococcus			
α-Hemolytic	2/6	6/6	4/6
Nonhemolytic	0/6	2/6	1/6
Neisseria sp.	0/6	5/6	0/6

*Patients correspond to those listed in Tables 9-2 and 9-3.
†Number of sputa with $\geq 10^6$ CFU/ml/number tested at monthly intervals.

Table 9-5
Comparison of Culture of 97 Sputa from Patients with Cystic Fibrosis by Streaking Sputum on Agar (Qualitative Culture)* or Dilution of Homogenized Specimen (Quantitative Culture)†

	Recovered from		
	Both	*Qualitative only*	*Quantitative only*
S. aureus	37	2	3
H. influenzae	11	2	29
Ps. aeruginosa	65	3	4
Oral commensal flora	68	24	1

*Present or absent.
†Present: $\geq 10^6$ CFU/ml, absent $< 10^6$ CFU/ml.

Table 9-6
Aerobic Bacterial Flora Recovered from 97 Homogenized Sputa from Patients with Cystic Fibrosis

	No. Present		Mean
	$\geq 10^4$	$\geq 10^6$	Concentration
S. aureus	40	18	7.1*
S. epidermidis	20	11	6.4
Ps. aeruginosa	69	30	7.4
H. influenzae	40	26	8.3
H. parainfluenza	6	4	6.8
Streptococcus			
α-Hemolytic	61	31	6.6
Nonhemolytic	17	9	6.6
Neisseria sp.	27	15	6.5
Other	20	13	6.4

*Log_{10} CFU/ml.

flora by qualitative culture, such as α- and nonhemolytic streptococci, *S. epidermidis, Neisseria* species, and diphtheroids, were present in 69 cultures from 35 patients. These usual inhabitants of the upper respiratory tract were often present at concentrations exceeding 10^6 CFU/ml. Histologically, microfoci of organisms have also been observed in sputum from which only these organisms have been cultured. *Pseudomonas aeruginosa* was recovered from 69 sputa, while *S. aureus* and *H. influenzae* were each isolated from 40. *Pseudomonas aeruginosa* was present at a geometric mean concentration of 3×10^7 CFU/ml, and *S. aureus* was present at a mean concentration of 1×10^7 CFU/ml. When present, *H. influenzae* was recovered at a geometric mean concentration of 2×10^8 CFU/ml, and ranged in concentration up to 7×10^{10} CFU/ml. Of 25 isolates of *H. influenzae* recovered by the quantitative method at concentrations of $> 10^6$ CFU/ml, only one isolate was typable (type b). *Hemophilus parainfluenza* was recovered six times.

The repetitive and frequent recovery of high concentrations of species of *Hemophilus, S. epidermidis,* α-hemolytic streptococci, nonhemolytic streptococci, *Neisseria* species, and diphtheroids by us (Tables 9-3 to 9-6) and others[6,12,13] suggests that the ecology of the lower respiratory flora of patients with cystic fibrosis is complex. It seems unlikely that these organisms always represent contamination with oropharyngeal secretions as the concentrations of these organisms in saliva, after rinsing the mouth with water, is usually substantially less than that which is found in sputum (Table 9-2),[6] and these organisms may repetitively be recovered from some patients (Table 9-4).

Patients with cystic fibrosis who were treated with long-term antibiotics have been observed to improve clinically without corresponding alterations of the qualitative sputum bacterial flora.[19-23] This apparent lack of correlation between the observed clinical results and sputum bacteriology may reflect culture methodology and failure to recognize some organisms, which may be present in high concentration, as potential lower respiratory pathogens. Thus, qualitative culture of expectorated sputum may underestimate the frequency with which *H. influenzae* is present in the sputum of patients with cystic fibrosis (Table 9-5),[6,18] and may not distinguish variations in the frequency and concentration of other organisms, including those usually considered to be normal inhabitants of the mouth flora. Employing quantitative culture of sputum, we have reported alterations in the concentrations and frequency of *S. aureus, S. epidermidis,* and *Hemophilus* species during periods of treatment with cephalexin as compared to placebo.[15] In addition, we have observed the emergence of resistant organisms in sputum during oral antimicrobial therapy[15] and also observed the emergence of β-lactamase-producing (ampicillin-resistant) strains of *Hemophilus* during treatment periods with intravenous carbenicillin in almost 10% of patients (unpublished observation).

SPECIFIC MICROORGANISMS ASSOCIATED WITH LOWER RESPIRATORY ILLNESS

Staphylococcus aureus

The decreasing prevalence of *S. aureus* in cultures of sputum from patients with cystic fibrosis over the past four decades has been assumed to be a consequence of frequent use of antimicrobials. However, this may also reflect the changing pattern of infection with *S. aureus* which has occurred simultaneously.[24] Patients harboring *S. aureus* in their lower respiratory tracts have an excess number of illnesses and require hospitalization more frequently than patients who are not colonized with *S. aureus.*[15] di Sant'Agnese and Talamo[25] have suggested that *S. aureus* is the agent primarily responsible for the widespread pulmonary changes in cystic fibrosis. Indeed, it has been proposed[26] that prevention of pulmonary colonization with *S. aureus* might minimize the progressive lung damage and subsequent colonization with *Ps. aeruginosa.*[26] Whether *S. aureus* is the specific pathogen inducing bronchopulmonary damage or whether any one of a number of potential respiratory pathogens may be responsible,[27] it is clear that the improved prognosis in cystic fibrosis occurred coincidentally with the introduction of antimicrobial agents effective against this organism.[28] In general, phage typing has shown that strains of *S. aureus* associated with patients with cystic fibrosis are similar to those strains encountered in the community,[29] but colonization with the same phage types may persist for many years.[30]

Pseudomonas aeruginosa

Prior to the introduction of effective antimicrobial therapy, *Ps. aeruginosa* was not associated with cystic fibrosis.[1] The increasing prevalence of this organism in sputum from patients with cystic fibrosis is thus probably a consequence of antimicrobial ecologic pressures.[31] Thus, antimicrobial therapy appears to select for both mucoid and nonmucoid strains.[15] Alternatively, acquisition of this organism may reflect the natural history of pulmonary infection in patients who are now surviving longer.[32] The role of this organism in the pathogenesis of lung disease is not clear.[25]

The majority of patients in most cystic fibrosis clinics now harbor *Ps. aeruginosa* (Table 9-6). More than half the patients colonized with *Ps. aeruginosa* are colonized with a peculiar mucoid strain, rarely seen in other patients. It is interesting that the mucoid and nonmucoid strains of *Ps. aeruginosa* recovered from the same patient appear to be of the same O antigen type,[33] and production of the mucoid substance is related to the presence of a bacteriophage.[34] The mucoid exopolysaccharide, characterized as resembling alginic acid,[35] is immunogenic[36] and may be a virulence factor.[27,33,36-39] However, production of the mucoid material does not appear to affect the intrapulmonary survival of *Ps. aeruginosa* or the mortality rate in guinea pigs.[40] However, it is possible that a specific impairment of lymphocyte responsiveness to *Ps. aeruginosa* occurs in patients with cystic fibrosis,[41] and depression of serum complement may occur in patients with cystic fibrosis during acute viral respiratory infection.[42] Immune complexes to *Ps. aeruginosa* have been demonstrated in 29 of 32 patients colonized with mucoid strains, whereas no precipitins were found in patients not colonized with mucoid strains.[43] More than half the patients had circulating immune complexes, leading to the inference that tissue damage in patients colonized with *Ps. aeruginosa* may occur as a result of the inflammatory response initiated by activation of complement by immune complex formation. In another study, 10 of 20 clinically stable patients with cystic fibrosis had circulating immune complexes, while circulating immune complexes were found in 16 of 18 patients during an acute exacerbation of pulmonary infection.[44] (See Chapter 10 for further discussion of this topic.)

Once established, colonization with *Ps. aeruginosa* is rarely, if ever, eradicated from the lower respiratory tract of the patient with cystic fibrosis.[36,45,46] It appears that antimicrobial therapy is the selection factor responsible for colonization, especially with the mucoid strains. Since these strains persist and apparently adversely modify the clinical course, the selection and use of antibiotics in these patients should be judicious.

Hemophilus Species

Species of *Hemophilus* frequently colonize the lower respiratory tract of patients with cystic fibrosis (Table 9-4 to 9-6).[2,12,13,15,27,47] In addition, a high proportion of patients with cystic fibrosis have precipitins to *H. influenzae*[48] and this proportion increases with age[32] (see Chapter 12). Although *H. influenzae* recovered from patients with cystic fibrosis is usually not typable serologically, most strains belong to the more virulent biotype I.[47] Although the pathogenicity of *Hemophilus* species in patients with cystic fibrosis has not been established, we observed a beneficial clinical response to cephalexin treatment of patients colonized with this organism.[15] In addition, we have observed patients who had deteriorating pulmonary functions, fever, leukocytosis, and new pulmonary infiltrates coincident with the appearance of *H. parainfluenza* in the quantitative sputum culture.

Oropharyngeal Commensals

We infer that the lower respiratory flora of patients with cystic fibrosis is complex and includes organisms considered part of the normal oropharyngeal flora (Tables 9-3 to 9-6). Indeed, we observed decreased sputum colonization with nontypable *H. influenzae* and *S. epidermidis* during drug treatment periods in a placebo-controlled trial.[15] The contribution of these species, as well as other commensal oropharyngeal organisms, to the production of purulent sputum and exacerbation of chronic bronchitis and pulmonary disease due to cystic fibrosis is not clear. In the adult with chronic bronchitis, however, these organisms would appear to have a major role in the pathogenesis of lower respiratory exacerbation,[49] and thus, by implication, may also in the patient with cystic fibrosis.

Other Microorganisms

Although some studies of children with cystic fibrosis report frequent colonization by *Enterobacteriaceae,*[50] including mucoid strains of *E. coli,*[51] in most series they are infrequently observed. Although sought from sequential sputum cultures over a 6-year period, *Streptococcus pneumoniae* ($\geq 10^6$ CFU/ml) has not been recovered in our laboratory with the exception of a single patient with bacteremic pneumococcal empyema complicating cystic fibrosis. Species of *Candida* have been recovered ($\geq 10^6$ CFU/ml) from less than 1% of sputum cultures and never repetitively from any of our patients. Although in some geographic regions as many as one third of patients with cystic fibrosis may have *Aspergillus fumigatus* precipitins[52–55] and signs and symptoms of allergic bronchopulmonary aspergillosis have been reported in 5 of 46 patients at one center,[56] we have never found this organism or observed allergic bronchopulmonary aspergillosis in this group of patients. (See Chapters 10 and 12 for differing points of view.) Neither colonization nor infection with anaerobic organisms in patients with cystic fibrosis has been systematically studied.

The roles of the most frequently recognized lower respiratory pathogens of childhood (viruses, *Chlamydiae,* and *Mycoplasma*) have not been systematically evaluated in patients with cystic fibrosis. During one respiratory season,[57] serologic evidence of associated nonbacterial infection was observed in 19% of acute exacerbations. Interestingly, respiratory syncytial virus (RSV) accounted for almost half of these, and illness due to this agent had an increased association with chronic colonization with *Ps. aeruginosa*. Similarly, Wright et al[58] found that 39% of severe exacerbations were serologically associated with viral infection, almost all of which were RSV or influenza A.

Nosocomial Infection

The hospitalized patient with cystic fibrosis, harboring an antibiotic-resistant organism, represents a management dilemma. On the one hand, these patients with chronic illness need to be encouraged in social interactions and vigorous physical therapy during hospitalizations that are often two to three weeks in duration. On the other hand, the nosocomial exchange of multiply antibiotic-resistant organisms within the hospital setting has been well established for patients with diverse diseases. Fortunately, with the possible exception of *S. aureus*, the expectorated flora of the patient with cystic fibrosis is relatively avirulent for the majority of normal individuals and even most hospitalized patients. However, those patients colonized with multiply antibiotic-resistant organisms may represent a substantial nosocomial risk to other patients with cystic fibrosis and also to patients who are immunologically compromised and housed on the same ward.

There are no carefully collated epidemiologic studies allowing an assessment of the true risks of nosocomial spread of organisms either by or to the patient with cystic fibrosis. However, strains of *S. aureus* from patients with cystic fibrosis are indistinguishable from those in the community at large,[29] and at least some family members, both with and without cystic fibrosis, may be colonized with strains of *Ps. aeruginosa* of the same pyocine type as the patient.[59] Recovery of *Ps. aeruginosa* has been recorded up to 4 feet from the bedside and from about a quarter of samples obtained during community activities on the ward.[60] Although not confirmed by pyocine typing, transmission of a strain of *Pseudomonas* has been suggested between two patients occupying the same cabin at summer camp.[61] Thus, the patient with cystic fibrosis would appear to have the potential to both acquire and spread organisms, especially within the hospital setting. Prudence would seem to dictate, therefore, that the hospitalized patient with multiply antibiotic-resistant organisms be separated from those at greatest risk.

ANTIMICROBIAL THERAPY FOR LOWER RESPIRATORY INFECTION

With the advent of the "antibiotic era," it quickly became apparent that antimicrobial agents could alter the outcome of acute lower respiratory exacerbations in patients with cystic fibrosis.[62,63] The importance of antibiotic therapy in modifying the long-term prognosis of patients with cystic fibrosis would also seem to have been established.[23,28,64] Less well established are indications for antibiotic use, preferred antimicrobial agents for the patient with cystic fibrosis, pharmacodynamics of antibiotics in patients with cystic fibrosis, and criteria for antibiotic effectiveness.

Antibiotic treatment in cystic fibrosis differs little from the treatment of respiratory infections in other patients. In all patients, a stepwise approach to rational antibiotic selection (Table 9-7) begins with the diagnosis: acute or chronic lower respiratory infection. The symptoms associated with lower respiratory infection include increased cough, sputum production, malaise, easy fatigability, and poor weight gain (or weight loss), especially when not associated with the voracious appetite characteristic of pancreatic insufficiency. Low-grade fever and changes in the white blood cell count and roentgenogram are late signs which may be absent in many. Sequential measurements of pulmonary function provide a sensitive and objective means of identifying increasing airway obstruction, a concomitant of both acute and chronic infection. This is manifested as a decrease in the forced vital capacity, the one-second forced expiratory volume, and the various flow-rate measurements. The easily measured peak expiratory flow rate is a relatively insensitive indicator of small airway disease where much of the obstruction initially occurs. Optimal use of pulmonary functions includes the longitudinal assessment of the spirometric measurement of the vital capacity and one-second forced expiratory volume, the plethysmographic measurement of the functional residual capacity, residual volume, total lung capacity, and the ratio of the residual volume to the total lung capacity. In addition, the progression of airway obstruction leads to ventilation perfusion mismatching, resulting in varying degrees of relative hypoxia, often accompanied by accumulation of carbon dioxide. Thus, the measurement of blood gases provides another important measurement of pulmonary function, particularly in children too young to perform spirometry and plethysmography. If the need for treatment is identified because of an acute exacerbation of symptoms or progressive deterioration of pulmonary function, repeat measurements of pulmonary function during the course of treatment are helpful guides to the effectiveness and duration of treatment.

Table 9-7
Basic Principles of Antimicrobial Selection

1. What is the diagnosis?
2. What is the probable etiology?
3. Is an antimicrobial indicated?
4. What are the expected antimicrobial susceptibilities of the likely infecting organism(s)?
5. What is the distribution of the antimicrobial?
6. What are the toxicities of the antimicrobial?

Classically, *Ps. aeruginosa* and *S. aureus* have been considered to be the major pathogens for the lower respiratory tract of these patients. However, it is probable that this is naive, and we also need to consider the concentration, or burden, of organisms as well as the other potential lower respiratory pathogens, such as those of the oropharyngeal flora, anerobes, viruses, chlamydias, and mycoplasmas. Once the potential pathogens have been identified, it is essential to anticipate the probable antimicrobial susceptibilities of the organisms and the pharmacology of the drugs to be employed. Bacteriologic assessment of response to therapy must be interpreted with the knowledge that the patients are chronically colonized and that changes in lower respiratory flora do not necessarily accompany either exacerbations of lower respiratory illness or antimicrobial intervention.

Acute Lower Respiratory Exacerbations

Perhaps the area of least controversy is the use of high doses of parenteral antibiotics for the patient with cystic fibrosis experiencing an acute lower respiratory exacerbation. In randomized studies, patients with exacerbations who harbor *Ps. aeruginosa* respond to therapy directed against this organism more frequently than patients who are not treated for this organism,[65,66] although this has not been a consistent finding.[67] Patients experiencing exacerbation of lower respiratory symptoms are often colonized with the same organisms at the time of exacerbation as previously, for example, the patient exemplified in Table 9-8. Thus, initial antibiotic selection may be tailored to these expected organisms. Although the flora may be altered by therapy, this is usually only a transient response.[15,65–67] If the patient has recently received antibiotics, initial antibiotic selection needs to be modified by the premise that the organism may be specifically resistant to the recently employed drugs.

Table 9-8
Course of Treatment of a 9-Year-Old Girl with Acute Lower Respiratory Exacerbation

	Preillness	Treatment* Day 0	Treatment* Day 21
FVC (%)	78	48	89
FEV_1 (%)	68	40	67
Culture			
Ps. aeruginosa	7.0†	7.8	NO‡
α-Streptococcus	7.0	7.3	NO‡

*Treatment with carbenicillin, gentamicin initiated.
†Homogenized sputum, $\log_{10}$ CFU/ml.
‡Sputum not obtainable.

In patients where the usual lower respiratory flora is unknown, initial antibiotic selection will need to include a β-lactamase-resistant penicillin and an aminoglycoside in high dosage. We utilize parenteral methicillin 50 mg/kg/dose given every four hours, gentamicin (or tobramycin) 2.5 mg/kg/dose given every six hours, and often carbenicillin 50 mg/kg/dose given every two hours. For β-lactamase-producing strains of *Hemophilus*, we employ chloramphenicol 20 mg/kg/dose (up to 2 g/day) given every six hours. Standard dosage recommendations for the aminoglycoside and β-lactam antibiotics have generally produced inadequate blood levels in patients with cystic fibrosis (see section on pharmacodynamics, below). Because the aminoglycosides and chloramphenicol have a narrow therapeutic index, therapeutic drug monitoring is essential for their optimal safe use. In addition, to minimize the risks of selecting for multiply antibiotic-resistant organisms, therapy should be modified once culture results are available.

Antibiotics and Ambulatory Management of Patients with Cystic Fibrosis

The most controversial use of antimicrobials in patients with cystic fibrosis involves their administration to ambulatory patients. Traditionally, antibiotics have been utilized only in the presence of a deteriorating clinical condition because prolonged antibiotic administration may induce colonization with antibiotic-resistant organisms. The role of "suppressive" antibiotic therapy in the ambulatory management of patients with cystic fibrosis has been recommended by many authorities[23,26,64,68] but remains controversial in the absence of long-term controlled studies. In a double-blind placebo-controlled crossover study,[15] sputum culture-specific antibiotics improved the course of patients with mild to moderate pulmonary disease due to cystic fibrosis, while the use of antibiotics in the absence of colonization by sensitive organisms was associated with drug-related morbidity. For example, both nonmucoid and mucoid strains of *Ps. aeruginosa* were acquired by one patient, and six other patients colonized by nonmucoid strains prior to drug administration acquired a mucoid strain in the sputum by the completion of the study. Similarly, one young adolescent girl, in whom antibiotics were selected for their activity against her pretreatment sputum flora, altered her sputum flora by acquiring *Ps. aeruginosa* (Table 9-9). In another patient (Table 9-10), oral ampicillin regularly selected for β-lactamase-producing *Hemophilus* species and oral chloramphenicol have been ineffective in modifying either sputum flora or her pulmonary function testing (not shown).

Short-term courses of sputum culture-specific antibiotics may improve the course of some patients with mild to moderate

Table 9-9
Acquisition of *Ps. aeruginosa* During Ambulatory Treatment with Antibiotics of a 14-Year-Old Girl with Cystic Fibrosis

	Pretreatment	After 3 Weeks of Antibiotics*	3 Months after Stopping Antibiotics
FVC (%)	94	83	109
FEV_1 (%)	58	56	60
Culture			
S. aureus	8.0†	8.3	8.3
S. epidermidis	6.6	–	7.0
Ps. aeruginosa	–‡	7.0	–
H. influenzae	8.3	8.3	7.8
Neisseria sp.	6.4	–	–

*Ampicillin and dicloxacillin.
†Homogenized sputum, $\log_{10}$ CFU/ml.
‡$< 10^4$ CFU/ml.

pulmonary disease due to cystic fibrosis, but may also have important adverse effects by selecting for resistant organisms, which in some patients may be associated with a decrease in their measured pulmonary function. The use of oral antibiotics, in the absence of colonization with organisms sensitive to the drug, would appear to afford little potential benefit and may be associated with significant drug-related morbidity. The effects of the long-term administration of antibiotics upon the pulmonary disease of patients with cystic fibrosis have not been evaluated by controlled studies. However, the available data suggest that long-term therapy may be associated with an accelerated rate of colonization with mucoid strains of *Ps. aeruginosa* and the potential for deterioration of the general condition of the patient.[15] The evaluation of the effectiveness of antibiotic therapy in these patients requires the use of objective parameters, such as sequential pulmonary function testing and quantitative culture of the sputum.

The Slowly Deteriorating Patient

To pediatric residents, the most controversial use of antibiotics in the management of patients with lower respiratory disease due to cystic fibrosis is the "tune-up" for the patient who is slowly deteriorating. Some patients who have been quite stable, as determined by sequential pulmonary functions, have remarkable improvement (Table 9-11) during short-term courses of high-dose parenteral antimicrobial therapy, not infrequently without significant alteration in the sputum flora. However, in approximately 10% of patients, resistant organisms in the sputum may emerge, which in some may be associated with a deterioration in the clinical condition (Table 9-12).

The indications for antimicrobial therapy, means of selecting an antimicrobial agent, duration of therapy, and criteria for the cessation (or continuation) of antibiotics are outlined (Table 9-13) for patients with acute lower respiratory exacerbations, ambulatory management, and therapeutic trials ("tune-up").

PHARMACODYNAMICS OF ANTIMICROBIAL AGENTS IN PATIENTS WITH CYSTIC FIBROSIS

Frequently, the failure to eradicate organisms from the sputum of patients with cystic fibrosis may be related to lower blood and pulmonary drug levels due to different drug pharmacokinetics in these patients. Thus, lower peak serum levels and more rapid excretion, and consequently lower tissue antimicrobial activity, have been reported for

Table 9-10
Selection of β-Lactamase-Producing *Hemophilus influenzae* by Oral Ampicillin in a 5-Year-Old Girl with Cystic Fibrosis

	Treatment Month							
	2/79	*3/79*	*4/79*	*5/79*	*7/79*	*8/79*	*9/79*	*10/79*
S. epidermidis	7.6*	6.3	+†	—‡	—	—	—	—
Ps. aeruginosa	8.3	7.6	+	7.6	7.3	8.0	8.7	7.6
H. influenzae	8.6§	9.2	+§	8.8	8.0§	8.0	8.3	8.0§
α-*Streptococcus*	7.5	8.0	+	6.8	7.0	—	—	—

Treatment‖: . . . . Amp → Chloro → Amp → [Chloro Carb Gent] Amp → [Chloro Carb Gent] → Chloro → Amp → Chloro → . . .

*Log_{10} CFU/ml.
†Present, bronchoscopy culture.
‡$< 10^4$ CFU/ml.
§β-Lactamase-producing.
‖Amp = ampicillin, Chloro = chloramphenicol, Carb = carbenicillin, Gent = Gentamicin. Drugs administered by the oral route except where enclosed by bracket which indicates intravenous administration.

Table 9-11
Parenteral Antimicrobial Therapy for a 9-Year-Old Girl with Slowly Deteriorating Condition

	Treatment* Day		
	0	*11*	*18*
FVC (%)	60	94	105
FEV_1 (%)	38	61	69
RV/TLC	0.65	0.34	0.30
Culture			
S. epidermidis	7.0†		—‡
Ps. aeruginosa	7.2		8.6
α-Streptococcus	6.5		9.0
Neisseria sp.	6.0		8.2

*Treatment with intravenous carbenicillin, tobramycin.
†Log_{10} CFU/ml.
‡$< 10^4$ CFU/ml.

many β-lactam antibiotics, including penicillinase-resistant drugs and the carboxyaminopenicillins, cephalosporins, tetracyclines, and many aminoglycosides, presumably because of altered protein binding, increased renal clearance, and/or increased apparent volumes of distribution.[20,21,69-77] Antibiotics, particularly the aminoglycosides, penetrate across the blood–bronchus barrier into bronchial secretions poorly,[21,65,78,79] whether given by intermittent or continuous administration,[80] leading to the suggestion that, perhaps, delivery of antibiotics by inhalation might be more effective.[81] However, the delivery of antibiotics by aerosol has been associated with both deterioration in ventilatory function[82] and the emergence of antibiotic-resistant organisms.[83,84]

Both the volumes of distribution and the rates of excretion are different for these patients than patients without cystic fibrosis and are unpredictable for patients with similar pulmonary involvement.[70,85] The means by which the antimicrobials are administered may also alter the blood levels. Thus, while the oral route is convenient and may be of potential value for the ambulatory suppression of organisms such as *S. aureus, H. influenzae,* and the oral commensals, oral antibiotics may not attain therapeutic blood levels because of altered absorption from the gastrointestinal tract.[77] In addition, the manner in which drugs are injected parenterally may alter drug availability.[86] For these reasons, an optimal therapeutic trial of antimicrobial agents in patients with

Table 9-12
Acute Respiratory Exacerbation due to β-Lactamase-Producing *Hemophilus parainfluenza* Occurring During Parenteral Antimicrobial Therapy in an 11-Year-Old Girl with Previously Stable Clinical Condition

	6 Months Pretreatment	3 Months Pretreatment	Treatment Day			
			0	*8*	*17**	*22*
FVC (%)	63	68	68	75	59	79
FEV_1 (%)	52	47	38	40	24	36
Sputum culture						
S. aureus	7.6†	8.0	7.3		—‡	5.0
H. influenzae	7.3	7.6	7.3		—	—
H. parainfluenza	—	—	—		7.6§	—
Treatment‖:		Amp‖ Diclox →	[Amp Meth] →		[Chloro] →	

*Onset of fever, leukocytosis, new infiltrate on chest roentgenogram.
†Log_{10} CFU/ml.
‡$< 10^4$ CFU/ml.
§β-Lactamase-producing.
‖Amp = ampicillin, Diclox = dicloxacillin, Meth = methicillin, Chloro = chloramphenicol. Drugs administered by the oral route except where enclosed by bracket which indicates intravenous administration.

cystic fibrosis requires individualized dosaging with frequent monitoring of antimicrobial levels. (See Chapter 18 for another reason for altered bioavailability of drugs in cystic fibrosis.)

SUMMARY

Because of defective mucociliary transport, chronic bacterial lower respiratory infection is universal in patients with cystic fibrosis. The lower respiratory microbial ecology is complex and unique in the individual patient but is often associated with multiple organisms including those of the oropharynx. Lower respiratory exacerbations may be frequently induced by nonbacterial pathogens, especially those commonly associated with lower respiratory infection among normal patients of comparable age. However, therapy of lower respiratory exacerbation should be directed to the bacterial flora colonizing the patient, particularly *Ps. aeruginosa, S. aureus*, and *H. influenzae* when present. Short-term courses of antibiotics directed against specific organisms colonizing the patient may significantly improve the patient's clinical condition but may be associated with adverse reactions. Long-term antibiotic therapy has not been shown to alter the long-term morbidity of patients with cystic fibrosis. The pharmacodynamics of antimicrobial drug therapy in these patients is unpredictable for the individual and must be monitored to maximize drug effectiveness.

Supported in part by U.S. Public Health Service grants RR-59 and HD-10598.

Table 9-13
Antimicrobial Therapy for Patients with Cystic Fibrosis

Acute lower respiratory exacerbation		
	Indication	Increased cough and sputum production; decreased physical activity; ± fever, leukocytosis, x-ray changes
	Antimicrobial	Directed towards organisms present in sputum at $\geq 10^7$ CFU/ml
	Duration	Until no further objective signs of improvement (often 10–14 days)
	Criteria for cessation	Objective improvement in culture, sputum production, weight gain, and sequential PFTs
Ambulatory antibiotics		
	Indication	Presence of pulmonary infiltrates and/or bronchiectasis when colonized with an organism (especially *S. aureus* or *Haemophilus* species) sensitive to antibiotics which may be administered orally
	Antimicrobial	Oral; directed towards organisms present at $\geq 10^6$ CFU/ml
	Duration	Less than 4 months
	Criteria for cessation	Adverse reaction including emergence of resistant organism; no objective improvement over 4 months
	Criteria for continuation	Continued objective improvement in culture, sputum production, weight gain, PFTs
Therapeutic trial ("tune-up")		
	Indication	New patient whose best baseline is unknown; gradual deterioration in growth, cough, sputum production, exercise tolerance, or PFT
	Antimicrobial	Parenteral in maximum therapeutic dose directed towards organisms at $\geq 10^6$ CFU/ml
	Duration	Until no objective improvement has been observed (often 10–14 days)
	Criteria for cessation	Adverse reaction including emergence of resistant organisms; no objective improvement after 14 days
	Criteria for continuation	Continued improvement in culture, sputum production, weight gain, or PFTs

REFERENCES

1. Esterly JR, Oppenheimer EH: Observations in cystic fibrosis of the pancreas. III. Pulmonary lesions. *J Hopkins Med J* 1968; 122:94–101.
2. Mearns MV, Hunt GH, Rushworth R: Bacterial flora of respiratory tract of patients with cystic fibrosis, 1950–1971. *Arch Dis Child* 1972;47:902–907.
3. Huang NN, Loon ELV, Sheng KT: The flora of the respiratory tract of patients with cystic fibrosis of the pancreas. *J Pediatr* 1961;59: 512-521.
4. Iacocca VF, Sibinga MS, Barbero GJ: Respiratory tract bacteriology in cystic fibrosis. *Am J Dis Child* 1963;106:115–124.
5. Dixon JMS, Miller DC: Value of dilute inocula in cultural examination of sputum. *Lancet* 1965;2:1046–1048.
6. Monroe PW, Muchmore HG, Felton FG, et al: Quantitation of microorganisms in sputum. *Appl Microbiol* 1969;18:214–220.
7. May JR: The bacteriology of chronic bronchitis. *Lancet* 1953;2:534–537.
8. Thorsteinsson SV, Musher DM, Fagan T: The diagnostic value of sputum culture in acute pneumonia. *JAMA* 1975;233:894–895.
9. Lorian V, Khavari P, Gray N: Quantitative bacteriological analysis of sputum as a test of antibiotic efficacy. *Appl Microbiol* 1967;15: 564-565.
10. Loria DB: Uses of quantitative analyses of bacterial populations in sputum. *JAMA* 1962;182:1082–1086.
11. Hedberg N: Quantitative study of bacteria in mixed populations. *Am J Clin Pathol* 1964;41:332-336.
12. Kilbourn JP, Campbell RA, Grach JL, et al: Quantitative bacteriology of sputum. *Am Rev Respir Dis* 1968;98:810–818.
13. Pirtle JK, Monroe PW, Smalley TK, et al: Diagnostic and therapeutic advantages of serial quantitative cultures of fresh sputum in acute bacterial pneumonia. *Am Rev Respir Dis* 1969;100:813–838.
14. Bartlett JG, Finegold SM: Bacteriology of expectorated sputum with quantitative culture and wash technique compared to transtracheal aspirates. *Am Rev Respir Dis* 1978;117:1019–1027.
15. Loening-Baucke VA, Mischler E, Myers MG: A placebo-controlled trial of cephalexin therapy in the ambulatory management of patients with cystic fibrosis. *J Pediatr* 1979;95:630–637.
16. Lennette EH, Spaulding EH, Truant JP: *Manual of Clinical Microbiology,* 2nd ed. Washington, DC, American Society for Microbiology, 1974.
17. National Committee for Clinical Laboratory Standards: Standard methods for dilution antimicrobial susceptibility tests for bacteria which grow aerobically. PSM-7. Villanova, Pennsylvania, 1980.
18. Koontz FP, Maquire GF, Moore R, et al: Evaluation of quantitative sputum from children with cystic fibrosis. *78th Annual Meeting, American Society for Microbiology.* Las Vegas, 1978, p 286.
19. Boxerbaum V, Doershuk CF, Pittman S: Efficacy and tolerance of carbenicillin in patients with cystic fibrosis. *Antimicrob Agents Chemother* 1968:292–295.
20. Huang NN, Hiller EJ, Macri CM, et al: Carbenicillin in patients with cystic fibrosis: Clinical pharmacology and therapeutic evaluation. *J Pediatr* 1971;78:338–345.
21. Marks MI, Prentice R, Swarson R, et al: Carbenicillin and gentamicin: Pharmacologic studies in patients with cystic fibrosis and *Pseudomonas* pulmonary infections. *J Pediatr* 1971;79:822–828.
22. Phair JP, Tan JS, Watanakunakorn C, et al: Carbenicillin treatment of *Pseudomonas* pulmonary infection. *Am J Dis Child* 1970; 120:22–25.
23. Shwachman H, Redmond A, Khaw KT: Studies in cystic fibrosis. Report of 130 patients diagnosed under 3 months of age over a 20-year period. *Pediatrics* 1970;46:335–343.
24. Smith AL: Antibiotic therapy: Efficacy and assessment. *Proceedings of the Eighth International Cystic Fibrosis Congress.* Toronto, Canadian Cystic Fibrosis Foundation, 1980, pp 382–388.
25. di Sant'Agnese PA, Talamo RC: Pathogenesis and physiopathology of cystic fibrosis of the pancreas. *N Engl J Med* 1967;277: 1287–1294.
26. Lawson DN: Contribution to panel discussion on microbiology and chemotherapy of the respiratory tract in cystic fibrosis. *5th International Cystic Fibrosis Conference.* Cambridge, 1969, p 225.
27. May JR, Herrick NC, Thompson D: Bacterial infection in cystic fibrosis. *Arch Dis Child* 1972;47:908.
28. Warwick WJ, Munson S: Life table studies of mortality. *Mod Probl Pediatr* 1967;10: 353–367.
29. Hoff GE, Hoiby N: *Staphylococcus aureus* in cystic fibrosis: Antibiotic sensitivity and phage types during the latest decade. *Acta Pathol Microbiol Scand* 1975;83:219–225.
30. Pittman FE, Howe C, Goode L, et al: Phage groups and antibiotic sensitivity of *Staphylococcus aureus* associated with cystic fibrosis of the pancreas. *Pediatrics* 1959;24:40–42.
31. Kulczycki LL, Murphy TM, Ballant JA:

Pseudomonas colonization in cystic fibrosis: A study of 166 patients. *JAMA* 1978;240: 30–34.

32. Mearns MB: Natural history of pulmonary infection in cystic fibrosis. *8th International Congress of Cystic Fibrosis.* Toronto, Canadian Cystic Fibrosis Foundation, 1980, pp 325–334.
33. Diaz F, Mosovich LL, Neter E: Serogroups of *Pseudomonas aeruginosa* and the immune response of patients with cystic fibrosis. *J Infect Dis* 1970;121:269–274.
34. Martin DR: Mucoid variation in *Pseudomonas aeruginosa* induced by the action of phage. *J Med Microbiol* 1973;6:111–118.
35. Linker A, Jones RS: A new polysaccharide resembling alginic acid isolated from *Pseudomonas. J Biol Chem* 1966;245:3845–3851.
36. Hoiby N: *Pseudomonas aeruginosa* infection in cystic fibrosis. Relationship between mucoid strains of *Pseudomonas aeruginosa* and the humoral immune response. *Acta Pathol Microbiol Scand* 1974;82:551–558.
37. Doggett RG, Harrison GM, Stillwell RN, et al: An atypical *Pseudomonas aeruginosa* associated with cystic fibrosis of the pancreas. *J Pediatr* 1966;68:215–221.
38. Lam J, Chan R, Lam K, et al: Production of mucoid microcolonies by *Pseudomonas aeruginosa* within infected lungs in cystic fibrosis. *Infect Immun* 1980;28:546–554.
39. Thomassen MJ, Demko CA, Boxerbaum B, et al: Multiple isolates of *Pseudomonas aeruginosa* with differing antimicrobial susceptibility patterns from patients with cystic fibrosis. *J Infect Dis* 1979;140: 873–880.
40. Blackwood LL, Pennington JE: Influence of mucoid coating on clearance of *Pseudomonas aeruginosa* from lungs. *Infect Immun* 1981;32:443–448.
41. Sorensen RU, Stern RC, Polmar SH: Lymphocyte responsiveness to *Pseudomonas aeruginosa* in cystic fibrosis: The relationship to status of pulmonary disease in sibling pairs. *J Pediatr* 1978;93:201–205.
42. Strunk RC, Sieber OF, Taussig LM, et al: Serum complement depression during viral lower respiratory tract illness in cystic fibrosis. *Arch Dis Child* 1977;52:687–690.
43. Moss RB, Lewiston NJ: Immune complexes and humoral response to *Pseudomonas aeruginosa* in cystic fibrosis. *Am Rev Respir Dis* 1980;121:23–29.
44. Church JA, Jordan SC, Keens TG, et al: Circulating immune complexes in patients with cystic fibrosis. *Chest* 1981;80:405–411.
45. Doggett RG, Harrison GM, Carter RE: Mucoid *Pseudomonas aeruginosa* in patients with chronic illness. *Lancet* 1971;1:236–237.
46. Thomassen MJ, Demko CA, Boxerbaum B, et al: Multiple isolates of *Pseudomonas aeruginosa* with differing antimicrobial susceptibility patterns from patients with cystic fibrosis. *J Infect Dis* 1979;140:873–880.
47. Hoiby N, Killian M: *Haemophilus* from the lower respiratory tract of patients with cystic fibrosis. *Scand J Respir Dis* 1976;57:103–107.
48. Burn MW, May JR: Bacterial precipitins in serum of patients with cystic fibrosis. *Lancet* 1968;1:270–272.
49. May JR: *The Chemotherapy of Chronic Bronchitis and Allied Disorders.* London, The English University Press Ltd, 1968, pp 5–24.
50. Seidmon EJ, Mosovich LL, Neter E: Colonization by *Enterobacteriaceae* of the respiratory tract of children with cystic fibrosis of the pancreas and their antibody response. *J Pediatr* 1975;87:528–533.
51. Macone AB, Pier GB, Pennington JE, et al: Mucoid *Escherichia coli* in cystic fibrosis: *N Engl J Med* 1981;304:1445–1449.
52. Mearns M, Longbottom J, Batten J: Precipitating antibodies to *Aspergillus fumigatus* in cystic fibrosis. *Lancet* 1967;1:538–539.
53. Schwartz RH, Johnstone DE, Holsclaw DA, et al: Serum precipitins to *Aspergillus fumigatus* in cystic fibrosis. *Am J Dis Child* 1970;120:432–433.
54. Warren CPW, Tai E, Batten JC, et al: Cystic fibrosis—immunological reactions to *Aspergillus fumigatus* and common allergens. *Clin Allergy* 1975;1:1–12.
55. Bardana EJ, Sobti KL, Cianciulli FD, et al: Aspergillus antibody in patients with cystic fibrosis. *Am J Dis Child* 1975;129:1164–1167.
56. Nelson LA, Callerame ML, Schwartz RH: Aspergillosis and atopy in cystic fibrosis. *Am Rev Respir Dis* 1979;120:863–873.
57. Petersen NT, Hoiby, N, Mordhorst CH, et al: Respiratory infections in cystic fibrosis patients caused by virus, *Chlamydia* and *Mycoplasma*—possible synergism with *Pseudomonas aeruginosa*. *8th International Congress on Cystic Fibrosis.* Toronto, Canadian Cystic Fibrosis Foundation, 1980, pp 346–351.
58. Wright PF, Khaw, KT, Oxman MN, et al: Evaluation of the safety of amantadine-HCl and the role of respiratory viral infections in children with cystic fibrosis. *J Infect Dis* 1976;134:144–149.
59. Laray-Causay LR, Cundy KR, Huang NN: *Pseudomonas* carrier rates of patients with cystic fibrosis and of members of their families. *J Pediatr* 1976;89:23–26.
60. Blessing-Moore J, Maybury B, Lewiston N:

Spread of *Pseudomonas* from cystic fibrosis patients. I. Mucosal droplets spread by cough. *Cystic Fibrosis Club Abstracts* 1979;20:2.

61. Thomassen MJ, Root JM: Transmission of *Pseudomonas aeruginosa* among cystic fibrosis patients at summer camp. *Cystic Fibrosis Club Abstracts* 1979;20:37.
62. di Sant'Agnese PA, Andersen DH: Celiac syndrome. IV. Chemotherapy of infections of the respiratory tract associated with cystic fibrosis of the pancreas; observations with penicillin and drugs of the sulfonamide group, with special reference to penicillin aerosol. *Am J Dis Child* 1946;72:17-61.
63. Shwachman H, Crocker AC, Foley G, et al: Aureomycin therapy in the pulmonary involvement of pancreatic fibrosis (mucoviscidosis). *N Engl J Med* 1949;41:185-192.
64. Shwachman H, Kulczycki LL: Long-term study of 105 patients with cystic fibrosis. *Am J Dis Child* 1958;96:6-15.
65. Wientzen R, Prestidge CB, Kramer RI, et al: Acute pulmonary exacerbations in cystic fibrosis. A double-blind trial of tobramycin and placebo therapy. *Am J Dis Child* 1980; 134:1134-1138.
66. Hyatt AC, Chipps BE, Kumor KM, et al: A double-blind controlled trial of anti-*Pseudomonas* chemotherapy of acute respiratory exacerbations in patients with cystic fibrosis. *J Pediatr* 1981;99:307-311.
67. Beaudry PH, Marks MI, McDougall D, et al: Is anti-*Pseudomonas* therapy warranted in acute respiratory exacerbations in children with cystic fibrosis? *J Pediatr* 1980;97: 144-147.
68. Matthews LW, Doershuk CF, Stern R, et al: Comprehensive and preventive treatment of cystic fibrosis, in Mangos J, Talamo R (eds): *Fundamental Problems of Cystic Fibrosis and Related Diseases.* New York, Intercontinental Medical Book Corp., 1973, pp 303-317.
69. Huang NN, Laray-Cuasay L, Yasmin N: Efficacy of sisomicin in patients with cystic fibrosis. *Infection* 1976;4:S465-471.
70. Vogelstein B, Kowarski A, Lietman PS: The pharmacokinetics of amikacin in children. *J Pediatr* 1977;91:333-339.
71. Spyker DA, Sande MA, Mandell GL: Tobramycin pharmacokinetics in patients with cystic fibrosis and leukemia. *18th Interscience Conference on Antimicrobial Agents and Chemotherapy.* 1978, Atlanta, Georgia.
72. Giannamor EM, Gross PA, Homayouni H: Requirements for increased dose of aminoglycoside in cystic fibrosis. *18th Interscience Conference on Antimicrobial Agents and Chemotherapy.* 1978, Atlanta, Georgia.
73. Finkelstein E, Hall K: Aminoglycoside clearance in patients with cystic fibrosis. *J Pediatr* 1979;94:163-164.
74. Yaffe SJ, Gerbracht LM, Mosovich LL, et al: Pharmacokinetics of methicillin in patients with cystic fibrosis. *J Infect Dis* 1977;135:828-831.
75. Michaelsen H, Bergan T: Pharmacokinetics of netilmicin in children with and without cystic fibrosis. *Antimicrob Agents Chemother* 1981;19:1029-1031.
76. Jusko WJ, Mosovich LL, Gerbacht LM, et al: Enhanced renal excretion of dicloxacillin in patients with cystic fibrosis. *Pediatrics* 1975;56:1038-1044.
77. Guggenbichler JP, Kiene LG: Bioavailability of oral antibiotics in cystic fibrosis. *Monogr Paediatr* 1979;10:34-40.
78. McCrae WM, Raeburn JA, Hanson EJ: Tobramycin therapy of infections due to *Pseudomonas aeruginosa* in patients with cystic fibrosis: Effect of dosage and concentration of antibiotic in sputum. *J Infect Dis* 1976;134:S191-193.
79. Mobelli G, Coppens L, Thys JP, et al: Anti-*Pseudomonas* activity in bronchial secretions of patients receiving amikacin or tobramycin as a continuous infusion. *Antimicrob Agents Chemother* 1981;19:72-75.
80. Klastersky J, Thys JP, Mobelli G: Comparative studies of intermittent and continuous administration of aminoglycosides in treatment of bronchopulmonary infections due to gram-negative bacteria. *Rev Infect Dis* 1981;3:74-83.
81. Hodson ME, Penketh ARL, Batten JC: Aerosol carbenicillin and gentamicin treatment of *Pseudomonas aeruginosa* infection in patients with cystic fibrosis. *Lancet* 1981;2:1137-1139.
82. Dickie KJ, deCroot WJ: Ventilatory effects of aerosolized kanamycin and polymixin. *Chest* 1973;63:694-697.
83. Klastersky J, Huysmans E, Weerts D, et al: Endotracheally administered gentamicin for the prevention of infections of the respiratory tract in patients with tracheostomy: A double-blind study. *Chest* 1974;65:650-654.
84. Feeley TW, duMoulin GC, Hedley-White J, et al: Aerosol polymixin and pneumonia in seriously ill patients. *N Engl J Med* 1975;293: 471-475.
85. Kelly HB, Menendez R, Fan L, et al: Pharmacokinetics of tobramycin in cystic fibrosis. *J Pediatr* 1982;100:318-321.
86. Leff RD, Roberts RJ: Methods for intravenous drug administration in the pediatric patient. *J Pediatr* 1981;98:631-635.

10

Immunology of Cystic Fibrosis: Immunity, Immunodeficiency and Hypersensitivity

Richard B. Moss

The immune system, the protector of the self against intrusion and disruption from foreign substances, whether they arise from the external or the internal environment, is characterized by two remarkable features: specificity and memory. The ability to distinguish self from not-self and to recognize upwards of one billion different foreign molecular configurations gives the immune system a razor-sharp specificity to deal with virtually any individual discrete challenge successfully. The ability to "remember" each challenge and mount a faster and qualitatively and quantitatively superior response to subsequent challenges from the same offender gives the immune system a method to not merely retain but also improve its efficiency with time. In this chapter we shall consider the function of the immune system in cystic fibrosis, particularly with regard to the major obvious defensive deficiency in the disease, chronic pulmonary infection.

Various models have been advanced to dissect the immune system's great complexity into intelligible units capable of investigation. We shall distinguish between specific components—those cells and molecules which recognize differences, termed antigenic determinants, on foreign cells and molecules—and nonspecific components, which are usually either first-line defenses holding off the enemy until the specific response is generated or are later recruited by the specific components to amplify the overall response. We shall also distinguish between local and systemic compartments of immune function, as this bears special importance in cystic fibrosis when considering the mucosal immune system as at least partially autonomous from systemic immunity. Finally, many discussions of the immune system separate affector from effector components, but such a dissection is not necessary for fulfilling the purposes of this chapter.

SYSTEMIC IMMUNITY IN CYSTIC FIBROSIS

Specific Immunity

Specific immunity consists primarily of lymphocytes and immunoglobulins. Lymphocytes exist in structurally and functionally discrete subpopulations. One arm of specific lymphocyte immunity is termed the B-cell system. Mature B cells are identified by surface immunoglobulin molecules on their cell membranes and by receptors for complement components. Upon antigenic stimulation some B cells undergo blast transformation into plasmacytes and begin secreting antibody, immunoglobulin molecules with specificity for an antigen. Major properties of the five known immunoglobulin classes are shown in Table 10-1. A second arm of specific lymphocyte immunity is termed the T-cell system. These lymphocytes are usually identified by their ability to bind sheep erythrocytes to form rosettes, although recently monoclonal antibodies recognizing surface molecules on T cells and capable of distinguishing functional subsets of T cells have become widely available. Instead of secreting immunoglobulins after antigenic stimulation, T cells exert their effects primarily by secreting a wide variety of mediator molecules termed lymphokines, such as interferon and macrophage inhibition factor (Table 10-2). Studies using a number of methods have successfully defined at least two subpopulations of T cells, one of which contains cells which help B cells to produce antibody and in certain circumstances directly kill foreign cells; the other subpopulation suppresses the intensity of the immune response, hence the popular terms helper T and suppressor T cells.

Humoral immunity Systemic B lymphocyte function has been extensively studied in cystic fibrosis.

Hypergammaglobulinemia in CF was first noted by paper electrophoresis of serum in 1960.[1] With the advent of quantitation of immunoglobulin levels by radial immunodiffusion in the mid-1960s, a number of studies reported immunoglobulin levels for the IgG, IgA, and IgM classes in CF. In general these studies show increasing IgG and IgA levels with age, consistent with chronic antigenic stimulation.[2-9] Some interesting anomalies, however, have emerged. Low levels of IgG or IgA were reported in 8 of 50 patients, all less than 3 years old, in one study[6] and in at least 16 of 106 in another.[10]

A large survey in Boston using automated nephelometry found 22% of 154 CF patients under 10 years of age had low IgG levels in contrast to 1–2% in 265 patients over 10, and an increasing prevalence of hypergammaglobulinemia G from 6.5% in those less than 10 years of age to 47% in those over 20 years of age. Patients with low IgG tended to have lower IgA and IgM values than those with normal IgG levels. Hypogammaglobulinemia G was not associated with any consistent deficiency of immune function.[11] The significance of low IgG or IgA levels in a minority of younger patients is unclear, although a protective effect is suggested by better arterial blood gas values and decreased colonization with *Pseudomonas aeruginosa* in these patients (see section on type III hypersensitivity below for a further discussion of this point).

Another recently appreciated aspect of immunoglobulin levels in cystic fibrosis was reported by Turner et al,[10] who found that

Table 10-1
Chemical and Physical Properties of the Immunoglobulin Classes*

	Immunoglobulin Class				
Characteristic	*IgG*	*IgM*	*IgA*	*IgD*	*IgE*
Chains:					
Heavy	γ	μ	α	δ	ϵ
Light	κ,λ	κ,λ	κ,λ	κ,λ	κ,λ
Monomer units	1	5	1–3	1	1
Electrophoretic mobility	γ_2-α_2	γ_1-α_1	γ_1-α_1	γ_1-β	γ_1-β
Principle mobility	γ_2	γ_1	β	γ	β
Sedimentation coefficient (Svedberg units)	6.7	19	7–15	7	8
Molecular weight	150,000	900,000	160–500,000	180,000	200,000
Percent carbohydrate	3	12	7.5	12	12
Serum concentration:					
Adult mean (mg/dl)	1,200	150	300	3	.01
Percent of total	70–80	5–10	10–15	< 1	< .01
Solubility	Euglobulin	Euglobulin	Pseudoglobulin	Pseudoglobulin	Pseudoglobulin
Sensitivity to mercaptans	0	+	+	?	?
Heat lability	±	+ +	+	+ + + +	+ + +
Number of subclasses	4	2	2	0	0
Genetic factors	Gm,Km	Mm,Km	Am,Km	Km	Km

*From: Stiehm ER, Fulginiti VA: *Immunologic Disorders in Infants and Children, 2nd ed.* Philadelphia, WB Saunders, 1980, p 57, with permission.

Table 10-2
Lymphokines*

Name	Abbreviation	Action
A. Affecting macrophages		
Migration inhibition factor	MIF	Inhibits the migration of normal macrophages
Macrophage aggregation factor	MAF	Agglutinates macrophages in suspension
Macrophage chemotactic factor	MCF	Causes macrophages to migrate through micropore filter along gradient
Macrophage resistance factor (postulated)		Renders macrophages nonspecifically resistant to infection with certain bacteria and viruses
B. Affecting Lymphocytes		
Blastogenic or mitogenic factor	BF or MF	Induces blast transformation and tritiated thymidine incorporation in normal lymphocytes
Potentiating factor	PF	Augments or enhances ongoing transformation in mixed lymphocyte culture or antigen-stimulated cultures
Cell cooperation or helper factor		Produced by T cells, increases the number or rate of formation of antibody producing cells in vitro
Suppressor factor (postulated)		Inhibits activation of, and/or antibody production by B cells
C. Affecting granulocytes		
Inhibition factor		Inhibits the migration of human buffy coat cells or peripheral blood leukocytes from capillary tubes or wells in agar plates
Chemotactic factor		Causes granulocytes to migrate through a micropore filter along a gradient
D. Affecting cultured cells		
Lymphotoxin	LT	Cytotoxic for certain cultured cells, eg, mouse L cells or HeLa cells
Proliferation inhibition factor and cloning inhibition factor	PIF, CIF	Inhibit proliferation of cultured cells without lysing them
Interferon		Protects cells against virus infection
E. Producing effects in vivo		
Skin reactive factor	SRF	In normal guinea pig skin induces indurated skin reactions that are histologically similar to delayed-type hypersensitivity reactions
Macrophage disappearance factor		Injected intraperitoneally, causes macrophages to adhere to peritoneal wall

*Adapted from *Cell-mediated Immunity and Resistance to Infection.* World Health Organization Technical Report Series No. 519, Geneva, 1973.

IgG, IgA, and IgE levels were significantly higher in CF patients with recent exacerbations of lung disease than in stable patients.

Systemic antibody responses have received extensive attention. Most studies have looked at agglutinating or precipitating antibodies to the major microbial colonizers in cystic fibrosis, namely, *Staphylococcus aureus, Pseudomonas aeruginosa, Hemophilus influenzae, Aspergillus fumigatus,* and *Candida albicans*, and found appropriately impressive responses when compared to controls with other chronic lung disease or normal subjects (for *Pseudomonas aeruginosa*, reviewed by

Hoiby;[12] for other microbes, reviewed by Fick and Reynolds[13] and Peterson et al[14]). In addition, systemic antibody responses to immunization with influenza vaccine, tetanus toxoid, or *Pseudomonas* lipopolysaccharide are normal.[11,15,16] These findings, combined with increased absolute number of B cells in infected patients[17] and the extreme rarity of septicemia in CF indicate that the systemic B cell–antibody response is generally intact.

Before assuming specific humoral immunity in CF is normal, however, several questions need to be answered. What is the cause and significance of hypogammaglobulinemia in a significant minority of younger patients? Do CF antibodies, although produced in ample quantity, function normally? (See the discussion of opsonization of *Pseudomonas* in the immunodeficiency section below for further consideration of this key question.) Finally, what is the significance of the apparently impaired B-cell differentiation as assayed by the decreased appearance of hemolytic plaque-forming cells after stimulation with pokeweed mitogen?[18,19]

A separate consideration of the IgE class antibody response in CF is given in the section on hypersensitivity below.

Cell-mediated immunity The cellular immune system is based on antigen-specific stimulation of T cells to proliferate and secrete lymphokines. T-cell function has traditionally been assayed in vivo by delayed cutaneous reactivity to common antigens such as *Candida albicans*, streptokinase/streptodornase, and tetanus toxoid. In vitro evaluation consists of enumeration of sheep red blood cell-rosetting lymphocytes along with antigen- and mitogen-induced lymphocyte proliferation studies. Less often, lymphokine production by sensitized T cells after stimulation is measured. Recently, assays for T helper and suppressor cell populations have also been conducted.

Skin testing for delayed cutaneous responsiveness is a measurable in vivo expression of cell-mediated immunity, although it is heavily dependent upon such variables as subject age, concentration of antigen, and interpretation of the induration–erythema response. CF patients exhibit, with only relatively rare exceptions in primarily cachectic patients, intact delayed skin reactivity.[20-22] In vitro studies enumerating T-and B-cell numbers and measuring lymphocyte proliferation following mitogen stimulation confirm the in vivo impression of intact cell-mediated immunity.[6,17,22-26] Lymphokine production following antigen stimulation has received less attention, but available evidence also favors an intact response.[27,28] It is of some interest to note that both homozygous and heterozygous CF serum apparently contain a factor or factors that affect the levels of CF or normal lymphocyte acid hydrolase enzymes both before and after mitogen stimulation. Thus, lymphocyte culture conditions (eg, using autologous CF serum instead of fetal calf serum) may effect study results.[29]

The T lymphocyte subpopulations in CF have been only very recently and incompletely studied. Using concanavalin A, a T-cell mitogen known to generate suppressor cell activity, Harper et al[22] found no differences between 12 CF and 10 normal subjects. Using lymphocyte cell-surface G and M heavy-chain receptors to identify suppressor and helper cells, respectively (a probe that has been shown to be of limited utility in light of information gathered from use of monoclonal antibodies to T-cell subsets), Sorensen et al[30] found elevated suppressor cells in four of five hospitalized CF patients. Future studies defining T-cell subsets with monoclonal antibodies and correlating results with clinical status are required to address the question of a possible T-cell immunoregulatory imbalance in cystic fibrosis.

A limited, but potentially important, defect in lymphocyte responses to *Pseudomonas aeruginosa* and other gram-negative bacteria has been reported and is discussed separately in the section on immunodeficiency below.

Nonspecific Immunity

Complement The complement system consists of more than 20 plasma proteins. A complicated nomenclature somewhat disguises the simplicity of a biologic amplification system based on the principle of cascading zymogen (or precursor protein) activation to active proteolytic enzymes with restricted substrate specificity which act to amplify potent inflammatory activity as a means of natural and acquired resistance. This system is under exquisite and redundant control by virtue of the lability of the active enzymes and their restricted substrates, and by at least four modulatory proteins.[31,32]

Classical pathway The first cascade to be discovered, and hence termed the classical pathway, is mainly concerned with acquired resistance because it is usually triggered by the combination of antigen with specific IgM or IgG antibody. The recognition site is on the C1q plasma protein, itself a subunit of a naturally occurring trimer consisting of three proteins, C1q, C1r and C1s. After C1q is bound to the activator, the C1r subunit is activated and in turn activates the C1s subunit. The trimer then has activity towards C2 and C4, the next components in the classical pathway. These two proteins can then combine to form the $C\overline{142}$ complex capable of cleaving and thus activating the lynchpin protein of the complement system, C3. The activated form of C3, termed C3b, is capable of cleaving C5. Its active form, C5b, is capable of assembling a large macromolecular complex including C5b, C6, C7, C8, and C9 on cell membranes. This complex produces cell lysis by literally punching a hole in the membrane and creating a free ion channel (Figure 10-1).

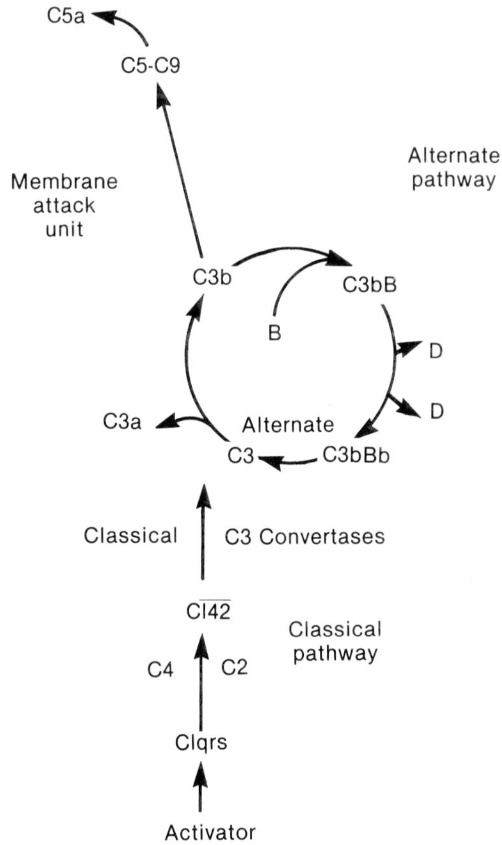

Figure 10-1 Reaction pathways of complement system.

Assays of the complement system are complicated by a necessary distinction between those assays measuring antigenic determinants, which may be shared by the precursor and active form of a given protein, and functional assays measuring certain parts or the entire cascade sequence.[33] The biological activity of the system is far more extensive than the well-known lytic function. Along the pathway various fragments and activated forms of complement proteins generate inflammatory responses by interacting with specific receptors on the surface of mast cells, leading to histamine and other anaphylactic mediator release; on the surface of polymorphonuclear leukocytes, leading to chemotaxis and activation of phagocytic mechanisms; and finally, by coating surfaces of target organisms such as bacteria or viruses to enhance their recognition by immune and inflammatory defense cells. Thus, the opsonic, chemotactic, and anaphylactic effects of complement activation may well be of greater biological significance than cell lysis.

Complement in cystic fibrosis The possibility that abnormalities of the complement system occur in CF was first suggested by Conover et al[34] following investigation of previously described ciliary dyskinesia activity in CF serum in rabbit tracheal and oyster gill bioassays. Using a rabbit tracheal bioassay, these workers reported dyskinesia activity in sera of patients with agammaglobulinemia, asthma, celiac disease, allergy, and systemic lupus erythromatosus as well as cystic fibrosis, and they suggested that a unifying abnormality in complement activity could account for such diversity. It was found that immunochemical but not lytic (functional) C3 was significantly elevated in CF patients and obligate heterozygotes compared to a control group.[35] The possibility that this increase reflected split products of C3 was considered, and further investigation led to the proposal that the observed increase being measured was actually the C3a fragment (C3 anaphylatoxin) detected in the bioassay and linked to IgG which presumably protected the C3a from degradation by its natural carboxypeptidase B-like plasma inactivator.[36] C3a was postulated to be the low-molecular-weight ciliary dyskinesia factor (CDF). This belief was supported by the conversion of normal sera having no CDF activity to a CDF-positive state by epsilon-aminocaproic acid, a known inhibitor of the carboxypeptidase B-like anaphylatoxin inactivator.[37] Conversely, incubation of CDF-positive CF sera with carboxypeptidase B produced reversion to a CDF-negative state. A deficiency or a defect in the function of the anaphylatoxin inactivator was suggested as an underlying defect in cystic fibrosis. However, subsequent studies showed that CF sera had normal levels of carboxypeptidase B-like activity.[38]

Other studies looking at complement components in cystic fibrosis have reported quite variable findings. Lieberman[39] found no significant elevation of C3 in CF patients compared to controls with other chronic lung diseases, although CF females had higher levels than CF men or control women. This study was criticized for using controls who were previously shown to quite possibly have ciliary dyskinesia activity in their serum and for neglecting the increased C3 levels previously found in heterozygotes.[40] Scanlin et al[41] pointed out that C3 levels must be age-matched as levels increase slightly from age 6 months to 14 years; they found that only 4 of 23 CF patients had raised C3 levels, and these were not localized to a specific age range.

Hann et al[42] reported elevations of immunochemical C3 and also C5 in patients and obligate heterozygotes compared to normal controls and controls with asthma, diabetes, or inflammatory bowel disease. These elevations were not correlated with age, sex, disease severity, sputum colonization, or therapy. Polley and Bearn[43] found ciliary dyskinesia activity in inactivated C3a (ie, after removal of C-terminal arginine) and elevated C3 levels in CF patients measured both immunochemically and by lytic (functional) assay. Holzhauer et al[44] found elevated immunochemical C3 in CF patients and heterozygotes compared to age-matched controls; in CF patients they reported a correlation of C3 levels with clinical status, lower clinical scores being associated with higher C3 levels. They also investigated C3 genetic polymorphism detected by electrophoretic mobility and found no significant changes in the gene frequencies. Another study of C3 polymorphism similarly found no variation in gene frequency for the fast and slow electrophoretic variants.[45]

Some studies have suggested that activation of complement commonly occurs in CF plasma. McFarlane et al[46] in a study concerned mainly with detection of immune complexes, noted that three fresh plasma samples of CF patients showed CF activation products when tested by two-dimensional immunoelectrophoresis. They reported that nearly half of 40 CF patients tested had low C3 levels. Age, sex, and clinical correlation were not provided. In four CF patients with documented viral lower respiratory infection, low levels of C3 and C4 were found which returned to normal after recovery; in contrast, such depressions were not found in CF patients without viral pneumonia.[47] Significantly lower mean C3 and C4 levels were reported in 30 CF patients compared to 40 healthy, age-matched controls in an Austrian study.[48]

The wide variation in reported results

might be ascribed to lack of correlation in most studies with each patient's clinical and infective status. We found normal or increased C3 levels immunochemically in both stable and acutely ill CF patients and could find no evidence for C3 activation in plasma using a counterimmunoelectrophoretic technique,[49] although more recent studies with a more sensitive two-dimensional immunoelectrophoretic technique indicate activation of C4 in plasma in some acutely infected patients (Moss, Hsu, and Milgrom, unpublished data).

There is, as yet, no clear reason for the finding of increased concentrations of C3 and sometimes C5 in obligate heterozygotes which suggest derangements more proximal to the CF genetic abnormality.[34,42,44] Wilson and co-workers[26,50] have shown that mononuclear cells from CF homozygotes and obligate heterozygotes secrete several ciliary dyskinesia factors, including a few that appear to be C3 and C5 activation fragments, suggesting a link between the CF genotype and mononuclear cell complement metabolism (possibly a defect in proteolytic enzymatic control of complement catabolism). The relation of a putative CF disease-specific ciliary dyskinesia factor ("cystic fibrosis protein") to the complement system is an area that needs further and intensive investigation. Perturbations in complement-mediated chemotactic activity have been suggested as a possible pathophysiologic mechanism in CF lung disease.[50]

Alternate pathway Over 25 years ago an alternate pathway of complement activation not requiring specific antibody was discovered. In biological importance this mechanism of natural resistance can scarcely be considered "alternative." Six distinct proteins have been identified, isolated, and reassembled in vitro to reproduce the function of this pathway. As in the classical pathway, C3 plays a pivotal role. Once C3 is split to generate C3b, the latter combines with factor B which has been activated to $\overline{Bb}$ by factor D. The active complex, called $\overline{C3bBb}$, is capable of cleaving more C3 to provide a positive feedback loop. This $\overline{C3bBb}$ complex is stabilized by the fourth protein, properdin. The remaining two components are regulatory β-globulin proteins, termed C3b inactivator and βIH. The biological activators of the alternate pathway appear to propagate the positive feedback loop by binding C3b in such a way as to decrease the usual regulatory activity of βIH.[51] An impressive array of apparently unrelated substances, prominently including microbial polysaccharides such as endotoxic lipopolysaccharide, can activate this pathway.[52]

Studies of the alternate complement pathway in CF have yielded results as variable as those for the classical pathway. Polley and Bearn[43] found decreased activation of factor B and C3 by inulin, an alternate pathway activator, in 10 of 11 CF patients. A more recent study found decreased serum factor B levels in one third of CF patients assayed.[48] In contrast, other studies using functional erythrocyte lytic assays under conditions blocking the classical pathway, but activating the alternate pathway, found no impairment in CF patients.[53,54] It should be noted that *Pseudomonas* lipopolysaccharide is a good in vitro alternate pathway activator.[54] The terminal common pathway (C3 to C9) activation by bacteria is intact[55] as is the ability of CF serum to generate C5a-related chemotactic factor when the alternate pathway is activated by zymosan.[56] A recent more extensive study supported a variety of functional abnormalities of the alternate pathway in a majority of CF patients studied with little evidence of classical pathway abnormalities. This study suggested the presence of serum inhibitors of alternate pathway function.[57] At present it is unclear whether these alternate pathway abnormalities are related to pulmonary infection and local pulmonary complement activation,[58] as one might expect, or represent a systemic disorder.

Phagocytosis The major cellular components of nonspecific systemic immunity are the peripheral blood granulocytes and monocytes.[59] The latter mature into tissue macrophages, where they acquire quite different structural and functional characteristics.[60] The functional capacity of peripheral blood CF granulocytes and monocytes has been assessed by several methods. The nitroblue tetrazolium (NBT) dye reduction test measures intracellular killing indirectly through assessment of the phagocytic cells' capacity to generate a metabolic burst spontaneously or during ingestion of latex or other particles. Increased hexose monophosphate shunt activity, oxygen consumption, and H_2O_2 and superoxide radical formation are involved in this metabolic burst. NBT reduction is normal or increased in CF patients, depending on infective status.[61-63]

Normal chemotactic responses to a variety of chemotactic factors, including zymosan-activated serum (which generates C5a by the alternate pathway), filtrates of bacteria, and lymphokine chemotaxins have been demonstrated in CF neutrophils and monocytes.[28,56,63] Acutely infected patients have normal or increased peripheral phagocytic chemotactic responsiveness.[63,64] Systemic phagocytosis in general, and NBT dye reduction in particular, seem normal or increased in acutely ill patients,[63,65,66] although one report found decreased CF granulocyte phagocytosis of *Staphylococcus aureus* despite normal NBT reduction,[61] and another found phagocytic deficiencies in some patients with a variety of chronic pulmonary infections, including CF, despite normal granulocyte enzyme activities and no evidence of serum inhibitors.[20] Finally, it should be noted that CF serum usually supports blood granulocyte phagocytosis of *Pseudomonas aeruginosa* as well as normal serum; this opsonic capacity diminishes or disappears when alveolar macrophages are employed as the phagocytic cell, as discussed more fully below in the section on immunodeficiency.[67]

PULMONARY IMMUNITY IN CYSTIC FIBROSIS

The primary function of the lung is gas exchange. However, recognition and the elimination of particles, toxins, and microbes at this huge delicate interface of body and world are essential to this function and are elaborately provided for by a network of mechanisms that in effect make the lung a complex and semiautonomous organ of immunity. The major components of this network have been slowly, and in many cases only recently, elucidated in studies going back to the earliest years of this century. Table 10-3 summarily lists these lung defense mechanisms; interested readers are referred to excellent recent reviews of respiratory immunology by Kaltreider,[68] Newhouse et al,[69] Green et al [70] and Brain et al.[71] In this section we shall consider pulmonary immunity as it relates to cystic fibrosis. To date, there is a dearth of information for most items on the list in Table 10-3 that is grossly disproportionate to the tremendous importance of pulmonary pathology in the natural history of cystic fibrosis.

Nonspecific Immunity

Impaction of particles, including microbes dispersed in droplets, on the nares, posterior pharynx, and carina prevents particles larger than 10–15 μm from entering the bronchi; most particles of 2–5 μm are deposited on the

Table 10-3
Defense Mechanisms of Respiratory Tract

- Nonspecific
  - Aerodynamic filtration
    - Impaction
    - Sedimentation
  - Airway reflexes
    - Cough
    - Bronchoconstriction
  - Mucociliary transport
    - Mucus blanket
    - Cilia
  - Soluble factors
    - Antiproteases
    - Complement
    - Lysozyme
    - Lactoferrin
    - Alveolar lining material
  - Cellular factors
    - Alveolar macrophage
    - Other: polymorphonuclear leukocyte, eosinophil, mast cell
- Specific
  - Humoral: Secretory IgA, IgG, IgE, ?IgM, ?IgD
  - Cellular: Lymphocytes

mucus blanket by sedimentation as velocity drops toward zero. Probably over 90% of particles greater than 2 μm thus do not reach the alveoli. The normal mucociliary blanket will remove these particles within an hour after deposition. Soluble antigens may be absorbed across the mucosal surface where they are likely to first encounter lymphoid cells in or below the epithelium. Particles less than 2–3 μm that penetrate beyond the bronchoalveolar junction (ie, to the respiratory bronchioles and alveoli) may be transported through lymphatic channels in a complex fashion over a period of one to over 100 days; but most substances reaching the alveoli are quickly detoxified in situ by alveolar macrophage phagocytosis. Alveolar macrophages, activated by this process, become potent secretory cells capable of recruiting inflammatory cells as well as carrying out their phagocytic function. Alveolar macrophage function, in turn, appears heavily dependent upon numerous soluble factors in the microenvironment, including alveolar lining material and specific and nonspecific opsonins (immunoglobulins and complement activation products). In addition, alveolar macrophages may leave the alveoli via the mucociliary transport system or migrate through lymphatic channels to regional lymph nodes where interactions with elements of the specific immune system may occur.

Clearly, something goes wrong—very wrong— very early in the course of cystic fibrosis which allows microorganisms to colonize the respiratory tract. Investigation of pulmonary immunity in CF is complicated by the need to determine, first, the initial defect or defects which allow colonization, and second, to discern the consequent changes which often interact with and compound each other. Because colonization occurs so early, usually within the first weeks or months of life,[72] separating causal from secondary changes is an extremely difficult, perhaps impossible, task. Virtually all of the work done to date suffers from this deficiency.

The classic hypothesis that a primary physicochemical abnormality of CF mucus is the basis for and precedes colonization and clinical respiratory infection must be seriously questioned in light of recent data on biochemical and rheologic properties of CF mucus which show no very early, or later disease-specific, changes. Although a molecular abnormality in mucus that alters the microenvironment significantly enough to cause selective binding and growth of certain bacteria such as *Staphylococcus aureus* and mucoid *Pseudomonas aeruginosa* is still a reasonable hypothesis for the origin of the respiratory infection, a gross primary change in mucus seems unlikely.[72-75] Thus, the catechism "obstruction of airways by thick tenacious CF mucus leads to infection" must be rigorously questioned. We must look at all aspects of pulmonary defense while continuing the analysis of CF mucus glycoprotein structure, state of hydration, ionic composition, and so on (See Chapter 6).

Lymphoid Tissue

Lymphoid tissue is found throughout the lung, organized in three structural levels: tracheobronchial and hilar lymph nodes, lymphoid nodules lacking capsules in the walls of the large and medium sized bronchi, and lymphoid aggregates and infiltrates distributed diffusely throughout peripheral lung tissue. The aggregates include specialized "lymphoepithelial organs" in the respiratory bronchioles which may act as primary antigen-intake points.[68] Until relatively recently, biopsy or autopsy specimens were the only method of assessing the structure and, to some extent the function, of lymphoid tissue in the lung. The advent of fiberoptic bronchoscopy in the last decade opened a new era in analysis of both cellular and acellular elements of the lower respiratory tract which has yielded invaluable insights into normal pulmonary immunity and the aberrations occurring across a broad spectrum of pulmonary disease.[76] Since the time the conventional histopathologic studies discussed immediately below were done, information relating to cellular elements of CF pulmonary immunity has become available by the use of such bronchoalveolar lavage techniques. Data on the acellular elements of the respiratory tract, on the other hand, are also available from studies of expectorated sputum due to the greater stability of at least some of these components in the harsh milieu of CF respiratory secretion.[77]

Martinez-Tello et al[78] studied autopsy lung tissue from subjects with a variety of bronchopulmonary diseases, including five cases of cystic fibrosis, and compared them to normal controls in regard to number of B cells and plasma cells reacting with fluoresceinated antisera to IgG, IgA, and IgM. Elevated numbers of cells staining for IgG and IgA were found in the interstitium and lymph nodes in the CF specimens, with a relatively greater increase in IgA-secreting cells in the interstitium and IgG-secreting cells in the nodes.

More recently, bronchoalveolar lavage studies of CF patients have been conducted. Normally, a lavage of 100 ml saline returns about half the volume, containing 5–10 $\times$ 10^6 cells, of which over 90% are alveolar macrophages, 5–10% are lymphocytes, and less than 1% are polymorphonuclear leukocytes.[76] In CF, a huge increase in the cell content to a mean of 3 $\times$ 10^6 cells/ml occurs, with about 70% of the cells being polymorphonuclear leukocytes, 20% alveolar macrophages, and 10% lymphocytes.[79,80] A greater proportion than normal of the cells are nonviable. As in normal peripheral blood and in normal lung lavage, a majority of the lymphocytes are T cells.[80]

These cellular changes are similar to those found in patients with other nontuberculous pulmonary infections.[81] There appears to be a correlation between clinical deterioration and the increase in the polymorphonuclear leukocyte-to-alveolar macrophage ratio.[82] To date, no studies of pulmonary T-cell function in CF have been done. The immunofluorescent data[78] suggest that the systemic hypergammaglobulinemia of the G and A classes in CF may be a reflection of increased pulmonary immunoglobulin secretion. A direct analysis of lavage fluid in comparison to serum for immunoglobulin content in cystic fibrosis patients and controls revealed a more complicated picture. Total immunoglobulin content of CF lavage fluid was increased approximately 40% over controls, but this increase was due to a rise in the level of secretory IgA, with IgG, IgM, and IgD levels not significantly higher than controls. In contrast, the rise of total immunoglobulin content of CF over normal serum was attributable to an increase in IgG.[83] One possible synthesis of these data is that the increased immunoglobulin found in CF lavage fluid originates from submucosal cells which are primarily secreting IgA, while the increased immunoglobulin found in serum originates in the regional lung lymph nodes, which contain primarily IgG-secreting cells.

Alveolar Macrophages

Alveolar macrophages obtained by bronchoalveolar lavage from CF and control lungs have been studied for morphology and phagocytic function. Ultrastructure, assessed by electron microscopy, reveals no differences between CF and normal alveolar macrophages; curiously, the CF alveolar macrophage seems, by this analysis, not to be activated or actively engaged in phagocytosis as would be expected.[82] The phagocytic function of the CF alveolar macrophage appears to be normal.[81,82,84] An apparently selective inhibition of both CF and normal alveolar macrophage phagocytosis of *Pseudomonas aeruginosa* by CF serum has been reported and is discussed separately in the section on immunodeficiency below.

The phagocytic function of the enormous numbers of polymorphonuclear leukocytes recruited to CF lungs and obtainable by bronchoalveolar lavage is preserved.[81,82]

Mucociliary Transport

Mucociliary transport (MT) is a major respiratory defense mechanism for removal of inhaled particulates, including microorganisms. It represents the net interaction of ciliary function and the viscoelastic properties of the overlying mucus.[85] There is a good deal of confusion in the literature regarding MT in CF, with some authoritative reviews concluding that it is defective[86] and others that it is normal.[75] Because of the variety of techniques used to measure MT, comparison of data is difficult. However, the only study finding uniformly slowed MT in CF, which visually measured movement of 0.6-mm Teflon disks across tracheal mucosa, may have had the results influenced by the technique, which included lidocaine anesthesia and possible local trauma from bronchoscopy. Other studies of MT in CF, most of which employed scintography of radioactively labeled particles on nasal or tracheobronchial mucosa, either found MT rates comparable to normal or reduced in proportion to the severity of underlying lung disease.[87-91] Ciliary structure and function appear to be normal unless secondarily and nonspecifically injured by advanced lung disease.[92,93]

Some have speculated that the well-known in vitro dyskinetic effect of homozygote and heterozygote CF serum on ciliated epithelium is operative in vivo and significant in the pathogenesis of pulmonary disease. The studies cited above, in addition to the obvious lack of effect in obligate heterozygotes, suggest this is not the case. A possible explanation for the discrepancy between in vitro bioassays and the in vivo situation with regard to the effect of CF serum was provided by the studies of Rossman and co-workers. They hypothesized that if CF serum factors are operative in the disease in vivo and MT is normal in stable CF, then CF serum must exert an effect only intermittently, most likely during episodes of increased inflammation when serum-derived molecules would have enhanced access to mucosal surfaces. They confirmed this hypothesis by showing that while CF serum had no effect on nasal MT in normal or CF subjects, pretreatment of the nasal mucosa with anti-IgE followed by local application of CF serum resulted in slowed MT in both normal and CF subjects. Thus, a requirement for prior inflammatory changes in the mucosa for the CF serum effect to be exerted was found. This effect of CF serum was also present (and more strikingly so) when isolated ciliary dyskinesia factor was used instead of whole CF serum.[89,94]

One may tentatively conclude that defective MT in CF is not a uniform primary aspect of the disease. When present, defective MT probably represents one of the myriad secondary effects of established respiratory disease in CF and may represent an effect of ciliary dyskinesia factors in CF serum operating in a mucosal microenvironment of inflammatory injury.

Pulmonary Humoral Immunity

Precipitating IgG antibodies are readily demonstrated in CF sputum against a variety of microbial, dietary, and autoantigens.[6,46,95] Sputum IgA and IgG antibodies to respiratory pathogens such as *Pseudomonas aeruginosa, Staphylococcus aureus,* and *Hemophilus influenzae* are ubiquitous in colonized patients. It is interesting to note that sputum IgA antibody titers are generally higher than sputum IgG antibody to the same antigen and sometimes higher than corresponding serum IgA titers, while IgG antibody titers are higher in serum than sputum.[4,96-99] These findings are consistent with the distribution of secretory cells, with greater numbers of IgA-secreting cells in the bronchial submucosa and IgG-secreting cells in the regional lung lymph nodes. The origin of the IgG antibody in bronchial fluid is unknown, but it seems reasonable to suspect the local nodes as the likely major source with arrival in the secretions via transudation of serum, and a variable fraction probably originating from IgG-secreting cells in the submucosa.[78]

The secretory IgA system is discussed separately in the immmunodeficiency section of this chapter.

Immunity to *Pseudomonas aeruginosa* In the preantibiotic era *Staphylococcus aureus* was the main respiratory pathogen in CF. Since then, there is little doubt that *Pseudomonas aeruginosa,* particularly in its atypical mucoid form, has become the major pathogen in the disease. This conclusion is based less upon the dramatic historical shift in the bacteriology of respiratory tract colonization to dominance by *Pseudomonas aeruginosa,*[100–105] which could merely reflect successful antistaphylococcal antibiotic therapy and the emergence of *Pseudomonas* as a benign opportunistic colonizer of damaged lungs, than upon the tremendous humoral immune response to *Pseudomonas,* a sine qua non of chronic infection, and the close relationship between mucoid *Pseudomonas* infection and poor clinical status and prognosis.[4,12,49,106–112]

Nevertheless, doubts about the pathogenicity of *Pseudomonas* in CF have persisted. These have been based upon the old question of the selection pressure of antistaphylococcal antibiotic therapy, the persistence of *Pseudomonas* colonization during and after acute exacerbations of pulmonary disease despite intravenous anti-*Pseudomonas* antibiotic therapy, and the impossibility of assuring specificity of presumptive anti-*Pseudomonas* therapy.[113,114] These doubts are certainly open to theoretical criticism and have been rebutted by studies linking *Pseudomonas* antibody responses to acute exacerbations of lung disease and by controlled studies of anti-*Pseudomonas* antimicrobial therapy.[14,115,116]

An understanding of normal immunity to *Pseudomonas* is a prerequisite to comprehending and combating *Pseudomonas* infection in CF. A breakthrough in this area, either in terms of antibiotic therapy or interruption of the pathogenetic sequence of infection, could revolutionize the clinical course of the disease.

A consideration of virulence factors associated with *Pseudomonas* is beyond the scope of this chapter. Suffice it to say that the basis for pathogenicity of *Pseudomonas aeruginosa* remains controversial, with much work in animals to implicate a wide variety of possible independent, additive, or synergistic elements including the following: cell-wall lipopolysaccharide, exotoxins, proteases, cellular pili (fimbriae), extracellular slime, phospholipase C, enterotoxin, and mucoid microcolony formation.[117–121] Human in vivo immune-response data provide suggestive evidence of pathogenicity for *Pseudomonas* lipopolysaccharide, exotoxin A, and several proteases.[122–125]

Systemic and pulmonary immunity to *Pseudomonas* show some important differences, yet similar underlying mechanisms. Systemic immunity requires polymorphonuclear leukocytes and is optimal when the organism is opsonized by specific antibody and complement.[126] IgM and IgG antibodies to cell-wall lipopolysaccharide are the chief immune opsonins.[127,128] Nonimmune opsonization of *Pseudomonas* by elements of the complement system, especially the alternate pathway, also occurs.[129,130] Direct activation of the alternate complement pathway by *Pseudomonas* extracellular slime glycoprotein has recently been demonstrated.[131]

Pulmonary immunity to *Pseudomonas* is adapted to key changes in compartmental defenses: the alveolar macrophage is the major phagocyte; there is virtually no IgM present in the normal lung while secretory IgA assumes an important role in humoral immunity; and complement components, while present, are in short and perhaps marginal supply.[132,133] The studies of Reynolds and co-workers have shown that pulmonary challenge with *Pseudomonas* results in a significant secretory IgA response in bronchial fluid which has specific agglutinative and inhibitory growth effects, along with an IgG response;[134] the local IgG response, however, provided superior opsonic activity for alveolar macrophages.[135,136] In addition, short-term T-cell activation occurs with lymphokine production detectable in bronchial lavage fluid.[137]

Recent investigations in animal models suggest that pulmonary and systemic immunity are in fact closely related in host defense against *Pseudomonas* respiratory infection. Parenteral vaccination of guinea pigs with *Pseudomonas* lipopolysaccharide results in killing of *Pseudomonas* in infected lungs, an effect due in major part to serum IgM antibodies which diffuse into bronchial fluids early in the course of acute inflammation and efficiently opsonize *Pseudomonas* for alveolar macrophages.[138] Deposition of *Pseudomonas* in mice lungs results in two-fold

fold greater growth of organisms when the animal is depleted of complement.[139] An even more dramatic increase to five times baseline levels is seen when the mice are rendered granulocytopenic.[140] Thus, intact immunity to *Pseudomonas* in the lung seems to include elements unique to local immunity (secretory IgA, alveolar macrophages) and key elements of systemic immunity (IgM, IgG, complement, neutrophils). The relative importance of these factors singly and in various combinations in the normal subject and CF patients has yet to be established.

It is also well worth pointing out that pulmonary immunity is very much dependent on the organism involved. For example, *Staphylococcus aureus*, another bacteria of great interest in CF, is efficiently phagocytosed by normal human alveolar macrophages in the absence of antibody or complement opsonins.[141] This ability was found to be dependent upon the expression of protein A on the cell wall of the staphylococcal strain. Staphylococcal protein A binds nonspecifically to the Fc region of IgG molecules, which in turn are found coating the surfaces of human alveolar macrophages as cytophilic antibodies.[142] Thus, different species of bacteria, and indeed different strains within a single species, can interact in quite different ways with the immune system.

A most interesting line of investigation has been pursued by Woods and co-workers. Building upon work showing that the ability of *Pseudomonas* to colonize the respiratory tract is correlated with the organism's ability to adhere to upper respiratory epithelial cells, they showed markedly increased adherence of *Pseudomonas aeruginosa* to CF buccal epithelial cells compared to controls. This increase correlated inversely with the amount of cell-surface fibronectin and directly with salivary proteases. They speculated that increased protease activity in CF respiratory secretions could lead to the measured loss of fibronectin.[143] Treatment of normal buccal cells with trypsin, which reduces surface fibronectin, results in increased bacterial adherence.[144] Fibronectin, a glycoprotein of about 400,000 mol wt, is found in plasma, connective tissue, and basement membranes, as well as on cell surfaces, and plays a major role in cell-cell and cell-connective tissue matrix interactions. Among the cells secreting it are lung fibroblasts and alveolar macrophages, and it is normally present in bronchial secretions.[145] The discovery of its possible role in prevention of bacterial adherence to respiratory tract epithelial cells represents a potentially key finding in the earliest stages of CF lung disease.

Other humoral factors The bronchial fluid is composed of 95% water to which is added an assortment of both locally produced and plasma-derived factors (Table 10-4). When mixed with upper respiratory secretion and saliva and expectorated, it is termed sputum. Although normal individuals may produce 100–350 ml of sputum a day, this does not lead to productive cough. Extensive studies of sputum or lavage fluid in CF have revealed numerous differences from normal stimulated mucus, but thus far no differences unique to CF in comparison with other chronic infective lung diseases have been found (See Chapter 6).

Lopez-Vidriero and Reid[146] make the important point that CF sputum must be compared to control sputum with similar degrees of purulence. When this is done, mucoid CF sputum (that is, less purulent sputum from the most mildly affected patients) is not more viscous than sputum from other diseases such as chronic bronchitis, asthma, and bronchiectasis. As CF sputum becomes more purulent, the DNA content becomes higher, and ultimately greater than in any of the other diseases. This striking increase appears mainly due to decomposition of leukocytes which have migrated in high numbers into the airway.[147] Mucoid CF sputum also appears to contain a greater serum component fraction in relation to locally produced components (as measured by serum and local glycoprotein markers) than the other diseases.[146]

Using crossed immunoelectrophoresis to quantitate soluble proteins in sputum, Brogan and co-workers[148] were able to distinguish two groups of CF patients. The first group

Table 10-4
Constituents of Bronchial Fluid and Their Origins*

Origin	Constituent
Airway epithelium (serous and mucous cells); Submucosal glands (mucous and serous cells)	Epithelial glycoprotein
Mucous cells (submucosal glands)	Secretory piece
Serous cells (submucosal glands)	Lactoferrin Lysozyme
Plasma component	Albumin Plasma glycoproteins: IgA (7S), IgG, IgM, IgE, α_1 acid glycoprotein, haptoglobin, β_1A globulin, β_2 globulin, α_2HS glycoprotein, hemopexin, α_1 antitrypsin, α_1 antichymotrypsin, α_2 macroglobulin, prealbumin, transferrin Electrolytes Water
Plasma cells	Immunoglobulins
Mast cells	Histamine Serotonin SRS-A,[†] etc
Type II pneumocyte	Alveolar surfactant

*From Lopez-Vidriero MT, Reid L: Bronchial mucous in health and disease. *Br Med Bull* 1978;34:63–74,[74] by permission of the British Council.
†SRS-A: slowly reactive substance of anaphylaxis.

had low levels of albumin, a plasma transudate, in sputum. Their sputum resembled sputum from patients with chronic bronchitis except for higher α_1-antitrypsin and somewhat lower IgA. The second CF group had high levels of albumin in sputum and resembled sputum from patients with acute asthma, who also showed increased transudation of plasma components, except for higher IgG levels in the CF patients. Secretory proteins with antimicrobial activity such as lactoferrin and lysozyme were present in CF sputum at levels similar to those in sputum from patients with asthma or bronchitis. Antiproteases such as α_1-antitrypsin and α_1-antichymotrypsin were also present at comparable or higher levels. These results have been confirmed.[149]

Use of bronchoalveolar lavage, which eliminates the problem of the mixing of lower and upper respiratory tract fluids, has produced very similar results. Spock and coworkers have shown that local pulmonary synthesis of the plasma proteins IgG, IgA, C3, C4, and transferrin also occurs.[150] When compared to normal, CF bronchial fluid showed increased immunoglobulin content attributable to secretory IgA, the presence of normally excluded large plasma proteins such as β_1-lipoprotein and α_2-macroglobulin, and relative reductions in transferrin, α_1-antitrypsin, and C4. Of note, levels of IgE and C-reactive protein exceeded levels in matched serum.[151] Histamine, bradykinin, and prostaglandin were also detected.[80] These findings of increased IgE, presence of mediators of immediate hypersensitivity, and evidence of increased capillary permeability are consonant with sputum studies showing IgE immunoglobulin and specific IgE antibodies and constituents of slow-reacting substance of anaphylaxis (leukotrienes D and B) in CF sputum.[152–154] CF lavage fluid also shows marked reduction of a low-molecular-weight protease inhibitor thought to provide 90% of the inhibitory activity of bronchial secretions.[155] Conversely, the proteolytic activity of CF bronchoalveolar lavage fluid is increased, but it is not known if this activity is due to endogenous or bacterial proteases or both.[156]

IMMUNODEFICIENCY

We have seen that the usual tests of global immunity reveal no major defects in patients with cystic fibrosis. Yet the major cause of morbidity and mortality in the disease, progressive pulmonary insufficiency, is primarily a result of chronic colonization of lung with a few restricted types of microorganisms, which manifests itself as chronic bronchitis and bronchiectasis with clear clinical exacerbations or frank bronchopneumonias. How do we reconcile apparently intact host defenses with this relentless infection?

The tools to answer this all-important question have only recently been added to the investigator's analytic weaponry. As our sophistication about the structure and function of the immune system grows, and the means to gain further knowledge become available, we are able to appreciate more subtle and compartmentalized defects that have gone undetected in the past. The key to colonization and chronic pulmonary infection may well be found in these areas.

Opsonic Deficiency

In 1971 Biggar et al[67] reported that the sera of six out of nine children with CF failed to support normal phagocytosis of *Pseudomonas aeruginosa* by rabbit alveolar macrophages. Normal peripheral blood polymorphonuclear leukocytes, in contrast, showed normal phagocytosis of *Pseudomonas* in the presence of the same CF serum. An opsonic deficiency was suggested by an improvement in alveolar macrophage phagocytosis of *Pseudomonas* when the cystic fibrosis serum was concentrated. A similar deficiency was noted in patients with hypogammoglobulinemia or selective IgA deficiency, or when normal serum was heated at 56°C for 30 minutes, or when the serum was decomplemented. However, none of the CF patients had subnormal immunoglobulin or hemolytic complement levels. Thus the implication of this study was that most CF serum lacked a component or components, possibly complement or immunoglobulin in nature, required for normal alveolar macrophage phagocytosis of *Pseudomonas aeruginosa.*

A second study by Boxerbaum et al[65] found similar results, in that CF serum was inferior to normal serum in supporting rabbit alveolar macrophage uptake and killing of *Pseudomonas aeruginosa*. No impairment was found when *Staphylococcus aureus* or *Serratia maracescens* were employed as phagocytic targets or when blood leukocytes were used as the killer cells. This study also found no impairment when CF heterozygote serum was used. Stored, frozen, or heated CF serum behaved normally, suggesting a labile inhibitor rather than a serum deficiency as the basis for the abnormality. These results were brought closer to the human in vivo conditions when the experiments were repeated in the same laboratory using human alveolar macrophages and a large number of CF serum samples. Of 49 CF patient serum samples, 46 inhibited alveolar macrophage phagocytosis of *Pseudomonas*, an effect that could be eventually overcome by serially diluting CF into normal serum but not by simple 1:1 mixing of CF and normal serum. In contrast to their earlier paper, the authors now found the inhibitory activity survived freezing and heating. The effect seemed to be a result of colonization by *Pseudomonas* in that the few patients with no inhibitory serum activity were not colonized with mucoid *Pseudomonas*, whereas all patients so colonized showed the inhibitory activity. Inhibition did not correlate with agglutinating antibody titers, which are primarily a function of IgM antibody.[84]

It is relevant to note here that mucoid *Pseudomonas aeruginosa* strains isolated from CF patients are usually sensitive to serum bactericidal activity, a process dependent on antibody and an intact complement pathway. Patients in poor condition may lose this serum bactericidal capacity for the autologous (but not heterologous) strain of *Pseudomonas aeruginosa*. Moreover, addition of these patients' serum to normal serum blocks the bactericidal activity against the autologous strain of *Pseudomonas*.[157,158] These inhibitory characteristics closely resemble blocking IgG antibody previously reported in chronic *Pseudomonas aeruginosa* infection.[159]

A decisive advance in the understanding of the opsonic deficiency of CF serum for *Pseudomonas aeruginosa* has been made by Fick and co-workers. They utilized the principle of affinity chromotography to design an immunoadsorbent gel to extract IgG antibodies specific for *Pseudomonas* lipopolysaccharide so that functional studies of isolated, purified *Pseudomonas*-specific IgG antibodies could be done.[160] In an elegant comparison of serum from CF patients with serum from patients with other chronic lung diseases, and with normal volunteers and patients with hematologic malignancies who had been immunized with *Pseudomonas* lipopolysaccharide vaccine, it was found that the CF antibody at equivalent agglutinating titers failed to support, and in fact somewhat inhibited, the uptake and killing of *Pseudomonas aeruginosa* by normal human alveolar macrophages. The CF antibodies did not appear complexed to antigen when analyzed by sucrose density gradient ultracentrifugation and appeared to qualitatively contain all four IgG subclasses. The antibody combining site—the Fab portion of the IgG molecule—showed a high affinity for *Pseudomonas*, whereas the antibody attachment site to the alveolar macrophage surface—the Fc portion of the IgG molecule—appeared to be defective.[161] Since the carbohydrate moieties of immunoglobulins are found exclusively in this region of the molecule, it is intriguing to speculate that a genetic defect in the biosynthesis of glycoproteins could manifest itself as such an immune deficiency. Prior to colonization, CF serum might then function as well as normal serum utilizing nonspecific serum bactericidal factors, but then induction of the strong IgG response would give rise to an apparent inhibitory activity as a result of its blocking activity in macrophage opsonization. The apparent restriction of this deficiency to *Pseudomonas aeruginosa* remains entirely unexplained. Teleologically, one could argue that such a preexisting defect woud exert strong selection pressure on this organism to colonize the CF lung.

Nor is the restriction of defective IgG-phagocytic interaction to alveolar macrophages, as opposed to peripheral blood leukocytes, explained. As this defect has now been demonstrated in at least three mammalian species—rat, rabbit, and man[84,162]—it seems clear that the physical, biochemical, and functional heterogeneity of phagocyte populations from different sites plays an important role in the opsonic defect.[163,164] Several lines of evidence suggest, however, that the major defect is in the immunoglobulin rather than the macrophage. First, as discussed in the preceding section, CF alveolar macrophages appear normal morphologically and functionally, although they do not appear to be activated as would normally occur in the presence of antigenic stimulation.[81,82] Activated macrophages are resistant to the inhibitory effect of CF serum.[165] Second, the restriction of the opsonic defect to *Pseudomonas* strongly mitigates against an abnormality in a nonspecific effector of host defense such as phagocytic capability and implicates a specific effector such as antibody. Third, studies which employ binding to lectin probes suggest a structural change in CF immunoglobulins, although conflicting results have been obtained.[166,167]

Clearly, more exacting work on the molecular structure, the class and subclass specificity, and the functional capacity of CF immunoglobulins is warranted, perhaps within the context of a unifying defect in glycoprotein metabolism.

Cellular Immunity to *Pseudomonas aeruginosa*

Although global cell-mediated immunity appears intact in cystic fibrosis, antigen-specific defects have been reported by Sorenson and co-workers. Using gentamicin-killed whole bacteria as antigens and culturing peripheral blood mononuclear cells in autologous plasma, they found a specific impairment of lymphocyte proliferative responses to *Pseudomonas aeruginosa* in CF patients with advanced disease.[25] Lymphocyte responses to antigens of gram-positive bacteria or mitogens were normal, but the defect extended to other gram-negative bacteria such as *Klebsiella pneumonia* or *E. coli.*[9,168] CF patients in good condition had supranormal responses. Incubation in normal plasma had a variable effect on lymphocytes from CF patients with defective responses. In some cases improvement of responsiveness was noted, whereas in other cases none was seen. These results suggested a specific acquired defect in cell-mediated immunity to *Pseudomonas aeruginosa* and other gram-negative organisms in cystic fibrosis.[25,169] When cystic fibrosis siblings were studied, the sibling in poorer condition invariably had poorer lymphocyte responses to *Pseudomonas* which were not correctable by normal plasma or plasma from the sibling in better condition.[170]

At present it is not clear whether the defect is at the cellular level or involves plasma factors which may adhere to lymphocytes tenaciously.[169] The possibility that humoral factors mediate this defect seems more likely in light of the demonstrable reversibility of the defect, as some patients with low lymphocyte responsiveness to *Pseudomonas* show dramatic improvement of that response after hospitalization and intensive treatment of exacerbation.[171] It is possible that humoral factors could modulate lymphocyte subpopulations and thereby indirectly mediate this defect.[30]

Further work on lymphokine production by CF lymphocytes and the interaction of antigen, antibody, immune complexes, and other humoral factors with normal and CF lymphocytes should help clarify the cause of this defect. For example, it is known that different antigens from *Pseudomonas aeruginosa* produce greatly different effects on human mononuclear cell preparations in vitro.[172,173] The dosage of the selected antigen employed in the in vitro experiment is also a critical determinant of the measured response.[174] Thus, much work needs to be done in defining the conditions for optimal and uniform responsiveness of lymphocytes to well-defined antigens before the complex questions of mechanisms can be addressed.

Secretory IgA

Secretory IgA plays a central role in mucosal immunity. The secretory IgA molecule is assembled in mucosal serous epithelial cells from precursors manufactured by two cell types. The immunoglobulin light and heavy chains and a third polypeptide, the J chain, are synthesized and secreted by plasma cells in the lamina propria of the bronchial and intestinal mucosa. The molecules of IgA are secreted primarily as dimers. These dimeric IgA immunoglobulins then bind to secretory component, a glycoprotein synthesized by serous epithelial cells, present probably as IgA receptors on the basal and lateral surfaces of the epithelial cells. The IgA-secretory component molecule is then endocytosed, transported across the epithelial cytoplasm in vesicles, and discharged onto the luminal surface.[175] IgA-secreting plasma cells and secretory component have been shown to be present in normal or increased amounts in CF patients in saliva, bronchial mucosa, and intestinal mucosa.[78,176–178]

Some provocative aspects of secretory IgA metabolism in CF have been presented. An early and increased stimulus to produce IgA immunoglobulin was suggested by the detection of IgA in CF but not control meconium[179] and by increased IgA synthesis by intestinal biopsies from CF patients as compared to patients with hereditary pancreatitis and controls.[178] The increased mucosal antigenic stimulus was confirmed by Hoiby and Hertz,[180] who showed increased serum precipitins to intestinal flora in CF patients. These results collectively implicate a supranormal mucosal antigenic entry in CF patients. If current concepts of secretory IgA function as primarily one of immune exclusion are correct, the implication is that there are prominent cracks in the "antiseptic paint" coating the mucosa of CF patients.

Some data in this regard have been presented by Wallwork and McFarlane.[181] In this study 7 of 22 CF saliva specimens lacked free secretory component, and 3 of those 7 specimens also lacked IgA. Free J chain was detected in CF sputum. Salivary secretory component in CF was immunochemically and electrophoretically altered. Free secretory component was found in an increased proportion of CF sera. This array of abnormalities suggests a derangement in the complex secretory IgA system. These results have not been confirmed. Further studies of IgA production by mucosal plasmacytes, secretory component production by epithelial cells, secretion of secretory IgA onto mucosal surfaces, and its biological function in CF are mandatory. The colonization of the lower respiratory tract in CF may be dependent on a functional deficiency of secretory IgA, which is known to play a crucial role in prevention of bacterial adherence to epithelial surfaces.[182] A defect in glycoprotein synthesis affecting immunoglobulin and/or secretory component function provides a possible underlying mechanism for involvement of the secretory IgA system in the overall pathophysiology of cystic fibrosis and seems a fruitful area for future investigation. An alternate or supplemental hypothesis is that damage to respiratory epithelium secondarily affects the assembly and secretion of intact, functional secretory IgA, leading to acceleration of the disease process.

HYPERSENSITIVITY

In 1905, Clemens Von Pirquet and Bela Shick noted the development of precipitating antibodies to horse serum proteins in individuals with horse serum sickness. From these observations, the term allergy was coined by Von Pirquet in 1906 to describe the state of acquired altered reactivity mediated by the immune system. This concept of deleterious altered immune reactivity has proved to be of enduring usefulness. With the subsequent growth in understanding of the immune response, the balance between host defenses and environmental challenges was seen to tilt now towards one side—insufficiency—and now towards the other side—hypersensitivity. In Von Pirquet's original language either could be considered "allergy," but the contemporary usage refers exclusively to a state of abnormally heightened responsiveness, and the term immunodeficiency has been applied to insufficient responsiveness. In recent years, the term allergy has increasingly been further restricted to one particular type of reaction discussed below as immediate hypersensitivity. Individuals possessing this type of hypersensitivity have been termed atopic.

In 1963, Gell and Coombs organized the mechanisms of hypersensitivity into four broad categories (Table 10-5). These categories have gained universal acceptance as tools for investigation and understanding of hypersensitivity phenomena, despite our awareness of extensive interactions and interdependencies of these conceptually discrete processes.[183] Since all types of hypersensitivity have been reported in cystic fibrosis, a brief discussion of each will be presented prior to a review of their role in the disease. Interested readers are referred to excellent reviews by Coombs and Gell,[184] Roitt,[185] and Wells.[186]

Mechanisms of Hypersensitivity

Type I—immediate hypersensitivity Immediate hypersensitivity, also termed anaphylactic or reaginic hypersensitivity, is a consequence of the release of a number of potent mediators from tissue mast cells and, to a lesser extent, blood basophils (Table 10-6). These cells have the unique ability to fix reaginic antibody to their cell membranes. The major reaginic immunoglobulin class in man is IgE, which is normally produced in extremely minute amounts, but in 10–20% of the population is produced in substantially greater (although still quite small) quantities. This genetic predisposition to produce IgE upon allergenic stimulation is the basis of the atopic state which underlies clinical allergy or type I hypersensitivity. It is also clear that under certain conditions some types of IgG antibody can act as reagins in

Table 10-5
Gell and Coombs Classification of Hypersensitivity Reactions

Type	Names Commonly Used	Antibody	Skin Test	Well-known Clinical Examples	Comment
I	Anaphylactic, reaginic, immediate	Primarily IgE; occasionally IgG (? IgG_4)	Immediate-type (10–30 min)	Pollen rhinitis; anaphylaxis; allergic asthma	Mediators released from reagin-sensitized mast cells produce tissue response
II	Cytotoxic Antibody	IgG or IgM	—	Transfusion reactions; hemolytic disease of newborn	May or may not involve complement or immune effector cells
III	Immune complexes, arthus type	IgG, sometimes IgM, ? other Ig	Arthus type: onset 3–8 hr, maximal 24 hr.	Serum sickness; lupus nephritis; rheumatoid vasculitis	Tissue damage dependent on complement and polymorphonuclear leukocytes
IV	Delayed, cell-mediated, tuberculin	Sensitized lymphocyte, no antibody requirement	Tuberculin type: onset 24–48 hr, maximal 48–72 hr	Tuberculin skin test; contact dermatitis (poison ivy, oak)	Mediators (lymphokines) released from antigen-sensitized lymphocytes produce tissue damage, mainly via recruitment of immune effector cells

man.[187] After synthesis in response to antigenic stimulation of IgE-producing lymphocytes, and fixation to mast cells (a process termed homocytotropism), a subsequent contact with an allergen capable of binding two cell-bound reaginic antibody molecules will lead to degranulation of the mast cell and release the mediators responsible for the pathophysiologic and clinical reactions of increased vascular permeability, edema, influx of inflammatory cells, and smooth muscle contraction.[188]

Type II – cytotoxic antibody When IgG or IgM antibody is produced to a cell-surface or cell-attached antigen, injury to the cell can occur through a variety of mechanisms. For example, the antibody can be directly cytotoxic through its ability to activate the complement cascade, which may result in cell lysis as well as recruitment of inflammatory

Table 10-6
Currently Recognized Mediators of Anaphylaxis*

Preformed mediators rapidly released from the granule		
Mediator	*Actions relevant to allergy*	
Histamine	Increased vascular permeability, pruritus, mucus secretion, prostaglandin synthesis, smooth muscle spasm, eosinophilotaxis, increased cyclic AMP and cyclic GMP	
ECF-A, NCF-A	Polymorphonuclear chemotaxis	
Superoxide	Toxicity, particularly to cell membranes	
Exoglycosidases	Unknown	
Preformed mediators that are slowly released from the granule or remain part of the granule matrix		
Mediator	*Actions relevant to allergy*	
Heparin	Polyanion, may act as absorptive surface, anticoagulant, inhibit complement	
Trypsin-chymotrypsin	Protease, proinflammatory	
Arylsulfatase	Destruction of SRS-A	
Peroxidase	Destruction of SRS-A, generation of singlet oxygen	
Superoxide dismutase	Dismutation of superoxide to hydrogen peroxide	
Inflammatory factor(s)	Generation of late-phase allergic reactions	
Secondarily formed mediators, generated by actions of primary mediators on target tissues		
Mediator	*Stimulant for formation*	*Primary actions*
Prostaglandins, thromboxanes, other arachinoids	Histamine, SRS-A, bradykinin, prostaglandin generating factor (PGF-A)	Many
SRS-A (Leukotriene C and D)	Unknown	Bronchoconstriction, vascular permeability
Bradykinin	Kallikrein of anaphylaxis	Bronchoconstriction, vasodilation
Potential mediators that may participate in allergic reactions		
Mediator	*Actions relevant to allergy*	
Acetylcholine	Bronchospasm, mucus secretion, increased immunologic mediator release, increased cyclic GMP	
Serotonin	Bronchospasm	
PAF (1-*O*-alkyl-2-acetyl-sn-glyceryl-3-phosphorylcholine)	Platelet aggregation and secretion	

*From Kaliner, 1980,[301] with permission.

cells to the area. Another mechanism is through opsonization, whereby the antibody-coated target cell is made an appetizing meal for phagocytes equipped with receptors for the free end of the antibody molecule. Still another mechanism, termed antibody-dependent cell-mediated cytotoxicity, involves killing of the antibody-coated target cell by several types of lymphoreticular cells which bind to the target cell via specific receptors for the free Fc end of the cell-fixed antibody molecule.

Type III – immune complex disease Most IgG and IgM antibodies, when combined with antigen, activate the classical complement cascade through fixation of C1q, which then triggers other complement proteins in sequence to activate and generate a variety of biologic effects (Figure 10-1). Probably the major inflammatory effect is exerted through small activation cleavage fragments of complement proteins C3 and C5, the anaphylatoxins C3a and C5a. Anaphylatoxin breakdown products in turn continue to exert biological effects. The anaphylatoxins and their by-products cause smooth muscle contraction, mast cell degranulation and, most importantly, are extremely potent chemotaxins, attracting predominantly polymorphonuclear leukocytes which not only phagocytose the antigen–antibody complexes but also release a variety of tissue-injuring proteolytic enzymes and products of the oxidative killing system such as superoxide anion and hydroxyl radicals. The fate of immune complexes once formed and their subsequent ability to result in tissue damage depends on a large number of variables such as valence, antigen–antibody ratio, affinity, the physicochemical properties of the antigen and antibody, the functional integrity of the reticuloendothelial clearance system, and interactions with humoral and cellular ligands.[189]

Type IV – cell-mediated (delayed) hypersensitivity The classic tuberculin skin reaction exemplifies this form of hypersensitivity which is mediated by sensitized T lymphocytes. Antigen-specific receptors are present on T cells sensitized by prior exposure to the antigen. On repeat contact with the antigen, which must be processed and presented by a macrophage, the lymphocyte secretes a variety of molecular mediators termed lymphokines. (Table 10-2). Lymphokines produce the effects of the type IV reaction directly or through secondary inflammatory cells in a manner analogous to the mast-cell mediators in the type I reaction.

Immediate (Type I) Hypersensitivity in CF

The earliest studies of allergic sensitivity in cystic fibrosis antedated the discovery of IgE as the major reaginic antibody of man, the development of in vitro assays for detection of IgE antibodies, and the elucidation of the pathophysiology of the type I reaction.[190] Thus, these studies relied on the classical combination of suggestive history, symptoms, and signs to derive a study population for immediate skin testing, which then yielded an overall prevalence of respiratory allergy of approximately 10–15% among CF patients.[191,192] After the advent of the IgE era in allergy, a somewhat higher prevalence of 24% was found when suggestive history was combined with skin testing, but additionally almost half of the "nonallergenic" CF group had elevated total IgE levels.[7] In the last decade many studies have been conducted on unselected CF populations to assess the prevalence of immediate skin test positivity, total IgE levels and, in some cases, the presence of specific IgE antibodies as determined by radioallergosorbent (RAST) testing. Table 10-7 lists the results of 23 such studies which have corrected the selection bias of earlier work and shown the prevalence of type I reactivity to be in the range of 50–75% in cystic fibrosis.

Specificity of allergic sensitization in CF Several of the studies listed in Table 10-7 have included various control groups, including nonaffected siblings, parents, non-CF atopics, subjects with a variety of other respiratory diseases, and healthy persons. These studies indicate that patients with cystic fibrosis have aggregate skin test reaction rates and total IgE levels comparable to

Table 10-7
Prevalence of Allergy (Type I Hypersensitivity) in Unselected CF Groups

Positive Skin Tests (%)	IgE Elevated (%) or Mean IgE	Reference
31/83 (38)*	ND	Mearns et al[193]
16/37 (43)*	ND	McCarthy et al[194]
ND	13/17 (76)	Spitz et al[195]
6/8 (75)	ND	Yohe[5]
ND	13/40 (33)	Wallwork et al[6]
ND	21/37 (57)	Rachelefsky et al[7]
30/43 (70)	ND	Warren et al[8]
23/30 (77)	17/30 (57)	Allan et al[196]
11/18 (61)*	Mean 160 units/ml	Bardana et al[197]
73/123 (59)	ND	Warner et al[198]
ND	11/22 (50)*	Galant et al[199]
20/26 (77)	14/26 (54)	McFarlane et al[152]
43/63 (68)	ND	Warner[200]
21/33 (64)	ND	Barron et al[201]
23/48 (48)	ND	Silverman et al[202]
80/81 (99)	ND	Mitchell et al[203]
17/44 (39)*	7/44 (16)	Carswell et al[204]
21/46 (46)	10/46 (22)	Nelson et al[205]
39/48 (81)	Mean 469 units/ml	Ormerod et al[206]
ND	7/31 (23)	Moss and Lewiston[49]
22/25 (88)	12/25 (46)	Tobin et al[207]
10/12 (83)	Mean 376 units/ml	Harper et al[22]
10/20 (50)	ND	Van Asperen et al[208]
Total 496/788 (63)	125/319 (39)	

**Aspergillus fumigatus* only.

atopic persons without cystic fibrosis (ie, allergic rhinitis, extrinsic asthma, and atopic dermatitis). The striking aspect of immediate hypersensitivity in CF is the distribution of allergen sensitization. When compared to other atopic groups, cystic fibrosis patients have a significant increase in sensitization to molds, especially *Aspergillus fumigatus*. Reaction rates to common allergens seen in atopic individuals—pollens, animal danders, house dust extract, and the house dust mite *Dermatophagoides pteronyssimus*—are of similar or lower frequency in CF than in other atopic groups.[152,198,200,202,204,205,207,209]

Aspergillosis This particularly high incidence of mold sensitivity seems to have practical consequences for the CF patient. In 1965, the first cases of allergic bronchopulmonary aspergillosis (ABPA) complicating CF were published.[210] Subsequently, the reported incidence of ABPA in CF has risen from a rarity to the neighborhood of 10–15% in recent studies.[205,206,211] This dramatic increase is a result of both the development of our understanding of the immunopathogenesis of ABPA and an increasing index of suspicion among physicians caring for CF patients. In his classic monograph, Pepys set forth the hypothesis that ABPA was the result of combined endobronchial type I and type III hypersensitivity reactions to *Aspergillus fumigatus*.[212] These sensitivities can be detected both by skin test bioassay for immediate (15–20 minutes) and late (4–6 hours) reactivity, and by in vitro detection of specific serum IgE and IgG antibodies to *A. fumigatus*. Subsequent investigations over the last decade, including the establishment of a primate experimental model of ABPA, have confirmed Pepys' hypothesis.[213]

A majority of CF patients show both skin test and serologic evidence of specific IgE production to *A. fumigatus* (Table 10-7).

Studies of IgG production as detected by precipitin formation in double-diffusion reactions or by radioimmunoassay show that at least one third of CF patients have increased levels of IgG antibody to *A. fumigatus*.[8,193,197,199,205,211,214] Thus, the immunologic prerequisites are set for the occurrence of ABPA in a sizable fraction of the CF population. The fact that the diagnosis remains a fairly uncommon occurrence may be ascribed in good part to the overlapping of certain diagnostic criteria for ABPA (Table 10-8) with the symptoms and signs of CF per se. The importance of establishing this diagnosis resides primarily in the fact that while the natural history of ABPA is often one of progressive pulmonary destruction,[215] the disease responds well to antiinflammatory therapy with corticosteroids but not to antiinfective therapy.[216] Furthermore, exacerbations of ABPA can be predicted serologically by following total IgE levels.[217]

Table 10-8
Operational Approach to Diagnosis of Allergic Bronchopulmonary Aspergillosis*

Suspect the diagnosis
- In patients with asthma who also have recurrent pulmonary infiltrations with eosinophilia, symptoms of pneumonia, or hemoptysis (particularly if infiltrations in upper lobes or hilar areas)

Confirm the diagnosis
- Either by
    1. Positive immediate and late skin test reactions with intradermal aspergillus antigen (approximately 5000 PNU)
    2. Positive aspergillus precipitins
    3. Elevated serum IgE level
    4. Positive *A. fumigatus* sputum cultures
- Or by
    - Bronchograms demonstrating proximal saccular bronchiectasis

Pitfalls
1. Sputum cultures not sensitive
2. Sufficient dosage and duration of corticosteroid therapy may suppress the laboratory abnormalities and the late skin test reaction
3. Several months after an acute episode, the IgE and precipitins may revert toward normal
4. Aspergillus antigen variability may produce false-negative results

*From Imbeau et al, 1978[217] with permission.

The propensity of CF patients to develop ABPA is, like their susceptibility to respiratory colonization with a restricted number of bacterial microorganisms, poorly understood. There are a variety of possible factors involved. There may well be elements of the endobronchial microenvironment that are conducive to colonization with *Aspergillus*, but what these elements, if any, may be is as yet entirely unknown. Second, iatrogenesis is also a distinct possibility, given the use of chronic antimicrobial therapy in many CF patients and mist therapy in some. Third, *Aspergillus* may not be the only mold capable of producing immunologic lung disease in CF, as increased IgG antibody to *Candida albicans* has been reported.[115,199] Fourth, most studies have suggested that the occurrence of hypersensitivity to *Aspergillus fumigatus* is a secondary consequence of the underlying progression of lung disease and thus occurs in older patients with poorer pulmonary function.[193,194,198,202,204,206] That acquisition of sensitivity to *Aspergillus* is a consequence of lung disease is buttressed by the finding that parental obligate heterozygotes for the CF gene have no greater evidence of skin sensitivity or serum IgE antibody to *Aspergillus* than controls.[202,204,209]

Inheritance The ability of CF patients to respond to inhalation of certain antigens with IgE antibody production is probably inherited, as are other forms of atopy.[218] Several lines of inquiry in this regard are of interest. First, Warner et al[209] have found an increased prevalence of atopy as determined by skin testing in CF obligate heterozygotes when compared to a control sample of the general population. They suggested that CF heterozygosity, by virtue of its high frequency, may be a significant factor in the pathogenesis of atopy. Their findings have been supported by studies of several other groups,[219,220] but strongly disputed by others.[202,207,221] The question of the relation of the CF gene to the inheritance of atopy thus remains unsettled. This question may acquire some further practical importance if screening for the CF carrier state becomes feasible. Rapid screening for atopy by skin testing or RAST determination for IgE antibodies could be used, if the association is genuine, to provide a high-risk group for the presumably more expensive and technically difficult CF carrier testing.

A second consideration in regard to inheritance of reaginic reactivity in CF relates to studies of histocompatibility antigens in CF subgroups (atopic versus nonatopic), CF homozygotes, and CF heterozygotes, since complex but discernible HLA patterns have been described in other atopic groups.[218] Studies in this area have consistently failed to turn up significant HLA associations with any of the above CF-related categories.[10,207,222–224]

In summary, immediate hypersensitivity in cystic fibrosis appears to be a common finding secondary to disruption of respiratory epithelial integrity. The genetic basis for IgE responsiveness to inhaled allergens remains obscure but seems, on balance of available evidence, independent of the genetic mechanisms operative in other atopic individuals. High rates of type I reactivity to *Aspergillus fumigatus* set the stage for the development of allergic bronchopulmonary aspergillosis in a significant minority of patients. Other practical consequences of immediate hypersensitivity in CF will be considered next.

Impact of atopy on clinical status and course Since the first reports associating allergy with cystic fibrosis,[225–227] the possible ameliorative or exacerbating effect of the former on the course of the latter has been disputed. Some reports indicate that atopic CF patients fared better than their nonatopic counterparts,[7,191] while others have found the opposite.[194,196,198,204–206] Turner and coworkers[10] related differences in total IgE levels to the number of recent pulmonary exacerbations, suggesting a greater effect of clinical condition on IgE production than hitherto appreciated. In all of these studies, failure to properly control for factors other than allergy influencing clinical status has stymied efforts to resolve this question.

Recently Pitcher-Wilmott et al[228] clarified the issue by using analysis of variance to control for important confounding factors. They showed that the major factor associated with status and prognosis was colonization with *Pseudomonas aeruginosa*; when this factor was controlled, atopy did not significantly influence either pulmonary status, general clinical condition, or prognosis. In the absence of an important complication such as ABPA, therefore, atopy in CF is probably significant in terms of symptomatic management rather than as a determinant of current overall status or as a prognostic factor.

Bronchial hyperreactivity Even more vexing is the question of the relationship between atopy, bronchial hyperreactivity, and clinical status. When we consider the role of asthma in CF, we first have to grapple with the problem of defining asthma itself. As recently pointed out, "We all know what it is, but who would trust anybody else's definition?"[229] Because of the diversity of etiologies, mechanisms, presentations, symptoms, and signs, the neat, simple, and true definition of asthma may be impossible to state. Probably the best we can do is agree with the phenomenological characterization of asthma as wide variability over short periods of time in resistance to flow in intrapulmonary airways.[230] This raises immediate problems in the CF patient. Is such variability—perhaps due to shifting mucoid impactations, perhaps due to smooth muscle spasm, perhaps due to inflammatory edema—asthma? The question is important because of the obvious practical implications it bears for therapy.

With recent technical advances in administering and standardizing bronchoprovocation testing,[231] the demonstration of bronchial hyperreactivity—defined as a greater degree of bronchoconstriction in response to a wide variety of physical, chemical, and pharmacologic stimuli than in normal subjects—has come to be considered diagnostic of asthma.[232] Application of these provocation tests to CF patients has helped clarify the role of asthma in cystic fibrosis. In part, this development was necessary because prior work had shown that the use of inhaled bronchodilators to assess bronchial lability yielded variable and inconsistent results.[233-237] The variability of response to inhaled bronchodilators has been ascribed to a number of factors: lack of uniform dose, delivery method, and time of testing; lack of controlled evaluation by repeat testing without bronchodilator; effect of repeated forced expiratory maneuvers on pulmonary function; lack of comparative data on static and dynamic lung volume changes to accompany expiratory flow data; and bronchodilator-induced increases in airway compliance which produce increased transmural pressure and dynamic compression of airways.[238,239] Some of these problems are circumvented by bronchoprovocation testing (BPT).

Results of studies employing BPT in CF are shown in Table 10-9. These studies indicate a prevalence of bronchial hyperreactivity of about 25–50% depending on the method employed. No conclusions regarding the relationship between bronchial hyperreactivity and atopy to underlying pulmonary function can be drawn from these studies. This may be due in some part to intrapatient as well as interpatient variability of bronchial lability over time.[244] One would not intuitively expect atopy to be a critical determinant of bronchial hyperreactivity, since it is well established that bronchial hyperreactivity is the final common pathway of numerous mechanisms, including decreased baseline airway size, smooth muscle alterations, disorders of parasympathetic or sympathetic regulation, and epithelial damage, as well as allergen-induced type I hypersensitivity reactions.

Strong evidence linking bronchial hyperreactivity to allergic sensitization has therefore been difficult to come by in any group of subjects.[232] That type I reactions do play a significant role in CF bronchial hyperreactivity is suggested not only by the association between atopy and bronchial hyperreactivity in some of the studies cited in Table 10-9, but also by specific antigen-induced bronchoconstriction in BPT of CF subjects,[194,245] and by the findings of mediators of type I reactions in sputum of CF patients.[153,154] Evidence of a significant cholinergic mechanism for bronchial hyperreactivity in CF, presumably vagally mediated, is supported by the bronchodilator efficacy of anticholinergic agents such as atropine and ipratropium bromide.[238,239,246] Finally, the relationship of bronchial hyperreactivity to underlying lung disease cannot be satisfactorily isolated from its relation to asthma. Longterm prospective studies are needed to properly assess the impact of bronchial hyperreactivity and of bronchodilatory therapy on the course of lung disease in cystic fibrosis.

Bacterial allergy The concept that specific IgE to bacteria could mediate type I reactions fell into disfavor in the 1960s when several double-blind studies of immunotherapy with bacterial extracts for infection-related wheezing showed no beneficial effect, in contrast to the beneficial effect of specific pollen or dust immunotherapy for allergen-induced asthma.[247] More recently, the major role of viruses (as opposed to bacteria) in triggering infection-related wheezing has been appreciated and specific IgE antibody to pathogenic viruses demonstrated.[248] In the recently recognized syndrome of extremely elevated serum IgE, chronic dermatitis, and recurrent staphylococcal abscesses and/or chronic mucocutaneous candidiasis, specific IgE antibody to *Staphylococcus aureus* and *Candida albicans* has been demonstrated.[249] Thus, in certain circumstances specific IgE antibodies to bacteria and viruses as well as fungi have been shown. As we have already seen, IgE antibodies to fungi, especially *Aspergillus fumigatus,* are a frequent finding in cystic fibrosis. Could there be IgE antibodies to bacteria or viruses also, and could these play a role in disruption of mucosal integrity?

Surface antigens of *Pseudomonas aeruginosa* have been shown to stimulate reaginic antibody production in mice.[250] Two recent

Table 10-9
Nonspecific Bronchoprovocation Tests in Cystic Fibrosis

Provocation	Results	Reference
Exercise—free range running	24/52 (46%) postexercise bronchoconstriction; associated with more severe lung disease	Day and Mearns[240]
Methacholine inhalation	11/23 (48%) positive in atopic (by history) group	Rothstein et al[241]
Exercise—treadmill running	14/35 (40%) postexercise bronchoconstriction	Counahan and Mearns[221]
Histamine inhalation	15/22 (68%) positive	Haluszka and Scislicki[242]
Exercise—treadmill running	8/36 (22%) postexercise bronchoconstriction; associated with more severe lung disease	Silverman et al[202]
Histamine inhalation	12/50 (24%) positive, associated with poorer baseline pulmonary function; no association with atopy	Mellis and Levison[243]
Methacholine inhalation	58/113 (51%) positive; associated with poorer baseline pulmonary function and history of wheezing, but not atopy; methacholine found superior to histamine [7/33 (21%) positive to histamine]	Mitchell et al[203]
Histamine inhalation	9/25 (36%) positive; no association with baseline pulmonary function	Tobin et al[207]
Histamine inhalation	10/25 (40%) positive; associated with more severe lung disease; responsiveness varied in some patients over time	Holzer et al[244]
Histamine inhalation	8/20 (40%) positive in a group with normal baseline pulmonary function; associated with atopy and history of asthma	Van Asperen et al[208]
Total	169/401 (42%) overall evidence of bronchial hyperreactivity	

studies suggest this occurs in CF patients. In our laboratory, using a sensitive and specific solid-phase radioimmunoassay,[251] we demonstrated IgE antibody to *Pseudomonas aeruginosa* in serum of 5 of 11 CF patients under 10 years of age, 7 of 27 between 10 and 20 years, and 4 of 17 of those over 20 years. In contrast, only 4 of 53 patients had IgE specific for *Staphylococcus aureus.*[115] Shen et al[252] demonstrated *Pseudomonas*-specific IgE by calculating reduction of total serum IgE after adsorption with various bacteria and found significantly greater activity for *Pseudomonas aeruginosa* in CF serum compared to asthmatic serum. Basophil histamine release has been shown after challenge with *Pseudomonas aeruginosa* antigen by complement-dependent and also independent (presumably IgE-mediated) processes in CF patients colonized with *Pseudomonas*[253] (Hoiby, personal communication.)

The clinical significance of these IgE antibodies to *Pseudomonas* remains to be determined. Certainly, the occurrence of type I reactions involving *Pseudomonas* on respiratory mucosa could have important consequences for epithelial integrity to entrance of antigens and subsequent development of significant systemic IgG response with formation of antigen-antibody complexes, activation of complement, and recruitment of tissue-damaging polymorphonuclear leukocytes. The possibility that viruses such as respiratory syncytial virus and *Mycoplasma* might also provoke reaginic responses in CF patients is worthy of investigation.

IgG_4 Although IgE is the major reaginic antibody in man, it is not the only one. Heat-stable, short-term sensitizing IgG antibodies (IgG-STS) capable of sensitizing skin and lung mast cells and basophils have been demonstrated and shown to be clinically relevant in a variety of diseases including allergic bronchopulmonary aspergillosis.[254] Currently, the IgG_4 subclass seems the best candidate for IgG-STS.[187] Elevated levels of serum IgG_4 were reported in 7 of 16 CF patients in one study,[255] and 43% of 37 CF patients as compared to 17% of 63 heterozygotes and 36% of 36 controls in a second study.[204]

Increases in IgG_4 are found principally in older CF patients.[207] On the other hand, abolition of the ability of CF sputum to passively transfer cutaneous anaphylaxis by incubation at 56°C for 30 minutes suggests that the reaginic activity is IgE-mediated.[152] Elevated levels of specific IgG_4 antibody to *Pseudomonas aeruginosa* have been recently demonstrated in colonized patients in our laboratory by enzyme immunoassay.[256] The clinical significance of this finding awaits further investigation. IgG_4 antibodies do not activate complement, are poor opsonins, and may be blocking antibodies in allergen immunotherapy and chronic infection.[257-259] It is possible that a pronounced IgG_4 response to *Pseudomonas* could account for the reported blocking activity.[157-159,161]

Allergy to pancreatin Several groups have reported cases of clinical allergic sensitization to pancreatic extracts in parents of children with cystic fibrosis.[260-262] The lack of reactivity of CF patients has been ascribed to the immunogenic character of pancreatin therapy, with the production of IgG antibody to trypsin in at least 80% of CF patients.[263] This IgG antibody may block IgE-mediated reactions much as allergen-specific IgG blocks IgE reactivity in allergic patients on immunotherapy.

Autoantibodies (Type II Hypersensitivity) in CF

Evidence of circulating antibodies to pancreatic tissue in patients with chronic pancreatic disease including cystic fibrosis[264] led Stein et al[265] to look for antibodies to lung and pancreas in a larger group of CF patients. They found that CF but not normal mucus contained precipitating antibodies to CF but not normal lung extract. Serum antibodies, however, were not found. Extending these findings to a broad range of antigens, McFarlane and co-workers found precipitins in CF sputum to saliva, colostrum, seminal fluid, urine, and serum, as well as serum antibodies to reticulin fiber.[6,46] Antinuclear antibodies have been found with increased frequency in CF patients, whereas classic IgM rheumatoid factor appears no more frequently than in controls.[266] Rheumatoid factors of the IgG class have been detected both frequently[267] and rarely.[268]

None of these studies has evaluated the biologic function, if any, of these antibodies (eg, complement-fixing ability or cytotoxicity). Nor has it been clearly shown that any of the autoantibodies detected is specific to cystic fibrosis. Similar types of autoantibodies are well known in various other chronic diseases.[269] It seems likely that these antibodies are an epiphenomenon reflecting the degree of tissue damage and are unlikely to be pathogenic. One instance of induced autoantibody formation that may be of clinical significance is the finding by Romeo and co-workers of IgG antibody formation to porcine trypsin in patients receiving exogenous pancreatic enzyme therapy.[270] These antibodies cross-react with human trypsin.[271] The possibility that such antibodies interfere with host proteolytic activity[272] or decrease efficacy of pancreatic enzyme therapy needs exploration.

Antibodies to CF-specific antigens The search for an antigen or antigens unique to cystic fibrosis which can be used to develop immunoassays for the cystic fibrosis phenotype or even genotype has been pursued for many years. With one generic exception, no unique antigenic features of cystic fibrosis at the molecular, cellular, or tissue level have been found (reviewed by Halbert[273] and by Talamo et al[274]). The exception relates to the various CF factors and their immunologic detection and characterization which are considered in Chapter 7 of this text. Two groups have reported preliminary success in raising antisera to an immunogenic factor or factors which may be unique to the CF genotype.[275,276] Confirmation in other laboratories is awaited along with extension of the assay to larger groups in blinded series. To date, no evidence of autologous immunogenicity of the CF factors has been documented; although several groups have claimed CF factors are associated with IgG in vivo, this is apparently not an antigen–antibody reaction.[277]

Immune Complexes (Type III Hypersensitivity) in CF

The presence of a strikingly florid yet ineffective humoral immune response to persistent microbial antigens provides a logical setting for immune complex formation in cystic fibrosis. Only recently, however, has the technology for detection, quantitation, and analysis of immune complexes supplied adequate research tools to investigate what may be an important link between microbial lower respiratory tract colonization and the debilitating and ultimately lethal clinical result. In 1975, McFarlane and co-workers[46] found deposition of immunoglobulin and complement by immunofluorescent staining techniques in the lung, trachea, and pancreas of necropsy specimens from two patients with CF. Lesser deposits were also noted in gut, lymphoid tissue, and liver. It should be noted that a similar deposition was also seen in lung tissue from autopsies on adults with other lung diseases, although elution of complexes was achieved only from CF lung tissue. Antibody specificity for staphylococcal α-hemolysin was found but the presence of other antigens was not clearly demonstrated. Surprisingly, these important but at best suggestive findings have not been pursued.

Recently, a number of laboratories using a wide variety of techniques for detecting soluble immune complexes have found a high incidence in CF serum and respiratory tract secretions.[49,278–281] Incidence and levels of serum immune complexes are significantly higher than in age-matched patients with other respiratory diseases.[49] The major questions that arise from these reports are, first, what is the relationship of immune complexes to the disease process—are they pathogenic or an epiphenomenon?—and second, are there therapeutic modalities which affect their presence, and if so, are other aspects of the disease process in CF thereby affected?

Evidence is accumulating that immune complexes play a pathogenic role in CF lung disease and are amenable to specific therapy.

1. The immune complexes are composed in part of antigens from microbes colonizing the respiratory tract, particularly *Pseudomonas aeruginosa*, and corresponding IgG or IgM complement-fixing antibody.[282] Complement activation is easily demonstrated in respiratory secretions but not in plasma, further implicating a compartmental origin and possible pathogenic mechanism.[49,58] Complement activation provides a powerful amplification mechanism for pulmonary inflammation.[283] In addition, immune complexes bound to macrophages may exert a suppressive as well as a stimulatory effect on immune function.[284] It is intriguing to speculate that immune complexes could be playing a role in the acquired humorally induced alveolar macrophage opsonic defect for *Pseudomonas aeruginosa* discussed in the preceding section on immunodeficiency.

2. There is a striking association between the appearance of circulating immune complexes and exacerbations of pulmonary disease.[115,281] In a longitudinal study of 96 patients at Children's Hospital at Stanford conducted over a two-year period, both the incidence and levels of circulating immune complexes correlated strongly with clinical

respiratory exacerbations and decreases in pulmonary function (Tables 10-10 and 10-11). Conventional treatment of exacerbations by hospitalization, intravenous anti-*Pseudomonas* antibiotics, intensive chest physiotherapy, and nutritional supplementation decreased levels of circulating immune complexes in two thirds of the patients when tested at follow-up one month later.

3. Those patients most likely to have significant immune complex formation are those chronically colonized with *Pseudomonas aeruginosa* who have high titers of specific antibody.[278] These CF patients are in poorer clinical condition than those who are not so colonized and those without strong antibody responses.[4] As the antibody titers and specificities increase, the prognosis worsens[285] and inflammatory acute-phase serum reactants increase.[286] Conversely, patients with hypogammaglobulinemia (most of whom are under 10 years of age) are in better pulmonary status than age-matched patients with normal or elevated immunoglobulin levels.[11]

4. Some CF patients do have symptoms and signs of systemic immune complex disease such as arthralgias or arthritis not attributable to hypertrophic pulmonary osteoarthropathy or hyperuricemia, recurrent or prolonged fevers, or cutaneous vasculitis.[287–289] In this subgroup with systemic manifestations decreased serum hemolytic complement activity is often found along with circulating immune complexes.[290] One might speculate that in this group immune complexes may arise from systemic antigen-antibody interactions or the immune complexes may have characteristics that increase systemic pathogenicity (eg, complement-activating ability is higher or reticuloendothelial clearance is decreased).

5. Immunologic studies, as in so many other areas of CF research, have often been stymied by the lack of a suitable animal model. Recently Cash and co-workers developed an animal model of chronic *Pseudomonas* bronchitis by use of bacterial inoculum in an agar-bead matrix which creates histologic lesions closely resembling those seen in CF lungs.[291] This model has been adapted by Pennington et al[292] to study the relationship of immunologic to histopathologic features. Guinea pigs infected by the *Pseudomonas* agar-bead method developed immunologic aberrations identical to those seen in CF (including hypergammaglobulinemia, high levels of specific antibody, and circulating immune complexes) concomitantly with histopathologic changes very closely resembling those found in CF lung tissue. Further boosting of *Pseudomonas*-specific antibody levels by active parenteral immunization with *Pseudomonas* lipopolysaccharide vaccine after the infection had been established had no protective effect and in some animals simultaneously exacerbated both the histologic and the humoral immunologic pathology.

6. Specific antiinflammatory therapy with corticosteroids in selected patients with clinically suspected systemic immune complex disease and circulating immune complexes resulted in appreciable clinical and pulmonary improvement as well as abolition

Table 10-10
Incidence of Increased ^{125}I-C1q Binding in Cystic Fibrosis Clinical Groups

Group (No.)	Samples	↑C1qBA (%)	χ^2	P
Acute (52)	84	39 (46)		
			11.1	<0.001
Stable (56)	103	23 (22)		
			8.6	<0.01
Convalescent (30)	46	22 (48)		
Total	233	84 (36)		

Table 10-11
Pulmonary Function and C1q Binding in CF Clinical Groups

	C1qBA (%)		VC (% of normal)*		PEFR (% of normal)†	
Acute	16.5 ± 12.5 N = 84		42.1 ± 13.7 N = 62		41.7 ± 18.6 N = 61	
		$P \cong 0.005$		$P < 0.0005$		$P < 0.0005$
Stable	11.9 ± 9.7 N = 103		63.4 ± 19.9 N = 62		60.9 ± 22.5 N = 62	
		$P = 0.005$		$P = 0.05$		$P < 0.05$
Convalescent	17.8 ± 15.0 N = 46		54.3 ± 20.9 N = 28		48.7 ± 27.9 N = 29	

*VC, vital capacity.
†PEFR, peak expiratory flow rate.

of circulating immune complexes.[293] We would caution that this work needs to be extended to broader categories of patients and the results assessed by well-designed controlled trials before its use can be recommended.

7. Direct evidence for a complement-independent pathogenic mechanism for *Pseudomonas*–anti-*Pseudomonas* immune complexes has been provided by the demonstration that human platelets exposed to such complexes are stimulated to release [^{3}H]serotonin.[294]

In summary, type III hypersensitivity reactions occur commonly in CF patients; usually arise in, but are not limited to, the pulmonary compartment; are strongly associated with pulmonary disease activity and deterioration of pulmonary function; are likely, but not proven, to have a pathogenic role; and appear to be amenable to specific antiinflammatory therapy.

Cell-Mediated (Type IV) Hypersensitivity in CF

Normal adaptive cell-mediated immunity and deleterious type IV cell-mediated hypersensitivity reactions are virtually indistinguishable in vitro, as both are characterized by antigenic activation and proliferation of lymphocytes followed by lymphokine production. In type IV hypersensitivity, the effects mediated by lymphokines are, on balance, harmful to the host. This may result from lymphocyte sensitization to host tissue antigens which normally do not stimulate an immune response or to prolonged or pronounced lymphokine production caused by a continuing antigenic stimulus. One must look to tissue damage in the form of granulomas or dermatitis to clearly differentiate hypersensitivity from cell-mediated immunity. Cell-mediated immunity in CF is discussed in the prior sections on immunity and immunodeficiency. The histologic hallmarks of delayed hypersensitivity are rarely seen in CF,[295] and their absence is presumptive evidence against type IV hypersensitivity reactions playing a significant role in the pathophysiology of the disease. Lymphokine production by CF leukocytes in the presence of lung and pancreatic tissue antigens, however, suggests that cell-mediated autoimmune sensitization to damaged tissue may be occurring.[27] These interesting findings have not been confirmed. CF patients with overt liver disease may show evidence of lymphocyte sensitization to liver cell membrane antigens, again suggesting that tissue damage may lead to delayed hypersensitivity to host tissues. In some of these patients, a dense lymphocytic infiltrate similar to that seen in chronic active hepatitis was found on liver biopsy, raising the question of participation of hypersensitivity in progression of organ damage.[296]

CONCLUSION

We have seen how CF lung disease involves aspects of normal immunity, potentially crucial areas of immune deficiency, and striking degrees of several types of hypersensitivity. How do these pieces of the CF puzzle fit together? We do not know. But in a disease where speculation has always run far ahead of proof, the author feels under no obligation to be circumspect. Figure 10-2 outlines a hypothesis concerning the pathogenesis of CF lung disease which is consistent with the known facts and arranges them in a sequence that could explain them.

In this hypothesis the inherited molecular defect—perhaps in glycoprotein metabolism—alters the lining of the respiratory tract in such a fashion as to permit binding and proliferation of microbes in the normally sterile bronchial tree. Two possible mechanisms for this binding are shown, namely an alteration in the functional ability of secretory IgA and changes in the surface-binding properties of respiratory epithelial cells, such as those observed with a deficiency of fibronectin. Thus, in this schema colonization of the respiratory tract by potential pathogens precedes gross changes in respiratory secretions such as purulence and increased viscosity. However, there is no doubt that, once colonized, primary and secondary changes may mutually aggravate and accelerate each other.

Once colonized, the next stage in the process could involve several mechanisms of potentiating an IgG antibody response, including stimulation of an early reaginic (IgE) response which would allow entry of large amounts of antigen below the mucosa. Again, defective mucosal antigen exclusion by defects in secretory IgA and/or other surface molecules would have the same result. Virulence factors of the colonizing agents could also play a significant role in facilitating antigen penetration to the submucosal line of the immune defenses.

The next step would, as a result of such abnormal penetration, involve an early massive and continuing stimulation of the IgG antibody response. At this point, two further complicating factors may occur. One is a dysfunction in the ability of IgG antibodies reaching the airway to effectively opsonize the microorganisms for alveolar macrophage phagocytosis. The second factor would be an increasingly destructive immune complex hypersensitivity reaction which would, by direct complement activation and perhaps also by alveolar macrophage activation, release potent chemotactic factors and trigger a massive influx of polymorphonuclear leukocytes. In this scenario, the major cause of lung damage is not microbial virulence factors—although they certainly would provide a share of the damage[297]—but release of leukocyte proteolytic enzymes and oxidative metabolites. During this period, a selection process possibly based on antiphagocytic capacity for mucoid strains of *Pseudomonas aeruginosa* would be occurring.

In such a scenario, a three-tiered approach to therapy seems ideal.

1. Prevention of colonization—this is the area requiring most intensive and fundamental research. The clues are there: we need to continue to investigate CF mucus, but also to closely examine the structure and function of CF immunoglobulins and other proteins of the bronchial fluid such as fibronectin and complement components. Bronchial alveolar lavage studies will likely be helpful in this regard particularly in infants being operated upon for meconium ileus.

2. Suppression of infection—by continuing development of better antimicrobial and especially anti-*Pseudomonas* chemotherapy, and reexamination of optimal administration of such therapy.[298]

3. Suppression of inflammation—interrupting the influx of polymorphonuclear leukocytes to the airways may result in a decisive contribution to the well-being of the patient, if our assumptions about the relatively low virulence of the colonizing agents and the relatively high toxicity of massive leukocytic influx to the airway lumen and walls are correct. This modality of therapy requires further research in animal models such as the agar-bear *Pseudomonas*

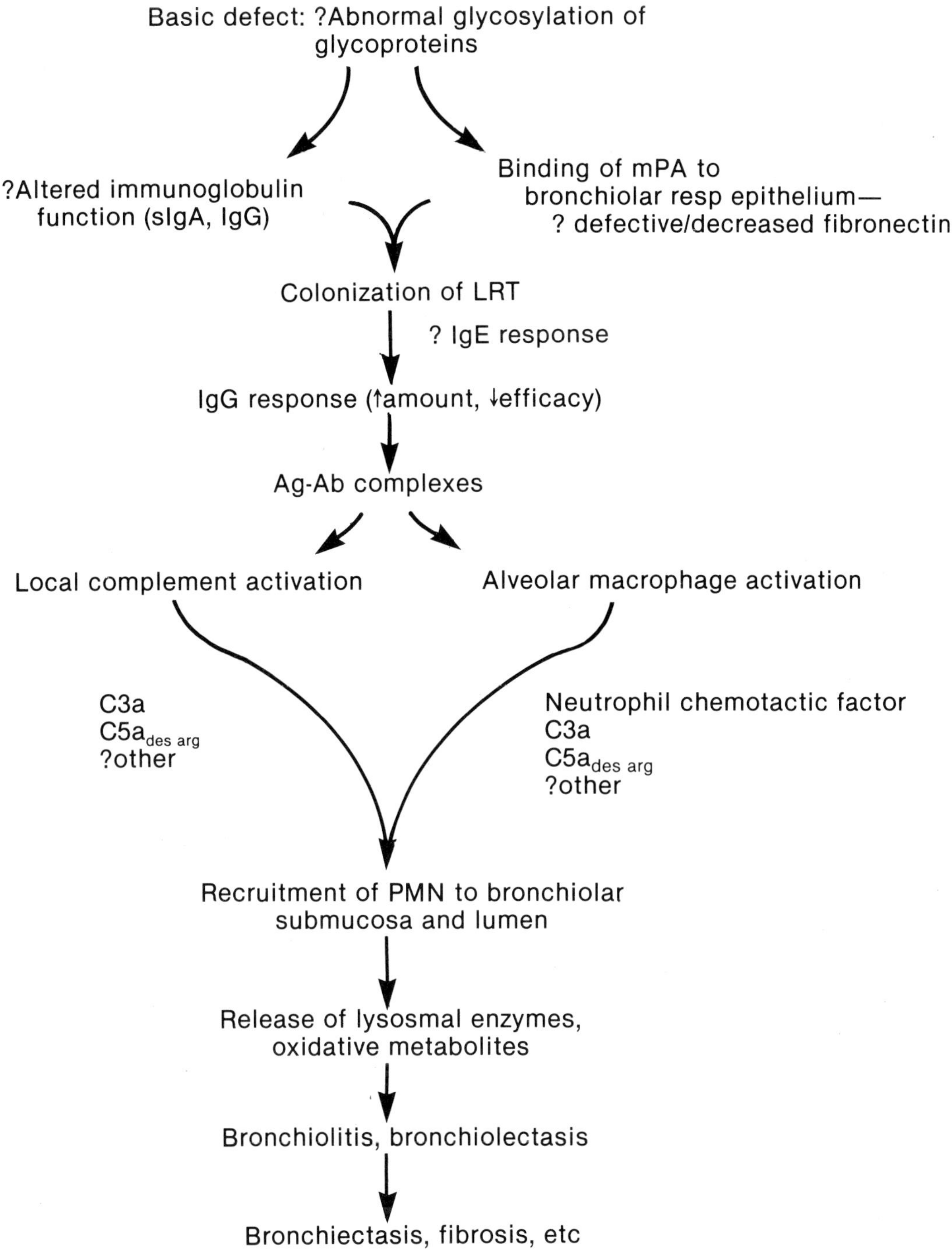

Figure 10-2 Pathogenesis of cystic fibrosis lung disease: A hypothesis. Abbreviations: mPA, mucoid *Pseudomonas aeruginosa;* LRT, lower respiratory tract; des arg, without arginine; PMN, Polymorpho-neutrophil.

bronchitis,[291] as well as controlled trials of such therapy in CF patients. The pharmacology of the 1980s will prominently feature an entirely novel series of both steroidal and nonsteroidal antiinflammatory agents characterized by potency and specificity.[299,300] These agents offer great promise to the CF patient of today and tomorrow. If we cannot slay the beast, let us at least capture it long enough to extract the fangs.

REFERENCES

1. Green MN, Kulczycki LL, Shwachman H: Serum protein paper electrophoresis in patients with cystic fibrosis. *Am J Dis Child* 1960;100:365–372.
2. Schwartz RH: Serum immunoglobulin levels in cystic fibrosis. *Am J Dis Child* 1966;111: 408–411.
3. Collins-Williams C, Thachyk SJ, Toft B, et al: Quantitative immunoglobulin levels (IgG, IgA, and IgM) in children with intractable asthma. *Ann Allergy* 1967;25:177–182.
4. Doggett RG, Harrison GM: *Pseudomonas aeruginosa*. Immune status in patients with cystic fibrosis. *Infect Immun* 1972;6:628–635.
5. Yohe RM: Allergy in patients with cystic fibrosis. *Ann Allergy* 1972;30:627–631.
6. Wallwork JC, Brenchley P, McCarthy J, et al: Some aspects of immunity in cystic fibrosis. *Clin Exp Immunol* 1974;18:303–320.
7. Rachelefsky GS, Osher A, Dooley RE, et al: Coexistent respiratory allergy and cystic fibrosis. *Am J Dis Child* 1974;128:355–359.
8. Warren CPW, Tai E, Batten JC, et al: Cystic fibrosis—immunological reactions to *A. fumigatus* and common allergens. *Clin Allergy* 1975;5:1–12.
9. Hoiby N, Andersen V, Bendixen G: *Pseudomonas aeruginosa* infection in cystic fibrosis. Humoral and cellular immune responses against *Pseudomonas aeruginosa*. *Acta Pathol Microbiol Scand Sect C* 1975;83: 459–468.
10. Turner MW, Warner JO, Stokes CR, et al: Immunological studies in cystic fibrosis. *Arch Dis Child* 1978;53:631–638.
11. Matthews WJ, Williams M, Oliphant B, et al: Hypogammaglobulinemia in patients with cystic fibrosis. *N Engl J Med* 1980;302:245–249.
12. Hoiby N: *Pseudomonas aeruginosa* infection in cystic fibrosis. Diagnostic and prognostic significance of *Pseudomonas aeruginosa* precipitins determined by means of crossed immunoelectrophoresis. A survey. *Acta Pathol Microbiol Scand Sect C* 1977(suppl); 262:1–96.
13. Fick RB, Reynolds HY: Immunoprophylaxis and immune responses in cystic fibrosis, in Sturgess JM (ed): *Perspectives in Cystic Fibrosis*. Toronto, Canadian CF Foundation, 1980, pp 335–345.
14. Peterson NT, Hoiby N, Mordhorst CH, et al: Respiratory infections in cystic fibrosis patients caused by virus, *Chlamydia*, and *Mycoplasma*. Possible synergism with *Pseudomonas aeruginosa*, in Sturgess JM (ed): *Perspectives in Cystic Fibrosis*. Toronto, Canadian CF Foundation, 1980, pp 346–351.
15. Modlin JF, Smith DH, Harding L: Clinical trials of bivalent A/New Jersey/76-A/Victonal/75 influenza vaccines in high-risk children. *J Infect Dis* 1977;136:S626–S631.
16. Pennington JE, Reynolds HY, Wood RE, et al: Use of a *Pseudomonas aeruginosa* vaccine in patients with acute leukemia and cystic fibrosis. *Am J Med* 1975;58:629–636.
17. Hoiby N, Mathiesen L: *Pseudomonas aeruginosa* infection in cystic fibrosis. Distribution of B and T lymphocytes in relation to the humoral immune responses. *Acta Pathol Microbiol Scand Sect B* 1974;82:559–568.
18. Götz M, Achmad R, Zielinski C, et al: Antibody production on the cellular level in patients with cystic fibrosis. *Monogr Paediatr* 1981;14:151–155.
19. Sorensen RU, Ruuskanen O, Miller K, et al: Abnormal B-cell differentiation in vitro in cystic fibrosis patients with advanced disease. *Cystic Fibrosis Club Abstr* 1981;vol 22:158.
20. Genin C, Gilly R, Touraine JL, et al: L'Immunité dans la mucoviscidose. *Arch Fr Pediatr* 1977;34:717–729.
21. McCarthy M, Spock A: In vivo assessment of cell-mediated immunity in patients with cystic fibrosis. *Cystic Fibrosis Club Abstr* 1979;20:58.
22. Harper TB, Gaumer HR, Waring W, et al: Cell-mediated immunity and suppressor T cell function in children with cystic fibrosis. *Lung* 1980;157:219–228.
23. Braunstein M, Van Ess J, Schwartz RH: T-lymphocytes in cystic fibrosis. *Cystic Fibrosis Club Abstr* 1975;16:28.
24. O'Grady, LR, Ray CG: Cellular immunity in cystic fibrosis. *Cystic Fibrosis Club Abstr* 1975;16:16.
25. Sorensen RU, Stern RC, Polmar SH: Cellular immunity to bacteria. Impairment of in vitro lymphocyte responses to *Pseudomonas aeruginosa* in cystic fibrosis patients. *Infect Immun* 1977;18:735–740.
26. Wilson GB, Bahm VJ: Synthesis and secretion of cystic fibrosis ciliary dyskinesia substances by purified subpopulations of leu-

kocytes. *J Clin Invest* 1980;66:1010–1019.
27. Gibbons A, Allan JD, Holzel A, et al: Cell-mediated immunity in cystic fibrosis. *Br Med J* 1976;1:120–122.
28. Berlow B, Catanzaro A, Jalowayski A, et al: Lymphocyte-mediated neutrophil chemotaxis in cystic fibrosis. *Cystic Fibrosis Club Abstr* 1980;21:52.
29. Lieberman J: Lymphocyte acid hydrolases in cystic fibrosis. *Chest* 1979;75:S221-S223.
30. Sorensen RU, Birch RE, Chase PA, et al: Lymphocyte subpopulations and functional abnormalities in cystic fibrosis, in Sturgess JM (ed): *Perspectives in Cystic Fibrosis.* Toronto, Canadian CF Foundation, 1980, p 35a.
31. Müller-Eberhard HJ: Chemistry and function of the complement system. *Hosp Prac* 1978; 12:33–43.
32. Ruddy S: Function of the control proteins of the classical and alternative complement activation pathways, in Thompson RA (ed): *Recent Advances in Clinical Immunology,* Vol 2. London, Churchill Livingstone, 1980, pp 91–111.
33. Cooper N: Laboratory evaluation of complement activation, in Nakamura RM, Dito WR, Tucker ES III (eds): *Immunoassays. Clinical Laboratory Techniques for the 1980's. Laboratory and Research Methods in Biology and Medicine.* New York, Alan R. Liss, 1980, pp 393–410.
34. Conover JH, Conod EF, Hirschhorn K: Ciliary dyskinesia factor in immunological and pulmonary disease. *Lancet* 1973;1:1194.
35. Conover JH, Conod EJ, Hirschhorn K: Complement components in cystic fibrosis. *Lancet* 1973;2:1501.
36. Conover JH, Conod EJ, Hirschhorn K: Studies on ciliary dyskinesia factor in cystic fibrosis. *Life Sci* 1974;14:253–259.
37. Hugli TE, Müller-Eberhard HJ: Anaphylatoxins: C3a and C5a. *Adv Immunol* 1978;26: 1–53.
38. Lieberman J: Carboxypeptidase B-like activity and C3 in cystic fibrosis. *Am Rev Respir Dis* 1975;111:100–102.
39. Lieberman J: Complement components in cystic fibrosis. *Lancet* 1974;1:1230.
40. Conover JH, Conod EJ: Complement in cystic fibrosis. *Lancet* 1975;1:47–48.
41. Scanlin TF, Norman ME, Rosenlund ML: C3 in cystic fibrosis. *Lancet* 1974;1:1382.
42. Hann S, Holsclaw DS, Shin HS. Complement components in cystic fibrosis. *Lancet* 1974;2:520–521.
43. Polley MJ, Bearn AG: Cystic fibrosis. Current concepts. *J Med Genet* 1974;11:249–252.
44. Holzhauer RJ, Van Ess JD, Schwartz RH: Third component of complement in cystic fibrosis. *Am J Hum Genet* 1976;28:602–606.
45. Lederberg S, Sackett D: Distribution of complement C3 variants in individuals with cystic fibrosis. *Am J Hum Genet* 1976;28:597–601.
46. McFarlane H, Holzel A, Brenchley P, et al: Immune complexes in cystic fibrosis. *Br Med J* 1975;1:423–428.
47. Strunk RC, Sieber OF, Taussig LM, et al: Serum complement depression during viral lower respiratory tract illness in cystic fibrosis. *Arch Dis Child* 1977;52:687–690.
48. Götz M, Lubec G: Complement in cystic fibrosis. *Eur J Pediatr* 1978;127:133–139.
49. Moss RB, Lewiston NJ: Immune complexes and humoral response to *Pseudomonas aeruginosa* in cystic fibrosis. *Am Rev Respir Dis* 1980;121:23–29.
50. Wilson GB, Fudenberg HH, Panse MT, et al: Cystic fibrosis ciliary dyskinesia substances and pulmonary disease. *J Clin Invest* 1981; 68:171–183.
51. Schreiber RD, Müller-Eberhard HJ: New developments in the activation of the alternate pathway of complement, in Nakamura RM, Dito WR, Tucker ES III (eds): *Immunoassays. Clinical Laboratory Techniques for the 1980's. Laboratory and Research Methods in Biology and Medicine.* New York, Alan R. Liss, 1980, pp 411–431.
52. Wilson MR, Salvaggio JE: Activation of the alternative pathway of complement. *J Allergy Clin Immunol* 1980;65:319–321.
53. Lyrene RK, Polhill RB, Guthrie LA, et al: Alternative complement pathway activity in cystic fibrosis. *J Pediatr* 1977;91:681–682.
54. Harper BL, Fine DP, Barnett DR: Complement function in cystic fibrosis. *Cystic Fibrosis Club Abstr* 1977;18:2.
55. Buescher ES, Winkelstein JA: The ability of bacteria to activate the terminal complement components in serum of patients with cystic fibrosis. *J Pediatr* 1978;93:530–531.
56. Church JA, Keens TG, Wang CI, et al: Normal neutrophil and monocyte chemotaxis in patients with cystic fibrosis. *J Pediatr* 1979;95:272–274.
57. Swender PT, Spitzer RE, Stitzel AE, et al: Abnormalities of the complement system in children with cystic fibrosis. *Cystic Fibrosis Club Abstr* 1980;21:94.
58. Schiotz PO, Sorensen H, Hoiby N: Activated complement in the sputum from patients with cystic fibrosis. *Acta Pathol Microbiol Scand Sect C* 1979;87:1–5.
59. Stossel TP: How do phagocytes eat? *Ann Intern Med* 1978;89:398–402.
60. Cline MJ, Lehrer RI, Territo MC, et al: Monocytes and macrophages: Functions and diseases. *Ann Intern Med* 1978;88:78–88.

61. Böhme B: Phagozytosedefekt der Granulozyten bei Zystischer Fibrose. *Helv Paediatr Acta* 1972;27:602–612.
62. Böhme B: Untersuchungen zur Zellularen Abwehr gegen *Pseudomonas aeruginosa* bei Mukoviszidose. *Z Erkr Atmungsorgane* 1975;143:66–69.
63. Hill HR, Warwick WJ, Dettloff J, et al: Neutrophil granulocyte function in patients with pulmonary infection. *J Pediatr* 1974; 84:54–58.
64. Church JA, Keens TG, Wang CI: Neutrophil and monocyte chemotaxis in acutely infected patients with cystic fibrosis. *Ann Allergy* 1980;45:217–219.
65. Boxerbaum B, Kagumba M, Matthews LW: Selective inhibition of phagocytic activity of rabbit alveolar macrophages by cystic fibrosis serum. *Am Rev Respir Dis* 1973;108: 777–783.
66. Bozkowa K, Nowakowska A, Siwinska-Golebiowska H, et al: Studies of humoral and cellular immune response in children with cystic fibrosis, in Sturgess JM (ed): *Perspectives in Cystic Fibrosis.* Toronto, Canadian CF Foundation, 1980, p 5a.
67. Biggar WD, Holmes R, Good RA: Opsonic defect in patients with cystic fibrosis. *Proc Natl Acad Sci USA.* 1971;68:1716–1719.
68. Kaltreider HB: Expression of immune mechanisms in the lungs. *Am Rev Respir Dis* 1976;113:347–379.
69. Newhouse M, Sanchis J, Beinenstock J: Lung defense mechanisms. *N Engl J Med* 1976;295:990–997, 1045–1052.
70. Green GM, Jakab GH, Low RB, et al: Defense mechanisms of the respiratory membrane. *Am Rev Respir Dis* 1977;115:479–514.
71. Brain JD, Proctor DF, Reid LM (eds): *Respiratory Defense Mechanisms, Part I, II.* New York, Marcel Dekker, 1977.
72. Oppenheimer EH: Similarity of the tracheobronchial mucous glands and epithelium in infants with and without cystic fibrosis. *Hum Pathol* 1981;12:36–48.
73. Lamb D, Reid L: The tracheobronchial submucosal glands in cystic fibrosis. A qualitative and quantitative histochemical study. *Br J Dis Chest* 1972;66:239–247.
74. Lopez-Vidriero MT, Reid L: Bronchial mucous in health and disease. *Br Med Bull* 1978;34:63–74.
75. Sturgess JM: Mucus secretion and clearance in the pathogenesis of cystic fibrosis. *Monogr Paediatr* 1981;14:60–74.
76. Hunninghake GW, Godek JE, Kawanami O, et at: Inflammatory and immune processes in the human lung in health and disease. Evaluation by bronchoalveolar lavage. *Am J Pathol* 1979;97:149–206.
77. Schiotz PO, Clemmensen I, Hoiby N: Immunoglobulins and albumin in sputum from patients with cystic fibrosis. *Acta Pathol Microbiol Scand Sect C* 1980;88:275–280.
78. Martinez-Tello FJ, Braun DG, Blanc WA: Immunoglobulin production in bronchial mucosa and bronchial lymph nodes, particularly in cystic fibrosis of the pancreas. *J Immunol* 1968;101:989–1003.
79. Sahu S, Lynn WS: Lipid composition of airway secretions from patients with asthma and patients with cystic fibrosis. *Am Rev Respir Dis* 1977;115:233–239.
80. Spock A: State of the art of lung lavage in patients with cystic fibrosis, in Warwick WJ (ed): *1000 Years of Cystic Fibrosis. Collected Papers.* Minneapolis, University of Minnesota, 1981, pp 113–116.
81. Cassino RJJ, Sordelli DO, Macri CN, et al: Pulmonary nonspecific defense mechanism in cystic fibrosis. *Pediatr Res* 1980;14:1212–1215.
82. Thomassen MJ, Demko CA, Wood RE, et al: Ultrastructure and function of alveolar macrophages from cystic fibrosis patients. *Pediatr Res* 1980;14:715–721.
83. Bell D, Spock A: Immunoglobulins of the distal airways of the lung in cystic fibrosis, in Sturgess JM (ed): *Perspectives in Cystic Fibrosis.* Toronto, Canadian CF Foundation, 1980, p 3a.
84. Thomassen MJ, Boxerbaum B, Demko CA, et al: Inhibitory effect of cystic fibrosis serum on *Pseudomonas* phagocytosis by rabbit and human alveolar macrophages. *Pediatr Res* 1979;13:1085–1088.
85. Wanner A: Clinical aspects of mucociliary transport. *Am Rev Respir Dis* 1977;116:73–125.
86. Wood RE, Boat TF, Doershuk CF: Cystic Fibrosis. *Am Rev Respir Dis* 1976;113:833–878.
87. Sanchis J, Dolovich M, Rossman C, et al: Pulmonary mucociliary clearance in cystic fibrosis. *N Engl J Med* 1973:288:651–654.
88. Yeates DB, Sturgess JB, Kahn SR, et al: Mucociliary transport in trachea of patients with cystic fibrosis. *Arch Dis Child* 1976;51: 28–33.
89. Rossman C, Dolovich J, Dolovich M, et al: Cystic fibrosis-related inhibition of mucociliary clearance in vivo in man. *J Pediatr* 1977;90:579–584.
90. Kollberg H, Mossberg B, Afzelius BA, et al: Cystic fibrosis compared with the immotile cilia syndrome. *Scand J Respir Dis* 1978; 59:297–306.
91. Antonelli M, Marcolini P, Lucarelli N, et al: Nasal mucociliary transport in cystic fibrosis. *Monogr Paediatr* 1981;14:89.
92. Katz SM, Holsclaw DS: Ultrastructural fea-

tures of respiratory cilia in cystic fibrosis. *Am J Clin Pathol* 1980;73:682–685.

93. Rutland J, Cole PJ: Nasal mucociliary clearance and ciliary beat frequency in cystic fibrosis compared with sinusitis and bronchiectasis. *Thorax* 1981;36:654–658.
94. Rossman C, Dolovich J, Dolovich M, et al: Effect of purified cystic fibrosis mucociliary inhibitor (CFMI) on nasal mucociliary transport in man. *Cystic Fibrosis Club Abstr* 1979;20:79.
95. Schiotz PO, Egeskjold EM, Hoiby N, et al: Autoantibodies in serum and sputum from patients with cystic fibrosis. *Acta Pathol Microbiol Scand Sect C* 1979;87:319–324.
96. Schiotz PO, Hoiby N: Precipitating antibodies against *Pseudomonas aeruginosa* in sputum from patients with cystic fibrosis. *Acta Pathol Microbiol Scand Sect C* 1975; 83:469–475.
97. Hann S, Holsclaw DS: Interactions of *Pseudomonas aeruginosa* with immunoglobulins and complement in sputum. *Infect Immun* 1976;14:114–117.
98. Schiotz PO, Hoiby N, Permin H, et al: IgA and IgG antibodies against surface antigens of *Pseudomonas aeruginosa* in sputum and serum from patients with cystic fibrosis. *Acta Pathol Microbiol Scand Sect C* 1979;87: 229–233.
99. Schiotz PO, Hoiby N: Precipitating antibodies against *Hemophilus influenzae* and *Staphylococcus aureus* in sputum and serum from patients with cystic fibrosis. *Acta Pathol Microbiol Scand Sect B* 1979;87: 345–351.
100. Huang NN, Van Loon EL, Sheng KT: The flora of the respiratory tract of patients with cystic fibrosis of the pancreas. *J Pediatr* 1961;59:512–521.
101. Iacocca VF, Sibenza MS, Barbero GH: Respiratory tract bacteriology in cystic fibrosis. *Am J Dis Child* 1963;106:315–324.
102. Doggett RG, Harrison GM, Stillwell RN, et al: An atypical *Pseudomonas aeruginosa* associated with cystic fibrosis of the pancreas. *J Pediatr* 1966;68:215–221.
103. Mearns MB, Hunt GH, Rushworth R: Bacterial flora of respiratory tract in patients with cystic fibrosis. 1950–1971. *Arch Dis Child* 1972;47:902–907.
104. May JR, Herrick NC, Thompson D: Bacterial infection in cystic fibrosis. *Arch Dis Child* 1972;47:908–913.
105. Hoiby N: Prevalence of mucoid strains of *Pseudomonas aeruginosa* in bacteriological specimens from patients with cystic fibrosis and patients with other diseases. *Acta Pathol Microbial Scand Sect B* 1975;83(6): 549–552.
106. Burns MW, May JR: Bacterial precipitins in serum of patients with cystic fibrosis. *Lancet* 1968;1:270–272.
107. Young LS, Yu BH, Armstrong D: Agar-gel precipitating antibody in *Pseudomonas aeruginosa* infections. *Infect Immun* 1970; 2:495–503.
108. Diaz F, Mosovich LL, Neter E: Serogroups of *Pseudomonas aeruginosa* and the immune response of patients with cystic fibrosis. *J Infect Dis* 1970;121:269–274.
109. Habboushe C, Iacocca V, Braddock L, et al: *Pseudomonas* agglutinins in patients with cystic fibrosis. *Pediatrics* 1971;48:973–974.
110. Hoiby N, Axelsen NH: Identification and quantitation of precipitins against *Pseudomonas aeruginosa* in patients with cystic fibrosis by means of crossed immunoelectrophoresis with intermediate gel. *Acta Pathol Microbiol Scand Sect B* 1973;81:298–308.
111. Harrison GM, Doggett RG. Terminal sputum flora in CF patients. *Cystic Fibrosis Club Abstr* 1975;16:42.
112. Clarke CW: Precipitating antibody to antigens of *Pseudomonas aeruginosa* in chronic obstructive lung disease. *Clin Allergy* 1977; 7:527–537.
113. Kulczycki LL, Murphy TM, Bellanti JA: *Pseudomonas* colonization in cystic fibrosis. *JAMA* 1978;240:30–34.
114. Beaudry PH, Marks MI, McDougall D, et al: Is anti-*Pseudomonas* therapy warranted in acute respiratory exacerbations in children with cystic fibrosis? *J Pediatr* 1980;97: 144–147.
115. Moss RB, Hsu YP, Lewiston NJ: ^{125}I-C1q binding and specific antibodies as indicators of pulmonary disease activity in cystic fibrosis. *J Pediatr* 1981;99:215–222.
116. Wientzen R, Prestidge CB, Kramer RI, et al: Acute pulmonary exacerbations in cystic fibrosis. A double-blind trial of tobramycin and placebo therapy. *Am J Dis Child* 1980; 134:1134–1138.
117. Liu PV: Biology of *Pseudomonas aeruginosa. Hosp Pract* 1976;January:139–147.
118. Baltimore RS, Mitchell M: Immunologic investigations of mucoid strains of *Pseudomonas aeruginosa*. Comparison of susceptibility of opsonic antibody in mucoid and nonmucoid strains. *J Infect Dis* 1980;141:238–246.
119. Young LS: The role of exotoxins in the pathogenesis of *Pseudomonas aeruginosa* infections. *J Infect Dis* 1980;142:626–630.
120. Lam J, Chan R, Lam K, et al: Production of mucoid microcolonies by *Pseudomonas aeruginosa* within infected lungs in cystic fibrosis. *Infect Immun* 1980;28:546–556.
121. Fick RB: *Pseudomonas* in cystic fibrosis. *Clin Chest Med* 1981;2:91–102.

122. Pollack M, Callahan LT, Taylor NS: Neutralizing antibody to *Pseudomonas aeruginosa* exotoxin in human sera. Evidence for in vivo toxin production during infections. *Infect Immun* 1976;14:942–947.
123. Klinger JD, Straus DE, Hitton CB, et al: Antibodies to proteases and exotoxin A of *Pseudomonas aeruginosa* in patients with cystic fibrosis. *J Infect Dis* 1978;138:49–58.
124. Pollack M, Young LS: Protective activity of antibodies to exotoxin A and lipopolysaccharide at the onset of *Pseudomonas aeruginosa* septicema in man. *J Clin Invest* 1979; 63:276–286.
125. Cross AS, Sadoff JC, Igiewski BH, et al: Evidence for the role of toxin A in the pathogenesis of infection with *Pseudomonas aeruginosa* in humans. *J Infect Dis* 1980; 142:538–546
126. Young LS, Armstrong D: Human immunity to *Pseudomonas aeruginosa*. I. In Vitro interaction of bacteria, polymorphonuclear leukocytes, and serum factors. *J Infect Dis* 1972;126:257–276.
127. Young LS: Human immunity to *Pseudomonas aeruginosa*. II. Relationship between heat-stable opsonins and the type-specific lipopolysaccharides. *J Infect Dis* 1972;126: 277–287.
128. Young LS: Role of antibody in infections due to *Pseudomonas aeruginosa*. *J Infect Dis* 1974;130:S111–S118.
129. Bjornson AB, Michael JG: Factors in human serum promoting phagocytosis of *Pseudomonas aeruginosa*. I. Interaction of opsonins with the bacterium. *J Infect Dis* 1974;130:S119–S126.
130. Peterson PK, Kim Y, Schmeling D, et al: Complement-mediated phagocytosis of *Pseudomonas aeruginosa*. *J Lab Clin Med* 1978;92:883–894.
131. Lambris J, Papamichail M, Ioannidis C, et al: Activation of the alternative pathway of human complement by extracellular slime glycolipoprotein of *Pseudomonas aeruginosa*. *J Infect Dis* 1982;145:78–82.
132. Reynolds HY, Newball HH: Analysis of proteins and respiratory cells obtained from human lungs by bronchial lavage. *J Lab Clin Med* 1974;84:559–573.
133. Robertson J, Caldwell JR, Castle JR, et al: Evidence for the presence of components of the alternative (properdin) pathway of complement activation in respiratory secretions. *J Immunol* 1976;117:900–903.
134. Reynolds HY, Thompson RE: Pulmonary host defenses. I. Analysis of protein and lipids in bronchial secretions and antibody responses after vaccination with *Pseudomonas aeruginosa*. *J Immunol* 1973;111: 358–368.
135. Reynolds HY, Thompson RE: Pulmonary host defenses. II. Interaction of respiratory antibodies with *Pseudomonas aeruginosa* and alveolar macrophages. *J Immunol* 1973; 111:369–380.
136. Reynolds HY, Kazmierowski JA, Newball HH: Specificity of opsonic antibodies to enhance phagocytosis of *Pseudomonas aeruginosa* by human alveolar macrophages. *J Clin Invest* 1975;56:376–385.
137. Reynolds HY, Thompson RE, Devlin HB: Development of cellular and humoral immunity in the respiratory tract of rabbits to *Pseudomonas* lipopolysaccharide. *J Clin Invest* 1974;53:1351–1358.
138. Pennington JE, Kuchmy D: Mechanism for pulmonary protection by lipopolysaccharide *Pseudomonas* vaccine. *J Infect Dis* 1980;142:191–198.
139. Gross GN, Rehm SR, Pierce AK: The effect of complement depletion on lung clearance of bacteria. *J Clin Invest* 1978;62:373–378.
140. Rehm SR, Gross GN, Pierce AK: Early bacterial clearance from murine lungs. Species-dependent phagocyte response. *J Clin Invest* 1980;66:194–199.
141. Hoidal JR, Schmeling D, Peterson PK: Phagocytosis, bacterial killing, and metabolism by purified human lung phagocytes. *J Infect Dis* 1981;144:61–71.
142. Verbrough HA, Hoidal JR, Nguyen BYT, et al: Human alveolar macrophage cytophilic immunoglobulin G-mediated phagocytosis of protein A-positive staphylococci. *J Clin Invest* 1982;69:63–74.
143. Woods DE, Bass JA, Johanson WG, et al: Role of adherence in the pathogenesis of *Pseudomonas aeruginosa* lung infection in cystic fibrosis patients. *Infect Immun* 1980; 30:694–699.
144. Woods DE, Straus DC, Johanson WG, et al: Role of fibronectin in the prevention of adherence of *Pseudomonas aeruginosa* to buccal cells. *J Infect Dis* 1981;143:784–790.
145. Rennard SI, Crystal RG: Fibronectin in human bronchopulmonary lavage fluid. *J Clin Invest* 1981;69:113–122.
146. Lopez-Vidriero MT, Reid L: Chemical markers of mucous and serum glycoproteins and their relation to viscosity in mucoid and purulent sputum from various hypersecretory diseases. *Am Rev Respir Dis* 1978;117: 465–477.
147. Barton AD, Ryder K, Lourenco RV, et al: Inflammatory reaction and airway damage in cystic fibrosis. *J Lab Clin Med* 1976;88: 423–426.
148. Brogan TD, Ryley HC, Neale L, et al: Soluble proteins of bronchopulmonary secretions from patients with cystic fibrosis,

asthma, and bronchitis. *Thorax* 1975;30: 72–79.
149. Pryjma J, Rudnik J, Zebrack J, et al: The local immune status in cystic fibrosis. *Monogr Paediatr* 1979;10:125–130.
150. Bell DY, Haseman JA, Spock A, et al: Plasma proteins of the bronchoalveolar surface of the lungs of smokers and nonsmokers. *Am Rev Respir Dis* 1981;124:72–79.
151. Bell DY, Spock A, Hook GER: Plasma proteins of the bronchoalveolar lining of the lung in cystic fibrosis. *Cystic Fibrosis Club Abstr* 1980;21:33.
152. McFarlane H, Allan JD, van der Zeil P: Passive cutaneous anaphylaxis (PCA) and specific IgE in cystic fibrosis and their heterozygotes. *Clin Allergy* 1977;7:279–284.
153. Lopez-Vidriero MT, Reid L: Chemical constituents of sol and gel phases of sputum from atopic and nonatopic cystic fibrosis, in Sturgess JM (ed): *Perspectives in Cystic Fibrosis.* Toronto, Canadian CF Foundation, 1980, p 26a.
154. Cromwell O, Walport MJ, Morris HR, et al: Identification of leukotrienes D and B in sputum from cystic fibrosis patients. *Lancet* 1981;2:165–175.
155. Spock A, Lanning CF, Kylstra JA, et al: Composition of lavage fluid from patients with cystic fibrosis. *Cystic Fibrosis Club Abstr* 1979;20:85.
156. Bell DY, Spock A: Unusual proteolytic activity in bronchoalveolar lavage fluid from the lungs of patients with cystic fibrosis. *Cystic Fibrosis Club Abstr* 1981;22:37.
157. Hoiby N, Olling S: *Pseudomonas aeruginosa* infection in cystic fibrosis. Bactericidal effect of serum from normal individuals and patients with cystic fibrosis on *P. aeruginosa* strains from patients with cystic fibrosis or other diseases. *Acta Pathol Microbiol Scand Sect C* 1977;85:107–114.
158. Thomassen MJ, Demko CA: Serum bactericidal effect on *Pseudomonas aeruginosa* isolates from cystic fibrosis patients. *Infect Immun* 1981;33:512–518.
159. Guttman RM, Waisbren BA: Bacterial blocking activity of specific IgG in chronic *Pseudomonas aeruginosa* infection. *Clin Exp Immunol* 1975;19:121–130.
160. Fick RB, Naegel GP, Reynolds HY: Use of *Pseudomonas aeruginosa* lipopolysaccharide immunoadsorbents to prepare high potency monospecific antibodies. *J Immunol Methods* 1980;38:103–116.
161. Fick RB, Naegel GP, Matthay RA, et al: Cystic fibrosis *Pseudomonas* opsonins. Inhibitory nature in an in vitro phagocytic assay. *J Clin Invest* 1981;68:899–914.
162. Boyd RL, Appell SV, Mangos JA: Pulmonary macrophage phagocytosis of *Pseudomonas aeruginosa* exposed to cystic fibrosis serum. *Clin Res* 1981;29:901A.
163. Nelson DS: Macrophages. Progress and problems. *Clin Exp Immunol* 1981;45:225–233.
164. Hocking WG, Golde DW: The pulmonary alveolar macrophage. *N Engl J Med* 1979; 301:580–587, 639–645.
165. Thomassen MJ, Demko CA, Sorensen RU, et al: *Pseudomonas aeruginosa* phagocytosis by normal human alveolar macrophages. Influence of in vitro activation on inhibitory effect of cystic fibrosis serum. *Cystic Fibrosis Club Abstr* 1981;22:163.
166. Shapira E, Menendez R: Increased binding of concanavalin A to α_2-macroglobulin, IgM and IgG from cystic fibrosis plasma. *Biochem Biophys Res Commun* 1980;93:50–56.
167. Hallinan F, Tempany E: Comparative analysis of lectin-binding properties of cystic fibrosis and control plasma glycoproteins. *Monogr Paediatr* 1981;14:40–45.
168. Sorensen RU, Stern RC, Chase P, et al: Defective cellular immunity to gram-negative bacteria in cystic fibrosis patients. *Infect Immun* 1979;23:398–402.
169. Sorensen RU, Chase PA, Stern RC, et al: Influence of cystic fibrosis plasma on lymphocyte responses to *Pseudomonas aeruginosa* in vitro. *Pediatr Res* 1981;15:14–18.
170. Sorensen RU, Stern RC, Polmar SH: Lymphocyte responsiveness to *Pseudomonas aeruginosa* in cystic fibrosis. Relationship to status of pulmonary disease in sibling pairs. *J Pediatr* 1978;93:201–205.
171. Sorensen RU, Stern RC, Chase PA, et al: Changes in lymphocyte reactivity to *Pseudomonas aeruginosa* in hospitalized patients with cystic fibrosis. *Am Rev Respir Dis* 1981;123:37–41.
172. Manthei U, Sieber OF, Jones JF, et al: Human lymphocyte response to *Pseudomonas aeruginosa* exotoxin and cell wall antigen. *Clin Res* 1978;26:187A.
173. Parmely M, Kanarek J, Fortado D, et al: Characterization of *Pseudomonas aeruginosa* antigens capable of eliciting in vitro cell-mediated immunity. *Cystic Fibrosis Club Abstr* 1981;22:49.
174. Sorensen RU, Rubin HR, Chase PA: Suppression of human lymphocyte proliferation by *Pseudomonas aeruginosa* in vitro. *Cystic Fibrosis Club Abstr* 1981;22:9.
175. Brandtzaeg P: Transport models for secretory IgA and secretory IgM. *Clin Exp Immunol* 1981;44:221–232.
176. South MA, Warwick WJ, Wollheim FA, et al: The IgA system. III. IgA levels in the serum and saliva of pediatric patients—evidence for a local immunoglobulin system. *J*

Pediatr 1967;71:645-653.

177. Gugler E, Pallavacini JC, Swerdlow H, et al: Immunological studies of submaxillary saliva from patients with cystic fibrosis and from normal children. *J Pediatr* 1968;73: 548-559.
178. Falchuk ZM, Taussig LM: IgA synthesis by jejunal biopsies from patients with cystic fibrosis and hereditary pancreatitis. *J Pediatr* 1973;51:49-54.
179. Rule AH, Lawrence D, Hager HJ, et al: IgA presence in meconium obtained from patients with cystic fibrosis. *J Pediatr* 1971;48: 601-604.
180. Hoiby N, Hertz JB: Precipitating antibodies against *Escherichia coli, Bacteroides fragilis ss thetaituomicron* and *Pseudomonas aeruginosa* in serum from normal persons and cystic fibrosis patients determined by means of crossed immunoelectrophoresis. *Acta Paediatr Scand* 1979;68:495-500.
181. Wallwork JC, McFarlane H: The SIgA system and hypersensitivity in patients with cystic fibrosis. *Clin Allergy* 1976;6:349-358.
182. Hanson LA, Brandtzaeg P: The mucosal defense system, in Stiehm ER, Fulginiti VA (eds): *Immunologic Disorders in Infants and Children, 2nd ed.* Philadelphia, WB Saunders, 1980, pp 137-164.
183. Lichtenstein LM: The interdependence of allergic and inflammatory processes, in Johansson SGO, et al (eds): *Molecular and Biological Aspects of the Acute Allergic Reaction.* New York, Plenum Press, 1976, pp 233-254.
184. Coombs RAA, Gell PGH: Classification of allergic reactions responsible for clinical hypersensitivity and disease, in Gell PGH, Coombs RRA, Lachmann PJ (eds): *Clinical Aspects of Immunology.* London, Blackwell, 1975, p 761.
185. Roitt I: *Essential Immunology, 4th ed.* London, Blackwell, 1980, pp 217-252.
186. Wells JV: Immune mechanisms in tissue damage, in Fudenberg HH, et al (eds): *Basic and Clinical Immunology, 3rd ed.* Los Altos, Lange Med Publ, 1980, pp 191-206.
187. Parish WE: The clinical relevance of heat-stable, short-term sensitizing anaphylactic IgG antibodies (IgG S-TS) and of related activities of IgG_4 and IgG_2. *Br J Dermatol* 1981;105:223-231.
188. Austen KF: Reaction mechanisms in the release of mediators of immediate hypersensitivity from human lung tissue. *Fed Proc* 1974;33:2256-2262.
189. Theofilopoulos AN, Dixon FJ: The biology and detection of immune complexes. *Adv Immunol* 1979;28:89-220.
190. Johansson SGO: The clinical significance of IgE, in *Clinical Immunology Update 1981.* Amsterdam, Elsevier/North Holland, 1981, pp 124-145.
191. Van Metre TE, Cooke RE, Gibson LE, et al: Evidence of allergy in patients with cystic fibrosis of the pancreas. *J Allergy* 1960;31: 141-150.
192. Kulczycki LL, Mueller H, Shwachman H: Respiratory allergy in patients with cystic fibrosis. *JAMA* 1961;175:358-364.
193. Mearns M, Longbottom J, Batten J: Precipitating antibodies to *Aspergillus fumigatus* in cystic fibrosis. *Lancet* 1967;1:538-539.
194. McCarthy DS, Pepys J, Batten J: Hypersensitivity to fungi in cystic fibrosis, in Lawson D (ed): *Proceedings of the Fifth International Cystic Fibrosis Conference.* London, Cystic Fibrosis Research Trust, 1969, pp 194-204.
195. Spitz E, Gelfand EW, Scheffer AL, et al: Serum IgE in clinical immunology and allergy. *J Allergy Clin Immunol* 1972;49: 337-347.
196. Allan JD, Moss AD, Wallwork JC, et al: Immediate hypersensitivity in patients with cystic fibrosis. *Clin Allergy* 1975;5:255-261.
197. Bardana EJ, Sobti KL, Cianculli FD, et al: *Aspergillus* antibody in patients with cystic fibrosis. *Am J Dis Child* 1975;129:1164-1167.
198. Warner JO, Taylor BW, Norman AP, et al: Association of cystic fibrosis with allergy. *Arch Dis Child* 1976;51:507-511.
199. Galant SP, Rucker RW, Grouncy CE, et al: Incidence of serum antibodies to several *Aspergillus* species and to *Candida albicans* in cystic fibrosis. *Am Rev Respir Dis* 1976; 114:325-331.
200. Warner JO: The variability of skin test hypersensitivity reactions in cystic fibrosis-immunological reactions to *A. fumigatus* and common allergens. *Clin Allergy* 1975;5: 1-12.
201. Barron R, Cotton E, Larsen G, et al: The prevalence of atopy in cystic fibrosis. *Cystic Fibrosis Club Abstr* 1977;18:38.
202. Silverman M, Hobbs FDR, Gordon IRS, et al: Cystic fibrosis, atopy, and airways lability. *Arch Dis Child* 1978;53:873-877.
203. Mitchell I, Corey M, Woenne R, et al: Bronchial hyperreactivity in cystic fibrosis and asthma. *J Pediatr* 1978;93:744-748.
204. Carswell F, Oliver J, Silverman M: Allergy in cystic fibrosis. *Clin Exp Immunol* 1979; 35:141-146.
205. Nelson LA, Callerame MLC, Schwartz RH: Aspergillosis and atopy in cystic fibrosis. *Am Rev Respir Dis* 1979;120:863-873.
206. Ormerod LP, Thomson RA, Anderson CM, et al: Reversible airway obstruction in cystic

fibrosis. *Thorax* 1980;35:768–772.
207. Tobin MJ, Maguire O, Reen D, et al: Atopy and bronchial reactivity in older patients with cystic fibrosis. *Thorax* 1980; 35:807–813.
208. Van Asperen P, Mellis CM, South RT, et al: Bronchial reactivity in cystic fibrosis with normal pulmonary function. *Am J Dis Child* 1981;135:815–819.
209. Warner JO, Norman AP, Soothill JF: Cystic fibrosis heterozygosity in the pathogenesis of allergy. *Lancet* 1976;1:990–991.
210. Mearns M, Young J, Batten J: Transient pulmonary infiltrations in cystic fibrosis due to allergic aspergillosis. *Thorax* 1965;20:385.
211. Brueton MJ, Ormerod LP, Shah KJ, et al: Allergic bronchopulmonary aspergillosis complicating cystic fibrosis in childhood. *Arch Dis Child* 1980;55:348–353.
212. Pepys J: *Hypersensitivity Diseases of the Lungs due to Fungi and Organic Dusts.* Basel, Karger, 1969.
213. Schatz M, Patterson R, Fink J: Immunologic lung disease. *N Engl J Med* 1979;300: 1310–1320.
214. Schwartz RH, Johnstone DE, Holsclaw DS, et al: Serum precipitins to *Aspergillus fumigatus* in cystic fibrosis. *Am J Dis Child* 1970;120:432–433.
215. Greenberger PA, Patterson R, Ghory A, et al: Late sequelae of allergic bronchopulmonary aspergillosis. *J Allergy Clin Immunol* 1980;66:327–335.
216. Wang JLB, Patterson R, Roberts M, et al: The management of allergic bronchopulmonary aspergillosis. *Am Rev Respir Dis* 1979;120:87–92.
217. Imbeau SA, Nichols D, Flaherty D, et al: Relationships between prednisone therapy, disease activity, and the total serum IgE level in allergic bronchopulmonary aspergillosis. *J Allergy Clin Immunol* 1978;62:91–95.
218. Marsh DG, Meyers DA, Bins WB: The epidemiology and genetics of atopic allergy. *N Engl J Med* 1981;305:1551–1559.
219. MacFarlane H, Allan JD: Cystic fibrosis heterozygosity in pathogenesis of allergy. *Lancet* 1976;1:1241.
220. Tacier-Eugster H, Wüthrich B, Meyer H: Atopic allergy, serum IgE and RAST specific IgE antibodies in patients with cystic fibrosis. *Helv Paediatr Acta* 1980;35:31–37.
221. Counahan R, Mearns MB: Prevalence of atopy and exercise-induced bronchial lability in relatives of patients with cystic fibrosis. *Arch Dis Child* 1975;50:477–481.
222. Polymenides Z, Ludwig H, Goetz M: Cystic fibrosis and HLA antigens. *Lancet* 1973;2: 1452.
223. Goodchild MC, Edward JH, Glenn KP, et al: A search for linkage in cystic fibrosis. *J Med Genet* 1976;13:417.
224. Säfwenberg J, Kollberg H, Lindblom JB: HLA frequencies in patients with cystic fibrosis. *Tissue Antigens* 1977;10:287.
225. Lowe CU, May CD, Reed SC: Fibrosis of the pancreas in infants and children. *Am J Dis Child* 1949;78:349–374.
226. Derbes VJ, Dent JH, White R: Intrinsic (non-allergic) bronchial asthma as a manifestation of fibrocystic disease of the pancreas. *J Allergy* 1957;28:287–291.
227. Lurie MH: Cystic fibrosis of the pancreas and nasal mucosa. *Ann Otol Rhinol Laryngol* 1959;68:748.
228. Pitcher-Wilmott RW, Levinsky RJ, Gordon I, et al: *Pseudomonas* infection, allergy, and cystic fibrosis. *Monogr Paediatr* 1981;14:157.
229. Gross NJ: What is this thing called love?— or defining asthma. *Am Rev Respir Dis* 1980;121:203–204.
230. Scadding JG: Definition and clinical categories of asthma, in Clark TJH, Godfrey S (eds): *Asthma.* Philadelphia, Saunders, 1977, pp 1–10.
231. Chai H, Farr RS, Froelich LA, et al: Standardization of bronchial inhalation challenge procedures. *J Allergy Clin Immunol* 1975;56:323–327.
232. Boushey HA, Holtzman MJ, Sheller JR, et al: Bronchial hyperreactivity. *Am Rev Respir Dis* 1980;121:389–413.
233. Featherby EA, Wenz TR, Levison H: The effect of isoproterenol in airway obstruction in cystic fibrosis. *Can Med Assoc J* 1970; 102:835–838.
234. Zaplatal A, Motoyama EK, Gibson LE, et al: Pulmonary mechanics in asthma and cystic fibrosis. *Pediatrics* 1971;48:64–72.
235. Landau LI, Phelan PD: The variable effect of a bronchodilating agent on pulmonary function in cystic fibrosis. *J Pediatr* 1973;82:863–868.
236. Shapiro GG, Bamman J, Kanarek P, et al: The paradoxical effect of adrenergic and methylxanthine drugs in cystic fibrosis. *Pediatrics* 1976;58:740–743.
237. Alidina L, Simon D, Palmer J, et al: Evaluation of aerosol agents in patients with cystic fibrosis. *Cystic Fibrosis Club Abstr* 1979; 20:23.
238. Larsen GZ, Parron RJ, Cotton EK, et al: A comparative study of inhaled atropine sulfate and isoproterenol hydrochloride in cystic fibrosis. *Am Rev Respir Dis* 1979; 119:399–406.
239. Kattan M, Mansell A, Levison H, et al: Response to aerosol salbutamol, SCH 1000, and placebo in cystic fibrosis. *Thorax* 1980;35:531–535.

240. Day G, Mearns MB: Bronchial lability in cystic fibrosis. *Arch Dis Child* 1973;48:355–359.
241. Rothstein RJ, Penney MA, Buckley JM, et al: Evaluation of reactive airway disease in atopic cystic fibrosis patients. *J Allergy Clin Immunol* 1974;53:100.
242. Haluszka J, Scislicki A: Bronchial lability in children suffering from some diseases of the bronchi. *Respiration* 1975;32:217–226.
243. Mellis CM, Levison H: Bronchial reactivity in cystic fibrosis. *Pediatrics* 1978;61:446–450.
244. Holzer FJ, Olinsky A, Phelan PD: Variability of airways hyperreactivity and allergy in cystic fibrosis. *Arch Dis Child* 1981;56:455–459.
245. Price JF, Weller PH, Harper SA, et al: Bronchial provocation tests in cystic fibrosis. *Monogr Paediatr* 1979;10:123–124.
246. Leupold W, Dietzsch HJ: Bronchial reactivity in children with cystic fibrosis and other recurrent or chronic bronchopulmonary diseases. *Monogr Paediatr* 1979;10:119–122.
247. Norman PS: An overview of immunotherapy. *J Allergy Clin Immunol* 1980;65:87–96.
248. Wellever RC, Wong DT, Sun M, et al: The development of respiratory syncytial virus-specific IgE and the release of histamine in nasopharyngeal secretions after infection. *N Engl J Med* 1981;305:841–846.
249. Berger M, Kirkpatrick CH, Goldsmith PK, et al: IgE antibodies to *Staphylococcus aureus* and *Candida albicans* in patients with the syndrome of hyperimmunoglobulin E and recurrent infections. *J Immunol* 1980; 125:2437–2443.
250. Danneman PJ, Michael JG: Reaginic antibody production to protein antigens of *Eschericha coli* and *Pseudomonas aeruginosa* by mice. *Infect Immun* 1976;14:694–702.
251. Reid MJ, Cheung NKV, Lewiston NJ: Microtiter solid-phase radioimmunoassay for specific immunoglobulin E. *J Allergy Clin Immunol* 1981;67:263–271.
252. Shen J, Brackett R, Fischer T, et al: Specific *Pseudomonas* immunoglobulin E antibodies in serum of patients with cystic fibrosis. *Infect Immun* 1981;32:967–968.
253. Skov PS, Norn S, Schiotz PO, et al: *Pseudomonas aeruginosa* allergy in cystic fibrosis. Involvement of histamine release in the pathogenesis of lung tissue damage. *Allergy* 1980;35:25–29.
254. Pepys J: IgG-STS antibodies as mediators of allergic reactions, in Steffen C, Ludwig H (eds): *Clinical Immunology and Allergology*. Amsterdam, Elsevier/North Holland, 1981, pp 349–355.
255. Shakib F, Stanworth DR, Smalley CA, et al: Elevated serum IgG4 levels in cystic fibrosis patients. *Clin Allergy* 1976;6:237–240.
256. Moss RB, Hsu YP, Leahy M, et al: IgG4 antibody to *Pseudomonas aeruginosa* in cystic fibrosis. *Cystic Fibrosis Club Abstr* 1982;23:13.
257. Iskander R, Das PK, Aalberse RC: IgG4 antibodies in Egyptian patients with schistosomiasis. *Int Arch Allergy Appl Immunol* 1981;66:200–207.
258. Moss RB, Hsu YP, Leahy M, et al: Enzyme immunoassay for honey bee venom specific IgG4. *Clin Res* 1982;30:165A.
259. Blessing J, Cheung NK, Reid M, et al: Specific IgE, IgG, and IgG4 in patients undergoing honeybee venom immunotherapy. *J Allergy Clin Immunol* 1982;69:S140.
260. Dolan TF, Meyer A: Bronchial asthma and allergic rhinitis associated with inhalation of pancreatic extracts. *Am Rev Respir Dis* 1974;110:812–813.
261. Bergner A, Bergner RK: Pulmonary hypersensitivity associated with pancreatin powder exposure. *Pediatrics* 1975;55:814–817.
262. Twarog FJ, Weinstein SF, Khaw KT, et al: Hypersensitivity to pancreatic extracts in parents of children with CF. *J Allergy Clin Immunol* 1977;59:35–40.
263. Romeo G, Parsons M, Bossen A, et al: Trypsin-binding IgG in cystic fibrosis. *Nature* 1978;274:909–911.
264. Murray MJ, Thal AP: The clinical significance of circulating pancreatic antibodies. *Ann Intern Med* 1960;55:548–555.
265. Stein AA, Manlapas FC, Soike KF, et al: Specific isoantibodies in cystic fibrosis. *J Pediatr* 1964;65:495–500.
266. Hoiby N, Wiik A: Antibacterial precipitins and autoantibodies in serum from patients with cystic fibrosis. *Scand J Respir Dis* 1975;56:38–46.
267. Schiotz PO, Egeskjold EM, Hoiby N, et al: Autoantibodies in serum and sputum from patients with cystic fibrosis. *Acta Pathol Microbiol Scand Sect C* 1979;87:319–324.
268. Moss RB, Hsu YP: IgM and IgG rheumatoid factors in cystic fibrosis compared to rheumatic diseases of childhood and controls. *Clin Res* 1982;38:96A.
269. Talal N: *Autoimmunity: Genetic, Immunologic, Virologic, and Clinical Aspects*. New York, Academic Press, 1977.
270. Romeo G, Parsons M, Bossen A, et al: Binding of ^{125}I-labeled proteinases to plasma proteins in cystic fibrosis. *Pediatr Res* 1979;13:1030–1036.
271. Denaro M, Romeo G: Antibodies cross-reacting with porcine and human trypsin in cystic fibrosis. *Pediatr Res* 1980;14:1086–1088.

272. Rao GJR, Nadler HL: Deficiency of arginine esterase in cystic fibrosis of the pancreas. Demonstration of the proteolytic nature of the activity. *Pediatr Res* 1975;9: 739–741.
273. Halbert SP: Immunological aspects of cystic fibrosis. *Mod Probl Pediatr* 1967;10: 144–157.
274. Talamo RC, Stiehm ER, Schwartz RH: Immunologic aspects of cystic fibrosis, in Mangos JA, Talamo RC (eds): *Cystic Fibrosis. Projections into the Future.* Miami, Symposia Specialists, 1976, pp 195–217.
275. Manson JC, Brock DJH: Development of a quantitative immunoassay for the cystic fibrosis gene. *Lancet* 1980;1:330–331.
276. Wilson GB: Monospecific antisera, hybridoma antibodies, and immunoassays for cystic fibrosis protein. *Lancet* 1980;2:313–314.
277. di Sant'Agnese PA, Davis PB: Research in cystic fibrosis. *N Engl J Med* 1976;295: 481–485, 534–541, 597–602.
278. Schiotz PO, Hoiby N, Juhl F, et al: Immune complexes in cystic fibrosis. *Acta Pathol Microbiol Scand Sect C* 1977;85:57–64.
279. Schiotz PO, Nielsen H, Hoiby N, et al: Immune complexes in the sputum of patients with cystic fibrosis suffering from chronic *Pseudomonas aeruginosa* lung infection. *Acta Pathol Microbiol Scand Sect C* 1978; 86:37–40.
280. Berdischewsky M, Pollack M, Young LS, et al: Circulating immune complexes in cystic fibrosis. *Pediatr Res* 1980;14:830–833.
281. Church JA, Jordan SC, Keens TG, et al: Circulating immune complexes in patients with cystic fibrosis. *Chest* 1981;80:405–411.
282. Moss RB, Hsu YP: Isolation and characterization of circulating immune complexes in cystic fibrosis. *Clin Exp Immunol* 1982; 47:301–308.
283. Daniele RP, Henson PM, Fantone JC, et al: Immune complex injury of the lung. *Am Rev Respir Dis* 1981;124:738–755.
284. Rabinovitch M, Manejias RE, Nussenzweing V: Selective phagocytic paralysis induced by immobilized immune complexes. *J Exp Med* 1975;142:827–838.
285. Hoiby N, Flensborg EW, Beck B, et al: *Pseudomonas aeruginosa* infection in cystic fibrosis. Diagnostic and prognostic significant of *Pseudomonas aeruginosa* precipitins determined by means of crossed immunoelectrophoresis. *Scand J Respir Dis* 1977; 58:65–79.
286. Hoiby N, Jacobsen L, Jorgensen BA, et al: *Pseudomonas aeruginosa* infection in cystic fibrosis. Occurrence of precipitating antibodies against *Pseudomonas aeruginosa* in relation to the concentration of sixteen serum proteins and the clinical and radiographical status of the lungs. *Acta Paediatr Scand* 1974;63:843–848.
287. Newman AJ, Ansell BM: Episodic arthritis in children with cystic fibrosis. *J Pediatr* 1979;94:594–596.
288. Soter NA, Mihm MC, Colten HR: Cutaneous necrotizing venulitis in patients with cystic fibrosis. *J Pediatr* 1979;95:197–201.
289. Goldsmith D, Schidlow D, Palmer J, et al: Rheumatic manifestations of cystic fibrosis, in Sturgess JM (ed): *Perspectives in Cystic Fibrosis.* Toronto, Canadian CF Foundation, 1980, p 17a.
290. Fick RB, Hen J, Dolan TF: Acute monoarticular arthropathies in cystic fibrosis. *Cystic Fibrosis Club Abstr* 1981;22:112.
291. Cash HA, Woods DE, McCullough B, et al: A rat model of chronic respiratory infection with *Pseudomonas aeruginosa. Am Rev Respir Dis* 1979;119:453–459.
292. Pennington JE, Hickey, WF, Blackwood LL, et al: Active immunization with lipopolysaccharide *Pseudomonas* antigen for chronic *Pseudomonas* bronchopneumonia in guinea pigs. *J Clin Invest* 1981;68:1140–1148.
293. Lewiston NJ, Moss RB: Circulating immune complexes decrease during corticosteroid therapy in cystic fibrosis. *Pediatr Res* 1982; 16:354.
294. Permin H, Norn S, Skov PS, et al: Platelet ^{3}H-serotonin release induced by *Pseudomonas aeruginosa* antigens in patients with cystic fibrosis. An in vitro model of immune complex disease. *Monogr Paediatr* 1981; 14:158.
295. Oppenheimer EH, Esterly JR: Pathology of cystic fibrosis. *Perspect Pediatr Pathol* 1975; 5:241–278.
296. Mieli-Vergani G, Psacharopoulos HT, Nicholson AM, et al: Immune response to liver membrane antigens in patients with cystic fibrosis. *Arch Dis Child* 1980;55:696–701.
297. Marks MI: The pathogenesis and treatment of pulmonary infections in cystic fibrosis. *J Pediatr* 1981;98:173–179.
298. Hodson ME, Penketh ARL, Batten JC: Aerosol carbenicillin and gentamicin treatment of *Pseudomonas aeruginosa* infection in patients with cystic fibrosis. *Lancet* 1981; 2:1137–1139.
299. Lewis RA, Austen KF: Mediation of local homeostasis and inflammation by leukotrienes and other mast cell-dependent compounds. *Nature* 1981;293:103–108.
300. Lee HJ, Soliman MRI: Anti-inflammatory steroids without pituitary-adrenal suppression. *Science* 1982;215:989–991.
301. Kaliner M: Is a mast cell a mast cell a mast cell? *J Allergy Clin Immunol* 1980;66:1–4.

11

Meconium

John D. Lloyd-Still

Meconium is a dark, greenish mass of desquamated cells, mucus, and bile that accumulates in the bowel during fetal life and is discharged shortly after birth. In healthy newborns the first postnatal passage of meconium occurs in 69% within 12 hours, 25% at 12–24 hours, and 5.8% at 24–48 hours.[1] Meconium is sterile, and the normal fecal flora appears by the second day. The amount of meconium passed by a full term, healthy newborn varies from 60–200 g.[2] Two excellent reviews of meconium in health and disease have been published.[3,4] About 70–75% of the total weight of meconium is water;[4–6] 70–80% of the dry mass of meconium is composed of mucous glycoproteins.[3] Meconium is rich in blood-group-specific substances which are the same as in the amniotic fluid and correspond with the blood type of the baby.[6] Table 11-1 summarizes data on the constituents of meconium in normal and in cystic fibrosis infants with and without meconium ileus.

Meconium abnormalities in CF are important in three clinical situations: (1) meconium ileus; (2) delay in the passage of meconium; and (3) screening purposes. The surgical management of meconium ileus is covered in Chapter 21. Screening tests for CF are analyzed in Chapter 2. Meconium abnormalities in CF are discussed below.

MECONIUM CONSTITUENTS

Viscosity and Water Content

Specimens from four infants with meconium ileus were five times more viscous than

Table 11-1
Major Differences in Constituents of Meconium from Controls and CF Infants With and Without Meconium Ileus*

	Control	CF	CF with Meconium Ileus	References
Viscosity			Increased × 5	7
Water content (%)	72.9		66	26
Minerals				
Sodium (mM/kg)	328 (86–640)	155 (63–230)	254 (163–336)	
Potassium (mM/kg)	93 (11–230)	67 (40–110)	33 (16–47)	
Magnesium (mM/kg)	84 (21–212)	65 (35–152)	37 (16–72)	
Zinc (μg/g)	230 (39–569)	157 (42–420)	138 (36–284)	
Copper (μg/g)	64 (22–152)	50 (16–128)	36 (21–61)	8
Iron (μg/g)	74 (28–172)	53 (32–98)	10 (2–21)	
Magnesium (μg/g)	20 (5–53)	10 (2–21)	11 (5–20)	
Calcium (mM/kg)	47 (7–174)	36 (19–59)	72 (20–204)	
Phosphorus (mM/kg)	20 (15–32)	21 (13–34)	36 (11–57)	
Proteins				
Protein (%)	9.5		61.0	26
Mucoprotein (%)	7.3		15.1	26
Albumin (%)	0.11	11.8		13
α_1-Antitrypsin	Present		Present	11
α_1-Antichymotrypsin	Present		Present	11
Transferrin	Absent		Present	11
β_{1C}-globulin	Absent		Present	11
IgA	Absent		Present	11
IgG	Absent		Present	11
Secretory IgA	Absent		Present	11
Proteolytic enzymes				
Trypsin	Present day 3	Absent in 75%		4
Glycoproteins				
Protein-bound carbohydrate (%)	50		10	18
Fucose	Normal		Increased	18
Sialic acid	Normal		Decreased	18
Disaccharidases				
Lactase		Increased × 100		24
Sucrase		Increased × 18		24
Maltase		Increased × 4.8		24
Isomaltase		Increased × 8.9		24
Total Reducing Sugars			Decreased × 4	6
Lysosomal enzymes				
α-D-Mannosidase			Decreased	25
β-Glucuronidase			Decreased	25
β-D-Fucosidase			Increased	25
Acid phosphatase			Normal	25
Alkaline phosphatase			Decreased	25
Lipids				
Phospholipids			?Increased	25
Cholesterol			?Increased	25
Cholesterol esters			?Increased	25
Bile acids				
No data in meconium ileus				
Increased in untreated CF infants				28

*Note that in a number of studies (4, 13, 24, 25) the data for CF infants with and without meconium ileus have been combined.

those from 46 full-term healthy infants.[7] It is thought the reduced water content in CF meconium accounts for the increased viscosity. The water content of meconium controls was 72.9% compared to 66.0% for meconium ileus infants.[26] Addition of albumin to normal meconium increases the viscosity,[9] while addition of pancreatic enzymes or normal duodenal fluid liquefies the sticky meconium in CF.[4]

Minerals

The mineral composition of meconium is high compared to amniotic fluid or urine. The mean concentrations of sodium, potassium, magnesium, zinc, copper, iron, and manganese are all higher in meconium from healthy infants and unaffected CF siblings compared with meconium from infants with CF.[8] In four specimens of meconium from meconium ileus patients there was an increase in calcium and phosphorus compared to normal. Levels of magnesium, zinc, copper, and iron were all decreased in meconium ileus compared to CF without meconium ileus or normal controls (Table 11-1). Assay of these elements for the diagnosis of CF is impractical owing to overlapping values and a wide range of distribution.

Plasma Proteins

Five to ten percent of the total dry weight of meconium is composed of plasma proteins and tissue debris.[10] Most plasma proteins are degraded by proteolytic enzymes except for the protease inhibitors α1-antitrypsin and α1-antichymotrypsin. Ryley et al[11] found approximately 5% of normal meconium specimens contain greater than 1 mg of albumin per gram dry weight. Figure 11-1 shows their results using a crossed immunoelectrophoresis technique. Note the large peak for albumin and the presence of other proteins including transferrin, β1C-globulin, immunoglobulin A (IgA), immunoglobulin G (IgG), and Gc globulin.

Amniotic fluid is considered to be the source of protein present in the meconium of infants with CF.[9] Pecau and Feigleson[12] demonstrated 7–17 proteins in meconium from CF, compared to 4 in normal meconium, 14 from normal amniotic fluid, and 18 from cord blood. It seems likely that the bulk of meconium ileus albumin represents unhydrolyzed and unabsorbed amniotic fluid protein.[3]

The albumin (as percentage of total soluble protein in meconium) in CF meconium was 11.8 compared to control values of

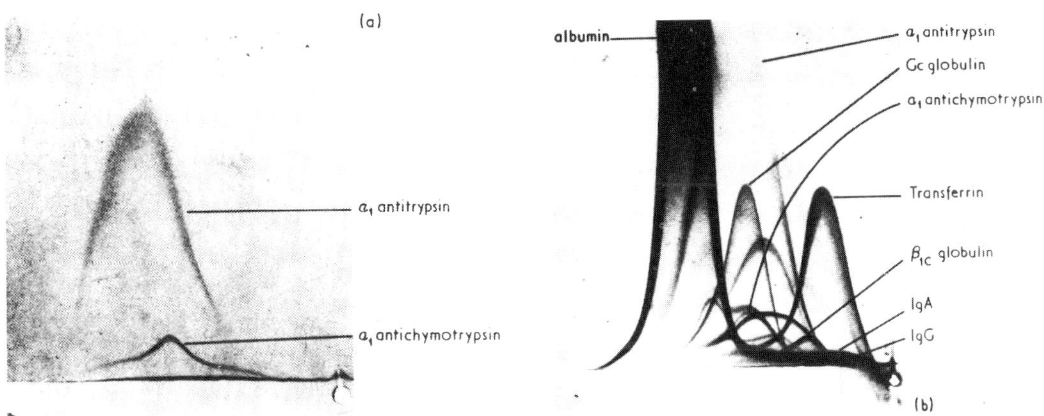

Figure 11-1 Crossed immunoelectrophoretic patterns of aqueous extracts of meconium against rabbit antihuman serum. The protein arcs were stained with Coomassie Blue. (a) Typical pattern produced by extract of normal specimen prepared from a 1% suspension of freeze-dried meconium showing peaks caused by α_1-antitrypsin and α_1-antichymotrypsin. (b) Pattern produced by aqueous extracts of specimen from CF patient (Case 1) prepared from a 1% suspension of freeze-dried meconium showing peaks caused by albumin, α_1-antitrypsin, α_1-antichymotrypsin, Gc globulin, transferrin, β_{1c} globulin, IgA, and IgG. Reproduced from Ryley et al: *Arch Dis Child* 1974;49:901 (reference 11), with permission.

0.11.[13] Rule et al[14] found IgA in 12 of 13 samples of meconium from patients with CF and in the amniotic fluid of CF mothers and mothers known to be heterozygotes for CF. Studies of normal amniotic fluid elicit little or no serum IgA and no secretory IgA. Rule et al[14] deduced that the meconium IgA was of fetal origin, although they could not exclude the possibility that the CF sample contained significant cross-reacting material. Secretory IgA is believed to be synthesized locally in mucous membranes shortly after birth in response to antigenic stimuli. Rule et al[14] suggested that secretory IgA synthesis may be associated with the disease process of CF, both prior to and after birth. See Chapter 10 for further discussion of this topic.

Proteolytic Enzymes (Trypsin, Chymotrypsin, Peptidases)

There is disagreement on the appearance of proteolytic activity in the normal neonate. Antonowicz and Shwachman[4] state that meconium from healthy infants lacks proteolytic activity until the third to fourth day of life. Lieberman[15] noted the appearance of proteolytic activity in 500-g fetuses (26–28) weeks) and found activity in 87% of full-term neonates. The concurrent appearance of tryptic activity with that of enterokinase suggests that the activation of zymogens by enterokinase is an essential factor in the appearance of tryptic activity in the fetal small intestine.[4] Proteolytic activity is absent in approximately 75% of infants with CF.[4] Fourteen different peptidases have been found in normal meconium,[16] but no data are available on peptidase activity in CF meconium.

Glycoproteins

Of the dry mass of meconium 70–80% is composed of mucous glycoproteins. Meconium predominantly consists of carbohydrate-containing substances that are resistant to proteolysis. The water-soluble fraction of meconium contains 80% of the total carbohydrate content. The monosaccharides detected were galactose, sialic acid, fucose, *N*-acetylglucosamine, and *N*-acetylgalactosamine with little or no mannose.[17] Whereas normal meconium contained about 50% protein-bound carbohydrate, the meconium from CF infants contained only about 10%.[18] Analysis of the mucous glycopolypeptides in CF showed greater amounts of fucose and lesser amounts of sialic acid than normal. These differences do not become apparent until the material has been purified to the mucous glycopolypeptide stage. Increased fucose concentration has important effects on the properties of mucous. Fucose has a hydrophobic group which, when present in excess, would reduce the water associated with the oligosaccharide unit. In addition, neighboring chains could associate through hydrophobic interaction. Both these effects would increase the gel-like properties of mucous and might be important in CF.[18] An abnormal distribution of α-L-fucosidase has been reported in CF with an increase in skin fibroblasts and a decreased activity in serum.[19] Interestingly, in fucosidosis, where the basic defect is a complete absence of α-L-fucosidase, the sweat electrolyte levels are in the CF range.[20] Further discussion of glycoprotein abnormalities is included in Chapter 6.

Glycosidases (Disaccharidases)

The development of the glycosidases in the normal fetus has been extensively studied.[21–23] The function of glycosidases is not only to hydrolyze disaccharides, but also to promote the synthesis of complex carbohydrates by transglycosidation.[24] Their origin is probably the intestinal mucosa, and they are susceptible to proteolysis.[3] The activities of sucrase and maltase were higher in fetal meconium than in the meconium of full-term infants. Lactase, trehalase, and cellobiose were low or undetectable in meconium. The gradual decrease in some enzyme activities in full-term as compared to premature infants is thought to be related to the appearance of other proteolytic enzymes in the fetal intestine.

In contrast, the activities (expressed as micromoles per gram of protein per minute) of lactase (×100), sucrase (×18), maltase (×4.8), and palatinase (×8.9) were significantly higher in CF meconium compared to healthy controls.[24] The reason for these increased glycosidase activities in CF is unknown but is thought to be related to the lack of proteolysis. It is relevant that there is a fourfold decrease in total reducing sugars in CF meconium compared to controls.[6] It has also been suggested that not only pancreatic proteases, but lysosomal enzymes may be necessary for the digestion of protein.[4] However, data on lysosomal protease activity in CF are lacking. The increased lactase activity in CF has been proposed as a screening test for CF in association with the increased albumin content.[24]

Lysosomal Enzymes

Lysosomal enzymes participate in the metabolism of polysaccharides and in the carbohydrate chains of glycoproteins, mucoproteins, mucopolysaccharides, and glycolipids. Antonowicz et al[25] confirmed the activity in lysosomal enzymes in the meconium from healthy neonates. They found considerable activity of α-D-mannosidase, *N*-acetyl-β-glucosaminidase, α-D-glucosidase and β-glucuronidase. The activities of α-L-fucosidase, β-D-fucosidase, and α-galactosidase were very low or absent. Acid phosphatase was present in lower concentration.

In CF meconium α-D-mannosidase and β-glucuronidase had significantly lower ($P<0.001$, $P<0.002$) activities compared to controls, while the activity of β-D-fucosidase was significantly increased ($P<0.001$). No difference was found in acid phosphatase activity.[25] The increased activity in β-D-fucosidase was also suggested as an alternative method for screening newborns for CF.[25]

Alkaline Phosphatase

This is a particulate enzyme and is distributed in several organelles. The activity of this enzyme in CF meconium was significantly decreased ($P<0.001$) compared to controls.[25]

Amylase

Some activity of amylase has been found in normal meconium.[4] However, data on amylase activity in CF meconium are lacking.

Lipids

Lipids comprise 12.3% of meconium solids and are important constituents of the glycolipids.[26] Lipids are present in normal meconium predominantly as fatty acids. Palmitic acid comprises 41%, stearic acid 18%, and arachidonic acid together with other fatty acids with more than 22 carbon atoms 41%. Preliminary investigations of lipids in CF meconium show an increase in phospholipids, cholesterol, and cholesterol esters when compared to controls.[25]

Bile Acids

Several investigators have analyzed the composition of bile acids in normal meconium.[27–29] Two primary (cholic and chenodeoxycholic) and two secondary (deoxycholic and lithocholic) bile acids have been identified in meconium.[27] Since meconium is sterile and secondary bile acids are synthesized by intraluminal bacterial enzyme systems, these observations suggest that the secondary bile acids are maternal in origin. The primary bile acids were predominantly unsulfated and comprised 40–60% of the specimens.[28] The transplacentally acquired secondary bile acids were sulfated compounds of which 60% were composed of lithocholic acid. Besides the four main bile acids of humans, several "atypical" bile acids were identified in meconium.[29] It is thought that these "atypical" bile acids reflect a special fetal bile acid metabolism and suggest that the fetal bile acid synthesis differs markedly from the adult. These findings are of interest as it appears that a resurgence of fetal biosynthetic pathways takes place under conditions of cholestatic liver disease, and cholestasis is a common feature in CF.

Data on bile acid composition in CF meconium is lacking, but excessive fecal bile acid loss is characteristic of untreated CF in the infant (see Chapter 18).

Steroids, Sterols, and Hemoglobin Metabolites

An extensive literature on the isolation of these compounds in normal meconium has been published.[3,4] Comparative data for CF meconium are lacking.

Summary

The abnormalities in CF meconium include increased viscosity, decreased water content, and an increased albumin content in association with numerous other plasma protein constituents. There is an absence of proteolytic enzymes, but the disaccharidases are increased. Some lysosomal enzymes are decreased, while others are increased. The total content of mucoprotein is considerably increased, while the protein-bound carbohydrate is decreased. The fucose is increased, while the sialic acid content is decreased. Analysis of mineral composition shows decreases in most constituents except calcium, which is increased in meconium ileus.

DIFFERENTIAL DIAGNOSIS OF MECONIUM ABNORMALITIES

A number of other conditions are characterized by increased albumin content in the meconium and include prematurity, intestinal atresia, melena neonatorum, pancreatic insufficiency with neutropenia (Shwachman-Diamond syndrome) and congenital atresia of the pancreatic ducts. These disorders may cause confusion if the increased albumin content of meconium is used as a screening test for CF. Shwachman et al[30] screened 2182 specimens of meconium for increased albumin content and found 46 positive results. Twenty-nine specimens came from infants with CF, and 12 yielded false-positive results (for further discussion, see Chapter 2).

CLINICAL SYNDROMES

Meconium Ileus

This subject is discussed in detail in Chapter 21. It has been postulated that the absence of pancreatic enzymes contributes to the development of meconium ileus. However, Oppenheimer and Esterly,[31] found no pancreatic lesions in 10 of 17 infants who died following meconium ileus. Thus, a defect in pancreatic enzyme production or secretion must precede the appearance of morphologic damage by reducing the intraluminal content of proteolytic enzymes. This reduction in proteolytic enzymes would also protect other enzymatic material in the meconium from digestion.[24]

It is mandatory to perform a sweat test in all newborn infants with intestinal obstruction or atresias, as CF accounts for over 30% of all newborns presenting with intestinal obstruction.

Meconium Plug Syndrome

The meconium plug syndrome is a common cause of low intestinal obstruction in the newborn infant and is usually a benign condition.[32] It has been reported with prematurity,[33] hypotonia,[34] following drug administration to the mother (eg, magnesium sulfate),[35] with Hirschsprung's disease,[33] in hypothyroidism, and in CF.[36] It has been postulated that the plug is related to impaired colonic motility and immaturity, or alternatively to abnormalities of the meconium itself.[32] Decreased trypsin concentration[4] and increased protein concentration have been described in the meconium plug, both of which subsequently return to normal.[37]

Rosenstein et al[38] reviewed the neonatal course of 87 infants with CF without meconium ileus and found 12 had clinical features consistent with the meconium plug syndrome. They postulated that meconium ileus and the meconium plug syndrome represent different gradations of the same pathogenic abnormality and suggested a sweat test should be performed in all infants with any type of meconium abnormality. Other authorities disagree with this interpretation and regard meconium ileus as being a specific abnormality associated with the presence of a microcolon; they regard the meconium plug syndrome as a distal obstruction quite unrelated to CF. (See Chapter 21 for our own data on the incidence of cystic fibrosis and the various meconium abnormalities.)

Meconium Ileus Unassociated with CF

This syndrome has now been well documented in at least 12 patients,[39–41] and we have personal experience of three patients. The clinical presentation and findings are similar to classic meconium ileus in association with CF. Moreover, a familial incidence has been reported.[40] Rickham[39] described 7 patients with this syndrome seen during a seven-year period during which there were 49 patients with meconium ileus and 58 patients with Hirschsprung's disease. Sweat electrolytes were reported in the normal range in 9 patients who survived, thus excluding CF. In the 3 patients who died sweat tests were not performed, and although the pancreases were normal on histology, CF could still have been present in view of the findings of a normal pancreas in 40% of CF infants who died from meconium ileus.[31] Tryptic activity was normal in all patients who survived. Three of the 5 survivors reported by Rickham et al[39] showed abnormalities in their glucose tolerance tests, 3 had abnormal gelatin absorption curves, and 1 had a flat glycine absorption curve. Fat absorption studies in 3 infants were normal. However, these findings could have been related to the "small-bowel contamination syndrome" in which fecal bacteria reside in the upper intestine following a motility disturbance, resulting in temporary impaired upper intestinal function with flat tolerance curves for glucose, amino acids and fat.[42]

It is important to follow these infants and repeat the sweat test if the clinical course is suggestive of CF. In our experience this is a more common error than the rare disorder of meconium ileus unassociated with CF.

Meconium Ileus Equivalent

Patients with CF, regardless of age, may develop obstruction of the intestine attributable to abnormal intestinal contents.[43] The name "meconium ileus equivalent" was originally coined by Jenson.[44] The obstruction by the viscous, sticky intestinal contents is most commonly found in the cecum and tends to occur in the older child with CF. The literature contains numerous case reports of patients with CF who developed meconium ileus equivalent and underwent a variety of surgical procedures. Since surgery is rarely necessary, and the condition is usually preventable, only brief mention will be made of this literature.

Jaffe et al[45] described 7 patients and summarized reports of 35 examples of meconium ileus equivalent that had developed in 34 patients. One of their 7 patients had an associated intussusception and another had acute appendicitis. The other 5 improved with medical therapy. Matsehe et al[46] described 12 patients with meconium ileus equivalent seen between 1950 and 1975. Two were operated on for fecal masses. They emphasized the triad of recurrent colicky abdominal pain, a mass in the right lower quadrant, and signs of mechanical intestinal obstruction in a patient with CF.

Meconium ileus equivalent is seen in over 10% of patients in any large CF clinic. It occurs more commonly in patients over 10 years of age and seems to have an increased incidence (35%) in black patients with CF.[47] The diagnosis can be suspected when a history of abdominal pain is elicited and physical examination reveals a mass in the right lower quadrant which may or may not be tender. If the patient is on antibiotics and the physician is unfamiliar with CF, the patient may be suspected of having appendicitis with appendix abscess, and this is probably the reason so many patients in the past were subjected to surgery. On rare occasions an associated intussusception, sometimes with a polyp as the lead point, may fail to respond to Gastrografin enema therapy and require laparotomy. We have personal

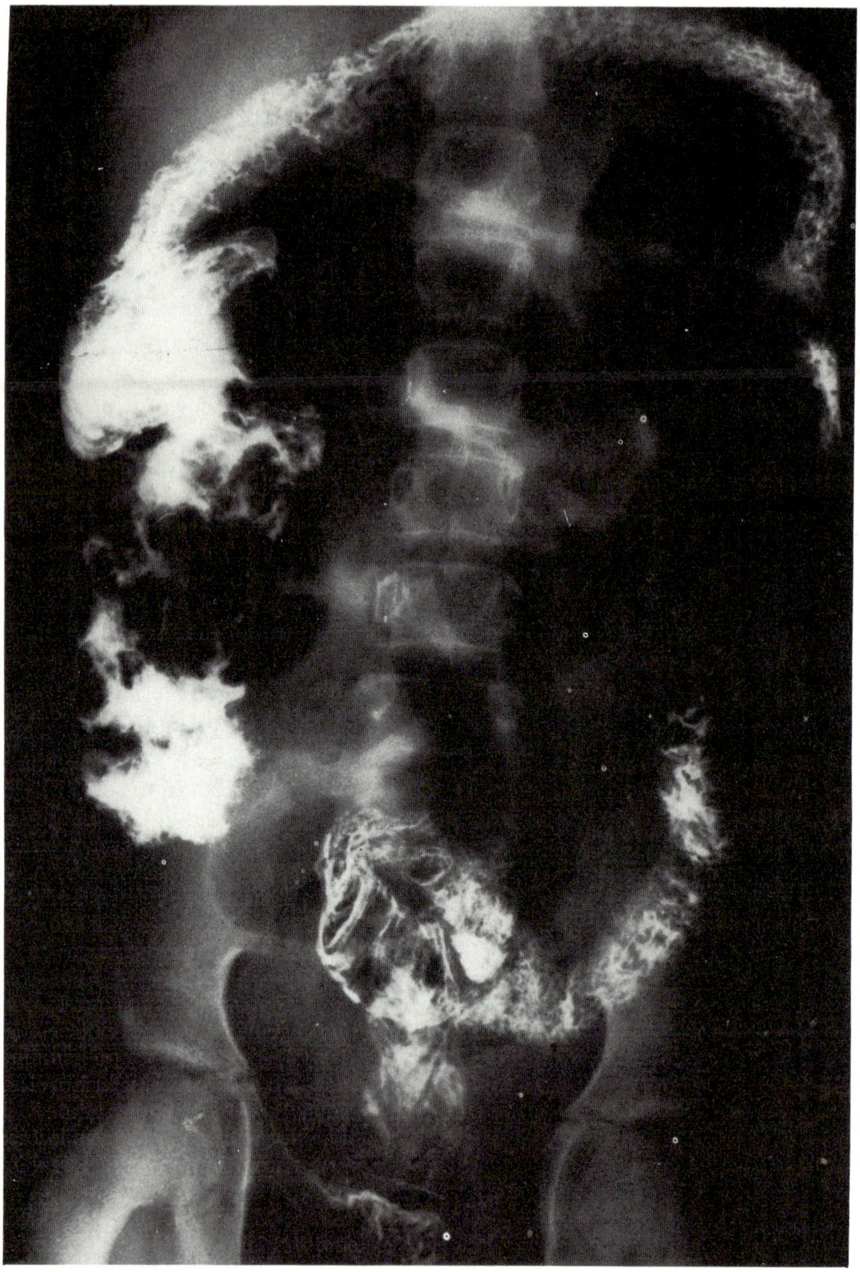

Figure 11-2 A 12-year-old female. Meconium ileus equivalent with obstructed small-bowel loops dilated with air. Irregular filling defects in the cecum and colon are the result of impaction by a mixture of thickened secretions and fecal debris. The hyperplastic mucosal pattern of the other portions of colon is a classical change of cystic fibrosis. (Courtesy of Dr. Sandra Fernbach.)

experience of two such patients. Small bowel volvulus has also been reported.[43]

Although meconium ileus equivalent is caused by the viscous fecal contents, it is difficult to explain why certain patients seem more prone to this complication than others. There seems to be some male predominance in the two large series reported.[45,46] While it is common to blame the condition on cessation of pancreatic enzyme replacement, dietary indiscretions, or intercurrent infections leading to dehydration, the precipitating event is usually unknown. In many ways the condition resembles intussusception where it has been hypothesized that hypertrophy of the Peyers patches occurs and an increased incidence of viral infections, including the rotovirus, has been reported.[48] The average age for intussusception in CF is 9 years, and this condition is considerably more common in CF patients than in the general population.[49]

TREATMENT

Treatment is largely preventive. All CF patients with palpable fecal masses should be questioned about abdominal pain. The condition should be explained to the patient and parents, and mineral oil in large doses (several tablespoons per day) prescribed until the masses have disappeared. Sometimes parents can be instructed to feel for the presence of abdominal masses. If abdominal pain is present or the pain is severe, the patient should be admitted to hospital for observation. If the plain and erect x-ray films of the abdomen show evidence of intestinal obstruction with fluid levels, then a Gastrografin enema (Gastrografin diluted 50% with normal saline) should be given (Figure 11-2). On occasions this may have to be repeated several times. Other treatments that have been given include a trial of *N*-acetylcysteine (Mucomyst) given orally (30 cc tid) or per rectum. The pulmonary status must be checked at this time as the presence of pain and anorexia may lead to deterioration. Surgery is required in those few patients who develop: (1) intestinal obstruction that cannot be relieved by medical measures; (2) persistent abdominal pain with continuing evidence of obstructive signs; or (3) the presence of an associated polyp.

REFERENCES

1. Sherry SN, Kramer I: The time of passage of the first stool and first urine by newborn infants. *J Pediatr* 1955;46:158–159.
2. Grulee CG, Bonar BE: *The Newborn; Physiology and Care.* New York, Appleton, 1926.
3. Harries JT: Meconium in health and disease. *Br Med Bull* 1978;34:75–78.
4. Antonowicz I, Shwachman H: Meconium in health and in disease. *Adv Pediatr* 1979;26: 275–310.
5. Hall IC, O'Toole E: Bacterial flora of first specimens of meconium passed by fifty newborn infants. *Am J Dis Child* 1934;47:1279–1285.
6. Rapoport S, Buchanan DJ: The composition of meconium: Isolation of blood group specific polysaccharides. Abnormal composition of meconium in meconium ileus. *Science* 1950;112:150–153.
7. Griffiths AD, Watkeys JEM: Meconium viscosity in healthy infants and those with meconium ileus. *Biorheology* 1976;13:225–230.
8. Kopito L, Shwachman H: Mineral composition of meconium. *J Pediatr* 1966;68:313–314.
9. Young DM, Schwert GW, Harris JS: Viscosity and origin of meconium in meconium ileus. *Proc Soc Exp Biol Med* 1958;99:673–675.
10. Schachter H, Dixon GH: A comparative study of the protein in normal meconium and in meconium from meconium ileus patients. *Can J Biochem* 1965;48:381–387.
11. Ryley HC, Neale L, Brogan TD, et al: Plasma proteins in meconium from normal infants and from babies with cystic fibrosis. *Arch Dis Child* 1974;49:901–904.
12. Pecau Y, Feigelson J: Compositions proteiques des meconiums et des selles de malade atteints de mucoviscidose et de sujets normaux. *Biol Gastroenterol* 1975;8:193–199.
13. Rule AH, Baran DT, Shwachman H: Quantitative determination of water-soluble proteins in meconium. *Pediatrics* 1970;45:847–850.
14. Rule AH, Lawrence D, Hager HJ, et al: IgA: Presence in meconium obtained from patients with cystic fibrosis. *Pediatrics* 1971; 48:601–604.
15. Lieberman J: Proteolytic enzyme activity in fetal pancreas and meconium. *Gastroenterology* 1966;50:183–190.

16. Grundig CA, Rumler W: Die aktivitat von enzymen des eiweiss-stoffwechsels in meckonium. *Acta Biol Med Ger* 1967;19:193–199.
17. Fraser D, Clamp JR: The glycoprotein content of meconium. *Clin Chim Acta* 1975;59: 301–307.
18. Clamp JR, Gough M: Study of the oligosaccharide units from mucus glycoproteins of meconium from normal infants and from cases of cystic fibrosis with meconium ileus. *Clin Sci* 1979;57:445–451.
19. Scanlin TF, Matacic SS, Glick MC: Abnormal distribution of α-L-fucosidase in cystic fibrosis: Decreased activitiy in serum. *Clin Chim Acta* 1979;91:197–202.
20. Durand P, Borrone C, Della Cella G: Fucosidosis. *J Pediatr* 1969;75:665–674.
21. Dahlquist A, Lindberg T: Development of the intestinal disaccharidase and alkaline phosphatase activities in the human foetus. *Clin Sci* 1966;30:517–528.
22. Auricchio S, Rubino A, Murset G: Intestinal glycosidase activities in the human embryo, fetus, and newborn. *Pediatrics* 1965;35:944–954.
23. Antonowicz I, Chan KS, Grand RJ: Development and distribution of lysosomal enzymes and disaccharidases in human fetal intestine. *Gastroenterology* 1974;67:51–58.
24. Antonowicz I, Ishida S, Shwachman H: Studies in meconium: Disaccharidase activities in meconium from cystic fibrosis patients and controls. *Pediatrics* 1975;56:782–787.
25. Antonowicz I, Ishida S, Shwachman H: Studies in meconium in cystic fibrosis: the activities of alpha-D-mannosidase, beta-glucuronidase, beta-D-fucosidase, acid and alkaline phosphatase. *Biol Neonate* 1978;34: 225–230.
26. Knauff RE, Adams JA: Meconium proteins and mucoproteins in meconium ileus. *Proc Soc Exp Biol Med* 1968;127:801–804.
27. Sharp HL, Peller J, Carey JB, et al: Primary and secondary bile acids in meconium. *Pediatr Res* 1971;5:274–279.
28. Watkins JB, Brown E: Conjugation and sulfation of lithocholic acid in fetal liver, in Paumgartner G, Stiehl A (eds): *Bile Acid Metabolism in Health and Disease*. London, MTP Press Ltd, 1977.
29. Back P, Walter K: Developmental pattern of bile acid metabolism as revealed by bile acid analysis of meconium. *Gastroenterology* 1980;78:671–676.
30. Shwachman H, Antonowicz I, Mahmoodian A, et al: Studies in meconium: An approach to screening tests to detect cystic fibrosis. *Am J Dis Child* 1978;132:1112–1114.
31. Oppenheimer EH, Esterly JR: Cystic fibrosis of the pancreas: Morphologic findings in infants with and without diagnostic pancreatic lesions. *Arch Pathol* 1973;96:149–154.
32. Clatworthy HW, Howard WHR, Lloyd J: The meconium plug syndrome. *Surgery* 1956; 39:131–142.
33. Mikity VG, Hodgman JE, Paciulli J: Meconium blockage syndrome. *Radiology* 1967;88:740–744.
34. Swischuk LE: Meconium plug syndrome: A cause of neonatal intestinal obstruction. *Am J Roentgenol Radium Ther Nucl Med* 1968; 103:339–349.
35. Sokal MM, Koenigsberger MR, Rose JS, et al: Neonatal hypermagnesemia and the meconium plug syndrome. *N Engl J Med* 1972; 286:823–825.
36. Rosenstein BJ: Cystic fibrosis presenting with the meconium plug syndrome. *Am J Dis Child* 1978;132:167–169.
37. Bruns T, Connell TR, Lacey JA, et al: Test strip meconium screening for cystic fibrosis. *Am J Dis Child* 1977;131:71–73.
38. Rosenstein BJ, Langbaum TS: Incidence of meconium abnormalities in newborn infants with cystic fibrosis. *Am J Dis Child* 1980; 134:72–73.
39. Rickham PP, Boeckman CR: Neonatal meconium obstruction in the absence of mucoviscidosis. *Am J Surg* 1965;109:173–177.
40. Dolan TF, Touloukian RJ: Familial meconium ileus not associated with cystic fibrosis. *J Pediatr Surg* 1974;9:821–824.
41. Shigemoto H, Endo S, Isomoto T, et al: Neonatal meconium obstruction in the ileum without mucoviscidosis. *J Pediatr Surg* 1978; 13:475–479.
42. Lloyd-Still JD, Shwachman H: Duodenal microflora: A prospective study in pediatric gastrointestinal disorders. *Am J Dig Dis* 1975;20:708–715.
43. Mullins F, Talamo R, di Sant'Agnese PA: Late intestinal complications of cystic fibrosis. *JAMA* 1965;192:741–746.
44. Jensen KG: Meconium-ileus equivalent in a 15-year-old patient with mucoviscidosis. *Acta Paediatr* 1962;51:344–348.
45. Jaffe BF, Graham WP, Goldman L: Postinfancy intestinal obstruction in children with cystic fibrosis. *Arch Surg* 1966;92:337–343.
46. Matseshe JW, Go VLW, DiMagno EP: Meconium ileus equivalent complicating cystic fibrosis in postneonatal children and young adults: Report of 12 cases. *Gastroenterology* 1977;72:732–736.
47. Stern RC, Doershuk CF, Boat TF, et al: Course of cystic fibrosis in black patients. *J*

Pediatr 1976;89:412–417.

48. Konno T, Suzuki H, Kutsuzawa T, et al: Human rotovirus and intussusception. *N Engl J Med* 1977;297:945.
49. Holsclaw DS, Rocmans C, Shwachman H: Intussusception in patients with cystic fibrosis. *Pediatrics* 1971;48:51–58.

SECTION TWO

CLINICAL MANIFESTATIONS

12

Pulmonary Manifestations

John D. Lloyd-Still

PATHOLOGY

Except for neonatal deaths resulting from meconium ileus, pulmonary complications are responsible for the great majority of the morbidity and almost all of the mortality in surviving patients with cystic fibrosis.[1] The earliest histologic changes in the respiratory tract are hyperplasia and obstruction of the submucosal glands of the trachea and major bronchi (Figure 12-1). These alterations precede infection since they are found in infants who succumb to meconium ileus and its complications and who have no inflammatory lesions in their lungs.[1] All patients who survived for 6 months or longer in their study had bronchiectasis present at autopsy.

Sturgess[2] quantified the development of the tracheobronchial submucosal glands in 22 infants with CF less than 4 months of age and 25 age-matched controls. In the lung no significant structural evidence exists for defective development of the submucosal glands in CF in the neonatal period. The earliest observed variable from normal is the enlarged lumen volume of the glandular acini that is apparent without cellular hypertrophy, gland enlargement, or proliferation. Sturgess[2] suggests that these changes may result from abnormal quality or hydration of the glandular secretions causing accumulation of mucus and dilatation of the ductular elements. Further discussion of the role of secretions in CF is included in Chapter 5.

Figure 12-2 illustrates the sequence of events in the lungs of patients with cystic

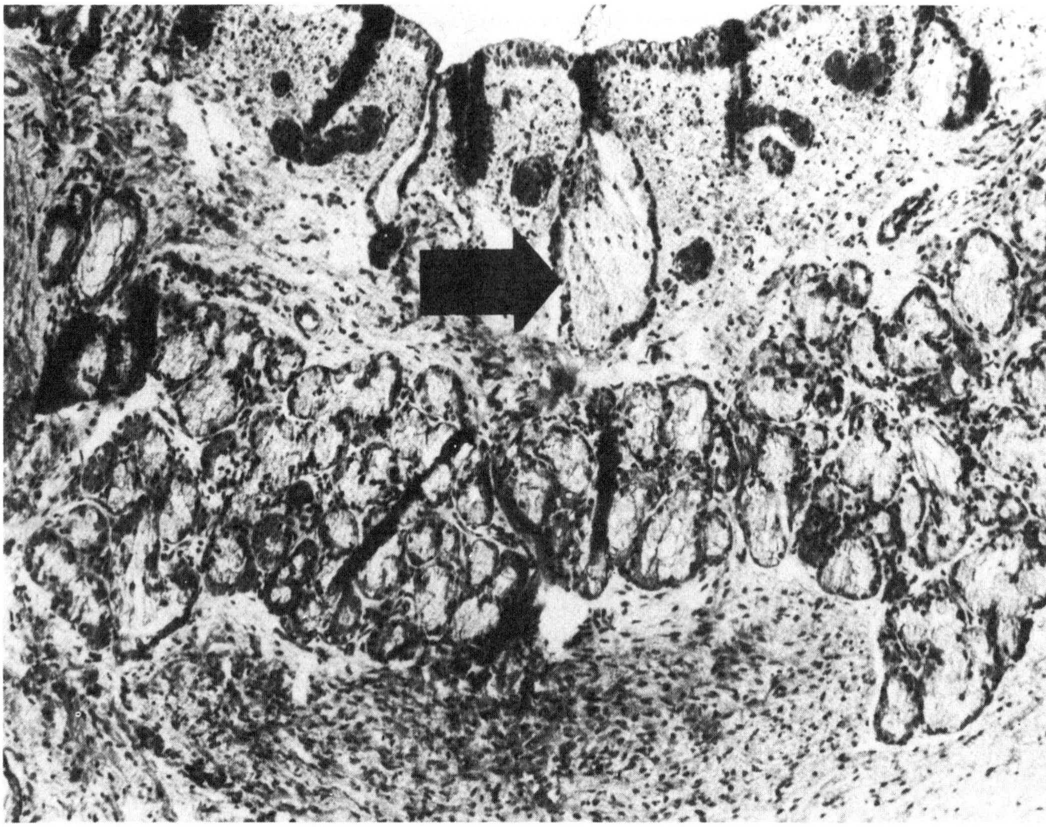

Figure 12-1 Mucous gland hyperplasia and obstruction of tracheal duct (arrow) with mucus in a 5-day-old infant with cystic fibrosis, but without infection in the upper respiratory tract or lungs. (Hematoxylin and eosin stain, × 100.) Reproduced from Oppenheimer at al: *Perspect Pediatr Pathol* 1975;2:241 (reference 1), with permission. Copyright 1975 by Year Book Medical Publishers, Inc, Chicago.

fibrosis. The earliest obstructive lesions occur in the bronchi and bronchioles in a nonuniform manner. Bedrossian et al[3] performed a quantitative study of the pathological findings in the lungs of 82 patients with CF who had autopsies performed between 1954 and 1972. Table 12-1 shows the pulmonary changes in the different age groups. Bronchial changes were more common and were almost universal, the most striking being noted in the epithelium and the submucosa. Epithelial alterations included loss of cilia, stratification, squamous metaplasia, and goblet cell hyperplasia. Squamous metaplasia (Figure 12-3) was noted even among infants and was progressively more common among older patients and at times affected peripheral bronchioles. The submucosa was usually infiltrated by acute and chronic inflammatory cells. Mucopurulent plugging of bronchi and bronchioli was almost universally present and filled the lumens of dilated proximal and distal airways as well as adjacent alveoli.

Figure 12-4 shows the scanning electron microscope appearance of a lobar bronchus from an older patient with CF and illustrates the obstructive mucous plugging, lack of cilia, and replacement with squamous epithelium. These types of changes occur early, as they were shown to be present in more than half the patients under 4 months of age in the Bedrossian et al[3] series. Figure 12-5 shows the changes in the epithelial surface from a child with CF secondary to inflammation and infection.[2] The cilia are disorganized, aggregated, and fused to form compound cilia or megacilia.

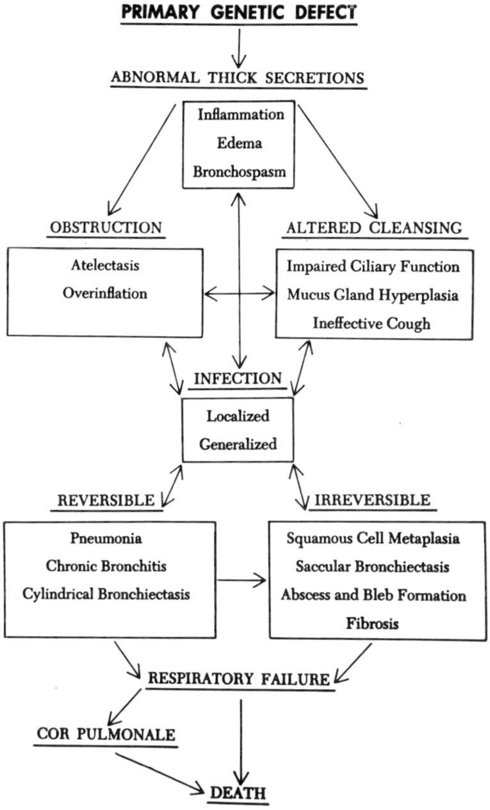

Figure 12-2 Sequence of events in CF lungs leading to different pathophysiological processes and ultimately respiratory failure. Reproduced from *Guide to Diagnosis and Management of Cystic Fibrosis,* Cystic Fibrosis Foundation, 1979 (reference 33), with permission.

Mucus and cellular debris are impacted among the cilia. Similar ultrastructural and functional changes occur in chronic bronchitis and asthma. Dysfunction of the mucociliary transport mechanism may result from defective cilia or from abnormal mucus secretion. A deficiency of the dynein arms of the microtubular doublets of cilia has been described as the basis of ciliary dysfunction in patients with Kartagener's syndrome (sinusitis, bronchiectasis, and situs inversus).[4] Sturgess et al[5] described three siblings with radial spoke defects in the cilia on electron microscopy, associated dysfunction of the mucociliary clearance mechanism, and one with immotile sperm. Sturgess [2] found no specific or fundamental defect in the cilia in cystic fibrosis.

Hypertrophy of the mucus-secreting glands occurs in CF[6] and is accompanied by hypersecretion of mucus.[7] Using in vitro and radiolabeling techniques, Sturgess and Reid[8] showed that the hypersecretion resulted from the increased population of secretory cells, increased basal rate of secretion by individual cells, and a greater response to cholinergic stimulation. In the epithelial mucus-secreting cells, no basic mechanism in secretion has yet been implicated in a specific abnormality in CF.[2]

Table 12-1
Pulmonary Changes in Patients with Pancreatic Cystic Fibrosis*

Pathological Findings	Group I (0–4 months) 15 pt.	Group II (4–24 months) 8 pt.	Group III (2–6 years) 28 pt.	Group IV (6–10 years) 14 pt.	Group V (10–24 years) 17 pt.
Bronchial changes					
Epithelial metaplasia	8 (53%)	6 (75%)	27 (96%)	13 (98%)	17 (100%)
Inflammatory infiltrate	11 (73%)	8 (100%)	28 (100%)	14 (100%)	17 (100%)
Bronchiectasis	3 (20%)	6 (75%)	28 (100%)	14 (100%)	17 (100%)
Mucopurulent plugging	10 (67%)	6 (75%)	27 (96%)	14 (100%)	17 (100%)
Parenchymal changes					
Pneumonia	11 (73%)	8 (100%)	27 (96%)	14 (100%)	14 (82%)
Emphysema	0 (0%)	0 (0%)	3 (11%)†	5 (36%)†	7 (41%)†
Hemorrhage	3 (20%)	0 (0%)	6 (22%)	2 (14%)	5 (29%)

*Reproduced from Bedrossian et al: *Hum Pathol* 1976;7:195 (reference 3), with permission.
†No more than minimal emphysema (< 10% of the lung is involved by point grid measurement).

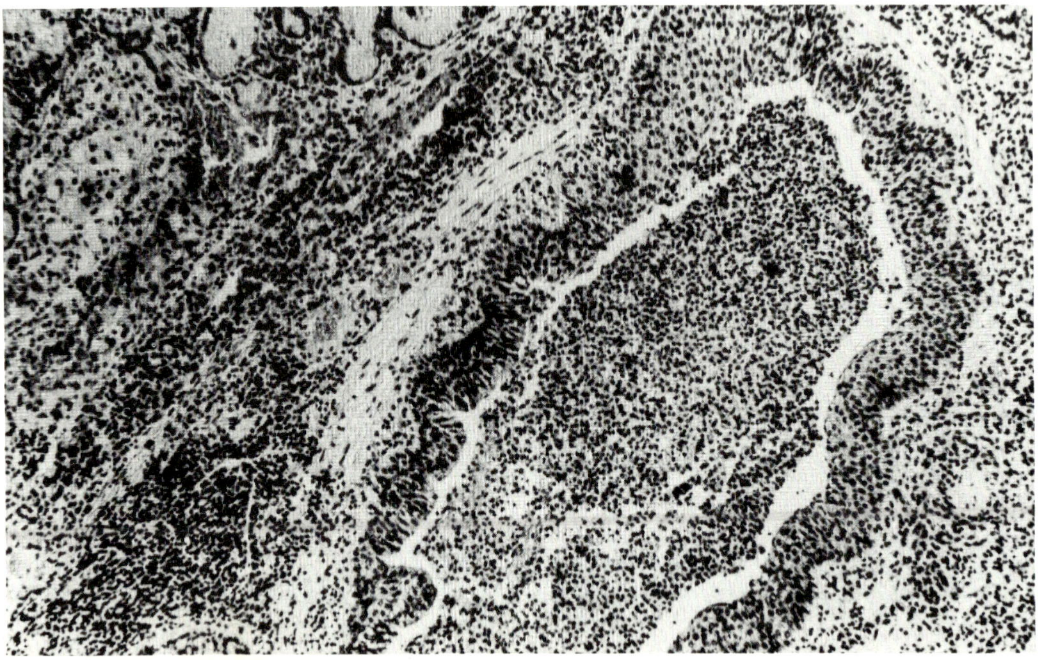

Figure 12-3 Microscopic section of a subsegmental bronchus with squamous metaplasia of epithelium. A mucopurulent plug fills the lumen, and the surrounding tissue shows extensive inflammation. (Hematoxylin and eosin stain, × 100.) Reproduced from Bedrossian et al: *Hum Pathol* 1976;7:195 (reference 3), with permission.

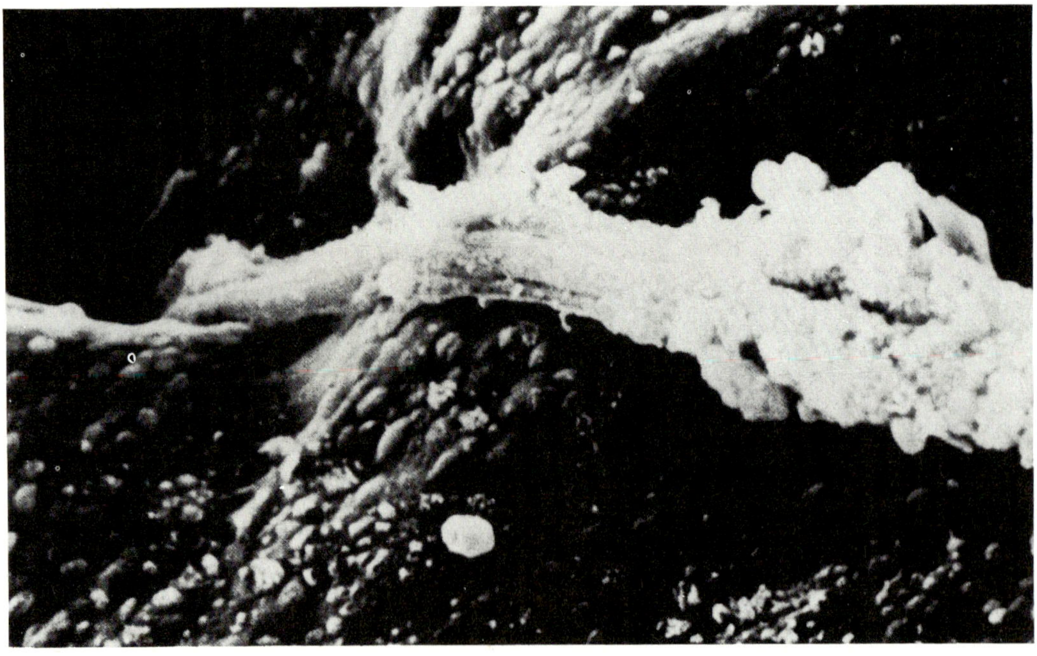

Figure 124 Scanning electron micrograph of lobar bronchus from an 18-year-old female with cystic fibrosis showing opening of smaller airway branch. Thick tenacious ropelike strands of mucus obstruct the airway lumen. Note the complete lack of cilia and replacement with a non-ciliated squamous-type epithelium. Reproduced from Sturgess JM: *Monogr Paediatr* 1981;14:66 (reference 2), with permission.

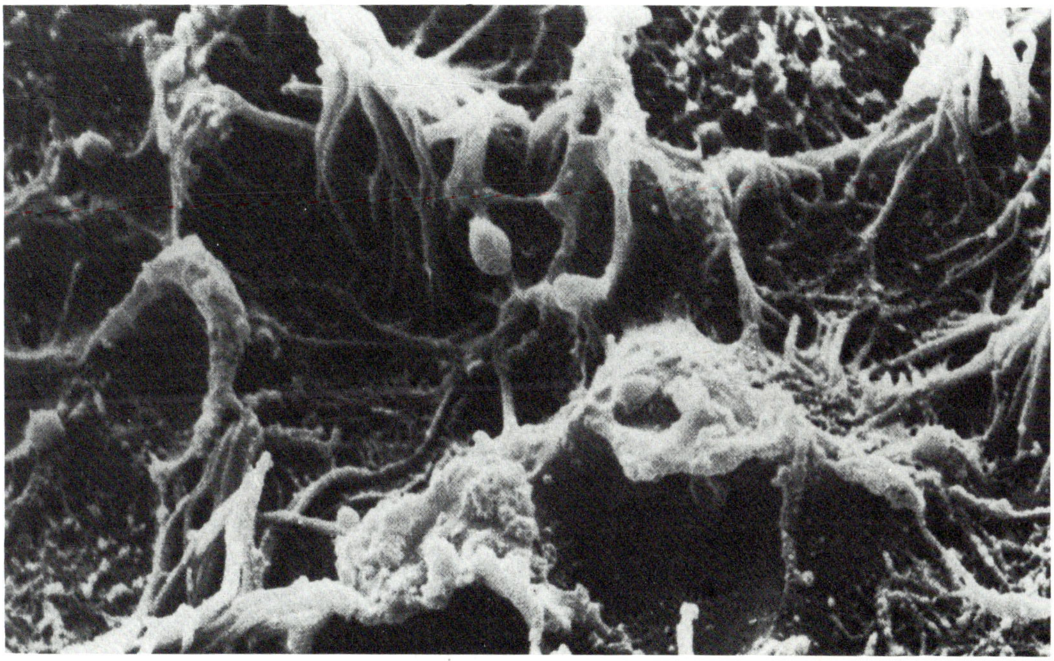

Figure 12-5 Scanning electron micrograph of epithelial surface from a child with cystic fibrosis showing changes secondary to inflammation and infection. The cilia are disorganized, aggregated, and fused to form compound cilia. Mucus and cellular debris are impacted among the cilia. Reproduced from Sturgess JM: *Monogr Paediatr* 1981;14:68 (reference 2), with permission.

A defect in the mucociliary transport mechanism has been implicated in the pathogenesis of lung disease in CF.[9] Several studies have reported conflicting results regarding the transport of radiolabeled or Teflon particles from the lungs of patients.[9-11] Each group of investigators has used a different tracer of mucociliary activity and therefore may have observed different physiological processes. The increased tracheobronchial clearance compared to healthy adult controls[10] can be attributed not only to normal clearance, but to more proximal deposition of labeled particles and to coughing. Slower tracheal transport rates than healthy subjects were reported by Wood et al,[11] who measured the rate of transport of 0.68-mm Teflon disks up the trachea by use of a fiberoptic bronchoscope. Data on clearance in the small airways (the site of initial involvement in CF) are unavailable.

A wide variation in transport rates from normal to abnormal was observed by Yeats et al.[9] The mean mucociliary tracheal transport rate increased with increasing maximum mid-expiratory flow. The results suggested that a higher serum factor activity, as measured by ciliary dyskinesia affect, was associated with faster mucociliary tracheal transport rates. This is contrary to the expectation that derangement in ciliary activity should result in decreased mucociliary function (see Chapter 10 for further discussion of mucociliary transport).

The earliest manifestation of pulmonary dysfunction is an abnormality in the distribution of ventilation, resulting in increased alveolar arterial oxygen differences.[12] Observations of pulmonary function testing in CF are consistent with the concept that the initial lesion is in the peripheral airways.[13]

Table 12-1 shows that the incidence of bronchiectasis rises from 20% under 4 months of age to 100% by 2 years. Emphysema was absent in patients under 2 years of age and occurred in 40% of patients older than 6 years, but never reached severe proportions. Most of the later complications of

CF (Figure 12-2) result from the combination of obstructive phenomena, impaired mucociliary clearing function, and infection by a variety of bacterial and nonbacterial agents. The right upper lobe and right middle lobe are especially prone to develop early involvement. Chronic infection results in bronchiolitis, bronchitis, peribronchial fibrosis, and bronchiectasis with the bronchial arteries becoming markedly dilated, resulting in hemorrhage (Table 12-1). The shunting of pulmonary capillary blood away from atelectatic alveolar areas, plus the loss of gas-exchange surface area leads to hypoxemia, hypercapnea, and cor pulmonale. The chapters on pulmonary function and cor pulmonale (Chapters 13 and 14) emphasize the irregular involvement of the lung in cystic fibrosis. Figure 12-6 shows the severe bronchiectasis mainly affecting the upper lobes in a patient dying of cystic fibrosis at 27 years of age.

INFECTION

Mearns[14] stated that pulmonary infection in CF requires consideration of the patient's age, year of birth, nature and age of the first pulmonary infection, and perhaps country of origin. The association of staphylococcal infection in the lungs of patients with CF is a feature of the earlier reports.[15-17] During the 1950s and 1960s, pulmonary infection with *Pseudomonas aeruginosa* (especially the mucoid variety) and *Hemophilus influenzae* were reported in increasing frequency. In the 1970s and 1980s, with the ability to isolate viral agents, the role of respiratory syncytial virus, the influenza virus, and others is being evaluated. Mearns[14] summarized a number of reported studies of pulmonary infections in CF from 1938 to 1978 and quoted the incidence for isolation of the following microorganisms: (1) *S. aureus* between 19 and 20%; (2) *P. aeruginosa* between 44 and 90%; (3) *H. influenzae* between 1 and 40%; and (4) *Escherichia coli* between 10 and 50%.

Tests for precipitins against *S. aureus, H. influenzae, P. aeruginosa, Streptococcus pneumoniae.* and *Klebsiella pneumoniae* were carried out on the serum of 195 patients with CF whose ages ranged from 3 weeks to 31 years.[18] Sputum was obtained for culture from 96 patients over 5 years of age. Their results are shown in Figure 12-7 for the antibacterial precipitins and in Figure 12-8 for the bacterial pathogens in the sputum. They made the following observations: (1) The prevalence of *S. aureus* precipitins increases more or less linearly with age. (2) The prevalence of *H. influenzae* precipitins also increases with age. (3) Precipitins to *P. aeruginosa* were more common than those to any other microorganisms between birth and 10 years, remained constant between 10 and 20 years, and showed a marked fall in the over-21-year-old group. The pattern for the sputum (Figure 12-8) shows trends similar to the serum precipitins. They interpreted the data to show that patients with CF are susceptible from birth to bronchial infections by any pathogen with which they come in contact.

However, the CF lung seems resistant to the tuberculin bacillus presumably because of the hypoxemia within the lungs. The prevalence of *P. aeruginosa* infection fell strikingly in the oldest patients, and they hypothesized that this might reflect the failure of many patients with *Pseudomonas* infection to survive into adult life. (See Chapter 20 for a different point of view.)

The mucoid *P. aeruginosa* isolated from the respiratory secretions of over 50% of patients with CF seems to be specific for the disease.[19,20] Kulczycki et al[21] investigated the role of *P. aeruginosa* colonization in the respiratory tract of 160 patients. They found that 70 (43.7%) of the 160 patients were free of *P. aeruginosa.* In the 54 patients with persistent *P. aeruginosa* the frequency of *P. aeruginosa* cultures was consistent for all ages from infancy through 30 years, suggesting that the frequency of *P. aeruginosa* cultures does not increase with age. The reason for the frequent colonization of patients with CF with *P. aeruginosa* and its change to a mucoid strain is not fully understood.[22] In 1961, Huang et al[23] found that 50% of hospitalized patients with CF who

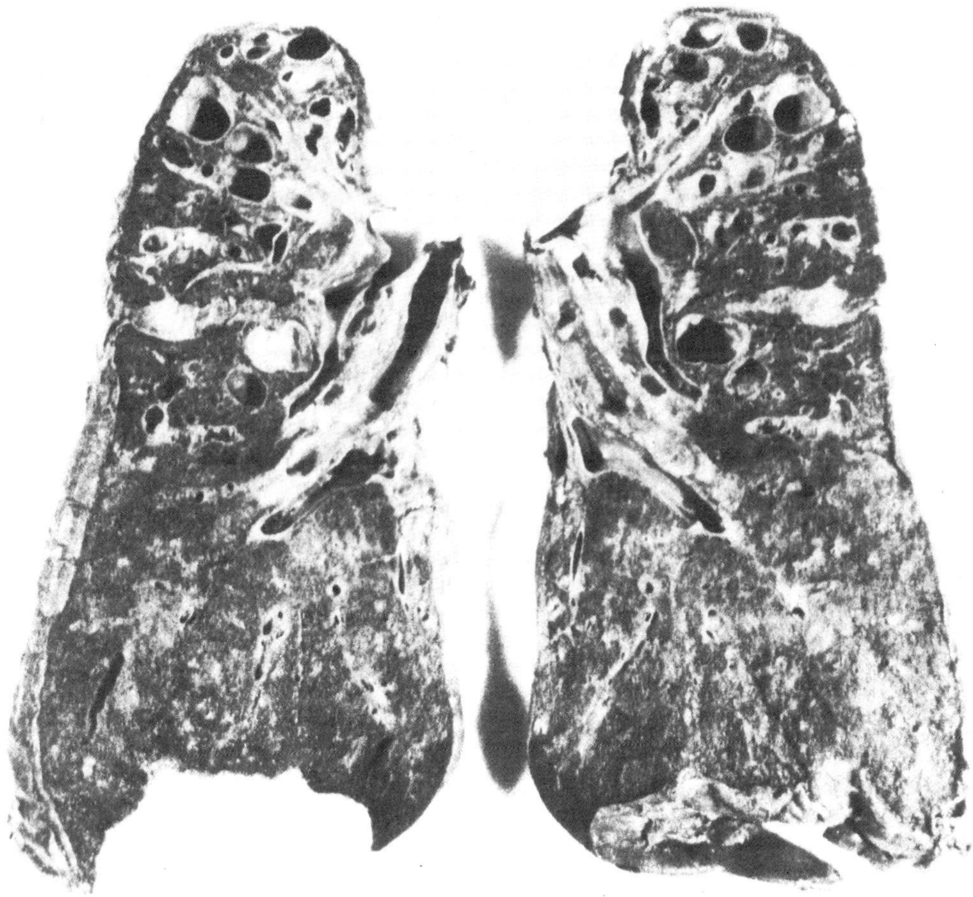

Figure 12-6 Severe bronchiectasis of upper lobe and chronic bronchitis and minimal bronchiectasis of lower lobe. Slab of lung fixed by endotracheal formalin at 25 cm H_2O pressure. Reproduced from Vawter et al: *Pathol Ann* 1979;14:357 (reference 121), with permission.

had received antibiotics before admission demonstrated *P. aeruginosa* on admission in cultures, whereas this was true in only 13% of those who did not receive antibiotics. Treatment with antibiotics, including the aminoglycosides, fails to eradicate *P. aeruginosa*. Kulczycki et al[21] suggested that the continuous use of antibiotics contributes to the persistence of *P. aeruginosa* and the appearance of mucoid strains. (Chapter 9 comes to the same conclusion.)

An alternative hypothesis is that patients with persistent *P. aeruginosa* and mucoid *P. aeruginosa* represent a more serious or "malignant" form of CF with more frequent complications, hospitalizations, and antibiotic therapy. There are infants and children with CF who pursue a rapid downhill course despite optimal therapy. In a report on 17 infants with CF and severe respiratory disease seen between 1968 and 1972, Lloyd-Still et al[24] found gram-negative microorganisms in every patient on tracheal culture (*P. aeruginosa* 11/17, *K. pneumoniae* 11/17, and *E. coli* 8/17). *S. aureus* was isolated in 6/17. The mortality rate was 65%, and cultures of the lungs at autopsy confirmed these findings. Viral cultures were not performed.

Recently Macone et al[25] reported mucoid strains of *E. coli* in the respiratory tract of 8 (11.8%) of 68 patients with CF whose

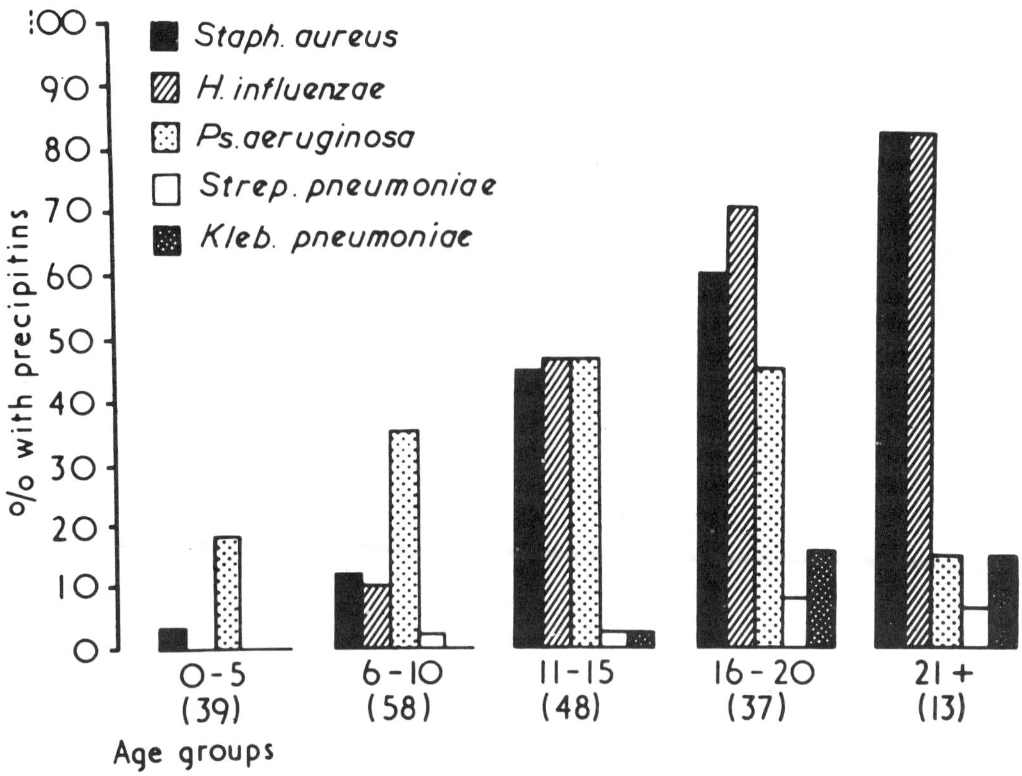

Figure 12-7 Prevalences of antibacterial precipitins in serum of patients with cystic fibrosis. Figures in parentheses indicate number of patients in each group. Reproduced from May et al: *Arch Dis Child* 1972;47:909 (reference 18), with permission.

sputum cultures yielded *E. coli,* as compared with none of 89 patients without CF who had *E. coli* in sputum. The mucoid substances purified from *E. coli* were biochemically and antigenically distinct from those of *P. aeruginosa.* They concluded that the respiratory tract in CF offers an environment conducive to the production of a mucoid colony, not only of *P. aeruginosa,* but other gram-negative bacilli as well.

The mucoid colonies of *Pseudomonas* in the CF lung are enclosed in a fibrous exopolysaccharide matrix which mediates their formation of microcolonies and may alter the efficacy of the normal defenses of the host (phagocytosis, antibodies, surfactants, etc) and of therapeutic agents (antibiotics).[26]

Viral infections account for the majority of respiratory infections in pediatrics.[27] Therefore, if the CF lung offers a favorable environment for bacterial microorganisms, one might expect similar susceptibility to damage from viral agents. In the older literature[17] chronic bronchopneumonia was often initiated by measles and pertussis. Despite widespread adoption of annual prophylactic influenza vaccination to children with CF, there are little data to document the incidence of this infection. Wright et al[28] performed a prospective study on 153 patients with CF for 60 days in midwinter in New England. An illness score was devised to detect a minor or major exacerbation of respiratory infection. Forty-eight patients experienced an episode of symptomatic respiratory illness during the study period. Paired sera were obtained for analysis of influenza A virus, influenza B virus, respiratory syncytial virus (RSV), parainfluenza viruses types 1, 2, 3, and 4, adenovirus, and *Mycoplasma pneumoniae.* Serologic evidence of viral infection was found in 7 of the

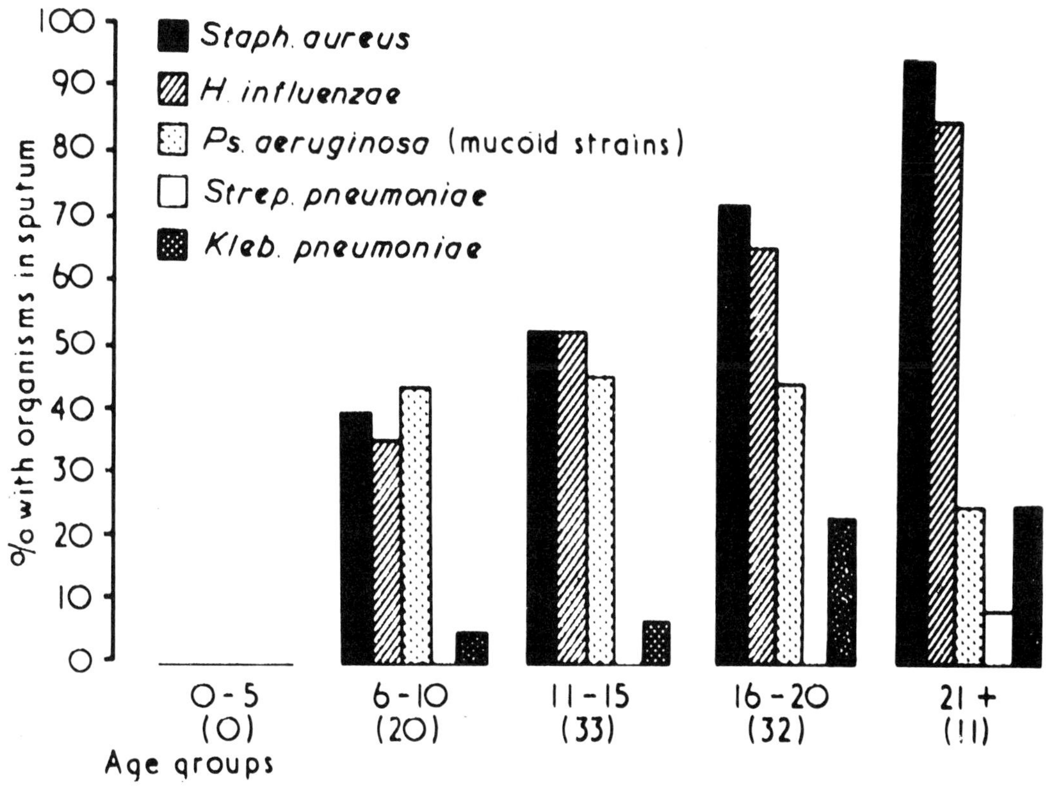

Figure 12-8 Isolation rates of bacterial pathogens from sputum of patients with cystic fibrosis. Figures in parentheses indicate number of patients in each age group. Reproduced from May et al: *Arch Dis Child* 1972;47:910 (reference 18), with permission.

18 patients with major exacerbations (39%), and 5 of the 18 patients with minor exacerbations of respiratory illness (28%). Influenza A virus and RSV accounted for these exacerbations. There was no serologic evidence of infection from *M. pneumoniae.* No tests were performed for rhinoviruses or coronoviruses, agents known to be important causes of respiratory illness. Similar data have been reported by Mearns.[14]

Another prospective study of respiratory infections performed on 116 patients with CF in Denmark[29] recorded 332 acute exacerbations during the 8-month study period. Bacteria alone accounted for 63% of exacerbations, viruses alone for 6%, a combination of bacteria and viruses for 13%, and unknown for 18%. Respiratory syncytial virus was the predominant viral agent, and RSV was significantly more frequently associated in patients who developed chronic *P. aeruginosa* infections during the period. A possible RSV/*P. aeruginosa* synergism was suggested by the rise in *P. aeruginosa* antibodies in relation to RSV infection. Although *M. pneumoniae* only accounted for 0.6% of their acute exacerbations, our recent experience and that of Mearns[14] suggests that this agent can be an important pathogen when prevalent in the community.

Holsclaw[30] reported that 30% of his patients had serologic evidence of past infection with *Legionella pneumophilia.* The accumulating data on viral isolations in CF add support to the hypothesis of May et al[18] that patients with CF are susceptible from birth to bronchial infections by any pathogen with which they come in contact (except the tuberculin bacillus). Infection due to *Aspergillus fumigatus* is discussed under clinical complications and in Chapter 10. Rarely other fungi, such as candidiasis, have been confirmed on lung biopsy.[31] Other opportunistic microorganisms, such as rapidly growing mycobacteria, have been reported in CF,[32] but are rare. Active tuberculosis only occurred in 2 patients of a total clinic population of 700 patients over an 18-year period[13] (for further discussion see Chapter 9).

DIAGNOSIS

Cystic fibrosis is a common disease, and in over 99% of patients the sweat test results will be diagnostic (see Chapter 4 for detailed discussion of sweat interpretation). In view of the serious prognosis and genetic implications of CF, one should not be reticent to perform large numbers of normal sweat tests in order to make the diagnosis. In our institution, over 600 sweat tests per year are performed to diagnose 15–20 new patients. All patients with intestinal obstruction in the newborn period are sweat tested, and these account for over 10% of the new patients. Seventy-five percent of our patients are now diagnosed under 2 years of age because a high index of suspicion is maintained. The major clinical presentations of CF are included in Table 12-2. Differential diagnostic criteria are summarized in the CF Foundation publication "Guide to Diagnosis and Management of Cystic Fibrosis."[33]

The physical findings on auscultation of the chest show a poor correlation with the chest radiography. It is essential to: (1) get the patient to take a deep inspiration to elicit the end respiratory rales, and (2) to auscultate the chest during coughing. Cystic fibrosis is frequently manifested by nonuniform involvement of the lungs. In severe disease air entry may be diminished but may clear with postural drainage. Waring[34] stressed four common errors in the diagnosis of CF: (1) failure to recognize clubbing; (2) failure to obtain a chest radiograph and sweat test in a child with a chronic cough; (3) misdiagnosis of chronic diarrhea (from pancreatic insufficiency) as food allergy; (4) poor technical performance of the sweat test. We would add two other common mistakes: (1) the patient looks too well to have the disease; and (2) failure to appreciate that the diarrhea in infants with CF is frequently watery in character.

Table 12-2
Important Clinical Manifestations and Physical Signs of Cystic Fibrosis in Different Age Groups

- Newborn
  - Meconium ileus, atresia, plug
  - Prolonged neonatal jaundice
- Infant
  - Pulmonary
    - Failure to thrive
    - Bronchiolitis, rhonci
    - Chronic cough, retractions, respiratory distress
    - Pulmonary infiltrates especially right upper and right middle lobe atelectasis
    - Clubbing
    - *Staphylococcus aureus* or *Pseudomonas* on culture
  - Gastrointestinal
    - Failure to thrive
    - Chronic diarrhea
    - Rectal prolapse
    - Abdominal distention
    - Edema, anemia
    - Vitamin deficiencies
  - Others
    - Salt loss
    - Bulging fontanelle
    - Gastroesophageal reflux, etc
- Older child
  - Pulmonary
    - Sinusitis, nasal polyps
    - Asthma, wheezing, rhonci
    - Bronchiectasis, rales
    - Hyperinflation
    - Clubbing, arthropathy
    - Hemoptysis
    - Pneumothorax
    - Cor pulmonale
    - Growth failure
  - Gastrointestinal
    - Malabsorption syndrome
    - Growth failure, delayed puberty
    - Meconium ileus equivalent
  - Others
    - Portal hypertension
    - Pancreatitis
    - Heat prostration
    - Intussusception, etc
- Adults
  - Glucose intolerance, diabetes
  - Sterility in males
  - Microgallbladder, gallstones, etc

Shwachman[35] enumerated the indications for a sweat test. A family history of the disease should make one suspicious, and once the diagnosis is made in the index patient, all siblings regardless of symptoms must be tested. The gastrointestinal and electrolyte manifestations are discussed in the appropriate chapters. In regard to pulmonary manifestations, sweat testing is recommended in all infants admitted to hospital with bronchiolitis, all children diagnosed with asthma, and all children with pneumonia and associated clubbing. The greater the number of abnormalities present in Table 12-2, the higher the chances of a child having cystic fibrosis. In the 10–15% of patients with intact pancreatic function, the index of suspicion will need to be higher as these patients tend to: (1) present later in life; (2) have milder disease; and (3) usually have normal growth patterns unless they have significant lung disease. Whenever in doubt, the sweat test should be performed as it is a minimum inconvenience to the child and will relieve anxiety. It is, of course, essential that one has confidence in the reliability of the technical aspects of the test. Referral to a specialized CF center is advisable when in doubt.

PULMONARY MANIFESTATIONS AND COMPLICATIONS

Upper Respiratory Tract, Nasal Polyposis, Sinusitis

The upper airway is often involved in CF.[13] The incidence of nasal polyposis ranges from 6.7% (50 of 742 patients)[36] to 20% (10 of 50 patients).[37] Rulon et al[38] stated that, in their experience, nasal polyps in persons less than 20 years of age were more common in persons afflicted with CF than in those without the disease. Polyps were noted in patients of all ages, the youngest being 2½ years old. Paranasal sinusitis was seen on x-ray in each case, while in 80 patients without nasal polyposis, 93% had x-ray involvement of their sinuses.[36]

Histologically, large mucous cysts and hyperplastic mucous glands are found in both CF and non-CF nasal polyps.[39] Three differences indicated an association with CF: (1) absence of basement membrane thickening; (2) absence of tissue eosinophilia; and (3) presence of predominantly acid mucin in cysts, mucous glands, and the surface mucous blanket of the polyp.

The polyps are often multiple, may cause complete nasal obstruction, and tend to give a characteristic facial appearance with depression and widening of the nasal bridge. Approximately 50% of the patients with nasal polyps were considered to be atopic on the basis of allergic symptoms and positive skin tests.[36] The severity of the pulmonary lesion is not reflected by the degree of involvement of the mucosal lining of the paranasal sinuses. Conservative management of nasal polyps in CF is suggested.[36] Simple polypectomy is carried out when nasal obstruction is complete. In some patients repeated polypectomies have been necessary over a number of years.[40] The unsatisfactory results of surgery are related to the high recurrence rate. Iodides are thought to increase the incidence of nasal polyps (see Chapter 23). Broad-spectrum antibiotics and local corticosteroid sprays are sometimes beneficial.

A number of investigators have reported a high incidence of deafness in patients with CF, but Taylor et al[37] considered these reports were related to the criteria for deafness. In their study they found 10% of 50 patients were transiently deaf in association with eustachian tube dysfunction; none had secretory otitis media. They considered the reported differences to be related to climate and seasonal variation.

Allergy

Skin hypersensitivity A high proportion of patients with CF have immediate skin hypersensitivity to multiple allergies. Warner et al[41] quoted a figure of 59% of 123 children in England. Higher figures were reported from Canada by Mitchell et al;[42] the commonest reactions were to house dust (99%),

June grass (87%), and ragweed (83%). Positive skin tests to molds were also common, especially to Dematiaceae (72%) and *Aspergillus fumigatus* (53%). These figures are higher than a control population.[43] Increased sensitization to these environmental antigens may indicate defects in the handling of antigens at mucosal surfaces. Mechanisms that have been postulated include poor clearance, increased absorption, and local immunodeficiency leading to a hyperimmune response and consequent lung tissue injury (see Chapter 10 for detailed discussion of this topic).

Respiratory allergies In contrast to the high incidence of skin reactivity in CF, the prevalence of respiratory allergies is similar to the normal population. Kulczycki et al[44] documented respiratory allergy in 44 (16.6%) of 266 living patients with CF with an age range of 1½–35 years. Van Meetre et al[45] reported similar findings in a retrospective study (19 out of 135 patients).

A more detailed study was performed by Rachelefsky et al,[46] who found 15 (24%) of 63 patients had evidence of respiratory allergies. Serum immunoglobulins on these 15 allergic and 22 nonallergic patients with CF were elevated when compared with those in normal age-matched controls. The allergic patients with CF had significantly higher IgE levels; IgG, IgM, and IgA levels were similar in the two groups. The clinical condition of the allergic patients, as noted by the Shwachman score, was better than the nonallergic, suggesting some modulating effect of respiratory allergy on the severity of the disease. They postulated that the respiratory secretions resulting from the allergic response might dilute and thin the viscid secretions commonly found in CF. However, contrary findings were reported by Warner et al.[41]

Bronchial hyperreactivity Wheezing is a major clinical feature of CF and resembles asthma. However, there are important differentiating features, and the response of patients with CF to bronchodilators is unpredictable. By means of a bronchial provocation test with histamine that depends on a basic functional abnormality of the asthmatic state, namely, heightened reactivity of the bronchial tree, the incidence of a positive response to inhaled histamine was 24% in patients with CF and more than 90% in the asthmatic patients.[47] With inhaled methacholine, positive responses occurred in 51% of patients with CF and 98% of those with asthma.[42] There was a significant correlation between a positive response to methacholine in CF and poor pulmonary function, but no relationship to positive allergic skin tests. Dose-response curves and time course to methacholine challenge differed in CF and asthma. These findings show that bronchial hyperreactivity is common in CF but is different from that in asthma.

Thus, patients with CF and patients with asthma share an increased frequency of atopy, increased sensitivity to inhaled methacholine, hypertrophy, and hyperplasia of the mucus-secreting apparatus in the upper and lower airways, and in addition a similar array of abnormal autonomic responses.[48] Davis et al[48] identified abnormal end organ responsiveness to exogenous agents, indicating that some lesion is present in α-adrenergic, β-adrenergic, and cholinergic systems at or beyond the level of the receptor (see Chapters 5 and 10 for further discussion of this topic).

Allergic bronchopulmonary aspergillosis (ABPA) The clinical features of ABPA include: (1) extrinsic or mixed-type asthma with episodes of symptomatic or silent fleeting pulmonary infiltrates; (2) immediate skin reactivity to *Aspergillus fumigatus;* (3) precipitating antibody against *Aspergillus fumigatus;* (4) eosinophilia; (5) elevated IgE concentration; and (6) central bronchiectasis on the chest radiograph. Specific IgE and IgG antibody against *Aspergillus fumigatus* are significantly elevated in children with ABPA. The total serum IgE declines with prednisone therapy and increases again with relapse.[49]

The incidence of ABPA during a two-year period in the CF population studied in Rochester, New York, was 11%.[50] Our experience confirms the importance of looking for ABPA in patients with CF and asthma (Figure 12-9), and we suspect these figures are not unusual. Although originally thought to affect mainly adolescents and older patients with CF, ABPA has recently been reported in young patients (the youngest being 2½ years old). The clinical manifestations range from total collapse of the lung or a lobe to extensive, but changing, areas of consolidation.[51] Five of the seven patients had recurrences. Contrary to other reports, these young children had mild disease and corticosteroids were not always required. On the basis of these reports, allergic bronchopulmonary aspergillosis must be considered in the differential diagnosis of any child with CF who develops asthma (see Chapter 10 which comes to the same conclusion).

Bronchiolitis

In 1953, di Sant'Agnese[52] described the dangers of lobar atelectasis in CF with 9 (49%) of 22 infants dying in the first year of life. However, other infants with CF may develop respiratory distress without evidence of lobar atelectasis. The diagnosis of CF in these infants is often delayed. Their clinical course is characterized by a bronchiolitis-like syndrome with marked respiratory distress, coughing, wheezing, poor air exchange, hyperinflation, cyanosis, hypoxemia, and a high mortality. Fever is rare. Failure to thrive and malnutrition result from feeding difficulties, vomiting, and pancreatic insufficiency.

Lloyd-Still et al[24] reviewed 17 such infants

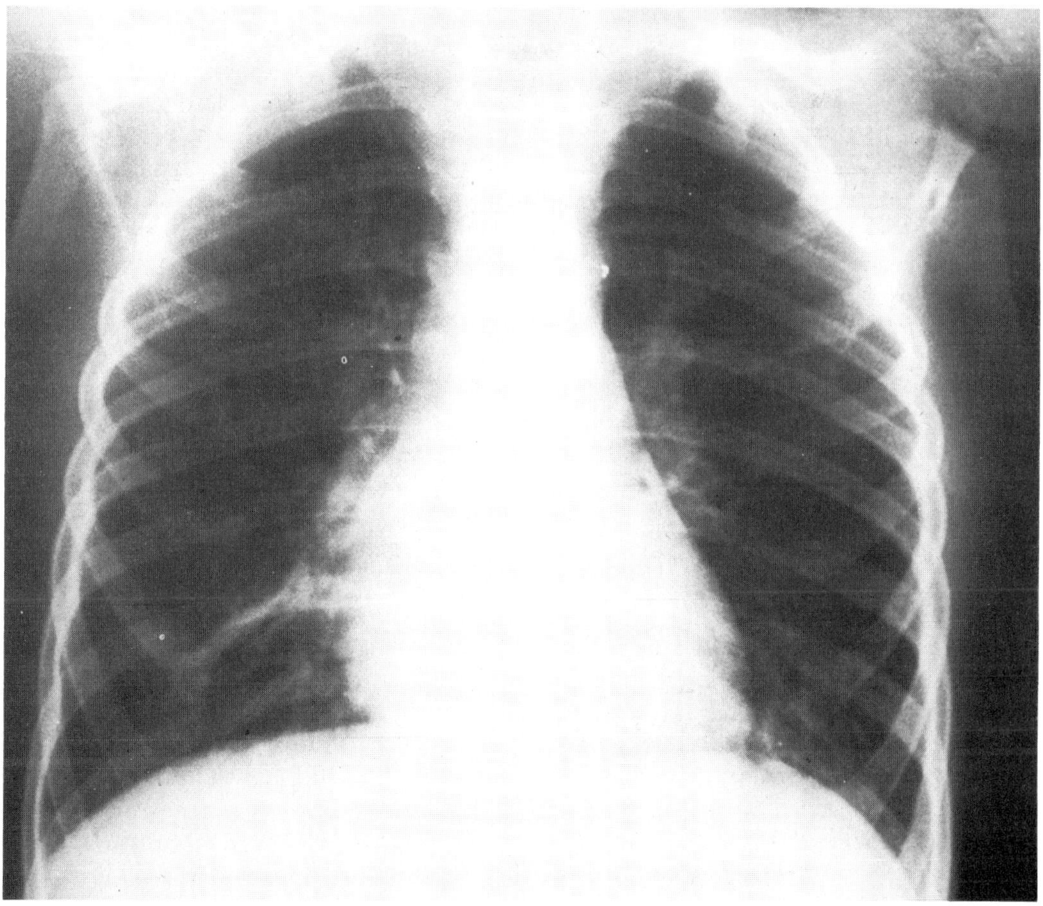

Figure 12-9 Chest radiograph of a 10-year-old patient with cystic fibrosis, asthma, and allergic bronchopulmonary aspergillosis. His serum IgE, specific IgE, and IgG to *Aspergillus* were all elevated. He responded to prednisone, but relapsed and required further courses.

admitted to the Children's Hospital Medical Center, Boston, between 1968 and 1972. Tracheal cultures showed a predominance of gram-negative microorganisms with *P. aeruginosa, K. pneumoniae,* and *E. coli* predominating. Severe abnormalities were ultimately noted on all chest radiographs; in 4 infants hyperinflation was the only abnormal finding on admission. Right upper lobe atelectasis was seen in 11 of 17 infants, left upper lobe (7/11), right middle lobe (5/17), lingular (4/17), and left and right lower lobes (4/17). The heart was enlarged from cardiac failure in the 10 infants who died (60% mortality). Blood gases showed severe hypoxemia (mean P_aO_2 37.5 mm/Hg). A combination of antibiotics, usually including aminoglycosides and chloramphenicol, were administered to all infants. The effect of corticosteroids was difficult to evaluate, but prolonged administration (average duration 102 days) was required in all infants who survived.

Although viral cultures were not performed on these infants, the authors stressed the clinical similarities between their patients and epidemic bronchiolitis caused by the respiratory syncytial virus. Bronchiolitis is considered by many authorities to be a manifestation of asthma, as over 50% of infants with proven viral bronchiolitis subsequently develop wheezing.[53] It is of interest that 4 of the 7 surviving children with CF developed subsequent wheezing. The poor response to antispasmodics and antibiotics in these severely ill infants supports a viral etiology for their bronchiolitis. In our experience, supportive care with oxygen, antibiotics, postural drainage, and careful nutritional management have made little difference to the mortality rate in these infants in the last few years. Even in surviving children, their clinical scores are significantly reduced as a result of the severe damage incurred during infancy.

Atelectasis, Mucoid Impaction

Plugging of the bronchi and bronchioles with secretions is the earliest pathological change in infants with CF at autopsy[54] and is invariably associated with atelectasis. If the patient died early in the course of the disease from asphyxia, no inflammatory changes or squamous cell metaplasia of the epithelium was found. More often the exudate becomes purulent with extension into the peribronchial alveoli. Finally, the bronchial lumen becomes dilated, the walls are destroyed, and bronchiectatic abscesses are formed.

The clinical importance of segmental or lobar atelectasis in infants with CF was emphasized by di Sant'Agnese.[52] In older children, Waring et al[55] detected so-called mucoid impaction of the bronchi at some time or another in 23 (33%) of their 70 patients. Mucoid impaction of the bronchi is diagnosed by the characteristic appearance of a "mucous bronchogram" on the chest radiograph. Waring et al[55] stressed that these changes are often misinterpreted as lobar pneumonia or lobular atelectasis, whereas, in fact, the intraluminal location of many of these opacifications has usually been overlooked. Atelectasis was rarely seen, and they thought this was due to subsegmental localization of the mucous plug which permits collateral ventilation and leads to hyperinflation. An understanding of this process is important as therapy should be directed to urgent relief of the bronchial obstruction, either by vigorous postural drainage combined with antibiotic therapy or, if this fails, by early bronchoscopy before secondary bronchiectasis occurs.

Figure 12-10A shows a typical right upper lobe lesion in an infant which cleared with therapy, only to be replaced by a similar process involving the right middle lobe (Figure 12-10B). Failure to reexpand these lobes will lead to the appearance shown in Figure 12-11A. This 12-year-old patient developed bronchiectatic cavities in her right upper lobe requiring resection to arrest the process (Figure 12-11B).

On occasion bronchoscopy will demonstrate that the obstruction is extrinsic to the bronchus (usually from enlarged hilar nodes involving the right middle lobe bronchus). Under these circumstances corticosteroids can be administered in combination with appropriate antibiotic therapy in an attempt to

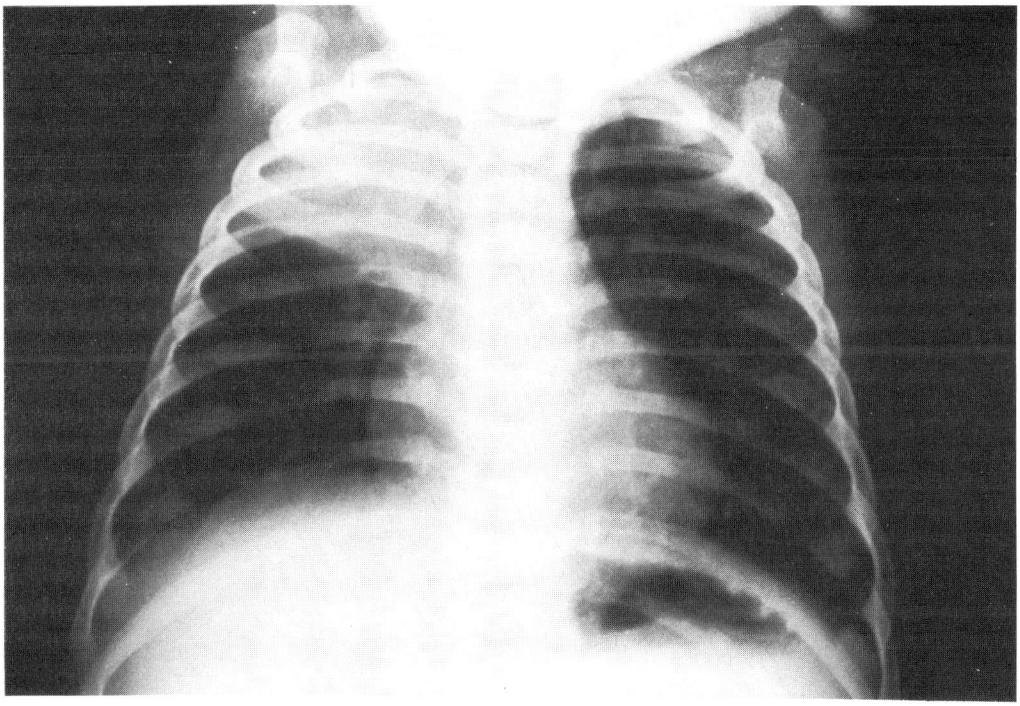

Figure 12-10A Three-month-old infant with cystic fibrosis. Opacification of right upper lobe. The upward displacement of the minor fissure indicates associated atelectasis. (Courtesy Dr. Sandra Fernbach.)

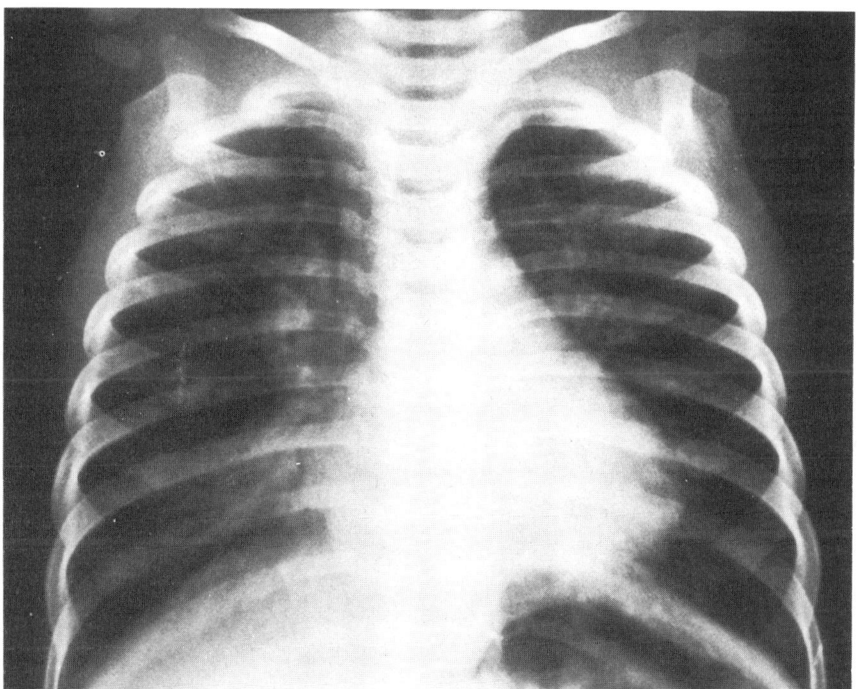

Figure 12-10B One month later the right upper lobe has reexpanded. Dense infiltrates have developed in the left lower lobe (retrocardiac) and right middle lobe. In addition, new infiltrates are present in the left upper lobe and the right perihilar region. (Courtesy Dr. Sandra Fernbach.)

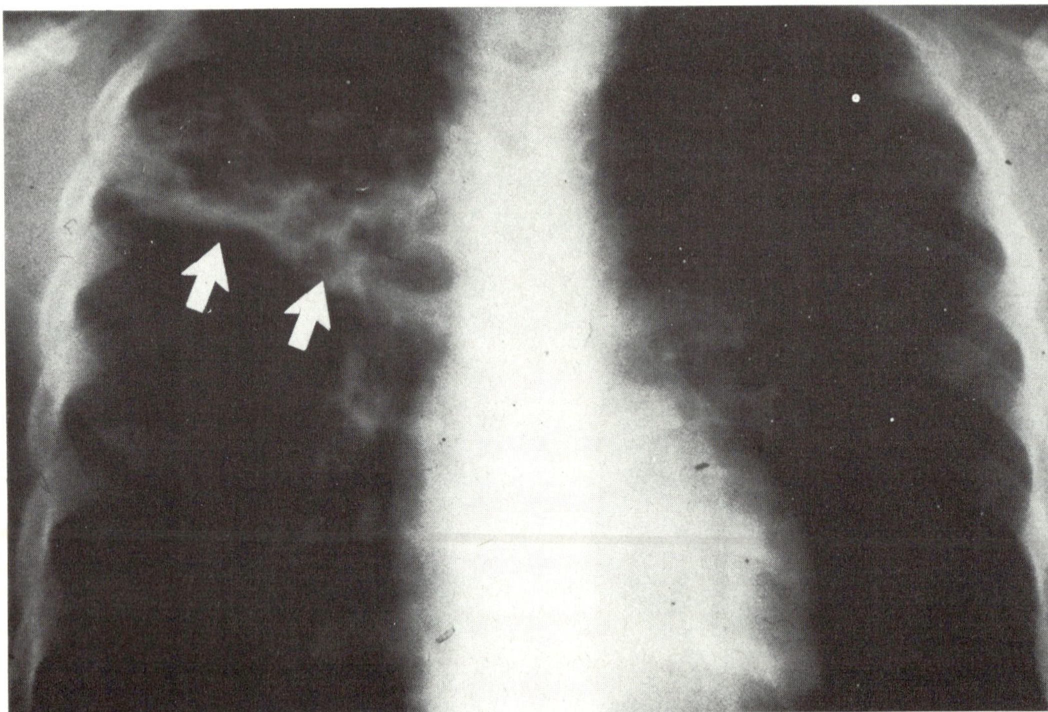

Figure 12-11A This 12-year-old female with cystic fibrosis had persistent fevers from the bronchiectasis in the right upper lobe. In view of the localized disease a right upper lobectomy was performed by Dr. Raffensperger. (Courtesy Dr. Susan Luck.)

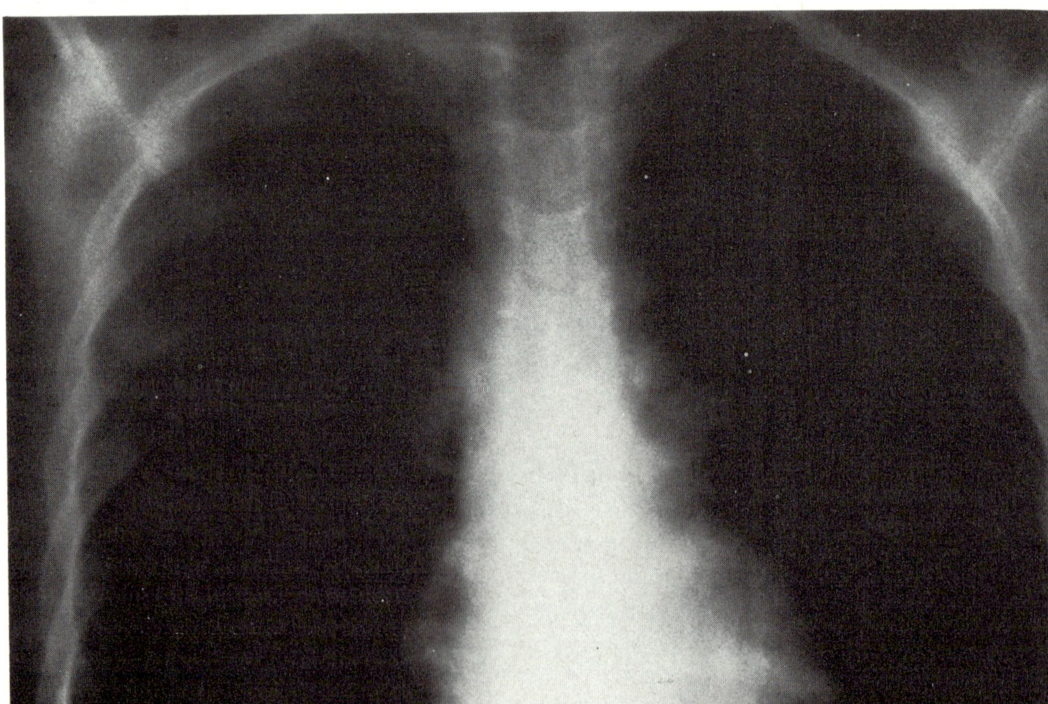

Figure 12-11B Postoperative appearance of the same patient. Hyperaeration is present. (Courtesy Dr. Susan Luck.)

shrink the hypertrophied lymphatic tissue, thus opening up the occluded bronchus. Complete obstruction of an entire lung has been reported in CF.[56] If the lobe fails to expand, large arteriovenous shunts may develop so that the lung tissue is poorly perfused as well as poorly ventilated. Under these circumstances surgery may be considered if feasible.

Figure 12-12 shows collapse of the left lower lobe in a 3-year-old patient with cystic fibrosis. Figure 12-13 is a bronchogram showing the appearance of fusiform bronchiectasis of the bronchi to the basilar segment of the left lower lobe. The incidence of abnormal findings on the chest radiograph in adults with CF has been reviewed by Davis in Chapter 20 (increased interstitial markings 98%, cystic bronchiectatic changes 68%, hyperinflation 66%, mucous plugging 32%, and lobar atelectasis 20%). Bronchography can be dangerous in CF and is being replaced by computerized tomography (CT scans).

Pneumothorax, Apical Bullae

As longevity increases in CF, pneumothorax is emerging as an increasingly common complication.[34] With rare exceptions, its appearance is related to spontaneous rupture of apical bullae in the lungs of older children and young adults. Surprisingly, pneumothorax was not encountered in the 146 autopsied cases reported by Oppenheimer and Esterly[1] or mentioned in their 82 autopsies by Bedrossian et al.[3] Pneumothorax has a significant mortality if left untreated.[56] Pneumomediastinum can occur with or without pneumothorax and can spread as subcutaneous emphysema.

Several large series of pneumothoraces in patients with CF have been reported,[56-60] and the following observations can be made: (1) The average age for the onset of pneumothorax is around 14 years. (2) Approximately 45% will recur. (3) Most patients have moderately severe disease at the

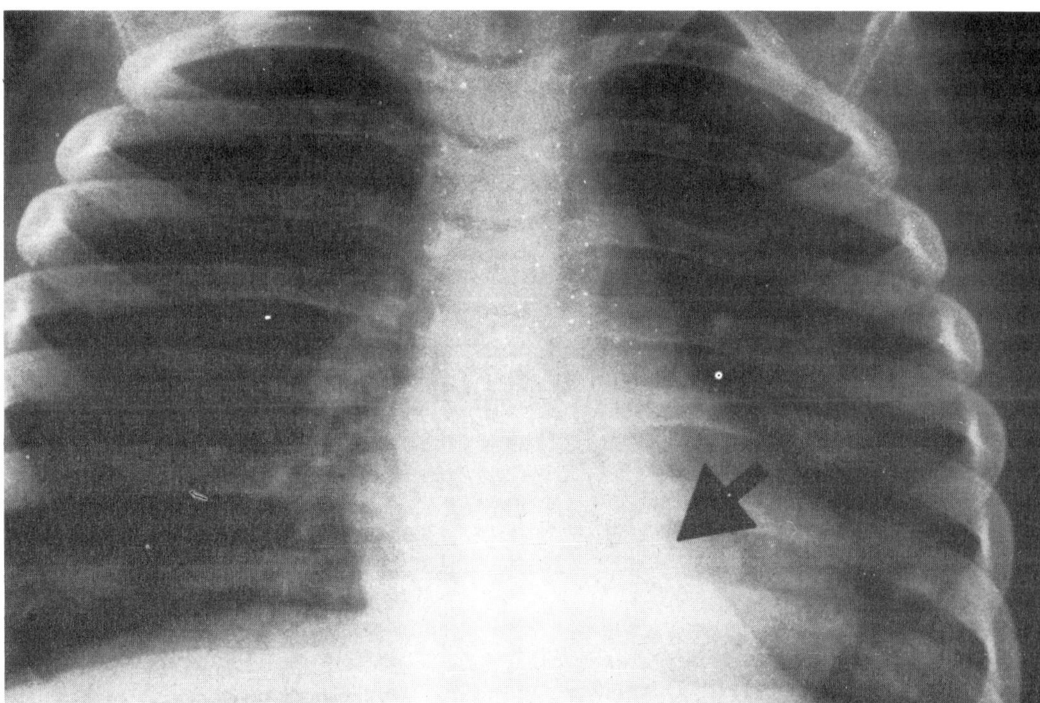

Figure 12-12 Three-year-old male with cystic fibrosis. Sharply demarcated collapse of left lower lobe segment causing wedge-shaped density behind the heart (arrow). No other parenchymal disease evident at this time. (Courtesy Dr. Sandra Fernbach.)

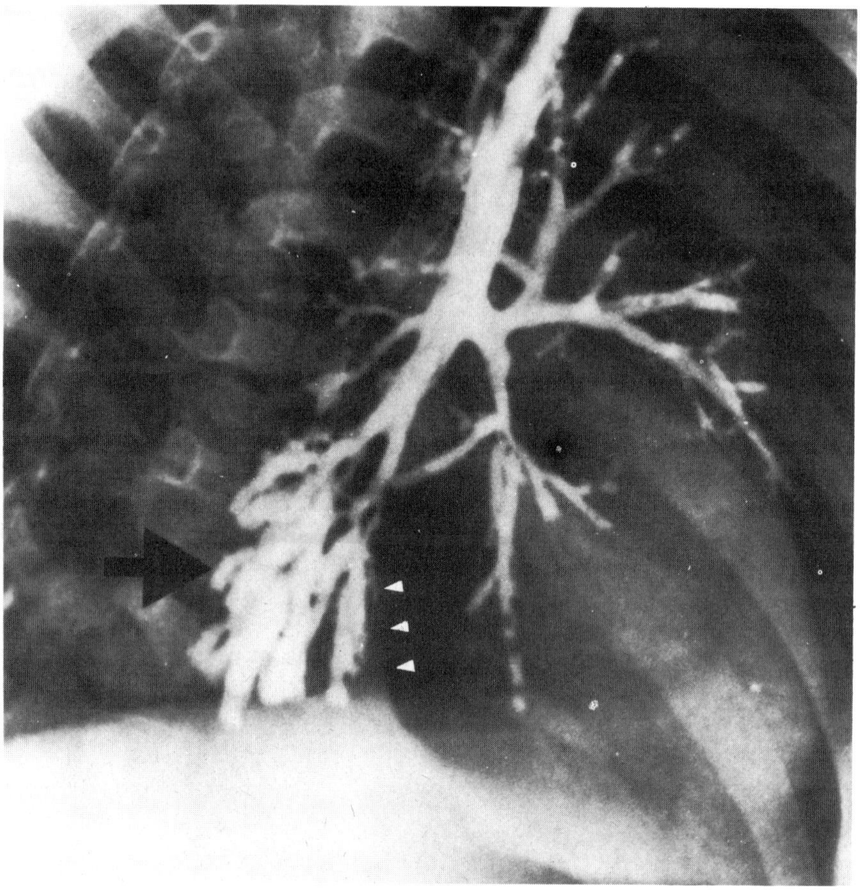

Figure 12-13 Fusiform bronchiectasis of the branches to the basilar segments of the left lower lobe (black arrows), sparing the superior segment. This bronchiectasis is associated with wedge-shaped atelectasis of these segments (white arrows). (Courtesy Dr. Sandra Fernbach.)

time of the pneumothorax (clinical score approximately 50). (4) The incidence of pneumothorax rises to 20% in adult patients. (5) Small pneumothoraces (detected on the chest radiograph) sometimes resolve spontaneously. (6) Chest tube insertion is required for symptomatic pneumothoraces, and sclerosing agents can be injected. Unfortunately, there is a 50% recurrence rate (see Chapter 21). (7) Some authorities now recommend that the majority of pneumothoraces should be treated with open thoracotomy and pleurectomy to prevent the high incidence of recurrence.

Symptoms suggestive of pneumothorax (Figure 12-14) are pleuritic pain, shoulder pain, and/or sudden onset of dyspnea in an older patient with moderately advanced disease. Precipitating factors include severe exertion, changes in altitude, and intermittent positive pressure breathing. Significant collapse of a lung due to pneumothorax may result in acute life-threatening respiratory failure and is a medical emergency requiring urgent efforts to reexpand the lung. Further discussion of pneumothorax and its treatment is included in Chapters 20 and 21. Travel restrictions for patients with a history of pneumothorax were advised by Boat et al,[57] in view of the dangers of altitude precipitating rupture of the bullae.

Hemoptysis

In the autopsy study of Bedrossian et al,[3] 16 (19.5%) of 82 specimens had areas of hemorrhage within the alveoli and the airways in association with bronchiectasis and prominence of the bronchial artery branches. Holsclaw et al[61] stressed the following reasons for the predisposition of the patient with CF to hemoptysis: (1) destruction of lung tissue with erosion of blood vessels from infection; (2) increased vascularity of the bronchial circulation in areas of bronchiectasis; (3) increased size and tortuosity of the bronchial arteries; (4) bronchopulmonary arterial anastomoses; and (5) engorgement and loss of elasticity of the pulmonary circulation because of pulmonary hypertension. Small amounts of hemoptysis are common in patients with bronchiectasis and usually respond to therapy of the pulmonary infection. The incidence of hemoptysis increases with age with over 75% of adults having this symptom at one time or another (see Chapter 20).

Massive hemoptysis is less common and is defined as either: (1) pulmonary hemorrhage resulting in death; (2) bleeding severe enough to warrant hospitalization; or (3) hemorrhage of such degree as to require blood replacement. A clinical estimate of at least 500 ml/episode was suggested.[61] The first blood streaking in the sputum in CF occurs at a mean age of 15 years, and the mean age

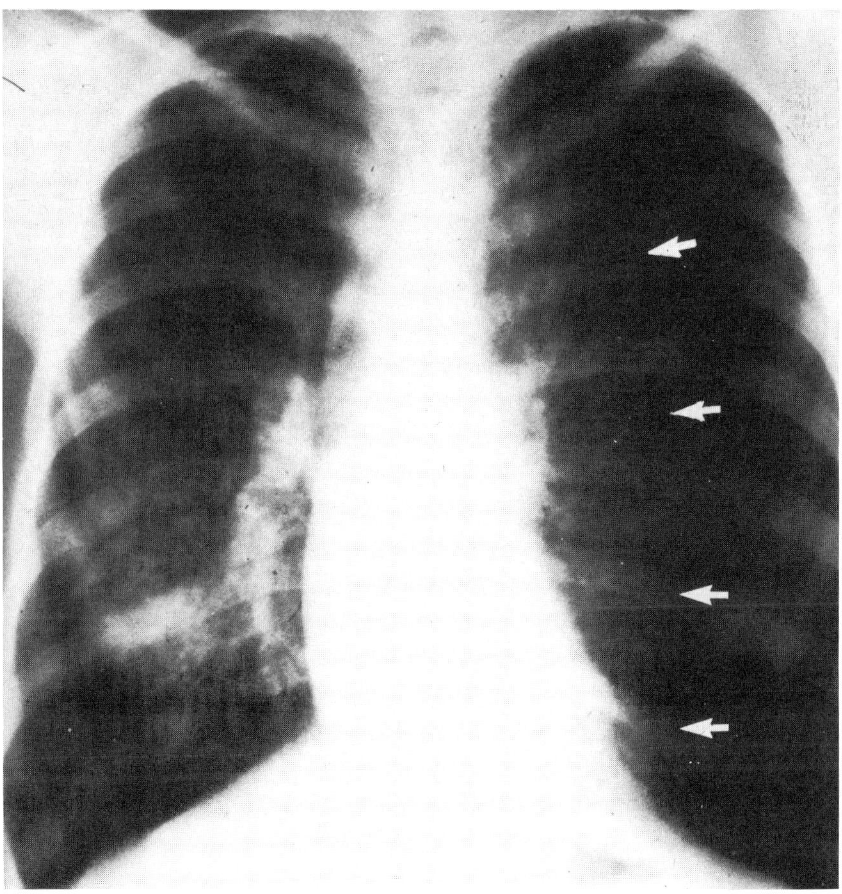

Figure 12-14 A left-sided pneumothorax (arrows) in a 15-year-old patient with cystic fibrosis. The flattened diaphragms and poorly defined heart borders are stigmata of advanced pulmonary disease.

of the initial massive hemoptysis was 18 years.[56] Holsclaw et al[61] emphasized the poor prognosis of massive hemoptysis with 13 (65%) of 19 patients dying within 6 months of the initial episode. By contrast, Stern et al[62] reported no deaths from hemorrhage in 38 patients treated with vigorous medical measures. However, there was a recurrence of massive hemoptysis in 17 patients (45%).

The therapy of massive hemoptysis is difficult. Postural drainage is temporarily discontinued, which leads to accumulation of secretions. Transfusions are given if there is shock or a fall in the hematocrit severe enough to precipitate dyspnea. Appropriate parenteral antibiotics are indicated. Vitamin K is administered if the prothrombin time is prolonged. Aspirin is contraindicated. Occasionally a patient is able to localize the source of the bleeding by a warm sensation over a specific area of the chest. Bronchoscopy is usually unhelpful, and surgical resection is rarely possible as these patients have severely impaired pulmonary function (see Chapter 21 for a discussion of options). At present the technique of bronchial artery embolization is being evaluated.[63,64] The latter authors reported cessation of bleeding in 12 of 13 patients (93%), although 5 of 13 patients (40%) had a recurrence of massive hemoptysis. Moreover they warned of the potential risks (transverse myelitis, esophagobronchial fistula, mesenteric infarction).

Cor pulmonale Heart failure secondary to chronic lung disease (cor pulmonale) ultimately develops in over 95% of patients with CF and is responsible for their death (Figure 12-15). The pathophysiology of this complication is discussed in Chapters 13 and 14.

Miscellaneous

Bacteremia Bacteremia in CF is rare except in infants. McCarthy et al[65] reported two cases with isolation of *S. aureus* and *Serratia narcescens.* Five of the 10 infants dying of respiratory failure[24] had identical microorganisms isolated from the blood and lung at autopsy (*E. coli, P. aeruginosa, Proteus,* and *Herrelia). Recently brain abscess was reported in three older patients;*[66] aerobic and anaerobic mouth microorganisms of low virulence were isolated, and the source was presumed to be bacteremia (see Chapter 22).

Botryomycosis This is a disease process characterized by granulomatous inflammation with the presence of granules bearing a resemblance to actinomycosis. The granules are composed of bacteria, fungi, or organic material surrounded by a hyaline substance. Katznelson et al[67] reported 7 patients with this complication of CF, of whom 5 died. *Micrococcus pyogenes* var *aureus* or *P. aeruginosa* were isolated singularly or in combination. The upper lobes are usually involved, and the ribs and mediastinum may also become involved by the suppurating process. Botryomycosis has not been reported since the advent of the aminoglycoside antibiotics.

Hypertrophic osteoarthropathy, arthritis Patients with severe pulmonary disease may develop gross clubbing and symptoms from hypertrophic osteoarthropathy. Indeed, we have seen patients with swellings over their wrists that were thought to be bone neoplasms and were biopsied. Pain may be intense and is improved with rest and oxygen. Clubbing can be quantitated by analysis of the shadowgraph.[120]

A different form of arthritis has been reported in less severely affected patients with cystic fibrosis. Newman and Ansell[68] reported 5 patients between 2 and 10 years of age. Attacks tended to be recurrent, usually affecting the large joints, and were associated with an erythematous rash. The duration was up to 10 days. There was no relationship between the attacks and the status of the disease. Laboratory studies were negative for rheumatoid factor and antinuclear antibody; only one of the 5 patients had an elevated sedimentation rate. Anemia and hyperuricemia (a complication of excessive administration of pancreatic enzymes) were absent. Radiological examination of the joints was normal. The arthritis may be due to immune complex disease[69] (see Chapter 10 for detailed discussion of this complication).

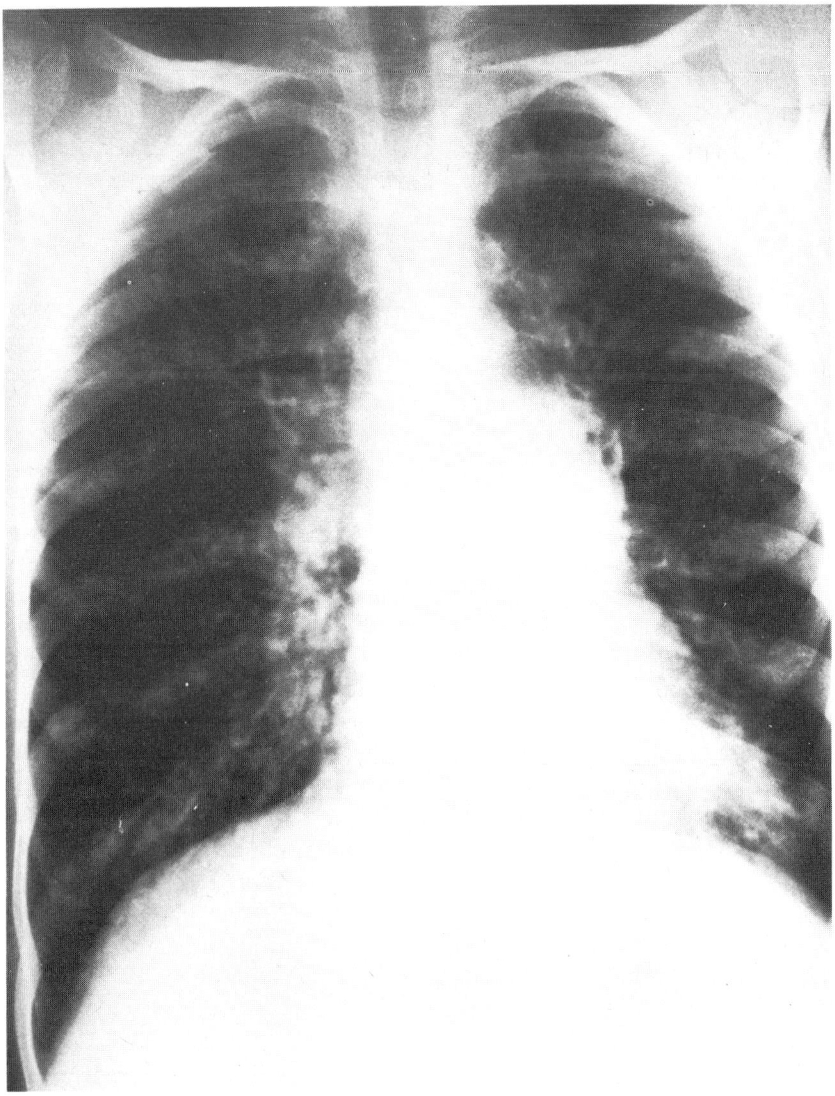

Figure 12-15 Eleven-year-old female with hallmarks of advanced lung disease in cystic fibrosis: air trapping, scattered parenchymal densities, and bronchiectasis. Prominence of the main pulmonary artery segment suggests pulmonary arterial hypertension. Note the shaggy heart border. (Courtesy Dr. Sandra Fernbach.)

Macroglobulinemia Rarely a purpuric skin rash involving the legs is seen in severely ill patients with greatly elevated levels of gammaglobulin. The disorder resembles Waldenstroms hypergammaglobulinemic purpura.[70]

Pneumatosis cystoides intestinalis This rare complication occurs in patients with severe pulmonary involvement (see the discussion of pneumatosis intestinalis together with the abdominal radiograph in Chapter 15).

Gastroesophageal reflux Gastroesophageal reflux is commonly present in infants with CF who are malnourished. Therefore, patients with vomiting, failure to thrive, and pneumonia in association with gastroesophageal reflux must be thoroughly investigated for all the common causes of this abnormality. Clinical evaluation should include sweat testing and exclusion of immunological deficiencies. Inadequate work-up of these patients may result in misdiagnoses.[71]

SCORING SYSTEMS

Methods for evaluating the severity of disease involvement (so-called clinical scoring systems) in CF are needed for: (1) assessment of current status; (2) assessment of previous status, especially at the time of the original diagnosis; (3) follow-up care to monitor the progression of disease and indications for therapeutic intervention; (4) as a prognostic indicator; and (5) research purposes. A number of different scoring systems have been devised and were the subject of a conference.[72] Cystic fibrosis is such a heterogenous disease and behaves in so many unpredictable ways, that it is unlikely that a single, universal patient scoring system will be devised to accommodate the requirements of clinicians, research workers, and others seeking prognostic indicators. Moreover, the standardization of many measures of patient status (eg, pulmonary function tests, nutritional parameters, and cardiovascular evaluation) are still unsatisfactory when applied to assess the severity of the disease process in cystic fibrosis. The following are some of the scoring systems in use.

Shwachman-Kulczycki score[73] This is the most widely used clinical scoring system and was originally developed to evaluate a therapeutic program. The score is detailed in Chapter 27. The system is based on four parameters that can all be assessed by the physician from the history and physical examination (general activity, physical examination, growth and nutrition, and chest radiograph). The disadvantages of the score include the lack of data concerning (1) pulmonary function tests; (2) the role of different infecting microorganisms; and (3) the complications of the disease.

Brasfield chest radiograph (roentgenogram) score[74] This system was an extension of the chest radiograph scoring system originally described by Chrispin and Norman.[75] Demerit points are scored and substituted from a perfect score of 25 points. Five different categories are scored, representing the most frequently occurring abnormalities seen on the chest radiograph, and include: (1) air trapping; (2) linear markings; (3) cystic-modular lesions; (4) large lesions; and (5) general severity (including complications such as pneumothorax). A high degree of reproducibility was found with different observers ($r = 0.91$), different institutions ($r = 0.81$), pulmonary function tests ($r = 0.81$), and the Shwachman-Kulczycki score ($r = 0.82$). In Figure 12-16 the relationship between the chest roentgenogram score and the Shwachman score is plotted to include values for baseline status, pulmonary exacerbations, hospitalizations, and death. This score has yet to find widespread acceptance in the various CF centers but has been widely endorsed.

Taussig-NIH score[76] This system is based primarily on pulmonary parameters of disease which account for 75% of the score points. Simple pulmonary function tests (vital capacity and forced expiratory volume) and complications such as pulmonary exacerbations, pneumothorax, and hemoptysis, which have been shown to have prognostic significance, are included. A curve depicting the probability of dying from CF within three years according to the prognostic score was determined. The authors claim that the score and mortality rate curve allow for rapid assessment of the patient's past and current clinical status and provide a rapid means of predicting life expectancy. Despite their statement that the score is simple to perform, in practice the Taussig-NIH score is more difficult to use than the Shwachman score. In our experience, few patients under 7 years of age are able to cooperate for reliable pulmonary function tests; in our clinic this would make this score impractical for 40% of our population. On the other hand, with adolescent and adult patients, this score may offer advantages over the Shwachman score. At present no study has compared the Brasfield chest radiograph score with the Taussig score.

Cooperman score[77] This is a simple scoring system that has not been adequately evaluated in a large number of patients.

Echocardiography An echocardiographic scoring system was developed by Lester et al[78] based on the sequence of echo abnormalities (see Chapter 14 for further details). This score correlated significantly with both the Shwachman-Kulczycki (r = 0.87) and Taussig-NIH (r = 0.86) clinical scoring systems, the Brasfield chest radiograph score (r = 0.86), and pulmonary function tests.

LONGITUDINAL STUDIES, PROGNOSIS

The annual reports from the data registry of the CF Foundation provide extensive data each year on survival. A life-table analysis of 95 patients with CF (Figure 12-17) compared patients with mild pulmonary disease (group 1) at diagnosis (chest radiograph score greater than 19 points out of a possible 25) with more severe pulmonary disease at diagnosis (group 2) and the total patient population.[79] Identical findings were shown when the life-table analyses were extended to 535 patients seen at the same Cleveland Cystic Fibrosis Center.[13] A similar trend for survival was shown by Shwachman et al,[80] who reported on 130 patients with CF diagnosed under 3 months of age and followed over a 20-year period. Thus, a better prognosis seems to be associated with (1) mild pulmonary disease at onset, and (2) the male sex.

There is some evidence that cumulative survival rates for patients with CF differ in different locales. Corey[81] noted the increased survival in the Toronto clinic patients when compared to survival for total Canadian clinics, which in turn were increased compared to the survival for total U.S. clinics. So far no explanation for these differences has been offered.

Another important observation from

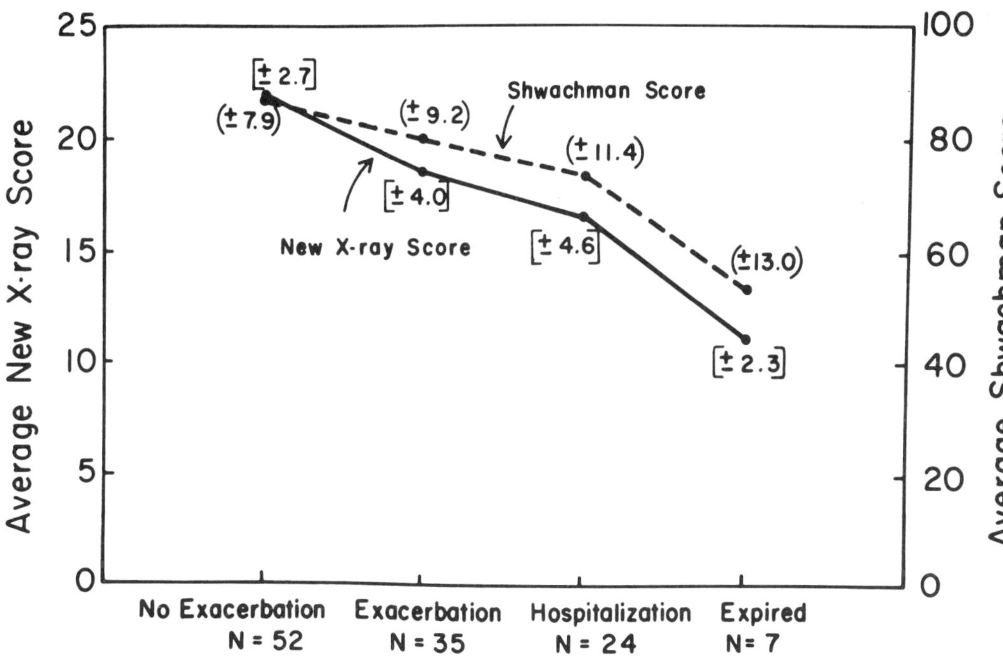

Relationship between average roentgenogram score, average total Shwachman score, and pulmonary exacerbations, hospitalizations, death. N = numbers of patients; [± 1 SD] = 1 SD of roentgenogram score, and (± 1 SD) = 1 SD of total Shwachman score.

Figure 12-16 Detailed on figure. Reproduced from Brasfield et al: *Pediatrics* 1979;63:24–29 (reference 74), with permission. Copyright American Academy of Pediatrics 1979.

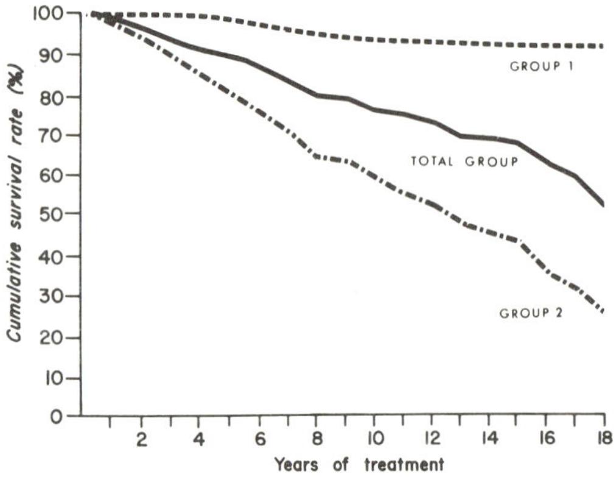

Figure 12-17 Life-table analysis of 95 patients with cystic fibrosis comparing patients with mild pulmonary disease at diagnosis (group 1), with more severe pulmonary disease at diagnosis (group 2), and the total patient population. These calculations are based on 1248 treatment years. Reproduced from Stern et al: *J Pediatr* 1976; 89:406–411 (reference 79), with permission.

longitudinal studies relates to the improved pulmonary function in patients without pancreatic insufficiency.[82] The Toronto group identified 51 patients with CF and normal pancreatic function. Patients without steatorrhea had significantly better pulmonary function in each age group beyond the age of 10 years compared to those with steatorrhea. They were unable to explain whether this was related to a mild genetic expression of the disease or to the presence of pancreatic function (see Chapters 3 and 15 for further discussion of this topic).

The chapter on pulmonary function (Chapter 13) emphasizes the enormous variability in the course of patients with cystic fibrosis. Thus, while some infants may pursue a rapid downhill course, some patients remain stable with almost normal pulmonary function studies for many years, and others may deteriorate at puberty. In some patients serial pulmonary function parameters are so variable that they cannot be classified into any particular clinical course.

Attempts to assess prognosis by statistical analysis of a large number of variables have been performed.[83] Six variables were found to have a significant predictive value in separating out those patients who died within the subsequent five years from those who remained alive. Five of the six variables were negative predictors (poor prognosis) and included the presence of *Pseudomonas, H. influenzae,* and/or other pathogenic microorganisms, and a low Shwachman-Kulczycki score on physical activity and chest radiograph. Gurwitz et al[84] summarized the factors associated with a poor prognosis in CF—the female sex, poor weight gain, multiple system (gastrointestinal and pulmonary) involvement, and abnormal chest radiograph findings in the first year of presentation.

INDICATIONS FOR HOSPITALIZATIONS

Some of the indications for hospitalization are shown in Table 12-3. If several of these problems are present, then the indications for hospitalization become more definitive. Complications requiring hospitalization that are related to other systems (surgery, nutritional, liver, endocrine, etc) are discussed in specific chapters.

Other relative factors influencing the decision to hospitalize include: (1) the age of

Table 12-3
Some Indications for Hospitalization of Cystic Fibrosis Patients

Diagnostic and educational (initial admission)
Increasing pulmonary infection
Fever
Weight loss
Increased coughing and/or spells
Increased respiratory rate
Rales increased sputum production
Worsening of the chest radiograph
Elevated white blood cell count
Deterioration of pulmonary function parameters
Hemoptysis
Pneumothorax
Cor pulmonale
Other system complications
Gastrointestinal
Electrolyte imbalance, etc

the patient—infants will require earlier admission, whereas a chronically ill adolescent can sometimes be treated at home with intravenous antibiotics by an indwelling heparin lock technique;[85] (2) the socioeconomic status of the family—facilities at home vary in terms of availability of food, number of siblings, paternal occupation, family stability, ability to perform postural drainage, etc; (3) psychosocial functioning of the family—patients will require earlier admission when the family has difficulty coping with the diagnosis or treatment (see Chapter 25). The duration of hospitalization for an acute pulmonary exacerbation varies between 10 and 14 days in most CF centers. Severely ill patients and infants may require a longer period of time. Little data are available to know the maximum period of benefit, or whether shorter courses of treatment would have similar beneficial results.

TREATMENT

The basic goals of treatment are to prevent progression of the pulmonary involvement and to maintain adequate nutrition, balanced by the need to allow the patient to lead as normal a life as possible.[30] Comprehensive care[13] includes parental and patient education and regular follow-up visits at intervals of 6–12 weeks, depending on clinical status. Complications must be anticipated and preventive measures instituted if possible.

In adults, Burrows and Earle[86] showed that chronic obstructive lung disease is a slowly progressive disorder that begins many years before the onset of clinical symptoms. The disease progresses in a more regular and predictable fashion than can be anticipated from clinical observations. Measurements of ventilatory capacity, resting heart rate, and carbon dioxide levels are the best indicators of prognosis. The erroneous assessment of the physicians is related to the relatively small yearly changes in pulmonary function tests, the tendency for clinicians to remember exceptional cases, and the optimistic attitudes of both patients and physicians. Unfortunately, much of the literature regarding therapeutic modalities in CF suffers from the same physician bias and is unsubstantiated by controlled trials as to efficacy. Therapies to prevent progression of lung disease will be discussed.

Treatment of Pulmonary Infection

The principles and approach to the therapy of pulmonary infections in CF are discussed in Chapter 9. Abnormalities in the immunologic system are closely related and are discussed in Chapter 10.

Physical Activity

Several authorities[13,30,34] have suggested that both increased physical activity and coughing are among the factors responsible for the increased survival of males with CF, whereas females are thought to be less active and to suppress their cough, presumably for psychological reasons. No data are available to support these statements (see Chapter 13 for further discussion of this topic), but if proven correct in subsequent studies, efforts must be directed to increase both physical activity and effective coughing mechanisms.

Postural Drainage, Breathing Exercises

The details of postural drainage can be found in the standard textbooks of respiratory therapy or the "Guide to Diagnosis and Management of Cystic Fibrosis."[33] Tecklin and Holsclaw[87] stated that chest physical therapy was one of the methods of pulmonary therapy accepted nearly everywhere. However, among older patients, compliance with postural drainage is notoriously poor. In view of the enormous time and energy required by patients, parents, and others, Wood et al[13] suggested that the following questions need to be addressed: (1) Which patients will benefit from postural drainage? (2) Can acute beneficial effects be translated into long-term improvement or arrest of progression? (3) Can the onset of significant obstructive lung disease be delayed by routine administration of postural drainage? (4) Can mechanical percussors be used effectively as manual percussors? (5) Can adolescent and adult patients effectively administer their own postural drainage?

The movement of mucus in the lungs is controlled by three factors: (1) the beating of the cilia; (2) gravity; and (3) the reversing air flow. In the normal lung, the ciliary beating is the most important function in mucus movement.[88] In a theoretical analysis of such a model, Blake[89] suggests that the importance of gravity increases with increasing thickness of the mucus. In CF where ciliary activity is deranged and hampered by the thickened mucus as a result of the increased secretions, gravity can become the dominant influence on mucus clearance, as was supported by the findings of Wong et al.[88] Furthermore, their observations suggest that in the presence of defective mucociliary function, coughing may replace ciliary activity as the more important lung clearance mechanism.

A number of studies in patients with CF have documented significant improvement in a variety of pulmonary function parameters and expectorated sputum volumes between 5 and 45 minutes following bronchial drainage.[87,90,91] All these studies used trained physiotherapists and continued treatment for at least 30 minutes. In the study of Wong et al[88] most patients with CF had defective mucus clearance, some had "normal" transport, and some did not respond to gravitational drainage. The role of pulmonary infection was stressed as, even in the normal subject, recovery was sometimes very prolonged after an acute pulmonary infection.

Other studies[92] using fewer positions for postural drainage were unable to confirm the improvement in pulmonary function. Moreover, results with the mechanical percussor have been shown to be as good as with the manual percussor.[93] A number of new approaches to improving pulmonary drainage by concentrating on effective coughing procedures have also been suggested,[94] and claim to be as effective as the standardized postural drainage treatments.

In summary, gravity can be used to enhance tracheal mucus clearance in many, but not all, patients with cystic fibrosis. In circumstances where the family or patient are able to perform bronchial drainage to a standard comparable to that done by a professional, there is evidence of significant improvement in most patients. In our experience a significant number of families and perhaps the majority of older patients do not continue postural drainage for the prolonged interval (30 minutes twice daily) that is recommended. Inadequate or faulty bronchial drainage may well be less helpful than increased physical activity and emphasis on the importance of coughing. Whether there is benefit from a prophylactic program of postural drainage in patients whose chest radiograph and pulmonary function parameters are normal remains unanswered. In practice most patients with CF have demonstrable impairment in one or other of these parameters.

Aerosols Before reviewing the effects of agents given by aerosol, one needs to know the distribution of the aerosol within the various parts of the lung. Alderson et al[95] investigated the efficiency of delivery of an aerosol in the form of an ultrasonic nebulizer to 22 children with CF aged between 8 months and 17 years. The children had ventilation studies with xenon-133 and radioaerosol studies with ^{113m} indium, ^{99m} Tc-albumin, or ^{99m} Tc-pertechnectate, allowing for comparison of the distribution of aerosol with regional ventilation. The results showed that only 0.8–6.4% of the dose reached the lungs, and the majority of the aerosol was deposited about the face, mouth, nasal passages, and pharynx. There was decreased aerosol entry to regions which were poorly ventilated. There was a positive correlation (r = 0.89) between increasing age and greater pulmonary deposition of the aerosol. They concluded that the efficiency of aerosol deposition is variable in children with CF, depending primarily on the age of the patient, whereas distribution within the lungs is related to regional variations in the severity of the pulmonary disease.

A critical assessment of the action of mucolytic agents and expectorants is difficult. Although mucolytic agents undoubtedly change the rheological properties of respiratory secretions in vitro, their effect on mucus secretion and mucociliary transport in vivo is not clear.[96] The demonstration of a beneficial effect of expectorants in patients with obstructive lung disease, including CF, has been based on subjective symptoms and rheologic studies of expectorated sputum, whereas the few studies which attempted actually to measure mucociliary transport in these patients have not convincingly demonstrated a beneficial effect.

N-Acetylcysteine (Mucomyst) is a mucolytic agent extensively used as an aerosol in the treatment of CF and can induce cough, irritation, and even bronchospasm. Although a number of reports claim benefits (decreased sputum viscosity and subjective improvement) from *N*-acetylcysteine therapy,[97,98] others remain unconvinced as to its efficacy.[99] Administration of antibiotics (neomycin, gentamicin, tobramycin, etc) by aerosol has been widely practiced[33] and not only carries the drug to the site of the infection, but allows the use of drugs that would be toxic if given systemically. Few studies have critically evaluated these claims.[100] Many authors[30,101,102] have suggested that pulmonary function testing be performed before and after inhalation of any agent to be delivered by the aerosol route to check for a possible detrimental effect. In practice this is a difficult policy to follow.

Intermittent positive pressure breathing (IPPB) There is no documented benefit for the use of intermittent positive pressure breathing therapy (IPPB) in CF.[13,30] Furthermore, it is expensive, time consuming, and can be detrimental by precipitating pneumothorax. Most authorities now seem agreed that its use is contraindicated in cystic fibrosis.

Mist Tent Therapy

The role of mist tent therapy in CF has been the subject of intense debate. Largely owing to the earlier reports of the Cleveland group[103,104] demonstrating significant improvement in pulmonary function parameters during controlled clinical evaluation, widespread adoption of mist tent therapy was practiced in the United States for many years. Wood et al[13] in their monograph on CF devoted more space to a discussion of the role of mist tent therapy than to any other therapeutic modality. Subsequently a number of controlled studies[105–107] found no significant differences in pulmonary function parameters. Rosenbluth and Chernick[108] found that mist tent therapy does not consistently influence sputum viscosity or volume in patients with cystic fibrosis. Further arguments against mist tent therapy include reports of deterioration in pulmonary function,[106] detrimental psychological effects,[105,109] and the added expense and time required for this form of therapy. Contamination of the tent by waterborne microorganisms is another potential side effect.

The subject of mist tent therapy was reviewed by Avery,[110] who pointed out that a normal temperate environment with 40–60% relative humidity seems to be the one most inhospitable to airborne viruses and most comfortable to the patient. In practice, the majority of cystic fibrosis clinics have discontinued routine mist tent therapy. There may be individual patients who may be improved by this form of treatment.

Bronchodilators

The role of bronchodilators in CF is controversial. Some authors have recommended their universal use to reduce airway obstruction if bronchospasm is present.[111,112] Others have found a reduction in expiratory flow rates in some patients after the administration of a bronchodilator aerosol and cautioned that this may be detrimental to the patient.[102,113,114]

Landau et al[102] found that 9 of 50 patients with CF had a measurable response to bronchodilators. Of these 9 patients, 5 improved and could be considered to have an associated asthmatic diathesis. The other 4 responded with a decrease in expiratory flow rate which was attributed to a reduction in tone of smooth muscle in the large airways, leading to their collapse in the presence of obstruction in the small airways.

Featherby et al[101] studied the effect of isoproteranol inhalation on 95 occasions in 47 patients. Spirometric and airway-resistance measurements showed small but statistically significant changes in maximum mid-expiratory flow rate, maximal breathing capacity, and airway resistance, although there was considerable variation from patient to patient. All these changes were small compared to those produced by bronchodilator administration to asthmatic children. Shapiro et al[114] examined the effect of aerosolized isoproteranol and oral theophylline (10 mg/kg three times daily) on pulmonary function in 12 patients with CF in a double-blind trial over 8 weeks. The responses to aerosolized bronchodilators were inconsistent from week to week. Ten of the 12 patients had adverse symptoms related to theophylline, and 6 of these had at least one theophylline level in excess of the therapeutic range of 10–20 μg/ml. The effect of isoproteranol on pulmonary function could not be used as a prognosticator for response to oral theophylline.

All these authors caution against routine administration of bronchodilators in CF and suggest that the response to these drugs should be measured in each individual patient. Plasma theophylline levels should be followed in those patients on oral bronchodilators, in view of the increased bioavailability of the drug which may be related to impaired clearance of the drug by the liver in cystic fibrosis.

Bronchopulmonary Lavage

Waring[34] reviewed the various types of bronchopulmonary lavage according to the method of instilling the liquid, the volume instilled, the duration of the procedure, and whether the goal is to fill the alveoli or not. He described five levels of increasing invasiveness in performing lavages: (1) transtracheal catheter lavage; (2) fiberoptic bronchoscopic lavage; (3) pertracheal catheter lavage; (4) rigid bronchoscopic lavage; and (5) total pulmonary lavage. The latter three methods require general anesthesia. Transtracheal catheter lavage is not used in CF except in those rare patients with a tracheostomy in place.

An extensive literature on bronchoscopic lavage has been published by those proponents of the procedure. The method used may be either the rigid bronchoscope under general anesthesia,[115] using volumes up to 400 ml/procedure or the fiberoptic bronchoscope under local anesthesia using smaller lavage volumes (100–150 ml/procedure).[116] Controversy exists over the benefits of the procedure as related to parameters such as clinical or chest radiograph score, blood gas measurements, pulmonary function tests, and long-term follow-up.

Subjective improvement is reported by most patients. Lavage with 10% and 5% *N*-acetylcysteine produced a significant increase in arterial carbon dioxide tension (P_aCO_2), and a decrease in arterial oxygen tension (P_aO_2) immediately after lavage.[115,117] Lavage with sodium chloride produced a decrease in P_aCO_2 and an increase in P_aO_2. Pulmonary function was impaired for 48–72 hours after lavage regardless of the agent used, and several patients developed postoperative pneumonia. Schidlow et al[118] compared parameters such as respiratory rate, temperature, white blood cell count, pulmonary function, and chest radiograph score in a large group of patients and concluded that lung lavage in CF is probably rarely indicated.

Other Preventive Measures

The National Center for Disease Control in Atlanta issues annual guidelines on influenza vaccination for high-risk patients. Immunization against influenza is recommended on an annual basis to all patients with CF over 6 months of age unless they are sensitive to egg protein or have had a previous reaction to the vaccine.

Atmospheric pollutants should be avoided. Smoking is contraindicated for the patient with CF and attempts should be made to dissuade other members of the family from smoking. Occupations involving contact with pollutants are especially detrimental to the patient with CF and anyone else with chronic lung disease.

Patients with severe pulmonary disease should be warned about the dangers of travel to high altitudes and by airplane. For example, the normal P_aO_2 goes down from 98 mm Hg at sea level to 67 mm Hg at 5000 feet. In a patient whose P_aO_2 runs in the 50s, there is a definite risk of producing severe anoxia and precipitating heart failure. Recommendations for airline travel of children with chronic pulmonary disease have been published.[119]

REFERENCES

1. Oppenheimer EH, Esterly JR: Pathology of cystic fibrosis. Review of the literature and comparison with 146 autopsied cases. *Perspect Pediatr Pathol* 1975;2:241–278.
2. Sturgess JM: Mucus secretion and clearance in the pathogenesis of cystic fibrosis, in Schoni M, Kraemer R (eds): *Current Problems and New Trends in Cystic Fibrosis, Monographs in Pediatrics, Vol. 14.* Basel, S Karger, 1981, pp 60–74.
3. Bedrossian CWM, Greenberg SD, Singer DB, et al: The lung in cystic fibrosis. A quantitative study including prevalence of pathologic findings among different age groups. *Hum Pathol* 1976;7:195–204.
4. Afzelius BA: A human syndrome caused by immotile cilia. *Science* 1976;193:317–319.
5. Sturgess JM, Chao J, Wong J, et al: Cilia with defective radial spokes—a cause of human respiratory disease. *N Engl J Med* 1979;300: 53–56.
6. Reid L, Haller R: The bronchial mucous glands. Their hypertrophy and change in intracellular mucus. *Mod Probl Pediatr* 1967; 10:195–199.
7. Sturgess JM, Reid L: Secretory activity of human bronchial mucous glands in vitro. *Exp Mol Pathol* 1972;16:362–381.
8. Sturgess JM, Reid L: An organ culture study of the effect of drugs on the secretory activity of human bronchial submucosal gland. *Clin Sci* 1972;43:533–543.
9. Yeates DB, Sturgess JM, Kahn SR, et al: Mucociliary transport in trachea of patients with cystic fibrosis. *Arch Dis Child* 1976;51:28–33.
10. Sanchis J, Dolovich M, Rossman C, et al: Pulmonary mucociliary clearance in cystic fibrosis. *N Engl J Med* 1973;288:651–654.
11. Wood RE, Wanner A, Hirsch JA: Measurement of mucociliary airway clearance in patients with cystic fibrosis and its stimulation by terbutaline. *Pediatr Res* 1974;8:471–476.
12. Lamarre A, Reilly BJ, Bryan AC, et al: Early detection of pulmonary function abnormalities in cystic fibrosis. *Pediatrics* 1972;50: 291–294.
13. Wood RE, Boat TF, Doershuk CF: State of the art—cystic fibrosis. *Am Rev Respir Dis* 1976;113:833–878.
14. Mearns MB: Natural history of pulmonary infection in cystic fibrosis. In *Proceedings Eighth International Congress Cystic Fibrosis.* Toronto, Canadian Cystic Fibrosis Foundation, 1980 pp 325–334.
15. Andersen DH: Cystic Fibrosis of the pancreas and its relation to coeliac disease. *Am J Dis Child* 1938;56:344–399.
16. Farber S: Pancreatic function and disease in early life. V. Pathologic changes associated with pancreatic insufficiency in early life. *Arch Pathol* 1944;37:238–250.
17. di Sant'Agnese PA: The pulmonary manifestations of fibrocystic disease of the pancreas. *Dis Chest* 1955;27:654–667.
18. May JR, Herrick NC, Thompson D: Bacterial infection in cystic fibrosis. *Arch Dis Child* 1972;47:908–913.
19. Doggett RG, Harrison GM, Stillwell RN, et al: An atypical *Pseudomonas aeruginosa* associated with cystic fibrosis of the pancreas. *J Pediatr* 1966;68:215, 221.
20. Reynolds HY, di Sant'Agnese PA, Zierdt CH: Mucoid *Pseudomonas aeruginosa*: A sign of cystic fibrosis in young adults with chronic pulmonary disease? *JAMA* 1976; 236:2190–2192.
21. Kulczycki LL, Murphy TM, Bellanti JA: *Pseudomonas* colonization in cystic fibrosis. A study of 160 patients. *JAMA* 1978;240: 30–34.
22. Zierdt CH, Williams RL: Serotyping of *Pseudomonas aeruginosa* isolates from patients with cystic fibrosis of the pancreas. *J Clin Microbiol* 1975;1:521–526.
23. Huang NN, Van Loon EL, Sheng KT: The flora of the respiratory tract of patients with cystic fibrosis of the pancreas. *J Pediatr* 1961;59:512–521.

24. Lloyd-Still JD, Khaw KT, Shwachman H: Severe respiratory disease in infants with cystic fibrosis. *Pediatrics* 1974;53:678–682.
25. Macone AB, Pier GB, Pennington JE, et al: Mucoid *Escherichia coli* in cystic fibrosis. *N Engl J Med* 1981;304:1445–1449.
26. Lam J, Chan R, Lam K, et al: Production of mucoid microcolonies by *Pseudomonas aeruginosa* within infected lungs in cystic fibrosis. *Infect Immun* 1980;28:546–556.
27. Glezen WP, Denny FW: Epidemiology of acute lower respiratory disease in children. *N Engl J Med* 1973;288:498–505.
28. Wright PF, Khaw KT, Oxman MN, et al: Evaluation of the safety of amantadine HCl and the role of respiratory viral infections in children with cystic fibrosis. *J Infect Dis* 1976;134:144–149.
29. Petersen NT, Hoiby N, Mordhurst CH, et al: Respiratory infections in cystic fibrosis patients caused by virus, *Chlamydia* and *Mycoplasma*—possible synergism with *Pseudomonas aeruginosa*. In *Proceedings Eighth International Congress Cystic Fibrosis.* Toronto, Canadian Cystic Fibrosis Foundation, 1980 pp 346–351.
30. Holsclaw DS: Cystic fibrosis: Overview and pulmonary aspects in young adults. *Clin Chest Med* 1980;1:407–421.
31. Jenner BM, Landau LI, Phelan PD: Pulmonary candidiasis in cystic fibrosis. *Arch Dis Child* 1979;54:555–556.
32. Boxerbaum B: Isolation of rapidly growing mycobacteria in patients with cystic fibrosis. *J Pediatr* 1980;96:689–691.
33. Guide to Diagnosis and Management of Cystic Fibrosis. Cystic Fibrosis Foundation, 6000 Executive Boulevard, Suite 309, Rockville, Maryland 20852, 1979.
34. Waring WW: Current management of cystic fibrosis. *Adv Pediatr* 1976;23:401–438.
35. Shwachman H: Cystic fibrosis, in Gluck L (ed): *Current Problems in Pediatrics, Vol. 8.* Chicago, Year Book Medical Publishing Inc, 1978, pp 5–72.
36. Shwachman H, Kulczycki LL, Mueller HL, et al: Nasal polyposis in patients with cystic fibrosis. *Pediatrics* 1962;30:389–401.
37. Taylor B, Evans JNG, Hope GA: Upper respiratory tract in cystic fibrosis. Ear-nose-throat survey of 50 children. *Arch Dis Child* 1974;49:133–136.
38. Rulon JT, Brown HA, Logan GB: Nasal polyps and cystic fibrosis of the pancreas. *Arch Otol* 1963;78:192–199.
39. Oppenheimer EH, Rosenstein BJ: Differential pathology of nasal polyps in cystic fibrosis and atopy. *Lab Invest* 1979;40: 445–449.
40. Jaffe BF, Strome M, Khaw KT, et al: Nasal polypectomy and sinus surgery for cystic fibrosis—a 10 year review. *Otolaryngol Clin N Amer* 1977;10:81–90.
41. Warner JO, Taylor BW, Norman AP, et al: Association of cystic fibrosis with allergy. *Arch Dis Child* 1976;51:507–511.
42. Mitchell I, Corey M, Woenne R, et al: Bronchial hyperreactivity in cystic fibrosis and asthma. *J Pediatr* 1978;93:744–748.
43. Godfrey RC, Griffiths M: The prevalence of immediate positive skin tests to dermatophagoides pteronyssinus and grass pollen in school children. *Clin Allergy* 1976;6:79–82.
44. Kulczycki LL, Mueller HL, Shwachman H: Respiratory allergy in patients with cystic fibrosis. *JAMA* 1961;175:358–364.
45. Van Metre TE, Cooke RE, Gibson LE, et al: Evidence of allergy in patients with cystic fibrosis of the pancreas. *J Allergy* 1960; 31:141–150.
46. Rachelefsky GS, Osher A, Dooley RE, et al: Coexistent respiratory allergy and cystic fibrosis. *Am J Dis Child* 1974;128:355–359.
47. Mellis CM, Levison H: Bronchial reactivity in cystic fibrosis. *Pediatrics* 1978;61: 446–450.
48. Davis PB, Shelhamer JR, Kaliner M: Abnormal adrenergic and cholinergic sensitivity in cystic fibrosis. *N Engl J Med* 1980; 302:1453–1456.
49. Wang JLF, Patterson R, Mintzer R, et al: Allergic bronchopulmonary aspergillosis in pediatric practice. *J Pediatr* 1979; 94:376–381.
50. Nelson LA, Callerame ML, Schwartz RH: Aspergillosis and atopy in cystic fibrosis. *Am Rev Respir Dis* 1979;120:863–873.
51. Brueton MJ, Ormerod LP, Shah KJ, et al: Allergic bronchopulmonary aspergillosis complicating cystic fibrosis in childhood. *Arch Dis Child* 1980;55:348–353.
52. di Sant'Agnese PA: Bronchial obstruction with lobar atelectasis and emphysema in cystic fibrosis of the pancreas. *Pediatrics* 1953;12:178–190.
53. Rooney JC, Williams HE: The relationship between proved viral bronchiolitis and subsequent wheezing. *J Pediatr* 1971;79: 744–748.
54. Zuelzer WW, Newton WA: The pathogenesis of fibrocystic disease of the pancreas. A study of 36 cases with special reference to the pulmonary lesions. *Pediatrics* 1949; 4:53–69.
55. Waring WW, Brunt CA, Hilman BC: Mucoid impaction of the bronchi in cystic fibrosis. *Pediatrics* 1967;39:166–175.
56. Shwachman H, Holsclaw DS: Pulmonary complications of cystic fibrosis. *Minn Med* 1969;52:1521–1528.
57. Boat TF, di Sant'Agnese PA, Warwick WJ, et al: Pneumothorax in cystic fibrosis. *JAMA*

1969;209:1498-1504.

58. Stowe SM, Boat TF, Mendelsohn H, et al: Open thoracotomy for pneumothorax in cystic fibrosis. *Am Rev Respir Dis* 1975;111: 611-617.
59. Luck SR, Raffensperger JG, Sullivan HJ, et al: Management of pneumothorax in children with chronic pulmonary disease. *J Thorac Cardiovasc Surg* 1977;74:834-839.
60. Rich RH, Warwick WJ, Leonard AS: Open thoracotomy and pleural abrasion in the treatment of spontaneous pneumothorax in cystic fibrosis. *J Pediatr Surg* 1978;13:237-242.
61. Holsclaw DS, Grand RJ, Shwachman H: Massive hemoptysis in cystic fibrosis. *J Pediatr* 1970;76:829-838.
62. Stern RC, Wood RE, Boat TF, et al: Treatment and prognosis of massive hemoptysis in cystic fibrosis. *Am Rev Respir Dis* 1977;117: 825-828.
63. White RI, Kaufman SL, Barth KH, et al: Therapeutic embolization with detactable silicone balloons. *JAMA* 1979;241:1257-1260.
64. Fellows KE, Khaw KT, Schuster S, et al: Bronchial artery embolization in cystic fibrosis; technique and long-term results. *J Pediatr* 1979;95:959-963.
65. McCarthy MM, Rourk MH, Spock A: Bacteremia in patients with cystic fibrosis. *Clin Pediatr* 1980;19:746-748.
66. Fischer EG, Shwachman H, Wepsic JG: Brain abscess and cystic fibrosis. *J Pediatr* 1979;95:385-388.
67. Katznelson D, Vawter GF, Foley GE, et al: Botryomycosis. A complication in cystic fibrosis. Report of 7 cases. *J Pediatr* 1964;65: 525-538.
68. Newman AJ, Ansell BM: Episodic arthritis in children with cystic fibrosis. *J Pediatr* 1979; 94:594-596.
69. Goldsmith D, Schidlow D, Palmer J, et al: Rheumatic manifestations in cystic fibrosis. In *Proceedings Eighth International Congress Cystic Fibrosis.* Toronto, Canadian Cystic Fibrosis Foundation, 1980 p 17a.
70. Nielson HE, Lundh S, Jacobsen SV, et al: Hypergammaglobulinemic purpura in cystic fibrosis. *Acta Paediatr Scand* 1978; 67: 443-447.
71. Frates RC, Cox KL: Cystic fibrosis mistaken for gastroesophageal reflux with aspiration. *Am J Dis Child* 1981;135: 719-720.
72. Cystic Fibrosis Conference Reports: Cystic fibrosis patient evaluations and scoring systems. Tucson, Arizona, March 15-17, 1978. Cystic Fibrosis Foundation.
73. Shwachman H, Kulczycki LL: Long-term study of one hundred five patients with cystic fibrosis. *Am J Dis Child* 1958;96:6-15.
74. Brasfield D, Hicks G, Soong SJ, et al: The chest roentgenogram in cystic fibrosis: A new scoring system. *Pediatrics* 1979;63: 24-29.
75. Chrispin AR, Norman AP: The systematic evaluation of the chest radiograph in cystic fibrosis. *Pediatr Radiol* 1974;2:101-106.
76. Taussig LM, Kattwinkel J, Friedewald WT, et al: A new prognostic score and clinical evaluation system for cystic fibrosis. *J Pediatr* 1973;82:380-390.
77. Cooperman EM, Park M, McKee J, et al: A simplified cystic fibrosis scoring system. *Can Med Assoc J* 1971;105:580-582.
78. Lester LA, Egge AC, Hubbard VS, et al: Echocardiography in cystic fibrosis: A proposed scoring system. *J Pediatr* 1980; 97: 742-748.
79. Stern RC, Boat TF, Doershuk CF, et al: Course of cystic fibrosis in 95 patients. *J Pediatr* 1976;89:406-411.
80. Shwachman H, Redmond A, Khaw KT: Studies in cystic fibrosis. Report of 130 patients diagnosed under 3 months of age over a 20-year period. *Pediatrics* 1970;46: 335-343.
81. Corey ML: Longitudinal studies in cystic fibrosis. In *Proceedings Eighth International Congress Cystic Fibrosis.* Toronto, Canadian Cystic Fibrosis Foundation, 1980 pp 246-255.
82. Gaskin K, Gurwitz D, Corey M, et al: Improved pulmonary function in cystic fibrosis patients without pancreatic insufficiency. In *Proceedings Eighth International Congress Cystic Fibrosis.* Toronto, Canadian Cystic Fibrosis Foundation, 1980 pp 226-230.
83. Knoke JD, Stern RC, Doershuk CF, et al: Cystic fibrosis: The prognosis for five-year survival. *Pediatr Res* 1978;12:676-679.
84. Gurwitz D, Corey M, Francis PWJ, et al: Perspectives in cystic fibrosis. *Pediatr Clin North Am* 1979;26:603-615.
85. Rucker RW, Harrison GM: Outpatient intravenous medications in the management of cystic fibrosis. *Pediatrics* 1974; 54:358-360.
86. Burrows B, Earle R: Course and prognosis of chronic obstructive lung disease. A prospective study of 200 patients. *N Engl J Med* 1969;280:397-404.
87. Tecklin JS, Holsclaw DS: Evaluation of bronchial drainage in patients with cystic fibrosis. *Phys Ther* 1975;55:1081-1084.
88. Wong JW, Keens TG, Wannamaker EM, et al: Effects of gravity on tracheal mucus transport rates in normal subjects and in patients with cystic fibrosis. *Pediatrics* 1977;60:146-152.

89. Blake J: On the movement of mucus in the lung. *J Biomed* 1975;8:179–184.
90. Denton R: Bronchial secretions in cystic fibrosis: The effects of treatment with mechanical percussion vibration. *Am Rev Respir Dis* 1962;86:41–46.
91. Lorin MI, Denning CR: Evaluation of postural drainage by measurement of sputum volume and consistency. *Am J Phys Med* 1971;50:215–219.
92. Levison H, Godfrey S: Pulmonary aspects of cystic fibrosis, in Mangos JA, Talamo RC (eds): *Cystic Fibrosis—Projections Into The Future.* New York, Intercontinental Medical Book Corporation, 1976, pp 3–24.
93. Maxwell M, Redmond A: Comparative trial of manual and mechanical percussion technique with gravity-assisted bronchial drainage in patients with cystic fibrosis. *Arch Dis Child* 1979:54:542–544.
94. Rossman C, Waldes R, Sampson D, et al: Does chest physiotherapy improve mucus removal in patients with cystic fibrosis. In *Proceedings Eighth International Congress Cystic Fibrosis.* Toronto, Canadian Cystic Fibrosis Foundation, 1980 p 32a.
95. Alderson PO, Secker-Walker RH, Strominger DB: Pulmonary deposition of aerosols in children with cystic fibrosis. *J Pediatr* 1974;84:479–484.
96. Wanner A: Clinical aspects of mucociliary transport. *Am Rev Respir Dis* 1977;116:73–125.
97. Reas HW: The effect of *N*-acetylcysteine on the viscosity of tracheobronchial secretions in cystic fibrosis of the pancreas. *J Pediatr* 1963;62:31–35.
98. Stamm SJ, Docter JM: Clinical evaluation of acetylcysteine as a mucolytic agent in cystic fibrosis. *Dis Chest* 1965;47:414–420.
99. Denton R, Kwart H, Litt M: *N*-Acetylcysteine in cystic fibrosis: Mechanical and chemical factors in treatment by aerosol. *Am Rev Respir Dis* 1967;95:643–651.
100. Holsclaw DS, Tecklin JS: A critical evaluation of bronchial hygiene in pediatric pulmonary disease. *Pediatr Ann* 1977;6:104–116.
101. Featherby EA, Weng TR, Levison H: The effect of isoproterenol on airway obstruction in cystic fibrosis. *Can Med Assoc J* 1970;102:835–838.
102. Landau LI, Phelan PD: The variable effect of a bronchodilating agent on pulmonary function in cystic fibrosis. *J Pediatr* 1973;82:863–868.
103. Matthews LW, Doershuk CF, Spector S: Mist tent therapy of the obstructive pulmonary lesion of cystic fibrosis. *Pediatrics* 1967;39:176–185.
104. Doershuk CF, Matthews LW, Gillespie CT, et al: Evaluation of jet type and ultrasonic nebulizers in mist tent therapy for cystic fibrosis. *Pediatrics* 1968;41:723–730.
105. Norman AP, Hall M: Nocturnal mist therapy in cystic fibrosis. *Practitioner* 1971;206:786–789.
106. Motoyama EK, Gibson LE, Zigas CJ: Evaluation of mist tent therapy in cystic fibrosis using maximum expiratory flow volume curve. *Pediatrics* 1972;50:299–306.
107. Chang N, Levison H, Cunningham K, et al: An evaluation of nightly mist tent therapy for patients with cystic fibrosis. *Am Rev Respir Dis* 1973;107:672–675.
108. Rosenbluth M, Chernick V: Influence of mist tent therapy on sputum viscosity and water content in cystic fibrosis. *Arch Dis Child* 1974;49:606–610.
109. McCollum AT, Gibson LE: Family adaptation to the child with cystic fibrosis. *J Pediatr* 1970;77:571–578.
110. Avery ME: Mist therapy—1973, in Mangos JA, Talamo RC (eds): *Fundamental Problems of Cystic Fibrosis And Related Diseases.* New York, Intercontinental Medical Book Corporation, 1973, pp 291–302.
111. Matthews LW, Doershuk CF, Wise M, et al: A therapeutic regimen for patients with cystic fibrosis. *J Pediatr* 1964;65:558–563.
112. Lifschitz MI, Denning CR: Assessment of bronchospasm in patients with cystic fibrosis. *Am Rev Respir Dis* 1969;99:399–405.
113. Zapletal A, Motoyama EK, Gibson LE, et al: Pulmonary mechanics in asthma and cystic fibrosis. *Pediatrics* 1971;48:64–72.
114. Shapiro GG, Bamman J, Kanarek P, et al: The paradoxical effect of adrenergic and methylxanthine drugs in cystic fibrosis. *Pediatrics* 1976;58:740–743.
115. Altman RP, Kulczycki LL, Randolph JG, et al: Bronchoscopy and bronchial lavage (BBL) in children with cystic fibrosis. *J Pediatr Surg* 1973;8:809–814.
116. Dahm LS, Ewing CW, Harrison GM, et al: Comparison of three techniques of lung lavage in patients with cystic fibrosis. *Chest* 1977;72:593–596.
117. Cezeaux G, Telford J, Harrison G, et al: Bronchial lavage in cystic fibrosis. A comparison of agents. *JAMA* 1967;199:73–76.
118. Schidlow DV, Simon D, Palmer J, et al: Tracheobronchial lavage in cystic fibrosis. In *Proceedings Eighth International Congress Cystic Fibrosis.* Toronto, Canadian Cystic Fibrosis Foundation, 1980 pp 231–235.
119. Report of the Cardiovascular Committee of

the Cystic Fibrosis Foundation: Airline travel for children with chronic pulmonary disease. *Pediatrics* 1976;57:408–410.

120. Bentley D, Moore A, Shwachman H: Finger clubbing: A quantitative survey by analysis of the shadowgraph. *Lancet* 1976;2:164–167.

121. Vawter GF, Shwachman H: Cystic fibrosis in adults. An autopsy study. *Pathol Ann* 1979;14:357–382.

13

Lung Function in Cystic Fibrosis

Hans U. Wessel

Beginning with the work of Andersen,[1] the early clinical and pathological descriptions of cystic fibrosis indicated that impairment of lung function associated with pulmonary disease of CF was to a large extent the result of small-airway obstruction by thickened secretions and purulent exudate. However, the first report on lung function in CF was not published until 1954, primarily because up to that time few patients survived to an age where they could successfully cooperate in such studies. Although this first study was based on observations in only 6 patients it is remarkable in that West et al[2] clearly identified most of the important features of impaired lung function in CF which have since been verified and expanded on in a large number of subsequent investigations. Notably these authors recognized the wide spectrum of functional impairment of the lungs. They showed that functional impairment correlates well with the clinical assessment of pulmonary involvement. They recognized that an increase of the residual volume and RV/TLC ratio are manifestations of early pulmonary involvement while a reduced TLC and CO_2 retention are late manifestations of severe chronic disease (see Glossary at end of chapter for list of abbreviations). They clearly demonstrated that abnormal intrapulmonary gas mixing and increased dead-space ventilation were the earliest signs of impaired lung function and concluded correctly that these changes were the result of abnormal ventilation-perfusion relationships primarily due to nonuniform distribution of alveolar ventilation as a result of bronchial obstruction.

These conclusions were supported by subsequent studies of intrapulmonary gas mixing in CF[3,4,5] and substantiated 18 years later more definitively by the elegant work of Lamarre et al.[6] These investigators demonstrated in 19 CF patients an increased alveolar–arterial (A–a) PO_2 gradient, decreased arterial PO_2 and increased V_D/V_T ratios even though lung volumes, flow rates, airway conductance, diffusing capacity, and mixing efficiency were still within normal limits. In retrospect these findings are not unexpected in CF since obstruction of small airways by thickened mucus is unlikely to be a uniform process. The precise matching of local pulmonary perfusion to local airway obstruction is equally unlikely. Therefore, small airway obstruction must result in more non-uniform distribution of ventilation-blood flow ratios within the lungs and thus to an increase in A–a PO_2 gradients.

Similar effects on gas exchange due to nonuniform distribution of ventilation as a consequence of small airway obstruction can be demonstrated for CO_2 and N_2. Thus, Battistini and Waring[7] showed increased ΔPCO_2 (10.9 mm Hg) in CF as compared to normals (5.1 mm Hg) and patients with asthma (6.2 mm Hg). Alveolar PCO_2 was estimated from end-tidal measurements and arterial PCO_2 by a rebreathing technique. They showed that in early pulmonary disease of CF end-tidal PCO_2 is reduced while arterial PCO_2 remains normal. As pulmonary disease progresses arterial PCO_2 increases until finally both alveolar and arterial PCO_2 are elevated above normal.

Similar to the changes of the A–a PO_2 and PCO_2 gradients, nonuniform distribution of ventilation–blood flow ratios are manifested also by an increase of the A–a PN_2 gradient, reflecting alveoli with low V_A/Q ratios.[8] In CF patients Corbet et al[9] showed that similar to Δ (A-a) PO_2, the alveolar-arterial PN_2 gradient is already abnormal when other parameters of lung function are still within normal limits.

ABNORMAL LUNG FUNCTION WITH PROGRESSION OF PULMONARY DISEASE

Lung Volumes and Capacities

Although small airway obstruction in early minimal pulmonary disease of CF may exist without measurable evidence of air trapping and abnormal lung volumes and lung mechanics, such findings are actually quite rare. Thus, of the 166 CF patients currently followed at the Children's Memorial Hospital with lung function studies, only two have entirely normal lung volumes and maximal airflow rates.

In most patients, even those with relatively mild pulmonary involvement, an increase in residual volume, RV/TLC ratio, and FRC can be demonstrated by the time they are old enough to undergo lung function studies. Clearly, increase of the RV and RV/TLC ratio are two of the earliest lung volume changes in CF.[1] In the presence of significant air trapping, the FRC measured by body plethysmography is greater than FRC measured by inert gas dilution, and the difference between the two provides an estimate of the trapped gas volume. Such differences are usually not found in normals.[10,11]

The vital capacity may remain within the lower limits of normal even when RV and FRC are significantly increased. As pulmonary involvement progresses, further reduction of the vital capacity occurs initially due to loss of expiratory reserve. Later on there is progressive decrease of the VC due to loss of inspiratory reserve. In mild to moderate pulmonary disease the total lung capacity is frequently maintained within normal limits. However, as lung tissue destruction progresses, there is eventually also progressive decrease of TLC.

Pulmonary Mechanics

The changes in lung mechanics which occur as a result of progression of pulmonary disease in CF have been studied in detail and are well understood. Frequency dependence of dynamic lung compliance, C_{dyn}, is one of the earliest of these changes.[12] C_{dyn} relates lung volume changes to corresponding changes in transpulmonary pressure (L/cm H_2O). Frequency dependence, ie, a decrease of C_{dyn} with increasing respiratory frequencies is not found in normal children and adolescents for measurements made above FRC within a range of frequencies of 80 breaths/min or less.[13] It develops, however, in the presence of non-uniform distribution of ventilation[14] and reflects small-airway obstruction, provided elastic recoil and resistance are within normal limits. As in the case of A–a O_2 differences, frequency dependence of C_{dyn} is a sensitive measure of small-airway obstruction and may be observed in CF when other lung function tests remain normal.

However, as airway disease progresses, other parameters of lung mechanics become measurably abnormal—notably maximal airflows—$\dot{V}_{max}$, which can be generated during forced expiration. $\dot{V}_{max}$ at a given lung volume is directly proportional to the elastic recoil pressure of the lungs ($P_{st\,l}$) and inversely related to the resistance of the upstream airway segment, R_{us}.[15] The resistance to airflow is determined by two components, frictional resistance, which is negligible at higher lung volumes and increased progressively as lung volume is reduced, and a component due to convective acceleration, which primarily reflects large airway dimensions and has its greatest effect at large lung volumes. The upstream airway segment as defined by Mead et al[15] includes the airways from the alveoli to the point of equal pressures (EPP). At EPP the pressure loss incurred along the airways during a forced expiration equals $P_{st\,l}$, and the pressure surrounding the airways (pleural pressure or less) equals intrabronchial lateral pressure. Consequently, transmural bronchial pressure, P_{tm}, is positive in the upstream segment and negative downstream of EPP. It follows that airway compression during forced expiration can only occur in the downstream segment. During a forced expiration, EPP is at the airway opening when pleural pressure reaches atmospheric pressure. As pleural pressure exceeds atmospheric pressure, EPP moves progressively upstream as long as airflow increases and becomes fixed when the resistance of the compressed downstream is sufficiently high to prohibit further increases in airflow.

Since early airways disease of CF is largely confined to small airways, $\dot{V}_{max}$ is initially reduced only at low lung volumes. Effort dependence of $\dot{V}_{max}$ at high lung volumes is maintained. In part this reflects the non-uniform distribution of airways disease and rapid emptying of non-involved or less involved airways which have fast emptying times. In CF reduction of $\dot{V}_{max}$ is primarily due to increased resistance of the upstream segment as a result of airways obstruction. Elastic recoil may remain remarkably normal despite prolonged hyperinflation and chronic bronchiolitis and bronchitis.[14] This finding is consistent with the usual absence of widespread destructive emphysema in CF patients who have died from their lung disease.[16] However, in other studies an exaggerated decrease in elastic recoil was noted as patients expired from maximum lung volume to 90% of TLC, indicating abnormally reduced $P_{st\,l}$ at lung volumes less than 90% of TLC.[17]

The increased resistance in the upstream segment, R_{us}, manifested by decreased $\dot{V}_{max}$ at low lung volumes in early CF lung disease contributes too little to overall airway resistance R_{aw}, to result in significant increases. Therefore, R_{aw} is not a sensitive measure of early CF lung disease. Increase of R_{aw} as pulmonary involvement progresses reflects either very extensive small-airways disease, obstruction of larger airways, or both.[14]

Diffusing Capacity

After death from the progressive pulmonary disease of cystic fibrosis, autopsy reveals the small and large airways to be obstructed with thick purulent mucus, and there is much destruction of alveolar tissue. It is evident that these changes must have greatly increased resistance to gaseous diffusion during the later stages of the disease. By contrast, when the resting CO diffusing capacity, $D_{L_{CO}}$, is measured early on in the disease, it is often found to be normal,[18-20] even when other indices of lung function such as maximal airflows at low lung volumes and FRC measured by body plethysmography are already distinctly abnormal. However, Zelkowitz and Giammona[21] have demonstrated that such patients with a normal resting $D_{L_{CO}}$ are unable to increase the diffusing capacity appropriately during exercise. These findings are different from those seen in patients with alveolar capillary block who have both a reduced resting and exercise $D_{L_{CO}}$ but usually show a normal rate of increase with exercise. However, they are similar to observations made in patients with severe pulmonary vascular disease,[22] suggesting that the inability to increase $D_{L_{CO}}$ with exercise is due to an inability to increase the area available for diffusion (impaired recruitment). The data on resting $D_{L_{CO}}$ in CF indicate that $D_{L_{CO}}$ is not a sensitive indicator of mild pulmonary disease.[23] However, in a large series[23] which included a wide spectrum of severity of pulmonary involvement, resting $D_{L_{CO}}$ correlated linearly with other parameters of lung function, notably FRC. However, none of the correlation coefficients were sufficiently high to permit prediction of $D_{L_{CO}}$ from these parameters.

Arterial Hypoxemia and CO_2 Retention

Arterial hypoxemia as a result of non-uniform distribution of ventilation is the earliest sign of impaired lung function and may exist in the absence of any other measurable abnormality.[5] As pulmonary involvement progresses, so does arterial hypoxemia which has been shown to correlate well with the clinical pulmonary status of these patients. In mild pulmonary involvement hypoxemia does not lead to clinical cyanosis since arterial O_2 saturation is minimally reduced because of the shape of the O_2 dissociation curve. With more advanced degrees of hypoxemia, cyanosis is usually clinically manifest. However, recognition of cyanosis in CF is rendered more difficult, since these patients as a rule have a diminished polycythemic response to hypoxemia, presumably because of chronic infection. It should be recognized that patients, in particular children, are frequently excited and hyperventilating immediately after arterial puncture. Therefore, arterial P_{O_2} measured under these conditions may be significantly higher than P_{O_2} measured in the undisturbed state (indwelling catheter, transcutaneous P_{O_2} electrode) or during sleep. Such measurements in the undisturbed state are essential when evaluating the need for ventilatory support by low flow O_2 at night designed to prevent or retard progression of pulmonary hypertension.[24]

The importance of these considerations is underlined by the results of a recent study[25] which demonstrated an average 7.4% decrease of S_aO_2 (range 1–22%) during REM sleep in 20 clinically stable CF patients. By comparison normal controls showed an average decrease of only 2% with a range of 1%–3%. It appears from such data that O_2, notably low flow O_2 at night, should not be withheld until it is required to relieve symptoms. Rather O_2 should be given much earlier in an attempt to forestall or retard the development of cor pulmonale. The rationale of this application of O_2 must be carefully explained to the patient since in our experience asymptomatic patients are often reluctant to use O_2 since they associate its use with end-stage disease and impending death.

In contrast to arterial hypoxemia which is an early finding, significant CO_2 retention is usually absent until the preterminal stage of pulmonary involvement.[2-4,26] These findings contrast with those in adults with chronic obstructive pulmonary disease. The absence of early CO_2 retention in CF is due to the patchy rather than diffuse pulmonary involvement which is readily discernible on physical examination of the lungs even in severe pulmonary disease. Since the CO_2 dissociation curve is nearly linear over the physiologic range, overall CO_2 retention is minimized by compensation of areas of high ventilation- blood flow ratios for areas with low $\dot{V}_A/\dot{Q}$ ratios. Moreover, CF patients tend to hyperventilate, even with relatively good lung function, such that their mean P_aCO_2 tends to be lower than normal. Since CO_2 retention is a late phenomenon, it correlates with poor lung function, evidence of cor pulmonale (pulmonary hypertension),[27] and poor prognosis.[28] Thus the data of Siassi et al[27] indicated that all patients with an arterial PO_2 of <50 torr and all with an arterial PCO_2 >45 torr had mean pulmonary artery pressures in excess of 30 torr, an indication of significant cor pulmonale. Moreover, with further arterial hypoxemia and CO_2 retention, mean pulmonary arterial pressure increased linearly with falling PO_2 and increasing PCO_2 (Figures 13-1, 13-2).

Response to Bronchodilator Challenge

Patients with CF have a higher than normal incidence of positive allergen skin tests and at least the same incidence of bronchial asthma as found in an age-matched control population. Moreover, patients with CF have altered airways reactivity in the absence of superimposed asthma. Thus, exercise challenge results in bronchodilatation rather than postexercise bronchoconstriction found in asthma.[29] Mellis[30] reported a 24% incidence of a positive response (bronchoconstriction) to inhaled histamine challenge of 50 CF patients. There was no correlation between the response to histamine and evidence of atopy, but all positive responders had more severe impairment of lung function than nonresponders, and a positive

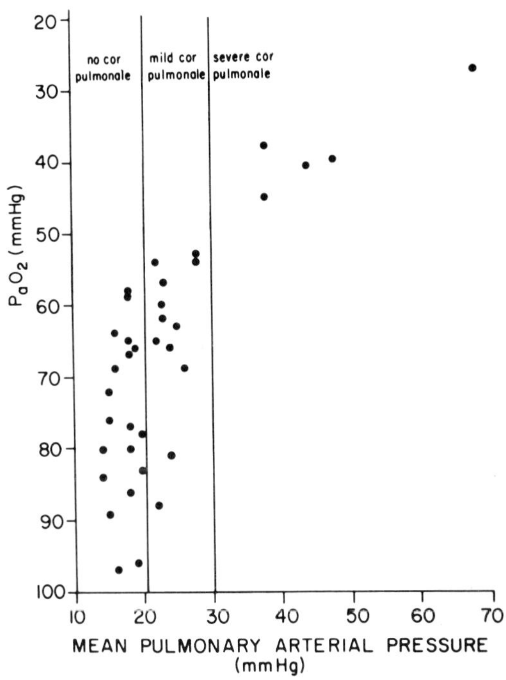

Figure 13-1 Graph showing the relationship between the severity of cor pulmonale and P_aO_2 in 34 patients with cystic fibrosis. Note that all patients with mean pulmonary arterial pressure greater than 30 mm Hg had P_aO_2 values less than 50 mm Hg. (Reproduced from Siassi B, et al: *J Pediatr* 1971;78:794 (reference 27), with permission.

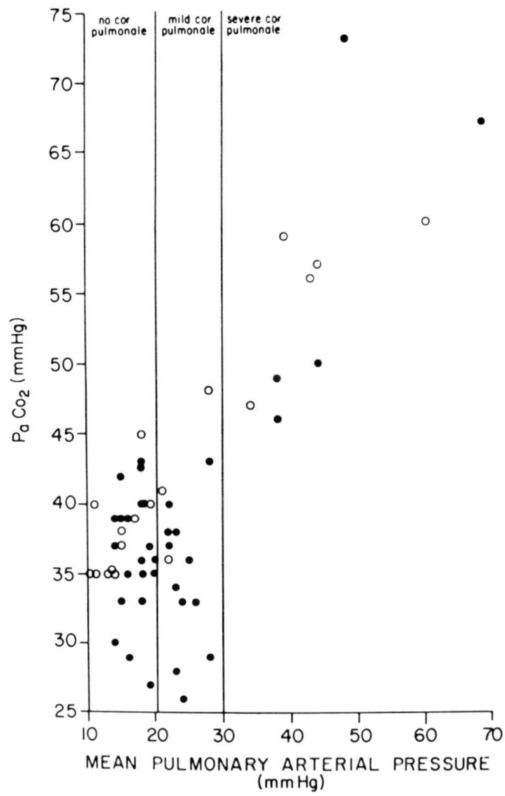

Figure 13-2 Graph demonstrating the relationship between the severity of cor pulmonale and P_aCO_2 in 52 patients with cystic fibrosis. In all instances except one, the patients with mean pulmonary arterial pressure greater than 30 mm Hg had P_aCO_2 greater than 45 mm Hg. The open circles represent patients collected from the literature. Reproduced from Siassi B, et al: *J Pediatr* 1971;78:794 (reference 27), with permission.

response was not seen in a patient with a normal $MEF_{25\%-75\%}$. The authors concluded that the abnormal bronchial reactivity was a reflection of the severity of their lung disease rather than the presence of asthma.

The response to bronchodilator challenge in CF patients is not predictable.[31,32] In the presence of superimposed asthma, there may be a significant component of reversible bronchoconstriction as indicated by increases in FEV, FEV_1, $MEF_{25\%-75\%}$, MVV, and PEF, and decreased R_{aw} and TGV. Similar changes may be seen in CF patients without asthma, although in our experience $\dot{V}_{max75\%}$ is rarely altered. Similarly TGV, FRC/TLC, and RV/TLC tend to remain unchanged following bronchodilator challenge. In other patients with moderately advanced pulmonary disease, bronchodilator challenge may result paradoxically in decreased maximal airflows and FEV, presumably owing to bronchial smooth muscle relaxation with a resulting tendency toward airway compression and collapse during the FEV maneuver.[31-33] These findings suggest that the bronchodilator response should be tested in all patients with CF and that bronchodilator therapy should not be instituted unless a beneficial effect on lung function can first be demonstrated.[30]

PROGRESSION OF PULMONARY CHANGES IN CYSTIC FIBROSIS

Once the diagnosis of cystic fibrosis has been established, two assumptions about the patient are almost always valid: (1) there is pulmonary disease, and (2) it is progressive. Since there is no cure for the pulmonary complications of CF, treatment is directed towards prolonging life by retarding the progressive destruction of the lungs which is ultimately the direct cause of death in the vast majority of these patients.

It follows that changes in survival rates and the rate of progression of impairment of lung function can provide important insights into the efficacy of treatment. Several long-term studies based on mortality tables have documented the marked improvement of survival in patients with CF witnessed over the past two decades.[34,35] Corey et al[36] examined the progression of pulmonary function impairment in 132 patients followed over periods of 5–7 years, in terms of the rate of change of FEV, FEV_1, and $MEF_{25\%-75\%}$.

Of the three variables, $MEF_{25\%-75\%}$ showed the greatest decline with time. Steeper rates of decline were seen in patients with more normal function at the time of the initial observations and in females at all levels of impairment, reflecting the poorer survival rates documented for females. The general patterns of these data suggested an exponential decay of lung function for this particular population. Similar observations have been reported by others.[37,38] However, the rate of decline of lung function parameters varied considerably between studies. It is noteworthy that in all studies significant numbers of patients showed no degradation of function over the span of observation and in some patients function actually improved. The marked divergence in the progression of lung disease between individuals indicates that models developed from population data cannot accurately predict the outcome in individuals. Moreover, clinical observations clearly indicate that in a given individual lung disease progresses frequently at markedly varying rates during the course of the disease.

Some patients develop significant lung disease early in infancy with unrelenting progression to death. In others pulmonary function impairment may be slight for many years followed by rapid decline at an alarming rate. Others show progression to moderate impairment of lung function followed by long periods of relative stability (Table 13-1).

LUNG FUNCTION STUDIES IN CF

Over the past 30 years lung function studies have increasingly contributed to our understanding of the pathophysiology underlying the pulmonary disease of CF and have become an integral part of patient care. Concomitant with the markedly increased interest in pediatric pulmonary physiology

Table 13-1
Female CF Patient with Evidence of Moderate Degree of Airway Obstruction at Age 9 Years, as Indicated by Reduced $MEF_{25\%-75\%}$ of 66% of Predicted*

Year	Age	FEV, ml (%)	MVV, liters/min (%)	$MEF_{25\%-75\%}$ liters/sec (%)
1967	9	1650 (84)	65 (108)	1.4 (66)
1968	10	1890 (84)	68 (96)	1.8 (73)
1969	11	1710 (68)	61 (78)	1.7 (62)
1970	12	1930 (74)	74 (90)	1.9 (66)
1971	13	2350 (82)	80 (90)	2.1 (68)
1972	14	2620 (75)	115 (111)	2.6 (73)
1973	15	2870 (76)	118 (107)	2.8 (74)
1975	17	3220 (81)	134 (118)	2.5 (65)
1976	18	3180 (79)	121 (107)	2.2 (56)
1977	19	3082 (78)	131 (116)	3.0 (78)

*Note that there are no significant changes during the next 10 years.
FEV, forced expired volume; MVV, maximum voluntary ventilation; $MEF_{25\%-75\%}$, maximal expired airflow during the midportion of the forced vital capacity.

and disease in general, there has been a proliferation of published lung function studies in CF. Thus, the comprehensive bibliography of the medical CF literature between 1813 and 1972[39] lists no references to pulmonary function before 1950. There were eight citations between 1950 and 1960, 114 between 1960 and 1970, and 70 references for 1971–1972 alone. The utility of this large volume of data has been somewhat diminished by the lack of standard approaches to pulmonary function testing (procedures, quality control, interpretation, and nomenclature). Similarly, pulmonary function equipment has lacked standardization with respect to performance specifications, calibration, etc.

In recognition of these deficiencies, the Cystic Fibrosis Foundation sponsored a GAP conference on standardization of lung function testing in 1978 to address these problems.[40] The conference developed a set of standards and recommendations to delineate minimal requirements for clinical, research, and epidemiologic studies of lung function in children. These recommendations include acceptance of the nomenclature proposed by the report of the ACCP-ATS Joint Committee on pulmonary nomenclature and embraced the recommendation of the Snowbird workshop on standardization of spirometry,[40] modified to address the special requirements of testing in children and expanded to include consideration of blood gas analysis, lung function tests other than spirometry, and exercise evaluation.

In the clinical care of patients with CF, lung function studies are important in the initial assessment of functional impairment, evaluation of short-term changes, exacerbation of infection, response to therapy, and determination of long-term trends.

In infants and small children who are unable to cooperate in the performance of pulmonary function studies, ie, those who cannot tolerate mouthpiece and nose clip and cannot perform breathing maneuvers on command, blood gas analysis (arterial, arterialized capillary, or transcutaneous) has remained the only method of assessing pulmonary function for routine clinical use. Although other lung function studies have shown feasibility in these age groups (body plethysmography, crying vital capacity, oscillatory resistance measurements), they have remained largely investigative tools because of technical difficulties, lack of standardization of methodology and equipment, and absence of standard reference data. However, routine pulmonary function studies, ie, spirometry, body plethysmography, maximal expiratory flow volume curves, can as a rule be obtained beginning with the sixth year of life. Occasionally, adequate cooperation can even be obtained in 4- and 5-year-old patients.

Methodology

Technically, the water-sealed 7- or 9-liter spirometer remains the simplest reliable instrument to use. Very little can go wrong; maintenance requires merely adjustment of the water level, replacement of CO_2 scrubber, and calibration of the recorder drum speed. The system permits measurement of minute ventilation, tidal volume, respiratory rate, and O_2 uptake. During FEV maneuvers, FEV, FEV_1, FEV_1/FEV, inspiratory capacity, expiratory reserve volume, and maximal mid-expiratory flow ($MEF_{25\%-75\%}$) can be reliably obtained. Maximum voluntary ventilation is readily measured. If a helium meter is included in the circuit, FRC by helium dilution can be readily determined, permitting computation of a residual volume and total lung capacity as well. However, all dilution techniques measure only the volume being ventilated. Therefore FRC so measured tends to be underestimated if there is a significant degree of air trapping, common in cystic fibrosis. As a result, successful treatment of airway obstruction due to purulent secretions and mucous plugs may result in a paradoxical apparent increase of the helium dilution FRC, when in fact the actual FRC has decreased or remained unchanged.

Since the $MEF_{25\%-75\%}$ is a relatively sensitive indicator of small-airway obstruction, the water-sealed spirometer provides sufficient quantitative information to follow lung function changes in the course of cystic fibrosis on a routine clinical basis. Owing to the simplicity of this device, data obtained with water-sealed spirometers in different laboratories are in all probability more readily comparable than data obtained with devices which are less standardized and where uniform quality control is therefore more difficult to achieve.

A case in point is the many commercially available devices to obtain maximal expiratory flow volume (MEFV) curves in order to examine instantaneous airflow at the mouth as a function of lung volume. This approach requires accurate measurement of instantaneous airflow for flows up to 12 liters/sec. The transducer must have adequate frequency response and linear output over the range of interest. Problems arise from the requirement to calibrate the flow transducer dynamically and to provide a faithful graphic representation of the flow volume data. The latter requirement must be met for two reasons: (1) flow volume curves provide important shape information; and (2) without graphic representation, numerical results may be misinterpreted. This is particularly true in children who frequently are unable to exhale to residual volume. If unrecognized, FEV will be underestimated and $\dot{V}_{max50\%}$, $\dot{V}_{max75\%}$, and mean $MEF_{25\%-75\%}$ will be overestimated.

In our laboratory we have implemented a computerized method which is part of a system designed for breath-by-breath analysis of ventilation pulmonary gas exchange.[41,42] Instantaneous flow and volume signals are obtained from a waterless spirometer (HiFi Spirometer, Med. Science, St. Louis, Missouri). After conditioning, the signals are digitized at a sampling rate of 50 samples/sec in the burst mode and stored on disk. The analysis program computes FEV, FEV_1, FEV_1/FEV, peak expiratory flow (PEF), $\dot{V}_{max50\%}$, $\dot{V}_{max75\%}$, and $MEF_{25\%-75\%}$. Numerical output is printed in terms of measured values, predicted values, and percent of predicted. The stored flow–volume curve is plotted by drum plotter with automatic scale adjustment for flow (y axis) and volume (x axis) and identification of PEF, $\dot{V}_{max50\%}$, and $\dot{V}_{max75\%}$ on the curves.

The use of a displacement spirometer to obtain flow signals has the advantage over pneumotachographs that flow measurements are independent of gas composition, a feature which is important when flow volume curves are obtained both during air and He/O_2 breathing. The system is calibrated by injection of a 4-liter air volume into the spirometer and acceptable when the direct measured volume (volume–transducer output) and the volume computed by integration of the instantaneous flow signal agree within 1% of the actually introduced volume. Another algorithm facilitates verification of the calibration at different volumes and flow rates.

The reproducibility of the MEFV parameters measured with this system was initially evaluated in terms of the mean ± 1 SD and the coefficients of variation of 25 consecutive MEFV curves obtained in three motivated, trained subjects over a 2-hour period (Table 13-2). In keeping with other studies, effort-dependent parameters such as FEV, FEV_1, and PEF have smaller coefficients of variation than $MEF_{25\%-75\%}$, $\dot{V}_{max50\%}$, and $\dot{V}_{max75\%}$, which are largely effort-independent. Moreover, the coefficient of variation tends to increase as flow decreases with measurements at smaller lung volumes, and in each case $\dot{V}_{max75\%}$ had the largest coefficient of variation.

There are several explanations for this behavior: (1) The flow transducer has the same absolute accuracy over the range of flow rates. As a result the measurement error becomes proportionally larger as absolute flow rates decrease. This finding can be substantiated by examining MEFV curves generated repetitively with a constant flow and volume source such as a volume controlled respirator. (2) The flow generated at the mouth becomes more "noisy" as large efforts are made to expel gas at low lung volumes and airway closure occurs. This is readily apparent from inspection of MEFV curves, particularly in patients with airways disease. The same phenomenon also explains the consistently smaller coefficients of variation for $MEF_{25\%-75\%}$ as compared to the $\dot{V}_{max50\%}$. The $MEF_{25\%-75\%}$ is obtained by measuring the volume change per unit time over the midhalf of the FEV, a process which filters random noise, whereas $\dot{V}_{max50\%}$ represents instantaneous flow at 50% of FEV. (3) The larger variability of flow at low lung volumes can also be related to measurements at different lung volumes in repetitive efforts. Considering the small coefficients of variation for FEV, the explanation can largely be discounted for the data shown in Table 13-2. However, this factor may be a significant source of variation in patient studies and, for purposes of comparison, flow rates should therefore be measured at the same lung volume. Such measurements can only be obtained in a body plethysmograph.

In order to evaluate the MEFV system in patients, we utilized as a measure of reproducibility the difference between the best (in

Table 13-2
Reproducibility of MEFV Curve Parameters in 3 Healthy Subjects*

	I		II		III	
	Mean ± 1 SD	*Coeff. var.%*	*Mean ± 1 SD*	*Coeff. var.%*	*Mean ± 1 SD*	*Coeff. var.%*
FEV, ml BTPs	6158 ± 132	2.1	4201 ± 98	2.3	2556 ± 84	3.3
FEV_1, ml BTPS	4898 ± 115	2.4	3211 ± 67	2.1	2313 ± 49	2.1
PEF, liters/sec	10.35 ± 0.32	3.1	6.45 ± 0.55	8.5	6.00 ± 0.26	4.3
MMEF, liters/sec	4.17 ± 0.24	5.8	2.65 ± 0.10	4.0	2.88 ± 0.20	6.8
$\dot{V}max_{50\%}$, liters/sec	5.22 ± 0.44	8.5	3.10 ± 0.18	5.7	3.82 ± 0.40	10.7
$\dot{V}max_{75\%}$, liters/sec	2.80 ± 0.31	11.1	1.41 ± 0.16	11.7	1.67 ± 0.30	18.1
N	25		25			

*25 consecutive determinations within 2 hours. I, male, 28 years, nonsmoker; II, female, 28 years, smoker; III female, 11 years, nonsmoker. Coefficient of variation % = (SD/mean) × 100.

terms of FEV) and the second best of three MEFV curves usually obtained during each patient evaluation within 5–10 minutes. Data obtained in 157 patients are shown in Tables 13-3 and 13-4. The patients were divided into four groups, ie, 20 normals and 40 patients with tetralogy of Fallot after intracardiac repair. None of these patients had evidence of airways disease. The other two groups were 50 asthmatics and 47 CF patients. Table 13-3 indicates age and height as well as the mean values of each MEFV parameter (± 1 SD), absolute and in percent of predicted to provide a measure of the range of observed values.

Tables 13-4 and 13-5 indicate the absolute values as well as the absolute and percent differences between the best and second-best effort of each MEFV parameter computed by paired comparison and expressed as mean difference ± 1 SD of the mean. In the normals none of the mean differences (absolute or percent) were statistically significant. With respect to FEV and FEV_1, the absolute differences of normals and tetralogy patients are smaller than in the patients with airways disease (asthma, CF). The absolute differences of the flow parameters are similar in all groups, but the percent changes are smaller in the patients without airways disease.

Table 13-3
Test Cohort, 157 Patients, 328 MEFV Curves Obtained in Duplicate

	Asthma	Cystic Fibrosis	Tetralogy of Fallot	Normal
No. patients	50	47	40	20
No. MEFVC (duplicate)	221	47	40	20
Age, years				
(mean ± 1 SD)	11.6 ± 2.6	13.3 ± 3.3	14.5 ± 3.9	15.6 ± 0.8
Height, cm				
(mean ± 1 SD)	114.5 ± 13.6	114.2 ± 15.6	156.1 ± 17.7	162.8 ± 8.2
Height, cm				
(range)	116 – 174	117 – 168	119 – 184	151 – 183

Table 13-4
Average ± 1 SD of MEFV Curve Parameters in Test Cohort, Breakdown by Diagnosis, Best MEFV Curves

	Asthma	Cystic Fibrosis	Tetralogy of Fallot	Normal
FEV	2378 ± 803	1686 ± 715	2705 ± 1043	3704 ± 547
FEV_1	1927 ± 626	1351 ± 593	2393 ± 890	3385 ± 492
PEF	3.89 ± 1.41	2.88 ± 1.23	5.12 ± 2.04	6.41 ± 1.15
MMEF	1.86 ± 0.72	1.29 ± 0.70	2.80 ± 1.34	4.06 ± 0.77
$\dot{V}max_{50\%}$	2.23 ± 0.97	1.59 ± 0.88	3.38 ± 1.70	4.70 ± 0.84
$\dot{V}max_{75\%}$	1.06 ± 0.44	0.70 ± 0.41	1.73 ± 0.92	2.56 ± 0.80
FEV%	87.7 ± 18.2	62.9 ± 19.1	76.8 ± 12.5	97.2 ± 12.0
FEV_1%	96.1 ± 23.6	69.8 ± 26.4	92.2 ± 15.3	131.7 ± 15.6
PEF%	70.5 ± 19.3	54.0 ± 20.0	77.2 ± 17.8	91.8 ± 15.0
MMEF%	66.9 ± 24.7	48.8 ± 25.8	80.1 ± 25.0	107.9 ± 17.8
$\dot{V}max_{50\%}$	70.1 ± 24.5	52.5 ± 28.6	84.8 ± 28.7	118.6 ± 19.7
$\dot{V}max_{75\%}$	61.9 ± 27.8	42.0 ± 23.2	81.1 ± 31.3	116.1 ± 30.4
No. patients	50	47	40	20

Table 13-5
Reproducibility of MEFV Curves*

	Asthma	Cystic Fibrosis	Tetralogy of Fallot	Normals
Δ absolute				
FEV, ml	133.8 ± 172†	93.5 ± 104†	41.9 ± 75†	49.8 ± 133
FEV_1, ml	83.6 ± 152†	68.3 ± 82†	44.9 ± 77†	42.6 ± 128
PEF, liters/sec	0.27 ± 0.47†	0.14 ± 0.37	0.16 ± 0.56	0.18 ± 0.59
MMEF, liters/sec	0.08 ± 0.25§	0.05 ± 0.18	0.01 ± 0.25	0.04 ± 0.30
$\dot{V}max_{50\%}$ liters/sec	0.11 ± 0.35§	−0.002 ± 0.30	−0.02 ± 0.58	−0.02 ± 0.45
$\dot{V}max_{75\%}$ liters/sec	0.03 ± 0.22	0.002 ± 0.02	−0.05 ± 0.29	−0.13 ± 0.43
N, patients	50	47	40	20
Δ Percent				
FEV	7.1 ± 10.3†	6.2 ± 6.2†	2.2 ± 3.8†	1.6 ± 4.2
FEV_1	6.6 ± 12.8†	6.1 ± 6.6†	2.3 ± 4.1†	1.8 ± 4.4
PEF	11.4 ± 19.1†	5.2 ± 13.6‡	4.1 ± 11.6§	3.5 ± 10.5
MMEF	7.3 ± 10.3‡	5.1 ± 16.5§	1.1 ± 10.0	−0.5 ± 7.0
$\dot{V}max_{50\%}$	7.8 ± 24.2§	3.8 ± 22.0	1.2 ± 15.7	0.1 ± 10.3
$\dot{V}max_{75\%}$	5.5 ± 26.5	6.9 ± 28.5	1.2 ± 17.0	−2.7 ± 13.8

*Difference between best and second best MEFV curve, absolute and in percent. Test cohort. Breakdown by diagnosis.
†P <0.001.
‡P <0.02.
§P <0.05.

The largest changes between best and second-best effort were seen in asthma patients. This is in part due to a change in airway resistance induced by the initial FEV maneuver itself.[43,44] An extreme example is shown in Table 13-6 for a patient in whom FEV maneuvers consistently induced significant bronchospasm such that all MEFV parameters were always largest when the FEV maneuver was first performed. The differences between first and second maneuver were highly significant for $MEF_{25\%-75\%}$, $\dot{V}_{max50\%}$, and $\dot{V}_{max75\%}$. The changes lasted for 20–30 minutes, if the patient was allowed to rest. Such behavior may also be seen in CF patients with superimposed asthma.

A consideration of the potential merit of pulmonary function studies in the clinical care of CF patients requires answers to two questions: (1) How sensitive are these tests as indicators of CF lung disease in relation to other clinical methods of evaluation, ie, primarily evaluation of symptoms, physical examination, and chest x-ray? (2) Which of the pulmonary function parameters are most useful to detect and quantitate the pulmonary involvement in CF and to follow its inevitable progression?

As to the first question; pulmonary function studies have the advantage of providing quantitative and reproducible (see above) numerical information rather than subjective or qualitative assessments. As a general rule they are more sensitive indicators of abnormality than clinical parameters of evaluation, the less pulmonary involvement has progressed. Patients with minimal or mild pulmonary disease frequently are asymptomatic, have scant physical findings, and normal or near-normal chest x-rays and yet will demonstrate significantly abnormal parameters of pulmonary mechanics and gas

Table 13-6
MEFV Curve Parameters in Male Asthmatic, Age 13, Determined on 8 Different Days over 2-Week Period*

		Absolute	Coeff. var. %	% Predicted	Δ%(absolute)	P
FEV, ml	1	2447 ± 129	5.3	71.1 ± 3.9	5.7 ± 15.9	NS
	2	2357 ± 324	13.8	68.4 ± 9.3		
FEV_1	1	2196 ± 76	3.5	85.3 ± 2.9	13.1 ± 13.5	.05
	2	1965 ± 239	12.2	76.0 ± 9.3		
PEF	1	4.98 ± 0.35	7.3	75.8 ± 5.2	8.5 ± 18.5	NS
	2	4.68 ± 0.63	13.5	71.1 ± 9.5		
MMEF	1	2.22 ± 0.21	9.5	63.0 ± 5.9	23.4 ± 20.5	.02
	2	1.82 ± 0.24	13.2	52.0 ± 6.7		
$\dot{V}max_{50\%}$	1	2.59 ± 0.24	9.3	65.0 ± 6.0	23.1 ± 13.2	.01
	2	2.12 ± 0.25	11.8	53.1 ± 6.3		
$\dot{V}max_{75\%}$	1	1.37 ± 0.18	13.1	63.9 ± 8.1	47.5 ± 4.26	.02
	2	0.97 ± 0.22	22.7	45.4 ± 10.2		

*Results indicate for each parameter mean ± 1 SD absolute and in percent predicted of first (1) and second (2) MEFV curve; Δ% mean ± 1 SD of absolute differences in % between (1) and (2). Coefficient variation (SD/mean) × 100, %.

exchange. Similarly, with moderately severe pulmonary involvement, lung function studies are frequently more sensitive indicators of change than clinical symptoms or findings. But as lung destruction nears its end, measures of lung function, with the exception of arterial P_{O_2} and P_{CO_2}, change little with further progression of disease, and careful physical examination of the chest may be a more useful indicator of pulmonary status.

The answer to the second question is implicit in the nature of the pulmonary lesion of CF which begins with small-airway obstruction. As we have seen, these changes may be so minimal in a few patients as to defy detection by currently available measurements of pulmonary mechanics. However, in the large majority of patients these changes are readily detectable by the time they are old enough to cooperate with pulmonary function studies. This is shown in Table 13-7 which represents data of 30 male patients with CF who were studied serially by spirometry which included FRC determination by helium dilution. The parameters, which are arranged in order of decreasing abnormality and expressed as percent of predicted for height, are shown for the first and last study obtained in this group. Column C indicates the average deviation from normal, ie, from 100% of predicted at the time of the first study, and column D the average rate of change between first and last study.

By these criteria the residual volume is the most sensitive indicator of listed parameters even though RV tended to be underestimated since FRC was determined by helium dilution. Note, however, that the $MEF_{25\%-75\%}$ is by far the most sensitive measure of abnormality that can be obtained during a forced expiration and showed almost twice the rate of change in this sample than FEV or FEV_1. The greater sensitivity of $MEF_{25\%-75\%}$ than FEV can also be demonstrated by comparing the incidence of abnormality (Table 13-8) of these two parameters shown for three sets of flow–volume curve parameters obtained in 69 CF patients.

Predictably the $\dot{V}_{max75\%}$ is the most sensitive indicator of abnormality, followed by $MEF_{25\%-75\%}$, $\dot{V}_{max50\%}$, PEF, FEV, and FEV_1. Note that the ratio FEV_1/FEV is the least sensitive of all parameters. The sensitivity of maximal expiratory airflow measurements can be enhanced by referencing the flow rates to TLC rather than FEV or by determining the isoflow–volume (as percent of TLC) where air and He/O_2 flow–volume curves have identical flow rates. However, this improvement of sensitivity is of little clinical importance, particularly as both methods require body plethysmography.

Considering the simplicity of the method, the sensitivity of the parameters, and the reproducibility of the results, it is apparent from the foregoing discussion and consistent with other data that the $MEF_{25\%-75\%}$ and FEV obtained with a water-sealed spirometer are the most useful and probably also most cost-effective parameters of lung function to follow the clinical progression of lung disease in most patients with CF. Certainly for routine clinical follow-up, volume displacement spirometry must be considered superior to flow-measuring devices unless they can be appropriately calibrated and a visual display or record of the MEFV curves is provided.

Routine Application of Lung Function Studies in Patients with CF

In the CF clinic we begin to obtain lung function studies at age 5–6 years. Once the patient has learned to perform forced expiratory maneuvers adequately, baseline

Table 13-7
First and Last Study of 30 Male CF Patients*

	A	B	C	D
RV	183.1 ± 72.7	202.3 ± 66.9	+83.1	+19.2
$MEF_{25\%-75\%}$	46.2 ± 38.4	32.9 ± 28.6	−53.9	−13.3
FEV_1	64.5 ± 30.4	56.7 ± 33.3	−35.5	− 7.9
FEV	68.0 ± 27.6	60.3 ± 27.2	−32.0	− 7.7
MVV	68.8 ± 24.8	61.3 ± 24.1	−31.2	− 7.5
FRC†	121.4 ± 28.2	125.4 ± 28.5	+21.4	+ 4.0
TLC	100.0 ± 15.4	94.7 ± 14.5	+0	− 5.3
N	30	30		
Age, years	10.2 ± 8.95	12.76 ± 3.4		
Height, cm	132.1 ± 14.6	144.0 ± 17.9		

*A: mean ± 1 SD of % of predicted, first study; B: mean ± 1 SD of % of predicted, last study; C: average deviation from 100% of predicted in percent of predicted at the time of the first study; D: average change between first and last study in percent of predicted.
†Determined by He dilution technique.

Table 13-8
Incidence of Grossly Abnormal, Moderately Abnormal, and Normal FEV and $MEF_{25\%-75\%}$ in 69 CF Patients

	Incidence (%)		
	A. first study	*B. last study*	Δ%*
FEV			
≤ 50%	13/69 (18.8)	25/69 (36.2)	+17.4
51–80%	31/69 (44.9)	24/69 (34.8)	−10.1
> 80%	25/69 (36.2)	20/69 (29.0)	−7.2
$MEF_{25\%-75\%}$			
≤ 40%	39/69 (56.5)	53/69 (76.8)	+20.3
41–80%	21/60 (30.4)	10/69 (14.5)	−15.9
> 80%	9/69 (13.0)	6/69 (8.7)	−4.3

*Δ% change represents percent in incidence between first and last study.

pulmonary function studies are obtained. Subsequently, MEFV curves are performed prior to each clinic vist. More complete pulmonary function studies are obtained at irregular intevals, most commonly at the end of a hospital stay for intravenous antibiotic therapy.

The more complete studies include spirometry, which serves primarily as a quality check, body plethysmographic studies, as well as MEFV curves and breath-by-breath ventilation during air and O_2 breathing. Spirometry includes ventilation, forced and slow maximal expirations, and maximum voluntary ventilation. Body plethysmography includes determination of thoracic gas volume, airway resistance, R_{aw}, and MEFV curves. MEFV curves obtained with the computerized system are done during air and He/O_2 breathing. Ventilation and pulmonary gas exchange is obtained during 3 minutes of air breathing followed by 3–7 minutes of N_2 washout during 100% O_2 breathing to determine FRC and anatomic dead space (Bohr equation) on a breath-by-breath basis.

The ventilation studies yield respiratory rate and period, inspiratory and expiratory timing events (T_I, T_E, T_I/T_{TOT}, and inspiratory and expiratory pause times), gas volumes (V_I, V_E, $\dot{V}_I$, $\dot{V}_E$), mean and peak flow rates (inspiratory and expiratory), gas uptakes and rates of uptake (O_2, CO_2, N_2), fractional concentrations, gas pressures (inspiratory, mean expiratory, end-tidal), and change in FRC based on analysis of N_2 exchange. Apart from the breath-by-breath variables, summary data at variable intervals (15–120 seconds) are generated for all above variables, and in addition for $V_{D\,anat}$, V_D/V_T, $\dot{V}_E/\dot{V}_{O2}$, $\dot{V}_A$, $\dot{V}_D$, $\dot{V}_{O2}$/kg, and $\dot{V}_{O2}/ht^2$.

Bronchodilator response to isoproterenol aerosol is tested if the patient has a history of wheezing, is a known asthmatic, or has bronchopulmonary aspergillosis. These studies include TGV, FRC by N_2 washout, R_{aw}, MEFV curves during air and He/O_2 breathing, and ventilation. If there is a question of post-exercise bronchoconstriction, the patient is exercised on a treadmill for 6 minutes at near maximal heart rates (> 170/min). Immediately following exercise, MEFV curves are obtained and repeated every 7 minutes during the next 35 minutes.

The technical aspects of arterial blood gas (ABG) studies have been discussed in detail.[40] In our institution ABG studies are usually done only in patients who have been admitted to the hospital. ABG studies are indicated in all patients who are noticeably cyanotic, particularly if O_2 is to be given. In such cases ABGs should be done before administration to obtain baseline data on hypoxemia and CO_2 retention. ABG studies should be repeated during O_2 therapy to determine the improvement of arterial oxygenation and the extent of CO_2 retention induced by O_2. If short-term (hours) serial studies are required, it is preferable to utilize either external monitoring by transcutaneous sensors or to install an arterial line, in order to obtain more reliable data in the undisturbed state and to avoid repeated punctures.

GLOSSARY

C	compliance, Δ volume/Δ pressure, ml/cm H_2O
D	diffusing capacity, ml/min/torr
P	pressure, torr or cm H_2O
$\dot{Q}$	blood flow/unit time, liters/min
R	resistance, pressure/flow, cm H_2O/liters/sec
T	time, min, sec, or msec
V	volume, liters or ml
$\dot{V}$	gas flow, volume/unit time, liters/sec

Subscripts

A	alveolar
a	arterial
aw	airway

dyn	dynamic
D	dead space
D anat	anatomic dead space
E	expiration
et	end-tidal
I	inspiratory
L	lung
max	maximal
st l	static recoil of the lungs
T	tidal
tm	transmural
TOT	total time, breath period, msec or sec

Lung volumes and capacities

FEV	forced expired volume = forced vital capacity, ml or liters BTPS
FEV_1	1-sec forced expired volume, ml BTPS
FRC	functional residual capacity, ml or liters BTPS
MVV	maximum voluntary ventilation
RV	residual volume, ml or liters BTPS
TGV	thoracic gas volume, ml or liters BTPS
TLC	total lung capacity, ml or liters BTPS

Airflow

$MEF_{25\%-75\%}$	average maximum expiratory flow during mid-50% of VC, liters/sec
PEF	peak expiratory flow, liters/sec
$\dot{V}max_{50\%}$	maximal expiratory airflow after expiration of 50% of VC, liters/sec
$\dot{V}max_{75\%}$	maximal expiratory airflow after expiration of 75% of VC, liters/sec
MEFV curve	maximum expiratory flow volume curve
EPP	equal pressure points where pressure surrounding the airways is equal to lateral intraairway pressure

REFERENCES

1. Andersen DH: Cystic fibrosis of the pancreas and its relation to celiac disease. *Am J Dis Child* 1938;56:344–399.
2. West JR, Levin SM, di Sant'Agnese PA: Pulmonary function in cystic fibrosis of the pancreas. *Pediatrics* 1954;13:155–164.
3. Harrison GM, Vallbona C, Murray J: Quantitative studies of intrapulmonary gas mixing and distribution in children with cystic fibrosis. *Am J Dis Child* 1960;100:530–531.
4. DeMuth GR, Howatt WF, Talner NS: Intrapulmonary gas distribution in cystic fibrosis. *Am J Dis Child* 1962;103:51–57.
5. Goldring RM, Fishman AP, Turino GM, et al: Pulmonary hypertension and cor pulmonale in cystic fibrosis of the pancreas. *J Pediatr* 1964;65:501–524.
6. Lamarre A, Reilly BJ, Bryan AC, et al: Early detection of pulmonary function abnormalities in cystic fibrosis. *Pediatrics* 1972;50: 291–298.
7. Battistini A, Waring WW: Arterial-alveolar carbon dioxide difference in cystic fibrosis. *Fracastoro* 1970;63:642 648.
8. Krauss AN, Soodalter JA, Auld PAM: Adjustment of ventilation and perfusion in the full term normal and distressed neonate as determined by urinary alveolar nitrogen gradients. *Pediatrics* 1971;47:865–869.
9. Corbet A, Ross J, Popkin J, et al: Relationship of arterial–alveolar nitrogen tension to alveolar–arterial oxygen tension, lung volume, flow measurements and diffusing capacity in cystic fibrosis. *Am Rev Respir Dis* 1975;112:513–519.
10. Weng TR, Levison H: Standards of pulmonary function in children. *Am Rev Respir Dis* 1969;99:879–894.
11. Kamel M, Weng TR, Featherby EA, et al: Relation of mechanics of ventilation to lung volumes in children. *Scand J Respir Dis* 1969;50:125–134.
12. Landau LI, Phelan PD: The spectrum of cystic fibrosis. *Am Rev Respir Dis* 1973;108: 593–602.

13. Macklem PT: Airway obstruction and collateral ventilation. *Physiol Rev* 1971;51: 368–436.
14. Otis AB, McKerrow EM, Bartlett RA, et al: Mechanical factors in the distribution of pulmonary ventilation. *J Appl Physiol* 1956;8: 427–443.
15. Mead J, Turner, JM, Macklem PT, et al: Significance of the relationship between lung recoil and maximum expiratory flow. *J Appl Physiol* 1967;22:95–108.
16. Wentworth P, Gough J, Wentworth JE: Pulmonary changes and cor pulmonale in mucoviscidosis. *Thorax* 1968;23:582–589.
17. Mansell A, Dubawsky C, Levison H, et al: Lung elastic recoil in cystic fibrosis. *Am Rev Respir Dis* 1974;109:190–197.
18. Strong LB: Measurements of pulmonary diffusing capacity in children. *Arch Dis Child* 1960;35:232–235.
19. Coork CD: Research on Cystic Fibrosis. In McIntosh R (ed): *Transactions of the Second International Conference on Cystic Fibrosis.* Baltimore, MD, French-Bray Printing Co, 1960, p 121.
20. Beier FR, Renzelti AD Jr, Mitchell M, et al: Pulmonary pathophysiology in cystic fibrosis. *Am Rev Respir Dis* 1966;94:430–440.
21. Zelkowitz PS, Giammona ST: Effects of gravity and exercise on the pulmonary diffusing capacity in children with cystic fibrosis. *J Pediatr* 1969;74:393–398.
22. Wessel HU, Kezdi P, Cugell DW: Respiratory and cardiovascular function in patients with severe pulmonary hypertension. *Circulation* 1964;29:825–832.
23. Featherby EA, Weng TR, Crozier DN, et al : Dynamic and static lung volumes, blood gas tensions and diffusing capacity in patients with cystic fibrosis. *Am Rev Respir Dis* 1970;102:737–749.
24. Hazinski TA, Hansen TN, Simon JH, et al: Effect of oxygen administration during sleep on skin surface oxygen and carbon dioxide tensions in patients with chronic lung disease. *Pediatrics* 1981;67:626–630.
25. Francis PWJ, Muller NL, Gurwitz D, et al: Hemoglobin desaturation: Its occurrence during sleep in patients with cystic fibrosis. *Am J Dis Child* 1980;134:734–740.
26. Doershuk CF: Observations of pulmonary function testing and blood gas analysis in children. *Bull NY Acad Med* 1972;48: 684–688.
27. Siassi B, Moss AJ, Dooley RR: Clinical recognition of cor pulmonale in cystic fibrosis. *J Pediatr* 1971;78:794–805.
28. Wagener JS, Taussig LM, Burrows B, et al: Comparison of lung function and survival patterns between cystic fibrosis and emphysema or chronic bronchitis patients. *Cystic Fibrosis Club Abstr* 1980;21:15.
29. Godfrey S, Mearns MB: Pulmonary function and response to exercise in cystic fibrosis. *Arch Dis Child* 1971;46:144–151.
30. Mellis CM, Crozier DN, Levison H: Heightened bronchial reactivity in cystic fibrosis. *Cystic Fibrosis Club Abstr* 1977;18:19.
31. Landau LI, Phelan PD: The variable effect of a bronchodilating agent on pulmonary function in cystic fibrosis. *J Pediatr* 1973;82:863–868.
32. Taussig LM, Landau LI: Cystic fibrosis seminars. *Respir Med* 1979;1:167–182.
33. Haluszka J, Scislicki A: Bronchial lability in children suffering from some diseases of the bronchi. *Respiration* 1975;32:217–226.
34. Warwick WJ, Pogue RE: Computer studies in cystic fibrosis, in Lawson D (ed): *Proceedings of the 5th International Cystic Fibrosis Conference.* London, Stuart House, 1969, p 320.
35. Huang NN, Macri CN, Girone J, et al: Survival of patients with cystic fibrosis. *Am J Dis Child* 1970;120:289–295.
36. Corey M, Levison H, Crozier D: Five-to-seven year course of pulmonary function in cystic fibrosis. *Am Rev Respir Dis* 1976; 114:1085–1092.
37. Menendez R, Mather F, Waring WW: Longitudinal patterns of obstructive lung disease in cystic fibrosis (CF). *Cystic Fibrosis Club Abstr* 1979;20:6.
38. Wagener JS, Taussig LM, Burrows B, et al: Comparison of lung function and survival patterns between cystic fibrosis and emphysema or chronic bronchitis. In *Proceedings Eighth International Cystic Fibrosis Congress,* Toronto, Canadian Cystic Fibrosis Foundation, 1980, pp 236–245.
39. Holsclaw DS Jr, Topham AL, (eds): *Cystic Fibrosis. A Comprehensive Bibliography of the Medical Literature 1813–1972.* Cystic Fibrosis Foundation, Atlanta, Georgia, 1977.
40. Taussig LM, Cherwick V, Wood R, et al: Standardization of lung function testing in children. Proceedings and Recommendations of the GAP Conference Committee. Cystic Fibrosis Foundation. *J Pediatr* 1980;97: 668–675.
41. Wessel HU, Stout RL, Paul MH: Minicomputer based system for breath-by-breath analysis of ventilation and pulmonary gas exchange. *Proceedings of the 5th Annual Conference on Computers in Cardiology,* IEEE Computer Society, Long Beach, California, 1979, pp 97–102.

42. Wessel HU, Stout RL, Bastanier CK, et al: Breath-by-breath variation of FRC: Effect on $\dot{V}O_2$ and $\dot{V}CO_2$ measured at the mouth. *J Appl Physiol* 1979;46:1122–1126.
43. Ferris BG Jr, Pollard DS: Effect of deep and quiet breathing on pulmonary compliance in man. *J Clin Invest* 1960;39:143–149.
44. Nadel JA, Tierney DF: Effect of a previous deep inspiration in man. *J Appl Physiol* 1961;16:717–719.
45. *Guide to Diagnosis and Management of Cystic Fibrosis.* Cystic Fibrosis Foundation, Suite 309, 6000 Executive Boulevard, Rockville, Maryland 20852, 1979.

14

Cor Pulmonale in Cystic Fibrosis

Thomas W. Riggs

Hans U. Wessel

Most patients with cystic fibrosis die ultimately with cor pulmonale.[1] Cor pulmonale, which is defined as right ventricular hypertrophy[2] is thought to develop secondary to pulmonary hypertension resulting from hypoxemia.[3,4] This hypoxemia has its genesis in ventilation–perfusion inequalities due to the focal and diffuse small-airways obstruction. Mild hypoxemia may occur on a chronic, intermittent basis, long before any right heart changes are apparent clinically. Studies of adults with chronic obstructive lung disease have shown that episodes of nocturnal arterial desaturation are associated with intermittent pulmonary hypertension on the basis of vasoconstriction.[5] Decreased nocturnal saturation has also been demonstrated in patients with cystic fibrosis.[6] Pathologic studies have established that medial thickening of the pulmonary arterioles and right ventricular hypertrophy exists in patients dying with cystic fibrosis.[3,4] Right ventricular hypertrophy and dilatation are an adaptation capable of maintaining normal function for a long period until clinical congestive heart failure appears. Therefore the clinical recognition of cor pulmonale represents a late event in the natural history of the patient's adaptation to a chronic, progressive hypoxemia that inexorably leads to pulmonary hypertension.[7]

The physical findings of cor pulmonale are often nonspecific because of the dominant pulmonary involvement of cystic fibrosis. When the disease is severe enough to cause clinical cor pulmonale, the cardiac signs may be completely masked by the pulmonary signs, making recognition of right ventricular involvement extremely difficult. Hyperinflation of the lungs leads to distant heart sounds, masking the accentuated pulmonic closure sound of pulmonary hypertension. Because of this masking effect and since pulmonary hypertension is frequently of a moderate degree, the distinct cardiac physical findings of severe pulmonary hypertension and right ventricular hypertrophy which are striking in the absence of pulmonary disease, are virtually never encountered in cystic fibrosis. Cyanosis and tachypnea are the hallmarks of severe pulmonary disease in advanced cystic fibrosis and neck vein distention is common. The diaphragms are flattened, suggesting hepatomegaly. However, when frank right heart failure supervenes, the liver may become tender and peripheral edema may make its appearance. Massive anasarca is rare, but occasionally edema of the eyelids may be the only manifestation of fluid retention. Sudden weight gain within days in patients with CF and severe pulmonary disease usually denotes right heart failure since weight gain due to increased muscle mass or subcutaneous fat is extremely unlikely in such patients.

ELECTROCARDIOGRAM AND CHEST ROENTGENOGRAMS

Standard electrocardiography and chest roentgenography often do not clearly indicate the onset and progression of changes in right ventricular status until considerable abnormalities exist. The increased residual volume and flattened diaphragms of cystic fibrosis result in a vertically oriented heart surrounded by tissue (overinflated lung) having a poor electrical conductivity as compared to blood or soft tissue. This results in a marked decrease in the voltage recorded by the surface ECG electrodes. Although the vectorcardiogram (VCG) is more sensitive than the standard electrocardiogram in detecting right ventricular hypertrophy (RVH) in patients with cystic fibrosis, clinical cor pulmonale can coexist with a normal ECG and VCG.[8,9] The chest roentgenogram may also be misleading. Cardiac dilatation may be masked by obstructive hyperinflation of the chest. Although serial evaluation may demonstrate a striking relative change, it is unusual for the cardiac shadow to appear enlarged, relative to the markedly hyperinflated lung fields.

ECHOCARDIOGRAPHIC EVALUATION

Echocardiography provides a more direct means of analysis of the right ventricular status than other noninvasive examinations. Both the internal dimension of the right ventricle (RVID) and the thickness of the right ventricular anterior wall (RVAW) can be measured and compared to normal values (Figure 14-1). In addition, the pulmonic valve echogram can be recorded simultaneously with the electrocardiogram, allowing measurement of the events of right ventricular systole or right ventricular systolic time intervals.[11] The right ventricular preejection period (RPEP) has been defined as the interval from the onset of right ventricular depolarization, as indicated by the Q wave of the ECG, to the opening of the pulmonic valve. The right ventricular ejection time (RVET) is the interval from opening to closure of the pulmonic valve (Figure 14-2). These intervals are each dependent upon the cardiac cycle length (heart rate), but their ratio, RPEP/RVET, is independent of heart rate; the RPEP/RVET ratio correlates well[12] with pulmonary artery diastolic pressure (Figure 14-3). Simply stated, increasing pulmonary artery diastolic pressure results in a lengthening of the time required by the right ventricle to open the pulmonic valve and a shortening of the time available for ventricular emptying. The use of the RPEP/RVET ratio accentuates these reciprocal changes. The normal range of RPEP/RVET is 0.20–0.30; a value greater than 0.35 almost always is associated with

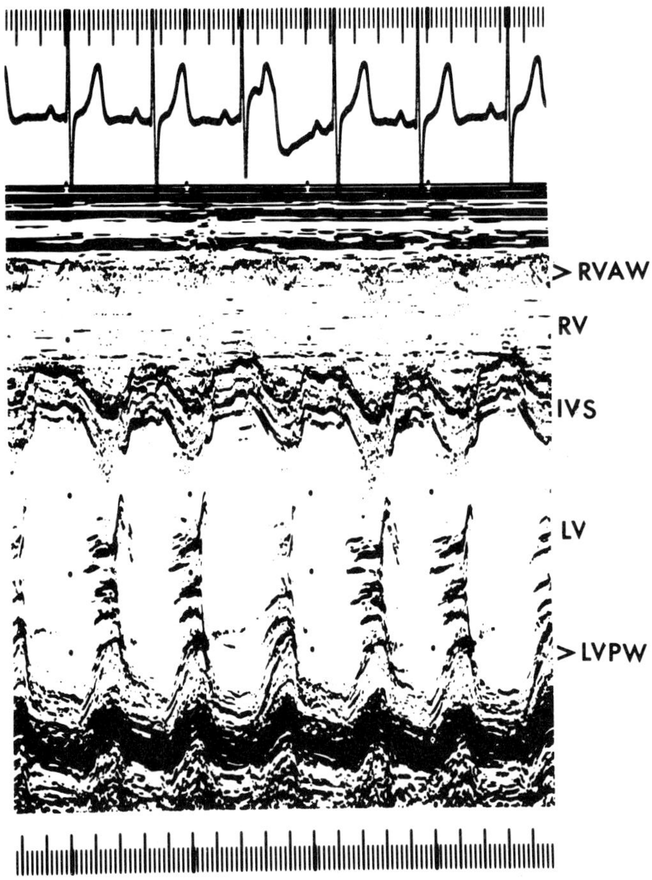

Figure 14-1 M-mode echocardiogram from a normal patient demonstrating the right and left ventricular internal dimensions and wall thickness measurements. IVS, interventricular septum; LV, left ventricle; LVPW, left ventricular posterior wall; RV, right ventricle; and RVAW, right ventricular anterior wall.

pulmonary hypertension. This ratio has also been used to assess pulmonary hypertension in normal neonates,[13] infants with persistent fetal circulation syndrome,[14] and patients with bronchopulmonary dysplasia.[15] Thus echocardiography can be used to assess the internal dimension and wall thickness of the right ventricle and to predict the presence of pulmonary hypertension from the pulmonic valve echocardiogram. Unfortunately, echocardiograms can be very difficult to obtain from children with cystic fibrosis. The hyperinflation and large residual lung volume limits the location (the so-called echo "window") on the chest wall from which the echocardiographic transducer is in acoustic continuity with the right ventricle and pulmonic valve. However, most patients can be examined and satisfactory images obtained.

Echocardiographic Studies in Cystic Fibrosis (Figure 14-4)

One of the first applications of echocardiography to cystic fibrosis was a study by Rosenthal et al,[16] in which the RVID was measured. The RVID was always enlarged in patients with severe (< 40) clinical score and infrequently in the excellent (> 85) score group. In the intermediate severity groups,

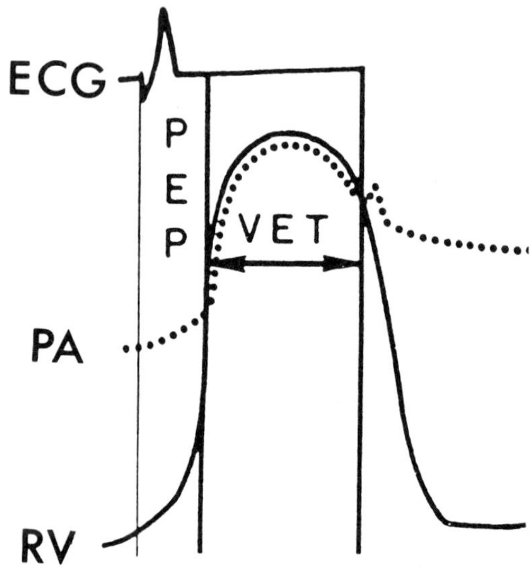

Figure 14-2 This drawing demonstrates the relationship between the right ventricular (RV) and pulmonary artery (PA) pressure and the simultaneous ECG. The period from the Q wave of the ECG to the opening of pulmonic valve is the preejection period (PEP), while the period from opening to closure of the pulmonic valve is the ventricular ejection time. (VET).

the RVID was usually (29/37) enlarged. There were significant correlations between RVID and clinical score ($r = -0.39$), vital capacity ($r = -0.33$), forced 1-second expiratory volume ($r = -0.35$), and residual volume ($r = +0.39$). However, these correlations were too low to allow accurate prediction of these parameters. Among 30 patients with RVH by ECG, 26/30 had an enlarged RVID. Conversely, among 30 patients with a normal ECG, 21/30 had a dilated RVID, thus a normal ECG was not a reliable indicator of whether the RVID was dilated or normal, while an abnormal ECG was usually associated with RV dilatation.

In a similar study by Gewitz et al,[17] 25 patients were examined. The RVID correlated well with the clinical score ($r = -0.73$), forced vital capacity ($r = -0.58$), and FEV_1 ($r = -0.61$). The RVAW also exhibited good correlation with clinical score ($r = -0.73$), FVC ($r = -0.58$), and FEV_1 ($r = -0.65$). Their patients also underwent ECG and VCG examinations. Only 10% of

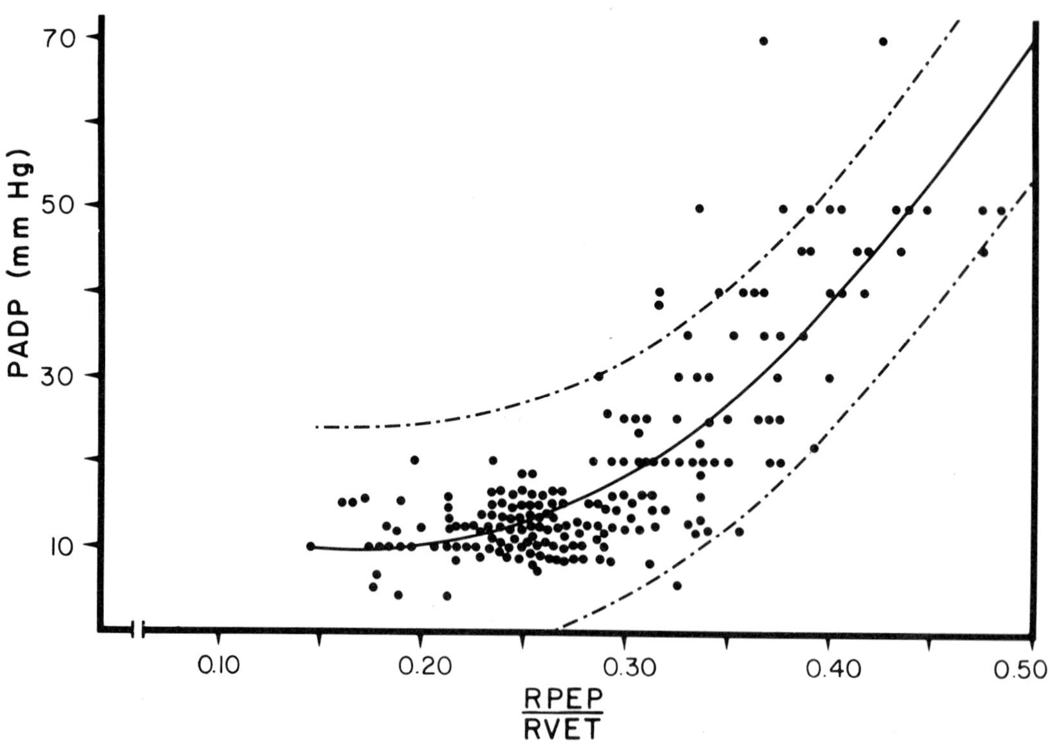

Figure 14-3 The relationship between the RPEP/RVET ratio and pulmonary artery diastolic pressure (PADP) in patients undergoing cardiac catheterization. The solid line describes a second-order polynominal regression equation, while the dashed lines encompass the 95% confidence limits.

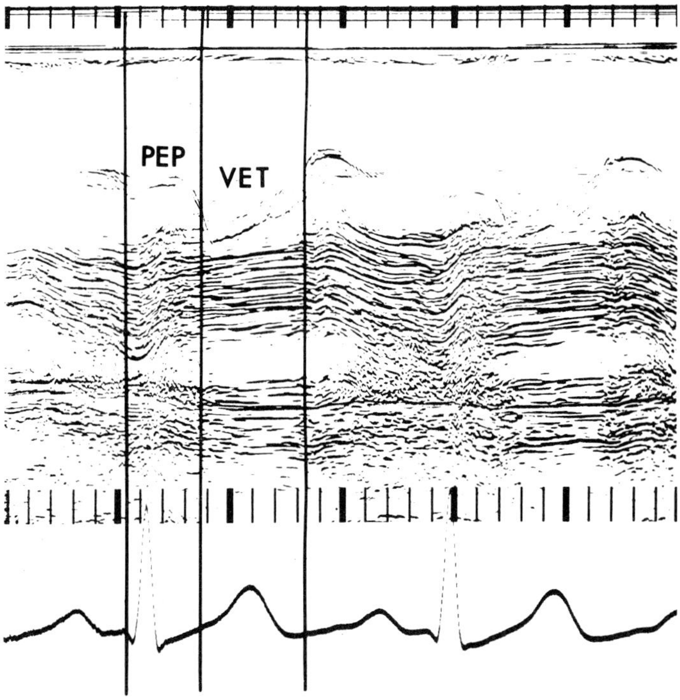

Figure 14-4 Pulmonic valve echocardiogram from a patient with clinical cor pulmonale and cystic fibrosis. The RPEP is prolonged and the RPEP/RVET is elevated (0.62), implying severe pulmonary artery hypertension. PEP, preejection period; and VET, ventricular ejection time.

their patients had RVH by ECG while 28% had RVH by VCG. An increased RVAW thickness was demonstrated in 52% of the patients with a normal ECG and in 43% of those with a normal VCG. Thus, the VCG was slightly more sensitive than the ECG in identifying RVH, but both were less sensitive than the echocardiogram.

Similar results were obtained by Ryssing[18] from an analysis of 31 patients. The RVID correlated with FVC ($r = -0.57$) and PEFR ($r = -0.62$). While 11 of their patients had an enlarged RVID, only four had an abnormal ECG. Included among their patients was one with clinical congestive heart failure (CHF) and a normal ECG.

Hirshfeld et al[19] used both simple and multiple regression analysis to correlate echocardiographic measurements with pulmonary function tests and clinical status. Among their 30 patients, 18 had clinical CHF and 9 died during the course of the study. The RVID correlated well with VC ($r = -0.51$), while the RVAW correlated well with RV ($r = 0.65$), VC ($r = -0.56$), and clinical score ($r = -0.56$). The RPEP/RVET was elevated to a mean value of 0.38 and showed excellent correlation with VC ($r = -0.73$), RV ($r = 0.72$), and clinical score ($r = 0.78$). Multiple correlation of RVAW, RVID, and RPEP/RVET allowed improved prediction of clinical score ($r = 0.84$), VC ($r = 0.80$), and RV ($r = 0.82$). The left ventricle was also examined in this study and found to be normal in size. Seven of 30 patients had evidence of LV dysfunction, however.

An echocardiographic profile of 34 patients with cystic fibrosis by Allen et al[20] demonstrated a dilated RVID and hypertrophied RVAW in most patients. The left ventricle appeared slightly smaller than normal, and there was LVH in some patients with advanced cor pulmonale.

Lester et al[21] proposed an echocardiographic scoring system for patients with cystic fibrosis. They evaluated 76 patients who were representative of the clinical spectrum of cystic fibrosis. Most of their patients (70%) had an increased RVAW and many (42%) had a dilated RVID. The RPEP/RVET was elevated in 9/34 patients. The frequency of abnormal findings progressively increased with decreasing clinical scores. The proposed scoring system assigns a perfect score of 25 points to a normal echocardiogram. An increasing number of points are accumulated corresponding to an increasing abnormality of each echo measurement, and the total number of demerit points accumulated in each section is subtracted from 25 to compute the echo score. This score correlated well with the Shwachman score (r = 0.88), the Brasfield roentgenogram score (r = 0.87), the Taussig-NIH score (r = 0.86), the FEV_1 (r = 0.76), the FRC (r = 0.77), and MMEF (r = 0.67).

RESPIRATORY VARIATION IN VENTRICULAR DIMENSIONS

Patients with cystic fibrosis exhibit characteristic respiration-related changes in right and left ventricular internal dimensions which may allow further insight as to right ventricular adaptation in cystic fibrosis (Figures 14-5, 14-6). During inspiration, there is augmented right ventricular filling

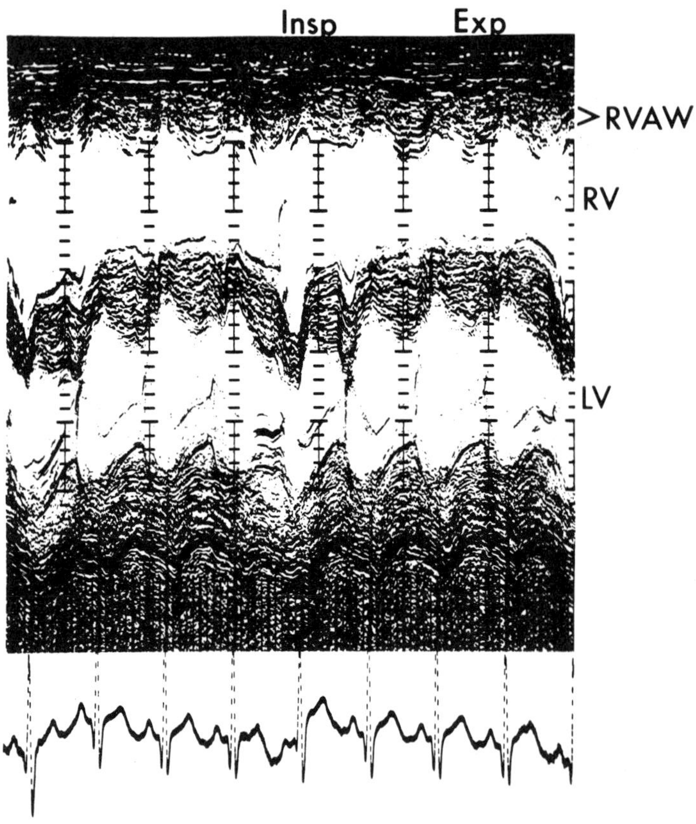

Figure 14-5 This M-mode echocardiogram, obtained from a child with moderately severe cor pulmonale and cystic fibrosis demonstrates increased thickness of the right ventricular anterior wall and phasic variation in ventricular dimensions with respiration. During inspiration, the right ventricle dilates and the left ventricle is compressed. Exp, expiration; Insp, inspiration; LV, left ventricle; RV, right ventricle; and RVAW, right ventricular anterior wall.

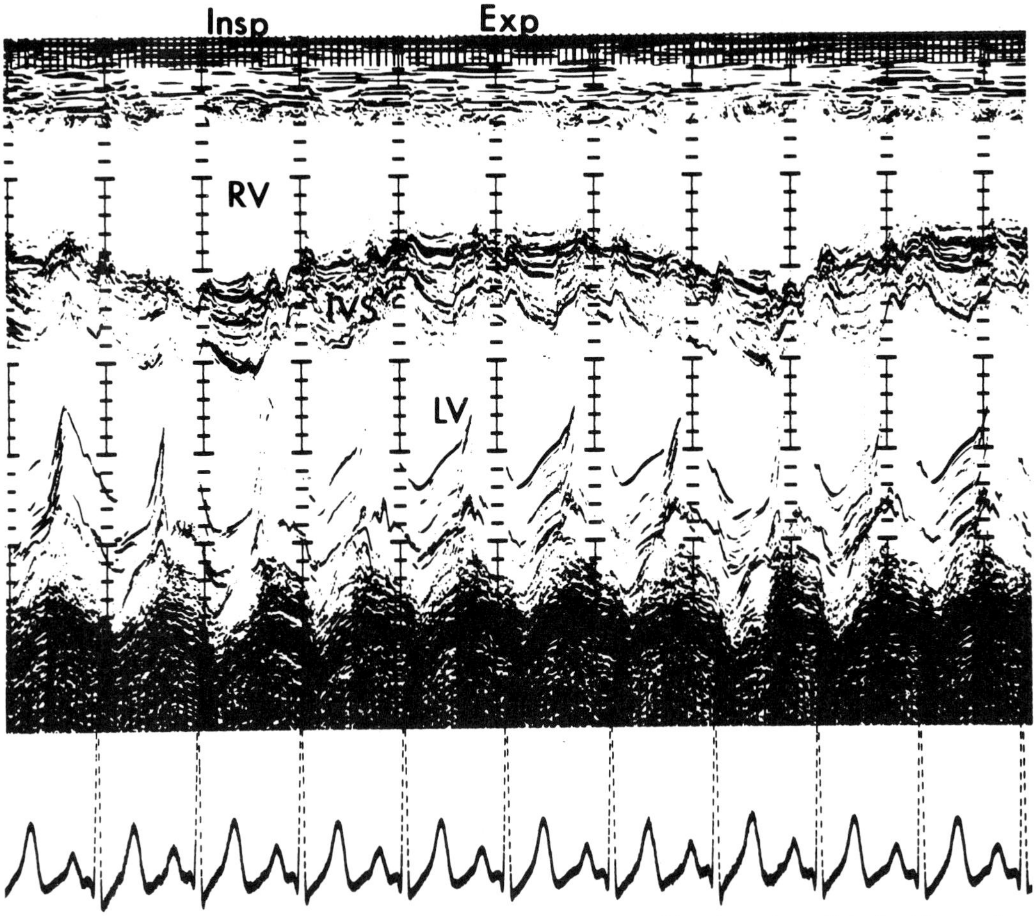

Figure 14-6 M-mode echocardiogram from a patient with cystic fibrosis and no clinical evidence of cor pulmonale. The ventricular septum exhibits respiratory variation in position, with right ventricular dilation and left ventricular compression during inspiration. Exp, expiration; Insp, inspiration; IVS, interventricular septum; LV, left ventricle; and RV, right ventricle.

and pulmonary venous pooling. This results in a slight increase in RVID and a trivial decrease in LVID during inspiration in normal patients.[22]

In cystic fibrosis, this cyclic variation in ventricular dimensions is exaggerated, presumably related to increased ventilatory effort.[23] These findings are identical to those described in adult patients with chronic obstructive pulmonary disease and pulsus paradoxus.[24] The increased right ventricular size that occurs in cystic fibrosis and is exaggerated during inspiration leads to flattening or compression of the left ventricle. This results in dyskinetic contraction which may contribute to diminished left ventricular stroke volume during inspiration.[25]

In patients with obstructive lung disease, the left ventricle is not only compressed during inspiration, but it is also subjected to an increased resistance to ejection. The transmural aortic pressure increases during the decrease in pleural pressure associated with inspiratory effort. The left ventricle's pressure is lowered during inspiration, while the pressure of the extrathoracic vascular beds is kept contant. Therefore, the left ventricle is facing an increased afterload during inspiration, since there is no difference as far as the left ventricle is concerned whether the pressure around the extrathoracic arterial bed is increased while the intrathoracic pressure is left constant or whether the extrathoracic vascular bed is left surrounded by a constant pressure and the pressure around the left ventricle is lowered.[26] The result is a decrease in left ventricular ejection time (LVET) and a decrease in aortic systolic blood pressure during inspiration.[24] This intermittent increase in left ventricular afterload and compression of LV size may explain the development of left ventricular dysfunction and fibrosis[27-29] observed in adults with chronic obstructive lung disease and occasional cystic fibrosis patients with advanced cor pulmonale.[19-21,30,31]

RADIONUCLIDE EVALUATION

Chipps et al[32] utilized radionuclide techniques to evaluate right and left ventricular ejection fractions (the latter were also evaluated during supine bicycle exercise) in 21 patients with cystic fibrosis. Most of their patients (72%) had decreased right ventricular ejection fractions. The left ventricular ejection fraction was abnormal at rest in four patients (total of 38%). During exercise, an additional three patients exhibited an abnormal left ventricular ejection fraction. Therefore, subclinical left ventricular failure was documented among some patients with cystic fibrosis who did not manifest clinical cor pulmonale. Similar results were found in adults with chronic pulmonary hypertension.[33]

These therapeutic failures are not surprising since severe pulmonary hypertension and right ventricular dysfunction does not occur until pulmonary disease is severe and associated with respiratory insufficiency.[9] However, since the underlying mechanism of cor pulmonale in cystic fibrosis is hypoxemia, early therapy to alleviate mild or intermittent hypoxemia offers hope to retard the development and progression of cor pulmonale and thus influence the natural history of this disease. In particular, low-flow oxygen administration during sleep in patients with cystic fibrosis may allow palliation of their hypoxemia and delay the onset of pulmonary vasoconstriction and pulmonary hypertension.[36,37]

CARDIAC CATHETERIZATION

Cardiac catheterization is an invasive, expensive procedure which cannot be used serially to assess cor pulmonale in cystic fibrosis. The data that are available[34] demonstrate: (1) elevated right atrial pressure, (2) pulmonary hypertension, (3) elevated pulmonary vascular resistance, and (4) preservation of a normal cardiac index.

TREATMENT OF COR PULMONALE

The treatment of cor pulmonale is not very effective, probably as a result of the late state in the natural history of the disease at which treatment is begun. In the recent description by Stern et al[34] of 61 patients with overt right-sided congestive heart failure, the mean survival was only 8 months after the onset of CHF. All of their patients received diuretics, which were found to offer some symptomatic relief. Digoxin can improve right ventricular function[35] but no improvement in survival was associated with digoxin administration. Tolazoline hydrochloride is a potent pulmonary and systemic arteriolar vasodilator and would theoretically be of some benefit to these patients. However, no clear symptomatic improvement or improved survival occurred. Alternatively, echocardiographic and/or radionuclide evaluation of these patients may allow identification of early stages of cor pulmonale when vasodilators and inotropic agents may still be of benefit.

REFERENCES

1. Royce SW: Cor pulmonale in infancy and childhood: Report on 34 patients with special reference to the occurrence of pulmonary heart disease in cystic fibrosis of the pancreas. *Pediatrics* 1951;8:255–274.
2. World Health Organization Expert Committee: Chronic cor pulmonale. *Circulation* 1963;27:594–615.
3. Symchych PS: Pulmonary hypertension in cystic fibrosis—a description and morpho-

metric analysis of the pulmonary vasculature. *Arch Pathol* 1971;92:409–414.

4. Ryland D, Reid L: The pulmonary circulation in cystic fibrosis. *Thorax* 1975;30: 285–292.
5. Boysen PG, Block AJ, Wynne JW, et al: Nocturnal pulmonary hypertension in patients with chronic obstructive pulmonary disease. *Chest* 1979;76:536–542.
6. Muller NL, Francis PWJ, Gurwitz D, et al: Mechanism of hemoglobin desaturation during rapid eye movements sleep in normal subjects and patients with cystic fibrosis. *Am Rev Respir Dis* 1980;121:463–469.
7. Fishman AP: Hypoxia on the pulmonary circulation—how and where it acts. *Circulation* 1976;38:221–231.
8. Liebman J, Doershuk CF, Rapp C, et al: The vectorcardiogram in cystic fibrosis. *Circulation* 1967;35:552–569.
9. Siassi B, Moss AJ, Dooley RR: Clinical recognition of cor pulmonale in cystic fibrosis. *J Pediatr* 1971;78:794–805.
10. Meyer RA: *Pediatric Echocardiography.* Philadelphia, Lea & Febiger, 1977.
11. Hirschfeld S, Meyer RA, Schwartz DC, et al: Measurement of right and left ventricular systolic time intervals in echocardiography. *Circulation* 1975;51:304–309.
12. Riggs T, Hirschfeld S, Borkat G, et al: Assessment of the pulmonary vascular bed by echocardiographic right ventricular systolic tissue intervals. *Circulation* 1978;57:939–947.
13. Riggs T, Hirschfeld S, Bormuth C, et al: Neonatal circulatory changes: An echocardiographic study. *Pediatrics* 1977;59:338–344.
14. Riggs T, Hirschfeld S, Fanaroff A, et al: Persistence of the fetal circulation syndrome: An echocardiographic study. *J Pediatr* 1977;91: 626–631.
15. Fouron JC, Le Guennec JC, Villement D, et al: Value of echocardiography in assessing the outcome of bronchopulmonary dysplasia of the newborn. *J Pediatr* 1980;65:529–540.
16. Rosenthal A, Tucher CR, Williams RG, et al: Echocardiographic assessment of cor pulmonale in cystic fibrosis. *Pediatr Clin North Am* 1976;23:327–344.
17. Gewitz M, Eshaghpour E, Holsclaw DS, et al: Echocardiography in cystic fibrosis. *Am J Dis Child* 1977;131:275–280.
18. Ryssing E: Assessment of cor pulmonale in cystic fibrosis by echocardiography. *Acta Paediatr Scand* 1977;66:753–756.
19. Hirschfeld SS, Fleming DG, Doershuk C, et al: Echocardiographic abnormalities in patients with cystic fibrosis. *Chest* 1979;75: 351–355.
20. Allen HD, Taussig L, Gaines JA, et al: Echocardiographic profiles of the long-term cardiac changes in cystic fibrosis. *Chest* 1979;75: 428–433.
21. Lester L, Egge AC, Hubbard VS, et al: Echocardiography in cystic fibrosis. A proposed scoring system. *J Pediatr* 1980;97: 742–748.
22. Raviele A, Riggs T, Garcia et al: Respiratory variations in frank vectorcardiography and echocardiography in children. *J Electrocardiol* 1981;14:73–79.
23. Morin DP, Cottrill CM, Johnson GL, et al: Effect of respiration on the echocardiogram in children with cystic fibrosis. *Pediatrics* 1980;65:44–49.
24. Settle HP, Engel PJ, Fowler NO, et al: Echocardiographic study of the paradoxial arterial pulse in chronic obstructive lung disease. *Circulation* 1980;62:1297–1307.
25. Jacobstein MD, Hirschfeld SS, Winnie G, et al: Ventricular interdependence in severe cystic fibrosis: A two-dimensional echocardiographic study. *Chest*, 1981;80:399–404.
26. Robotham JL: Cardiovascular disturbances in chronic respiratory insufficiency. *Am J Cardiol* 1981;47:941–949.
27. Rao S, Cohn KE, Eldridge FL, et al: Left ventricular failure secondary to chronic obstructive lung disease. *Am J Med* 1968; 45:229–241.
28. Baum GL, Schwartz A, Llamas R, et al: Left ventricular function in chronic obstructive lung disease, *N Engl J Med* 1971;285: 361–365.
29. Frank MJ, Weisse AB, Moschos CB, et al: Left ventricular function, metabolism and blood flow in chronic cor pulmonale. *Circulation* 1973;47:798–806.
30. Oppenheimer EH, Esterly JR: Myocardial lesions in patients with cystic fibrosis of the pancreas. *Johns Hopkins Med J* 1973;133: 252–261.
31. Michelson N: Bilateral ventricular hypertrophy due to chronic obstructive lung disease. *Dis Chest* 1960;38:435–446.
32. Chipps BE, Alderson PO, Roland JMA, et al: Noninvasive evaluation of ventricular function in cystic fibrosis. *J Pediatr* 1979; 95:379–384.
33. Krayenbuehl HP, Turine J, Hess O: Left ventricular function in chronic cor pulmonale. *Am J Cardiol* 1978;41:1150–1158.
34. Stern RC, Borkat G, Hirschfeld SS, et al: Heart failure in cystic fibrosis. *Am J Dis Child* 1980;134:267–272.
35. Smith DE, Bissett JK, Phillips JR, et al: Improved right ventricular systolic time intervals after digitalis in patients with cor pulmonale and chronic obstructive pulmonary

disease. *Am J Cardiol* 1978;41:1299–1304.

36. Francis PWJ, Muller NL, Gurwitz D, et al: Hemoglobin desaturation: Its occurrence during sleep in patients with cystic fibrosis. *Am J Dis Child* 1980;134:734–740.

37. Hazinski TA, Hansen TN, Simon JA, et al: Effect of oxygen administration during sleep on skin surface oxygen and carbon dioxide tensions in patients with chronic lung disease. *Pediatrics* 1981;67:626–630.

15

Growth, Nutrition, and Gastrointestinal Problems

John D. Lloyd-Still

There seems unanimous agreement that pancreatic insufficiency is the major cause of the growth failure and nutritional deficiencies that are so prominent a feature of most patients with cystic fibrosis. In the past, the term "pancreatic infantilism" was used.[1] Sproul and Huang[2] reported on 110 patients with CF ranging in age from 6 to 18 years, and found that the majority had substandard values for weight, height, and anthropometric measurements. The reduction in these parameters correlated with increasing severity of disease.

Kraemer et al[3] observed 117 patients between 1956 and 1976 and demonstrated that the relative underweight (weight loss corrected for height) was most pronounced in children with predominantly pulmonary symptoms. Moreover, the degree of underweight correlated inversely with survival. Gaskin et al[4] performed longitudinal pulmonary function studies on a large group of CF patients and showed that the decline in pulmonary function was greatly increased in those with steatorrhea. Those patients with intact pancreatic function (10% of the CF population) consistently had pulmonary function tests significantly better than those with impaired pancreatic function. They were unsure whether this was due to a mild genetic expression of the disease or related to the effects of malnutrition.

In contrast to the results in earlier studies,[2,3] recent data from the Toronto CF Center show that only a minority of their patients have deficits in their growth parameters.[5] Moreover, their cumulative survival figures are considerably better than those for Canada or the United States.[6] The highest mortality (Table 15-1) occurred in patients with meconium ileus, but those patients who survived the neonatal period had the same prognosis as those without meconium ileus. Patients with both pulmonary and gastrointestinal symptoms (53%) of the total group) had the next highest mortality. The mortality rates of patients presenting with gastrointestinal symptoms only (17%) or pulmonary symptoms only (18%) were half those of the combined pulmonary and gastrointestinal group. These findings would suggest that nutritional factors may be as important as lung disease in ultimate prognosis,[6] a statement that is contradictory to the commonly accepted criteria for prognosis in cystic fibrosis.

Two recent observations have relevance to the importance of nutritional factors in the prognosis of cystic fibrosis. Firstly, several studies[7-9] have shown that the recommended dietary allowance (RDA) in CF children was approximately 80% of the norm (range of 52–93%) in 40% of a clinic population. In the past, the statement was made that CF children had excessive appetites with RDAs between 100–150% of the normal, but it now appears that only 60% of the patients fall into this category. Secondly, studies of the nutritional intake of children and adolescents with chronic inflammatory bowel disease (Crohn's disease and ulcerative colitis) have shown that the majority of patients with growth failure consume an inadequate caloric intake and that this is a far more important determinant for their growth failure than the effects of malabsorption or steroid therapy which were blamed in the past.[10-12] Moreover, supplementary feeding regimens, either by intravenous hyperalimentation, constant infusion elemental diets, or nutritional supplements can frequently reverse this negative caloric balance, resulting in correction of the growth failure. These concepts offer new approaches to the therapy of the nutritional problems in cystic fibrosis.

Table 15-1
Classification of Diagnoses of Cystic Fibrosis and Deaths by Different Types of Presentations at The Hospital for Sick Children, Toronto, 1952–1978*

Symptoms at Presentation	Number Diagnosed	Number of Deaths	Deaths (%)
Meconium ileus	83	34	41
Pulmonary and gastrointestinal symptoms	387	113	29
Gastrointestinal symptoms only	121	18	15
Pulmonary symptoms only	128	17	13

*Modified from Gurwitz et al: *Pediatr Clin North Am* 1979;26:603 (reference 6).

DEVELOPMENT OF GASTROINTESTINAL FUNCTION

Several excellent reviews on this subject in the normal infant have been published.[13,14] The mean birth weight for CF infants is 2.9 kg,[15] lower than the mean for the United States (3.3 kg). Some authorities have suggested that this implies evidence of an intrauterine insult in cystic fibrosis. Specific information on how the development of gastrointestinal function in CF infants compares to the normal is limited. The development of the exocrine pancreas in infants with CF with and without meconium ileus diverges from the normal pattern. There is a constant lack of exocrine tissue, before or at full-term birth, which persists.[16] Cystic fibrosis infants above 42 weeks postconceptional age can be distinguished from controls on the basis of a quantitative assessment of acinar volume. Eighty-five percent of CF infants have absent proteolytic enzyme activity in their stools in the first few days after birth, and the lack of development of pancreatic function is probably the most significant deficit in the development of gastrointestinal function in cystic fibrosis.

PATHOLOGY

This is described in detail in Chapter 3, but some further comments are necessary in discussing the nutritional complications of cystic fibrosis.

Body Composition

Autopsy studies on the body composition of infants dying of CF show findings similar to those of malnourished infants dying from other causes.[17] Infants dying from meconium ileus showed more profound changes than CF infants without meconium ileus, presumably because the malnutrition in the former had been present since birth. These changes are illustrated in Figure 15-1, where the maximum reductions were found in percentage of body weight compared to normals. Less severe changes were found in brain weight and body length. These pathologic findings may have significance in view of the association between malnutrition and detrimental effects on brain structure and function. Studies to investigate whether malnourished infants with CF suffer from impaired intellectual development have been performed, and the results have been reassuring.[18] See Chapter 22 for further discussion of this topic.

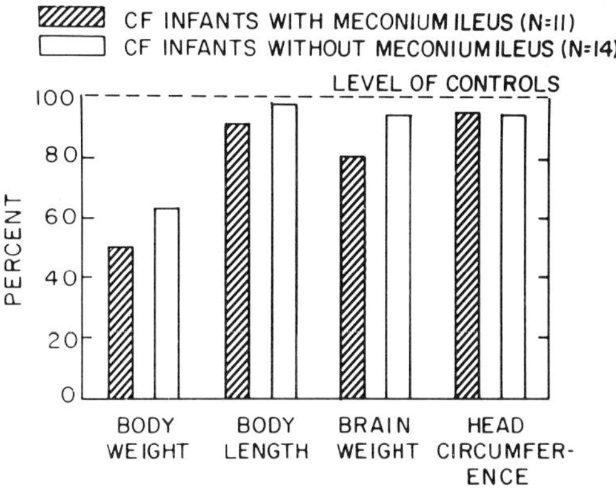

Figure 15-1 Percentage body weight, body length, brain weight, and head circumference in two groups of infants dying with cystic fibrosis (with and without meconium ileus). Reproduced from Lloyd-Still JD (ed): *Malnutrition and Intellectual Development,* Lancaster MTP Press Ltd., 1976, p 117 (reference 17), with permission.

Pancreas

Oppenheimer and Esterly[19] performed autopsies on 146 children who died from CF and reviewed the pathologic findings. They concluded that: (1) There is a spectrum of pancreatic changes among cases at any given age. (2) Diagnostic pancreatic lesions may be absent in an individual case irrespective of age. (3) There is generally a direct correlation between age and severity of findings in the pancreas.

The earliest pancreatic lesion in CF is focal inspissation of eosinophilic material in acini and ductules with flattening of the epithelium. Retention of secretions produces dilatation of acini and ducts and atrophy of acinar tissue. Fibrosis then ensues, and ultimately the exocrine pancreas may be entirely replaced by fat in which only the islets of Langerhans remain. Ultimately even the islets cease to function, with diminished production of insulin and glucagon and the development of diabetes. Remarkably, there is rarely any evidence of an inflammatory reaction to this destructive process (see Chapter 17 for a discussion of acute pancreatitis in CF). This is surprising, as in most other types of pancreatic obstruction proteolytic enzymes are liberated with considerable inflammatory reaction. Moreover, serum immunoreactive trypsin levels are elevated in the majority of CF infants under 10 weeks of age (see Chapter 2).

The pathogenesis of the pancreatic lesion is presumed to result from obstruction by the abnormal mucus. The concept that many patients with CF start off with a normal pancreas (and a normal lung) is an important one. Once the control of these abnormally thick secretions is understood, then the possibility of therapy to prevent further destruction of the pancreas will become the therapeutic goal. Farber[20] suggested that the nervous control of secretion in the pancreas and other glands of the body represented a logical and promising approach to an understanding of the nature of the disease.

Intestine

Meconium ileus Meconium ileus occurs in approximately 10% of newborns with CF and is discussed in detail in Chapters 11 and 21. Anatomic abnormalities including ileal and jejunal stenosis and atresia, reduplication, omphalocele, congenital bands, volvulus, and mesenteric defects are found in 50% of these infants and must have occurred in utero. Surgical correction of these defects may be incomplete, with the production of a short-bowel syndrome or blind-loop syndrome that will lead to additional malabsorptive and nutritional abnormalities.

Small intestine Bodian[21] in his classic monograph on 62 autopsies in CF attributed meconium ileus to the abnormal mucus secreted by the intestinal glands. He considered that it was unlikely that absence of pancreatic enzymes had more than a contributory effect since other pancreatic malformations associated with lack of enzymes during fetal life are not accompanied by meconium ileus. Support for this hypothesis was found by Thomaidis and Arey,[22] who studied clinical and pathologic data from 30 infants and children with CF without meconium ileus and from 9 infants with meconium ileus. Severe involvement of the intestinal glands of the small bowel was common in infants with meconium ileus compared with age-matched infants without meconium ileus.

Freye et al[23] performed more detailed examination of the small intestine in 21 children with CF who underwent peroral biopsy. Sections stained with hematoxylin and eosin appeared normal to light microscopy. Periodic acid–Schiff stains showed a thickened mucus cover in those patients with abnormal absorption. Electron microscopy revealed normal columnar and goblet cell structure. The microvilli, which were markedly altered in other malabsorption syndromes, were normal. A coarse fibrillar substance, probably mucus, covered large areas of the biopsy specimens from patients with CF who had steatorrhea. It was not observed in normal biopsies or in the patients with CF without steatorrhea. This substance occurred closely adherent to the fine fibrillar layer which is usually fused with the striate border of epitheleal cells.

The findings of Freye et al[23] supported the concept proposed by Dische et al[24] that a mechanical factor in the form of pathologic mucus may contribute to the absorption defect in patients with cystic fibrosis. Morin et al[25] confirmed the normal appearance of jejunal biopsies by light microscopy in 37 children with CF and found the uptake of lysine was normal, whereas that of phenylalanine and cycloleucine were reduced in CF compared to controls. They interpreted their findings as suggesting an intestinal component to the malabsorption of patients with cystic fibrosis.

Large intestine Neutra and Trier[26] applied quantitative stereological methods to biopsies of rectal mucosa from five CF patients, five sibling controls, and two normal controls to measure goblet cell numbers, crypt luminal volume, and volume of intraductular mucus. They found that CF crypt lumini were variably dilated, but the average relative volume of intracellular mucus and the numbers of goblet cells in CF mucosa were comparable to those of siblings and adult controls. In CF biopsies, lower surface columnar absorptive cells consistently contained putrative lipid droplets and rapidly accummulated large lipid droplets during short-term organ culture. Lipid droplets were not observed in the same cell types of control biopsies before and after short-term organ culture.

They were unable to explain whether these changes were related to essential fatty acid deficiency, defects in fatty acid membrane composition, or alterations in calcium metabolism. They disclaimed the possibility of unabsorbed fecal lipid being available to the CF absorptive cell, but were unable to exclude the possibility that the CF absorptive cells differ metabolically from controls. The physiological factors governing the release of mucus from intestinal goblet cells are poorly understood, and in experiments on the role of parasympathetic stimulation, it was found that much of the secreted radiolabeled mucus remained tightly adherent to the mucosa.[27]

GROWTH

Parameters

Accurate serial measurements of height, weight, and head circumference are essential components of the clinical examination of all infants and children. The growth chart allows comparison of an individual child with a large population in terms of percentile ranking for height, weight, and head circumference, and it provides a basis for calculations of growth velocity. The National Center for Health Statistics has published new standards for growth charts[28] that have replaced the previous growth charts which were based on data accummulated over 30 years ago. Growth velocity varies with age and sex and accelerates during adolescence.

Bone Age

Determination of the level of epiphyseal maturation or "bone age" is helpful in evaluating children with abnormal growth. The standards of Greulich and Pyle[29] are widely used. The bone age tends to be normal in genetic or familial short stature. A delayed bone age does not provide specific information as it is present in intrauterine growth retardation, psychosocial dwarfism, endocrine disorders, constitutional short stature, and nutritional abnormalities. The major value of the bone age is prognostic. Short children whose bone age is delayed have a much better prognosis for ultimate height than do children whose bone age is consistent with their chronologic age.

Differential Diagnosis of Growth Disorders

The major cause of growth retardation in CF is the result of pancreatic insufficiency. However, the spectrum of growth failure in pediatrics involves several complex factors which may potentiate the growth problems of children with cystic fibrosis. The differential diagnosis of some of the more important causes of growth failure are shown in Table 15-2. A detailed family history must enquire for genetic causes of short stature. The birth history and maternal complications must be obtained to exclude intrauterine growth retardation or the small-for-gestational-age infant. Endocrine causes for growth retardation, such as hypothyroidism or growth hormone deficiency, are treatable. This subject is discussed in detail in Chapter 19.

Another approach to the etiologic classification of failure to thrive or loss of weight includes the following six major groups of disorders[30]: (1) qualitative or quantitative inadequacy of food intake; (2) defects in assimilation of foods; (3) loss of food substances; (4) failure of utilization or increased metabolism; (5) neurologic and psychologic; and (6) undetermined.

Psychosocial deprivation or dwarfism This condition accounts for between 58 and 82% of children admitted to hospital for investigation of "failure to thrive."[31] Inadequate parenting or neglect will be

Table 15-2
A Simplified Approach to Differential Diagnosis of Growth Disorders

Genetic
Familial
Intrauterine
Chromosomal
Nutritional
Gastrointestinal disease
Other chronic disease (cardiac, renal, etc)
Psychosocial
Drugs
Constitutional short stature
Endocrine
Hypothyroidism
Growth hormone deficiency
Others
Chronic disease (pulmonary, cardiac, renal, etc)
Drugs
Miscellaneous
Bone disease, others

documented, and the disorder is a major component of the child abuse syndrome. A detailed psychosocial history is mandatory. These children are commonly apathetic, have delayed developmental milestones, and rapidly thrive when removed from the home environment. The underlying reason for failure to gain weight is inadequate caloric intake or nutritional deprivation.[32] In large CF centers there are always a number of problem families with the psychosocial deprivation syndrome. Unfortunately, once an organic disorder, such as CF, is diagnosed, there is a tendency to ascribe a poor response to treatment to the organic disorder. It is imperative to recognize these poorly functioning families and institute appropriate social service and nutritional support.

Constitutional short stature Constitutional short stature is defined as height two standard deviations or more below the mean for age, retarded skeletal maturation in relation to chronological age, but otherwise no abnormal tests, medical history, or physical examination findings and no family history of short stature.[33] It is the major cause of growth retardation referred to endocrinologists. In a series[33] of 263 children referred for short stature, 149 (56.7%) had consitutional short stature, 19 (7.2%) had isolated growth hormone deficiency, 16 (6.1%) had intrauterine growth retardation, 8 (3%) had maternal deprivation, 9 (3.4%) had chromosome abnormalities, 8 (3%) had hypothyroidism, and 54 (20.6%) had systemic disease.

Gastrointestinal disease In CF, pancreatic insufficiency leads to massive steatorrhea with symptoms such as excessive appetite, abdominal distention, and diarrhea suggestive of disease in the gastrointestinal tract. In a few patients with Crohn's disease and growth failure, gastrointestinal symptoms may be absent.

Drugs The role of drugs in growth is complex. Some drugs lead to gastritis and anorexia. Cytotoxic drugs, such as methotrexate, may directly damage the enterocyte and lead to a malabsorption syndrome. Others, such as corticosteroids and anabolic steroids, exert side effects on the endocrine glands and result in excessive weight gain. Antibiotics, such as the tetracyclines, may have a growth-promoting effect. Thus, a detailed history of the medications prescribed is essential in evaluating any growth problem.

Evaluation of Nutritional Status

Dietary assessment Carefully controlled studies have now defined the requirements for total energy intake, protein, fat, carbohydrate, and other nutrients for different physiological groups. For most nutrients known to be required by humans, a recommended dietary allowance (RDA) has been established by the Committee on Dietary Allowance of the Food and Nutrition Board.[34] A study of the nutritional status of preschool children in the United States, 1968–1970, utilized this method.[35] Dietary intake is also dependent on the dietary habits of the family. Apart from a few patients who are food faddists, or in instances such as the selenium controversy (when CF patients were advised to take selenium supplements by a veterinarian), there is no reason to believe that dietary habits in CF families are abnormal. Dietary assessment is best performed by a 3- to 7-day written record kept by the patient or parents. Clinical nutritionists can analyze the intake with a computer program which will give the percentage RDA for total calories, protein, fat, carbohydrate, vitamins, and minerals.

Prospective studies on the dietary intake of a large group of CF patients are limited, but ranges of energy intakes between 52 and 135% of the RDA have been reported.[7–9] By contrast, infants with CF in the phase of "catch-up growth" after diagnosis have energy intakes of 150–175 calories/kg/day.[1] Hubbard[9] found that of 22 patients surveyed for dietary intake, 10 had intakes less than 100% (mean 80%) of RDA, and 12 had intakes between 101 and 150% (mean 115%) of the RDA. These data contradict the oft-quoted statement that CF children consume an excessive amount of calories.

Metabolic Balance Studies

Metabolic balance studies performed on six CF patients by Khaw and Shen were quoted by Shwachman.[1] One subject had minimal disease, two subjects had predominantly gastrointestinal symptoms, and three had both pulmonary and gastrointestinal symptoms. The clinical scores ranged from 46 to 95. The caloric intake and excretion were determined by bomb calorimetry. The total caloric expenditure was calculated from serial sampling of oxygen consumption, carbon dioxide production, and urinary nitrogen excretion. The caloric intake varied from 61 to 86 kcal/kg/day. Fecal caloric loss increased with increasing severity of gastrointestinal symptoms (controls 4% of fecal caloric loss compared to 16% with pancreatic insufficiency). The patient with minimal disease had the highest total energy balance and had less body water than the severely affected patients. Total body fat as percentage of body water was 6.3–13.8% in the five affected subjects, and 27% in the minimally affected subject (controls 15–17%).

Another study[7] of 10 malnourished CF patients measured basal O_2 consumption, specific dynamic action of food (SDA), energy balance, and T_3 studies in the basal state. The patients were then placed on a supplement supplying 1000 more calories per day with 20% as dietary fat and 80% as carbohydrate for three weeks. Protein intake was fixed at 3 g/kg/day. Four normal children were studied as controls. The results showed the energy intake at the basal level was 77 calories/kg/day; at the increased energy level it was 116 calories/kg/day (controls 64 calories/kg/day). The CF patients showed a 30% higher basal energy expenditure expressed as basal metabolic rate (calories/m²/hr) or as oxygen consumption (ml/min/kg). The mean calculated energy balance for growth in CF was -3.7 ± 5, and in controls 17 ± 2 calories/kg/day. On the increased energy level patients were able to achieve a positive energy balance of 19 ± 3 calories/kg/day. This led to significant weight gain in the three-week supplement period (2.0 ± 0.3 kg).

The authors concluded: (1) CF patients had a higher basal energy requirement than normal controls. (2) They showed a negative energy balance in the basal state. (3) With increased caloric intake, the CF patients achieved a positive energy balance that is adequate for growth and possibly catch-up growth.

Clinical signs of malnutrition The following clinical signs have been listed as suggestive of protein–calorie malnutrition of early childhood[36]: edema, dyspigmentation of the hair, thin sparse hair, muscle wasting, depigmentation of the skin, psychomotor changes, moon face, hepatomegaly, and flaky-paint dermatosis. The two severe syndromes of kwashiorkor and marasmus are easy to identify. Marasmus is well recognized in CF infants prior to diagnosis. The clinical complication of hypoproteinemia is discussed later in this chapter and is rarely complicated by the classical dermatosis of kwashiorkor. The term protein–calorie malnutrition is preferred.

Anthropometry Measurements available for field surveys of protein–calorie malnutrition include weight, length, head circumference, triceps, and subscapsular skin folds. Measurements can then be compared with reference standards. Studies in CF (Figure 15-2) show poor weight gain in infancy prior to diagnosis, and improvement when therapy is instituted with an average weight about one standard deviation below the mean during the preadolescent years. During adolescence the weight tends to fall off again as the pulmonary condition worsens.[37] Similar findings for height and subscapsular skin-fold thickness were found, but there was less marked depression of head growth and triceps skin-fold thickness.[38] A positive correlation ($P < 0.0003$) was found between weight score and chest x-ray scores in 56 children.[38]

The importance of measurements of height or length is emphasized since the extent of height deficiency in relation to age can be regarded as a measure of the duration

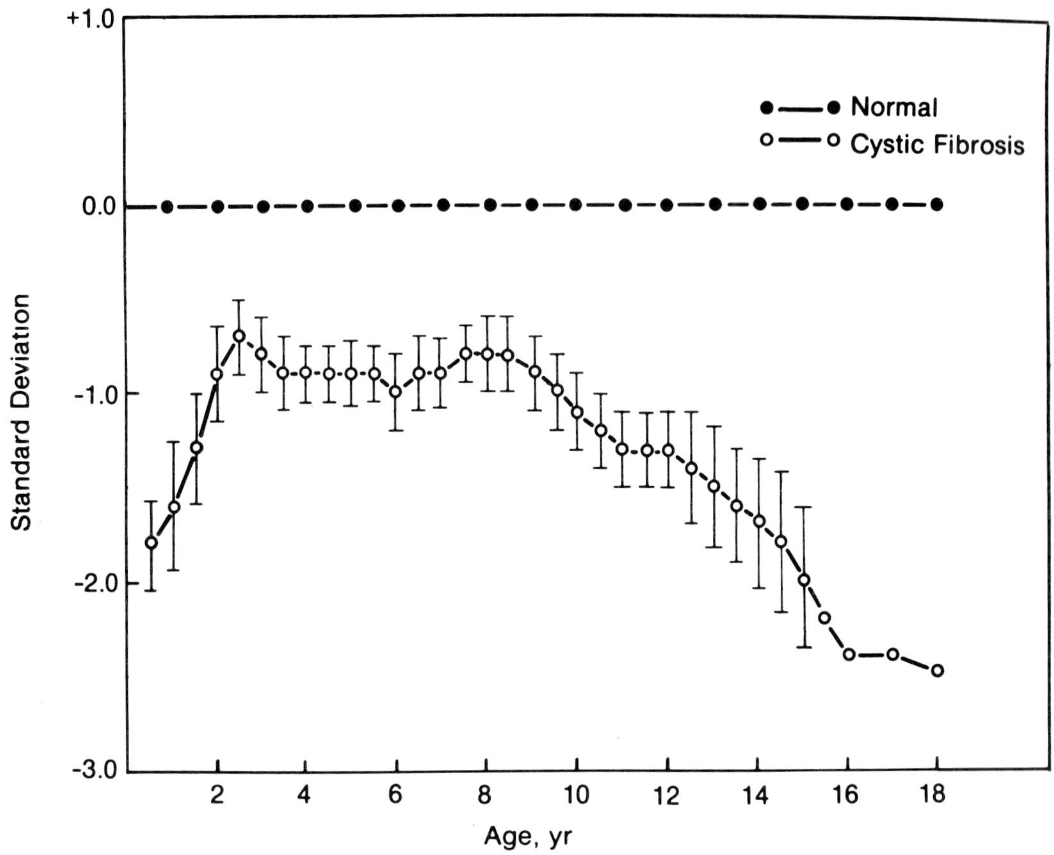

Figure 15-2 Weight growth, expressed as standard scores or SD from norms for age and sex. Normal children are represented by mean (SD = 0). Numbers of patients in each age group: 13 to 16 at ½ to 1½ years, 21 to 33 between 2 and 10 years, 12 to 19 between 10½ and 12½ years, 5 to 7 between 13 and 15 years, and 3 at age 15½ and older. Standard error of mean up to age 15 (vertical bars). From Berry HK, et al: *Am J Dis Child* 1975;129:165–171 (reference 37), with permission. Copyright 1975, American Medical Association.

of malnutrition.[39] Weight for height can be used as an index of current nutritional status, whereas height for age gives a picture of past nutritional history.[40]

In Figure 15-3 the growth chart of a patient with CF shows a fall off in both height and weight gain after the age of 13 years when her pulmonary function progressively deteriorated. In Figure 15-4 her weight is plotted against her pulmonary function values. Note how her pulmonary function flucuates widely in response to therapy, but over a 5-year period her pulmonary function shows significant deterioration. During the same interval there was no significant weight gain.

Bone age Delayed bone age is commonly seen in cystic fibrosis.[2]

Biochemical tests At present there is no satisfactory biochemical test of malnutrition suitable for use in all parts of the world. The following have been suggested:[36]

Total protein and albumin Reduction in these levels is largely confined to children with kwashiorkor but is also a frequent feature of infants with cystic fibrosis. However, severe marasmus can be present with a normal protein and albumin concentration.

Fasting urinary urea-creatinine ratio Low rates of urinary urea to creatinine are found in children eating small amounts of protein. Thus, this is a measure of dietary rather than nutritional state. It is likely these

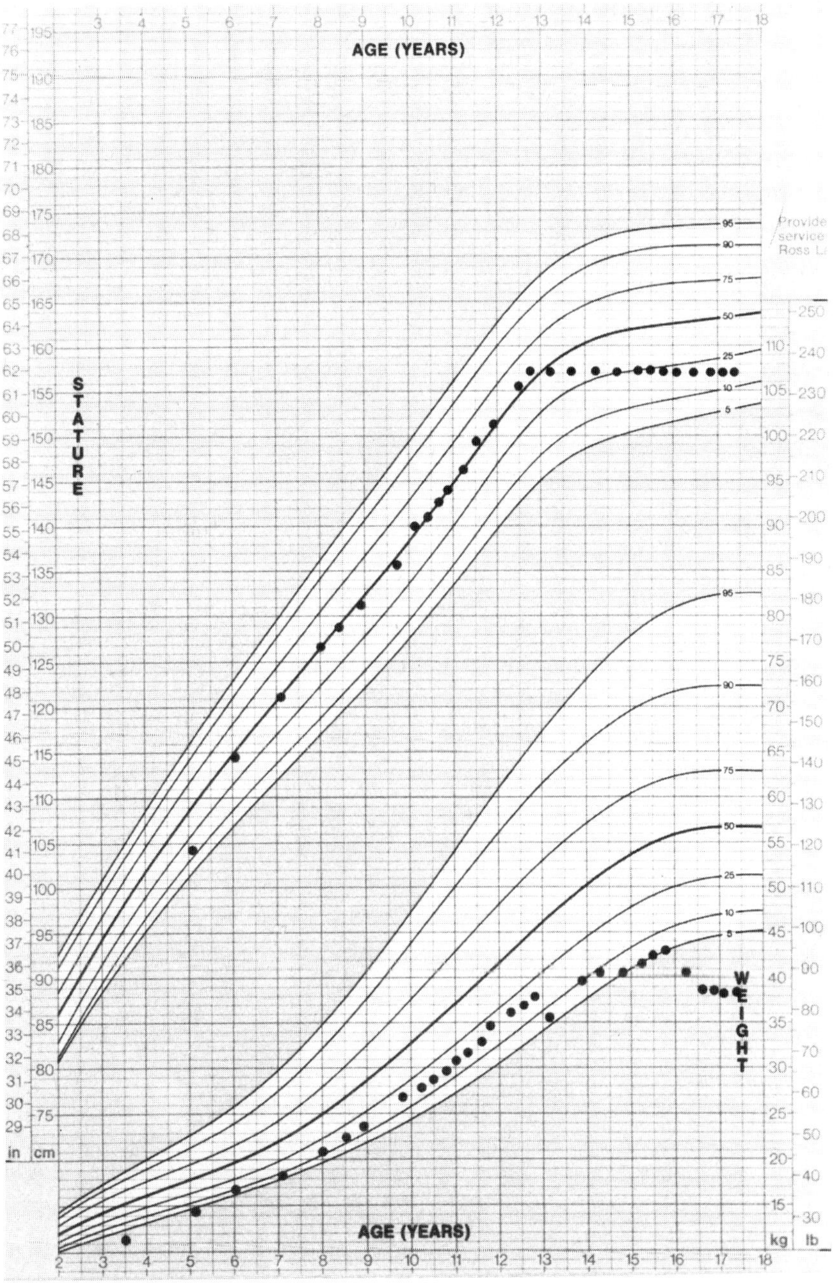

Figure 15-3 The growth chart of a CF patient who developed significant pulmonary deterioration after the age of 13 years. Note the lack of gain in height and weight during the next five years. (Courtesy Dr. Hans Wessel.)

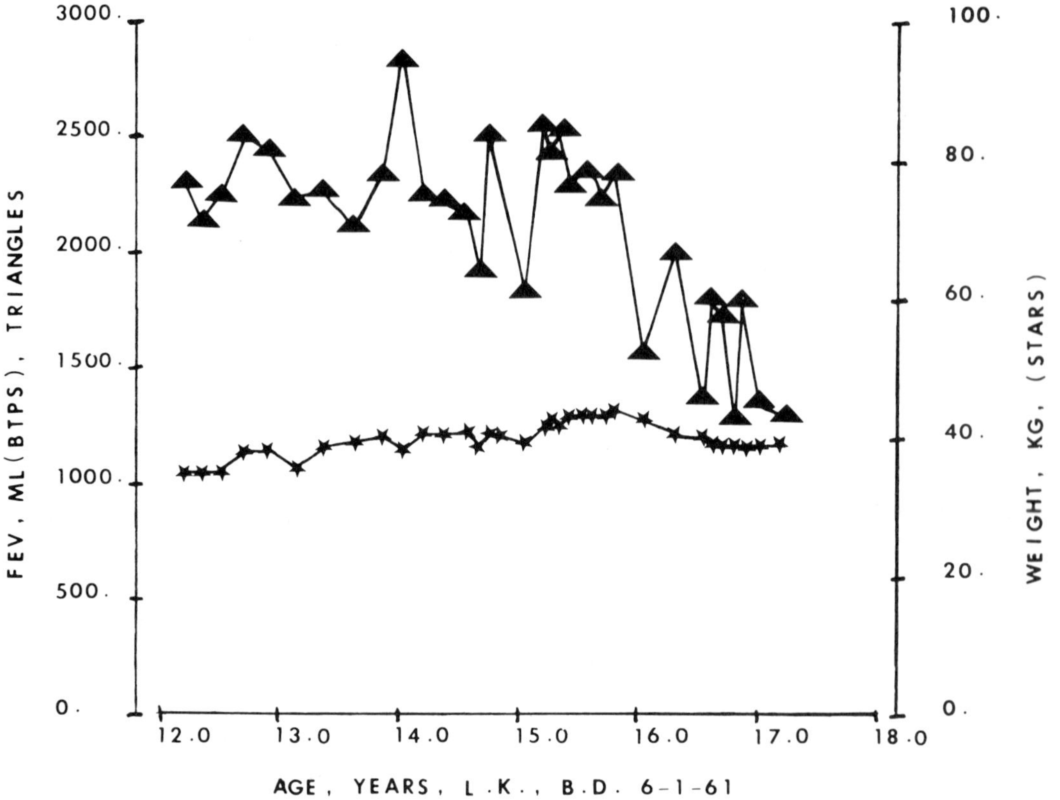

Figure 15-4 Pulmonary function plotted against weight for the same patient shown in Figure 15-3. Note the wide fluctuation in pulmonary function tests related to therapy. There is significant deterioration over the five-year period. During the same interval her weight remained unchanged. (Courtesy Dr. Hans Wessel.)

ratios could be applicable to CF infants where the dietary protein intake will be unavailable to the infant owing to the lack of proteolytic enzymes.

Urinary sulfur–creatinine ratio The basis of this test is similar to the urinary creatinine ratio, but it also reflects the dietary intake of high-quality protein as indicated by those with a high sulfur content.

Serum amino acid ratio The serum amino acid ratio is disturbed in kwashiorkor. This test is a good reflection of primary protein deficiency. A low valine–glycine ratio reflects a decrease in essential amino acids, and there is an increase in nonessential amino acids. Essential amino acid levels in serum generally were low in CF and nonessential amino acid levels were normal or slightly raised.[37]

Urinary hydroxyproline index This test depends on the fact that in nutritionally dwarfed children the excretion of hydroxyproline peptides is very low. However, intercurrent infections result in high excretions of hydroxyproline.

Urinary creatinine to height index This depends on the fact that loss of muscle in malnutrition results in a reduction of 24-hour creatinine excretion.

Few of these biochemical tests are likely to be helpful in the management of CF infants. Most abnormalities, such as alterations in protein or amino acid status, rapidly reverse with therapy.

Endocrine Adaptation to Malnutrition

Basal growth hormone levels are elevated in untreated subjects with kwashiorkor and return to control levels with dietary treatment. In addition, most observers agree that growth hormone is also elevated in marasmus.[41] Despite the elevated growth hormone levels, the bioassayable somatomedin is reduced.[42] The somatomedins are growth-hormone-dependent peripheral effectors of many of the anabolic activities of growth hormone, especially those causing skeletal growth. As the elevated growth hormone levels fall and albumin and transferrin levels rise with treatment, somatomedin increases to normal values. Fasting growth hormone levels are elevated in CF and show an unresponsiveness to hypoglycemia.[43] Data on somatomedin levels in CF are discussed in Chapter 19.

Protein–calorie malnutrition affects insulin levels and is characterized by failure to respond normally to both low and high blood sugar levels. The precise mechanisms for the defect in insulin secretion are unknown, but body potassium and/or chromium deficits, decreased gastrointestinal absorption, defective gut insulinotropic factors, and disordered insulin transport by the pancreas have been postulated. Pancreatic damage and decreased functional pancreatic mass have not been ruled out,[41] and pancreatic function is known to be decreased temporarily in protein–calorie malnutrition.[44] Glucagon levels initially increase and then decrease as fatty acids and ketones become the major fuel sources with more prolonged starvation.

The hypothalamic–pituitary–adrenal axis is not only intact and responds appropriately to various types of stimulation including stress, but it also may be in a state of slight hyperfunction.[45] The functional status of the thyroid is confusing, but there is probably decreased active thyroid hormone at the cellular level.[41]

Thus, the endocrine changes associated with malnutrition are complicated, with the end result being a state of growth arrest. Other endocrine changes alter body composition so as to conserve substrate for vital functioning, with protective adaptations to the deficiencies or imbalances in energy and protein.[41] Whether these changes are relevant to the subject with CF will require data from similar studies performed on a malnourished CF population and a well-nourished CF population and comparison of these results to normal controls. Certainly many of the hormone abnormalities found in CF bear similarities to those found in protein–calorie malnutrition.

Effects of Infection on Nutrition

The traditional principles for establishing dietary allowances must be reevaluated in the presence of acute and chronic infections because of anorexia, withdrawal of solid food, fever, adverse effects of treatment, impaired intestinal absorption, and increased nutrient losses in urine, skin, feces, or through internal sequestration.[46] Since acute and chronic pulmonary infection is present in the majority of patients with CF, it is relevant to consider the host nutritional responses to infection in some detail. These responses include prominent changes in nitrogen and protein metabolism, altered rates of carbohydrate and lipid production and utilization, and changes in mineral, electrolyte, trace element, and vitamin metabolism.[47]

In Figure 15-5, Beisel[48] has illustrated the sequence of nutritional responses during the course of a "typical" generalized febrile infectious illness. Although the exact series of events depicted in Figure 15-5 does not necessarily occur in every acute infection, many host nutritional responses follow predictable patterns. Other variables include the type of infecting microorganism, the severity of the disease, the occurrence of certain complications, or the predominant involvement of a certain organ system, which in the case of CF will be the lung.

Catabolic and anabolic changes The well-recognized catabolic response to infection develops and progresses in a stereotyped pattern.[49] This metabolic pattern of catabolic wasting is similar from illness to illness despite differing etiologies. Fever, impaired dietary intake, and duration of illness are the key factors determining the magnitude of the catabolic losses. It has been estimated that

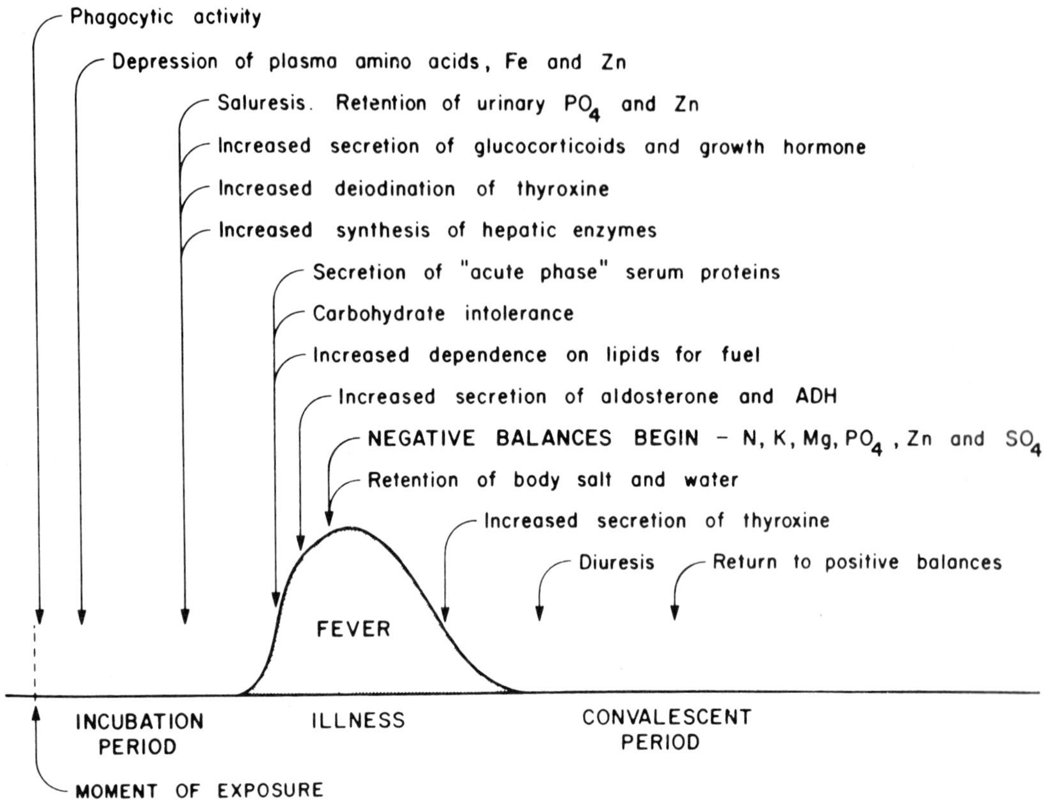

Figure 15-5 Schematic representation of the sequence of nutritional responses that evolves during the course of a "typical" generalized febrile infectious illness. Reproduced from Beisel WR: In McKigney JI, Munro HN (eds): *Nutrient Requirements in Adolescence,* MIT Press, 1976, p 257 (reference 48), with permission.

an 11–13% increase in caloric intake is necessary for each degree centigrade of fever.[50]

An anabolic response was identified during infection and manifested by an increased rate in the synthesis of new protein.[51] This anabolic effect is overshadowed during the incubation and febrile periods by the catabolic losses. Examples of anabolic responses to infection include increased production of new phagocytes and intestinal mucosal cells, an increase in protein synthesis by the liver, and the production of specific immunoglobulins.[49] It is of interest that in CF the levels of immunoglobulins correlate with disease activity.[52]

Protein and amino acid metabolism Alterations in patterns of host protein metabolism are the most important nutritional consequences of infection.[49] The evolution and resolution of an inflammatory response, as well as the repair of cellular and tissue damage, are all dependent upon protein-synthesizing mechanisms. In CF, the body weight has been shown to correlate well with the degree of pulmonary infection.[2,3,37]

All varieties of acute infectious illness (bacterial, viral, and parasitic) are accompanied by negative body nitrogen balances which begin after the onset of the febrile response. Changes in rates of both intake and loss of nitrogen contribute to the negative values. Anorexia is a prominent feature of infectious illness, including children with CF during acute exacerbations of pulmonary infection. The excessive loss of body nitrogen is derived from the protein component of skeletal muscle and can be lessened by normal or increased quantities of caloric intake and dietary protein.

During an acute infection the body will use its available amino acids in a variety of ways that exaggerate or modify their normal patterns of utilization and metabolism. The liver increases its output of acute-phase-reacting glycoproteins, such as haptoglobin, α_1-antitrypsin, α_1-acid glycoprotein, ceruloplasmin, complement, and others.[53] Concomitantly many individual amino acids, such as alanine, branched-chain amino acids in muscle, and tryptophan may be lost for future availability to the body because of their accelerated metabolic degradation.

Other nutrient metabolic changes Comparable negative balances of other important intracellular elements include magnesium, potassium, phosphate, sulfate, and zinc. If diarrhea plays an important role in the infectious process, direct fecal losses of sodium, chloride, bicarbonate, and potassium result.

Trace metals Zinc and iron rapidly disappear from the plasma in acute infection and accumulate in the liver.[47] The utilization of stored iron for incorporation into hemoglobin is blocked, and there is the progressive development of anemia. In contrast to the lowering of plasma zinc and iron, the copper in the plasma increases in infections and is thought to be related to the increased ceruloplasmin secretion by the liver.[53]

Vitamins The effect of an infectious process on vitamin metabolism is a largely unexplored area.[54] Overt symptoms of vitamin deficiency have been precipitated in some individuals by the occurrence of severe infectious illness.[46] Heightened metabolic activity stimulated by severe infection and fever accelerates the utilization of various vitamins. Moreover, if the infectious process leads to necrosis and repair, there will be an increased demand for nutrients, including vitamins which, if not present in sufficient amounts, might lead to deficiency states.

The best documented data are in relation to riboflavin metabolism which correlated well with nitrogen loss during the catabolic state.[55] Riboflavin deficiency is sometimes present in CF patients despite the fact that it is not a fat-soluble vitamin. Furthermore, riboflavin deficiency is closely related to lipid metabolism with reduced levels of linoleic, linolenic, and arachidonic acids in the serum and liver of rats.[56] Other vitamins reported to be decreased during the infectious process include vitamins A, C, and folic acid, but the documentation of consistent changes is controversial.

Carbohydrate changes and gluconeogenesis in infection Gluconeogenesis means the formation of glucose within the body from protein, fat, and substances other than carbohydrate. It is the mechanism by which lactate and amino acids are converted to glucose. It occurs in the liver and kidney, plays a major role in the control of the level of glycemia in the fasted patient, and allows the removal of large amounts of lactic acid from the blood. Gluconeogenesis is initially stimulated during infections and is abetted by the substrate amino acids derived from muscle protein, but with prolonged duration the body becomes hypoglycemic.[49]

All hormones that regulate carbohydrate metabolism participate in the host response to infection.[47] Fasting concentrations of glucagon and insulin are increased. The catecholamines help to stimulate gluconeogenesis during infections. However, despite the widespread changes in carbohydrate metabolism during infection, there have not been any specific enzyme aberrations identified in the carbohydrate metabolic pathways.[47] During a severe infection, the body depends primarily for its energy needs on carbohydrates and amino acids.

A glucose–alanine cycle has been proposed in man.[57] It was suggested that during fasting the maintenance of normal blood glucose is dependent upon hepatic gluconeogenesis, with alanine synthesized in muscle serving as the principal substrate. In early infection there is an increase in plasma glucose and a depression of plasma alanine. The enhanced activity of the hepatic gluconeogenic enzymes, together with an increased rate of uptake of alanine by the liver, bring about these changes.[49] In the terminal stages of overwhelming infection, the blood sugar values cannot be maintained, tissue carbohydrate stores are exhausted, and plasma amino acid concentrations are high. The measurements of glucose and alanine during early infection contradict the measurements done at a later time. These results illustrate the importance of serial measurements of nutrients during the progress of an infection.

Lipids The host responses involving lipid metabolism, unlike the responses of nitrogen, do not develop along stereotyped patterns, but vary instead with the infecting microorganism and with the presence or absence of a bacterial toxin.[49] Some of the changes in triglycerides, free fatty acids, ketone bodies, phospholipids, cholesterol, and lipid-displaced plasma activity during infection with a variety of microorganisms *(S. typhimurium, S. pneumoniae),* viruses, and endotoxemia have been summarized by Blackburn.[58] The most profound effects occur with gram-negative bacterial infections, endotoxemia, and sepsis. Despite similarities in free fatty acid kinetic data, there are important differences in the response of phospholipid moieties to infections with *S. pneumoniae, S. typhimurium,* and endotoxin.[49] Moreover, these differences vary with sequential measurements.

Dietary manipulations, particularly in the amount of glucose, may alter the contribution of free fatty acids to the total energy requirement. Similarly, ketogenesis and ketone body levels are influenced by dietary manipulations, insulin level, and severity of infection. Lipid-dependent, protein-sparing therapies are not effective where starvation ketonemia exists. Lipid alterations in infection are minor compared to those involving protein metabolism.[58]

Hormones Adrenal glucocorticoid production is increased two- to five-fold above normal during the first several days of an acute febrile infection, but may become subnormal if the infection becomes chronic.[47] This increase in adrenal cortical concentration is thought to be related to failure of deconjugation of the steroids by hepatic enzymes. The mineralocorticoid hormones follow similar changes to the glucocorticoids. The elevated glucagon and insulin have been mentioned previously. Catecholamines are also elevated and stimulate gluconeogenesis. The thyroid hormones are metabolized at an increased rate, but are thought not to play a primary role in initiating or sustaining the hypercatabolic response to fever.

Other substances Several biologically active substances, including serotonin, histamine, and prostaglandins, and a large variety of lysosomal enzymes are liberated by host cells in contact with an inflammatory reaction. These biologically active substances can initiate localized effects at the anatomical site of the invading bacteria, or they can affect more distant tissues or lead to generalized intravascular phenomenon such as activation of the kinin and complement systems or the clotting cascade.[47]

Effects of Malnutrition on Immune System

Immunologic abnormalities in CF are reviewed in Chapter 10. Immune system dysfunction can result from single-nutrient deficiencies or excess, alone or in combination with generalized protein–calorie malnutrition. Acquired immune dysfunction in man occurs with deficiencies of iron, zinc, vitamins A and B_{12}, pyridoxine, and folic acid.[59] The effects of essential fatty acid and vitamin E changes are more complicated. Defects or excess of many trace elements and single nutrients thus have potential for causing immune dysfunction in man. Since nutritionally induced immune dysfunction is generally reversible, it is important to recognize and identify any illness in which immunologic dysfunction is of nutritional origin.

DIGESTION AND MALABSORPTION

Stomach

The lumen of the stomach functions as a temporary reservoir in which food is subjected to the actions of gastric secretions.

The major functions of the stomach involve secretion and motility. The secretions consist of hydrochloric acid; mucus; digestive enzymes including pepsin, cathepsin, gelatinase, and lipase; and with R protein and intrinsic factor (a glycoprotein essential for the absorption of vitamin B_{12}). Three substances stimulate the oxyntic cells to produce hydrochloric acid—acetylcholine, gastrin, and histamine. Histamine is an important agent for the exogenous stimulation of gastric secretion but does not have an important physiologic role in acid secretion.[60]

Studies on gastric secretion and function in CF are limited. Roulet et al[61] studied five CF teenagers with pancreatic insufficiency. Gastric emptying time and gastric secretion rate were similar to controls. Gastric lipolysis is due to a pregastric lipase originating in von Ebners glands in the posterior third of the tongue. Lingual lipase activity was measured in eight other CF patients and eight controls. Lipase activity was higher ($P < 0.05$) in CF patients than controls. Intragastric lipolysis of a butterfat triglyceride test meal was fast in both groups, but more extensive ($P < 0.05$) in CF patients than in controls. The authors concluded that gastric function contributing to the first stage of fat digestion was present in CF and that the elevated intragastric lipase might reflect a compensatory mechanism.

Cox et al[62] performed basal and pentagastrin-stimulated gastric acid secretory studies on 40 patients with CF (11.6 ± 6.7 years) and 13 controls. All CF patients had steatorrhea. Fasting serum gastrin levels in 20 CF patients were normal. Significant elevations in mean basal acid output ($P < 0.05$), maximal acid output ($P < 0.001$), and peak acid outputs per hour per kilogram body weight ($P < 0.001$) were found in CF compared to controls.

Protein Absorption

Procedures to measure nitrogen balance include: (1) metabolic balance studies where diets of known composition are fed and fecal nitrogen measured; (2) timed blood or urine concentration curves (an indirect approach which may produce artifacts and does not produce quantitative absorption data); (3) intubation methods where test meals containing "markers" are fed and the intestinal contents sampled periodically with an indwelling tube; and (4) intestinal perfusion techniques, preferably employing a double-lumen tube. In CF, data from methods 1 and 4 have been obtained. Protein digestion is also discussed in Chapter 17.

Dietary protein accounts for 11–14% of the daily caloric intake and amounts to 70–100 g/day in adults. In addition to exogenous (dietary) protein which accounts for 65–90% of postprandial intraintestinal protein, there is a significant amount of endogenous protein from secretions and sloughed mucosal cells.[63] Since only 1–2 g/day of protein nitrogen is found in feces, the assimilation process is remarkably efficient. Protein digestion proceeds through the catalytic actions of gastric pepsin and then through the action of trypsin, chymotrypsin, elastase, and carboxypeptidases from pancreatic juice. Gastric pepsin liberates about 15% of the available amino-nitrogen, the rest being accounted for by the pancreatic enzymes. The proteases are synthesized in the pancreatic acinar cells as inactive proenzymes (or zymogens) and are secreted into the duodenum where initial activation by the proenzyme trypsinogen is catalyzed by enterokinase to convert it to the active trypsin.

The initial stage of digestion of dietary protein accomplished by sequential action of activated proteases within the intestinal lumen yields about 30% neutral and basic amino acids and 70% small peptides.[63] Enzymes hydrolyzing small peptides are present in the intestinal epithelial cell. Ten to 20% of intestinal dipeptidase activity is present in the brush border, the remainder being attributable to intracellular (soluble) peptidases. It seems probable that only the neutral and basic amino acids are normally transported into the cell in the form of amino acids and that the others enter the cell primarily as constituents of small peptides that are hydrolyzed by specific intracellular peptidases.

Dipeptidases are particularly prominent in the cytosal fraction, whereas trito octapeptidases are found at the brush border. The activity of L-alanyl-L-phenylalanine hydrolase, a cytoplasmic peptide hydrolase, was significantly reduced in 37 CF children compared to controls and was as low as in children with gluten-induced enteropathy.[25] Peptides may be more efficiently absorbed than free amino acids in the normal adult,[64,65] but this may not occur with pancreatic insufficiency as with cystic fibrosis.

Chase et al[8] were surprised that low serum protein levels were not found more frequently in CF children. Data on serum albumin levels in newly diagnosed infants and children with CF are limited. In our experience the serum albumin is frequently below normal in infants and younger children at diagnosis but rapidly returns to normal after the addition of pancreatic enzymes.

The association of hypoproteinemia, edema, and anemia is well recognized in infants with CF[66–69] and occurred in 5% of our clinic population. This complication is thought to be aggravated by feeding a formula containing soybean protein[68] with 80% of the undigested nitrogen being excreted in the feces. Shahidi et al[66] documented a fall in serum albumin from 4.0 to 2.56 g/dl over 30 days in a CF infant fed a soy formula. The normal half-life of ^{131}I-labeled albumin excluded an exudative enteropathy. These observations suggest that in the presence of pancreatic insufficiency, digestion, absorption, or both, of soybean protein is more affected than cow's milk protein. Albumin levels in 138 CF children less than 10 years of age under therapy with pancreatic enzymes were in the normal range.[52]

Albumin metabolism was investigated with [^{125}I]albumin and [^{51}Cr]albumin metabolic studies in 19 older CF patients with a mean age of 14 years (range 8–25 years).[70] Ten patients had hypoalbuminemia. The mean plasma volume of hypoalbuminemic patients was 57.4 ± 9.4 cc/kg, while that of normoalbuminemic patients and controls was 43.6 ± 3.1 cc/kg and 42.0 ± 4.4 cc/kg, respectively. Mean albumin synthetic rates, total circulating albumin, and fractional catabolic rates in the three groups did not differ significantly. Hypoalbuminemia in older patients with CF results primarily from dilution of a normal albumin mass by an enlarged plasma volume. Seven of the 14 patients with CF demonstrated slightly increased gastrointestinal clearance of [^{51}Cr]albumin. This was a contributory, but relatively minor, factor in the production of hypoalbuminemia. Two of six patients with liver involvement exhibited decreased albumin synthetic rates. In one of these two cases, hyposynthesis was a significant contributing factor to hypoalbuminemia. The authors concluded that hypoalbuminemia in patients with advanced CF is suggestive of severe cor pulmonale.

West et al,[71] in a classic paper, measured the changes in blood amino nitrogen levels in normal infants and CF infants following ingestion of whole proteins and protein hydrolysates. They found that protein hydrolysates were better absorbed in infants with CF than are whole proteins and recommended them as the formula of choice. Data on amino acid absorption in CF are limited. Morin et al[25] studied intestinal uptake of three ^{14}C-labeled amino acids in jejunal biopsy specimens from 37 children with CF, 16 with gluten-induced enteropathy, and 18 controls. Uptake of lysine was normal in CF patients, whereas that of phenylalanine and cycloleucine were reduced as compared to controls.

These studies were extended by Milla et al,[72] who performed in vivo perfusion studies in 11 CF patients, 3 patients with other forms of pancreatic insufficiency, and 12 controls. Net absorption rates of phenylalanine and glycine were significantly reduced in CF patients compared to controls. However, absorption of lysine and the dipeptide glycyl-L-phenylalanine was not significantly different from the controls. Absorption of glycine from the dipeptide solution was markedly increased in the CF patients compared with its absorption from the amino acid solutions.

These results demonstrated an in vivo defect in the absorption of neutral amino acids from the proximal jejunum in cystic fibrosis. The normal absorption of lysine and glycyl-L-phenylalanine suggests that in CF there exists a relative abnormality in the mucosal transport system responsible for absorption of neutral amino acids. Interestingly, the absorption of phenylalanine was impaired in other forms of pancreatic insufficiency, and the authors speculated that the exocrine pancreas might play a role in modulating phenylalanine transport and other mucosal transport systems. However, the abnormal gastrointestinal hormonal responses found in CF[73] and other structural abnormalities found on electron microscopic examination of the intestine in CF[26] could also be factors.

Two major classes of lipoproteins, low density and high density, are decreased in the serum of patients with CF.[74] Major apoproteins are also decreased. However, others[8] have been unable to confirm these findings. Since essential fatty acids and the fat-soluble vitamins A, E, and K depend on lipoproteins for transport in the serum, deficiencies of these proteins might have important consequences for the patient with cystic fibrosis.

Shmerling et al[75] performed studies of fecal fat and nitrogen in a large series of healthy children and in children with malabsorption. Normal infants below one year of age excrete up to 3–4 g of fat per day, whereas the upper limit in healthy children was 3 g/day and in adolescents up to 5 g/day (71 controls). Fecal nitrogen excretion in controls was 1 g/day for infants and 1.2 g/day for children. Figure 16-6 shows the correlation between fecal fat in grams per day and fecal nitrogen in grams per day in the controls and children with malabsorption. Fifty patients had untreated celiac disease, and 11 patients had untreated exocrine pancreatic insufficiency of whom 9 had cystic fibrosis. Figure 15-6 shows that the fecal nitrogen (azotorrhea) correlated with the steatorrhea, and the highest values for both were found in untreated CF children.

Similar data was reported in an older CF population (age 12–17 years) by Lapey et al.[76] The amount of steatorrhea and azotorrhea varied greatly between individual CF patients regardless of age at diagnosis, age at study, height, weight, or state of nutrition. In older patients, clinical symptoms, state of nutrition, and growth achieved did not correlate with the amount of steatorrhea and azotorrhea. Lapey et al[76] stated that the growth failure and state of nutrition correlated more closely with the pulmonary state than with pancreatic deficiency.

Studies on the fecal amino acid pattern of CF children show excess losses involving most of the amino acids found in proteins, together with some of their decarboxylation products, amines, and non-alpha amino acids compared to controls.[77] Seakins et al[78] proposed the following possible sources of fecal amino acids in CF: (1) impaired absorption of amino acids (transport defect, barrier of mucus, and interference by other malabsorbed materials); (2) excess secretion of amino acids; (3) pancreatic supplements; (4) effect of antibiotics; and (5) bacterial degradation of partially digested protein.

In a subsequent detailed study, Seakins et al[79] presented evidence that excess fecal amino acids in CF are derived from unabsorbed dietary protein. Changes in the absorption of fat and nitrogen had little effect on the amino acid patterns. The amino acid pattern improved following the introduction of a protein hydrolysate formula. The recent demonstration of altered intestinal amino acid absorption in CF[72] suggests that the situation is more complicated. The significance of this loss of fecal amino acids is difficult to assess. Seakins et al[79] used sulfonamides and streptomycin to detect changes in the fecal amino acid patterns. It is possible that other antibiotics could more effectively change the fecal flora and reduce this fecal amino acid loss secondary to bacterial proteolysis.[116]

Pancreatic extracts reduce fecal nitrogen excretion.[75] Forstner et al[80] showed that fecal nitrogen increases linearly with nitrogen intake in patients on pancreatic supplements at a rate of about twice normal. They concluded that the defect in nitrogen absorption was less severe than that seen with fat in cystic fibrosis. They also noted that the addition of cimetidine and bicarbonate to pancreatic enzymes failed to influence azotorrhea as strikingly as steatorrhea.

Summary The major abnormalities in protein metabolism in CF are found in untreated infants who present with edema, anemia, and hypoalbuminemia. The fecal nitrogen loss in CF children is about twice normal, but less than the loss of fat. In older patients hypoalbuminemia is related to a dilutional effect secondary to the increased plasma volume and cor pulmonale. An excessive loss of fecal amino acids is present in CF and is thought to be mainly the result of bacterial proteolytic action on unhydrolyzed protein. Some evidence for an intestinal mucosal defect for the absorption of certain amino acids has been reported. Most abnormalities in the protein status of CF patients reverse under treatment with pancreatic enzymes, but detailed analysis of serum amino acid metabolism is lacking.

Carbohydrate Absorption

Normal The pattern of carbohydrate ingestion changes with age. During infancy lactose accounts for 35–55% of the dietary carbohydrate.[81] The average adult in developed countries consumes 350 g of carbohydrate per day of which 60% is starch, 30% sucrose, and 10% lactose.[82] Starch is a polymer of glucose in the form of amylose and amylopectin, the principle dietary starch. The important disaccharides are lactose (glucose–galactose), sucrose (glucose–fructose), and maltose (glucose–glucose). Both salivary and pancreatic amylase act to break down the amylose to maltose and maltotriose, and the amylopectin to maltose, maltotriose, and limit dextrins.

Digestion of carbohydrates begins in the mouth with the action of salivary amylase on starch. Gastric acidity rapidly inactivates salivary amylase, and digestion of starch continues within the lumen of the small intestine by the action of pancreatic α-amylase. The disaccharides are hydrolyzed by disaccharidases (maltase, isomaltase, sucrase, and lactase) situated in the brush border of the mucosal cell, and the appropriate sugar substrate enters the intestinal cell.

The developmental pattern of the disaccharidases has been extensively studied in man.[13] Active transport of sugars requires Na^+ and is an energy-dependent mechanism, probably with sugar binding to a common carrier, but there is considerable controversy about the exact relationship between hydrolysis and transport.[83] Xylose is a pentose which is absorbed in the duodenum and proximal jejunum and is actively transported by the small intestine via the sugar transport mechanism but has a low affinity for the carrier. Xylose is used as a test of upper intestinal mucosal function and is sensitive to damage caused by gastroenteritis, gluten-induced enteropathy, and occasionally in milk-induced allergy.[84]

Cystic fibrosis Pancreatic amylase activity is very low in the duodenal fluid of healthy infants under 6 months old.[85] Pancreatic amylase is absent in the duodenum of the 85% of patients with CF without pancreatic function. However, in the 15% of CF patients with variable degrees of pancreatic function, amylase activity is detected.[86] Moreover, in these patients there may be a dissociation of activity of the different enzymes. Eventually all enzyme activity is lost, but this process varies considerably from patient to patient. The order of decreasing enzyme activity detected in CF patients by the pancreozymin–secretin test was carboxypeptidase A, trypsin, amylase, chymotrypsin, and lipase.[87]

Davidson et al[88] postulated that in CF the salivary amylase activity is increased and that this could compensate for the loss of pancreatic α-amylase. Presumably the normal maltase activity in the intestinal mucosa in CF is sufficient to complete starch digestion.[25] Data on starch absorption in untreated CF patients with steatorrhea shows marked impairment,[85] but once pancreatic supplements (which contain amylase) are given, starch is well tolerated.

Glucose absorption in CF appears to be normal until it is affected by pancreatic islet

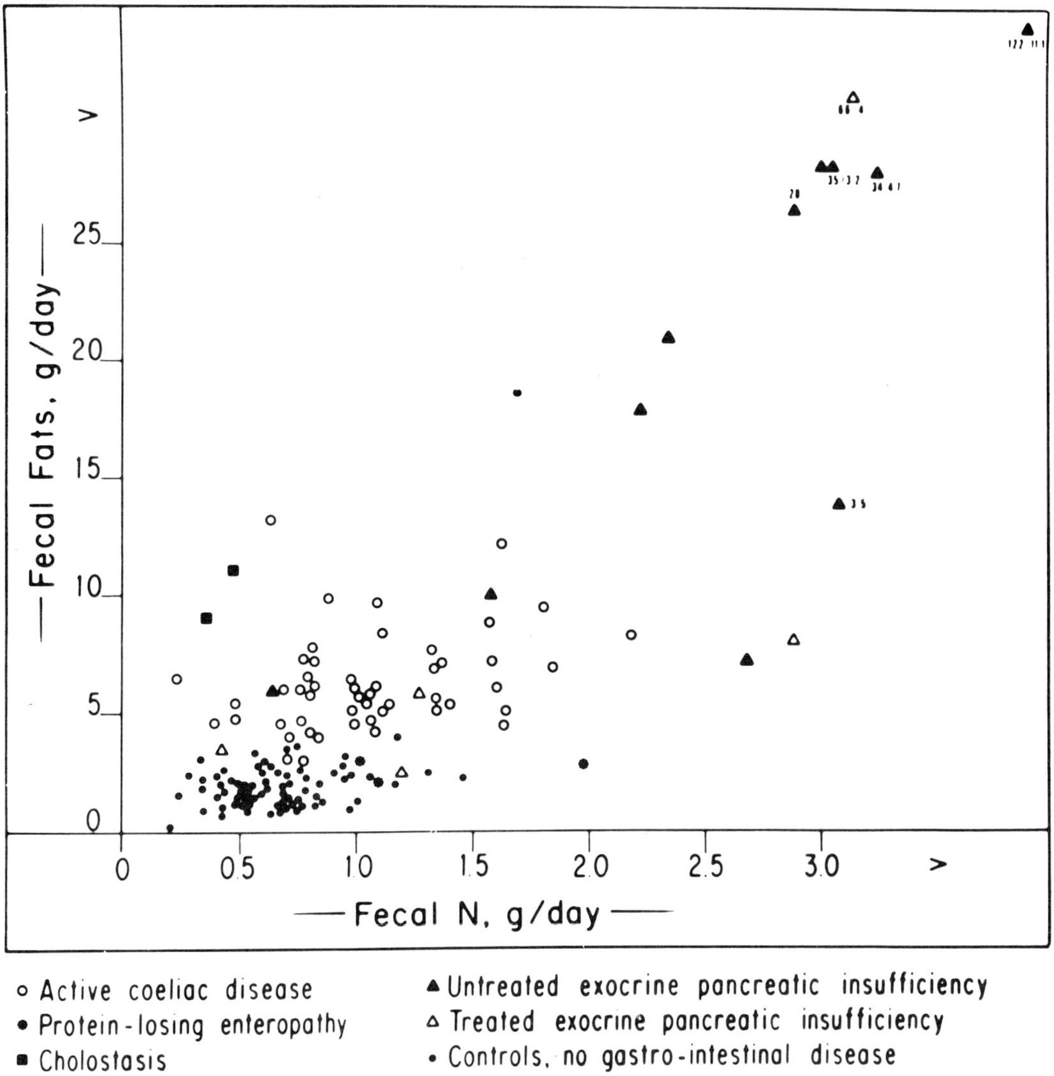

Figure 15-6 Correlation between fecal fat (g/day) and fecal nitrogen (g/day) in control subjects and in patients with malabsorption and maldigestion. Reproduced from Shmerling DH, et al: *Pediatrics* 1970;46:690 (reference 75), with permission. Copyright American Academy of Pediatrics 1970.

cell degeneration, when a diabetic glucose tolerance curve may be found.[89] Absorption of disaccharides in CF were studied by Gibbons[90] and found to be normal except in one patient who had had a bowel resection for meconium ileus. The activity of the disaccharidases was studied by small intestinal biopsy and found to be normal[25] or increased[91] for maltase and sucrase. The activity of lactase was depressed in 23% of one series of 37 children.[25]

In the other series of 63 patients,[91] those children under 5 years of age had normal activity, but in the older patients a group was found that had low lactase activity. However, none of the patients with depressed lactase activity had clinical symptoms following lactose ingestion. The lactase deficiency is considered a manifestation of a genetic deficiency and unrelated to cystic fibrosis.

Xylose absorption in CF appears to be increased above controls, both by the 1-hr blood absorption test[84,92] and in the urine.[76]

These findings indicate that the mucosal surface appears to be intact in CF for the absorption of small molecules such as xylose.

Fat Absorption

Normal Most diets provide 30–55% of calories from fat. The adult ingests 60–100 g of fat daily. The natural fats consist of 98–99% triglycerides containing three long-chain fatty acids (95% by weight) and a glycerol backbone (5% by weight). The remaining 1–2% includes phospholipids, free fatty acids, monoglycerides, diglycerides, cholesterol, and other nonsaponifiable matter. Phospholipids are essential components of cell membranes and other cellular components. They form a large percentage of the lipids of serum and are important in absorption and transport of fatty acids.

Naturally occurring fatty acids contain 4–24 carbon atoms in a molecule. Long-chain fatty acids contain 12 or more carbon atoms and of these, fatty acids with 16 and 18 carbon atoms predominate. About 51% of the fatty acids of breast milk and 43% of the fatty acids of cow's milk have 18 carbon atoms in the chain. Triglycerides with long-chain fatty acids yield 9 kcal/g on combustion. Medium-chain triglycerides contain 8–10 carbon atoms, yield 8.3 kcal/g, and are more readily absorbed than long-chain fatty acids. Short-chain fatty acids containing 4–6 carbon atoms are not abundant in food fats and yield only 5.3 kcal/g.[93]

Fatty acids are classified according to the number of reaction (unsaturated or "double bond") linkages between the carbon atoms. Saturated fatty acids are devoid of double bonds, are more stable, and account for the firmness of fats at room temperature. The most common fatty acids in natural fats are palmitic (16 carbon atoms) and stearic (18 carbon atoms). Monounsaturated fatty acids (monoenoic) have one double-bond linkage; oleic acid has one double-bond linkage and 18 carbon atoms and furnishes one third of all the fatty acids in human milk and cow's milk. Polyunsaturated fatty acids are classified as dienoic, trienoic, and tetraenoic, depending on the number of double-bond linkages. Of greatest interest are linoleic (18 carbon atoms, 2 double bonds), arachidonic (20 carbon atoms, 4 double bonds), and linolenic (18 carbon atoms, 3 double bonds).[93]

The most important steps in fat absorption are:[83] (1) intraluminal phase, requiring pancreatic lipase and bile salts; (2) passage into mucosal cell; (3) reesterification to triglyceride within the mucosal cell; (4) chylomicron formation; and (5) entry of chylomicron into lymphatics.

The details of fat absorption and the abnormalities in fatty acids and fat-soluble vitamins in CF are discussed in detail in Chapters 16 and 17. However, since pancreatic insufficiency is the major cause of the malabsorption and growth retardation in CF, it is important to discuss some of this information.

Triglyceride is insoluble in the intraluminal intestinal water but is acted on by secreted pancreatic lipase which functions at the oil–water interface to split off the two fatty acids from the alpha positions, leaving the single fatty acid combined with the glycerol as the beta monoglyceride (Figure 15-7). Colipase is also required for pancreatic lipase to become active. The released long-chain fatty acids and the monoglyceride are insoluble in water and are brought into the intraluminal solution by combining with the secreted bile acid in a physicochemical complex called the micelle. At sufficient intraluminal concentrations of secreted bile acids (the critical micellar concentration), bile acids become oriented to form a sphere. The fatty acids, monoglycerides, and fat-soluble vitamins (A, D, E, and K) become imbedded in the micelle. The diglycerides and triglycerides require hydrolysis by lipase to become monoglycerides of fatty acid for absorption. The micelle disintegrates at the intestinal surface membrane, allowing the released monoglyceride and fatty acids to enter the lipoprotein membrane of the intestinal cell. The bile acids remain within the lumen of the intestine for further micelle formation and are reabsorbed in the terminal ileum in the enterohepatic circulation.

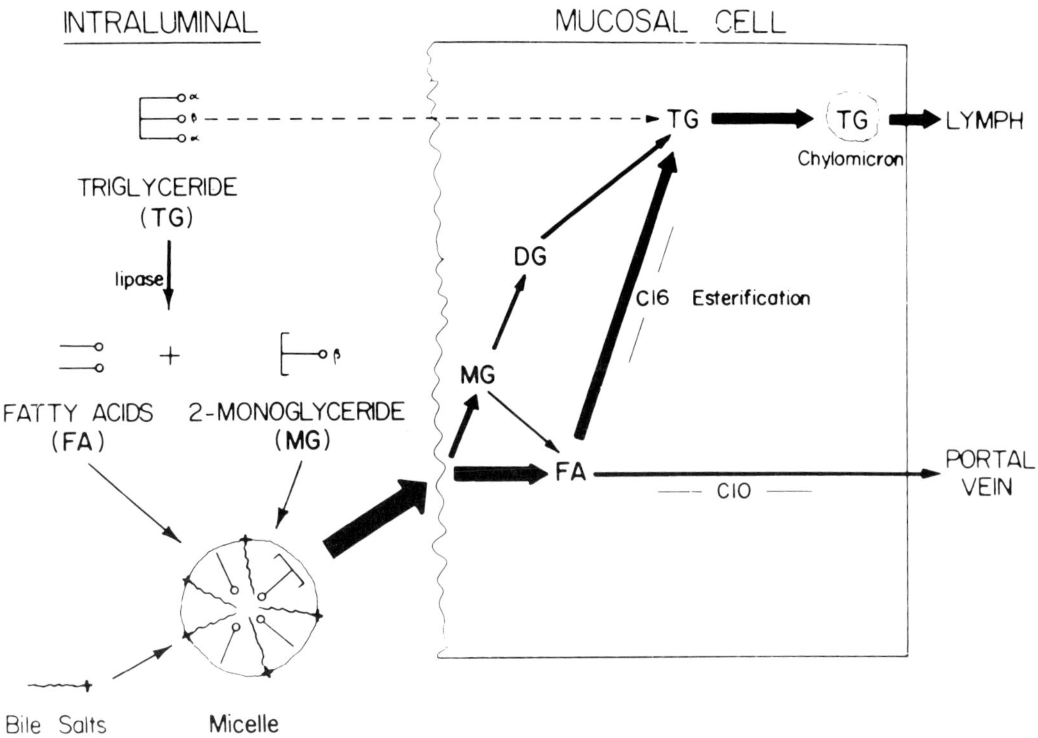

Figure 15-7 Fat digestion and absorption. Structures are represented diagrammatically as well as by name. See text for elaboration. Reproduced from Gray GM: In Sleisinger MH, Fordtran JS (eds): *Gastrointestinal Disease, Pathophysiology, Diagnosis, Management,* Philadelphia, WB Saunders, 1973, p 251 (reference 94), with permission.

This is a very efficient mechanism, with 95% of the bile acid being reabsorbed in a single recirculation. The fatty acids and monoglyceride in the intestinal cell are reesterified to triglyceride by intracellular enzymes and then combine into a large particle called the chylomicron, which is coated with protein, cholesterol, and phospholipid, and preferentially enters the lacteal to the thoracic duct and the venous system.[94]

A low-molecular-weight cytosolic protein, fatty acid binding protein, has been isolated from the intestine.[95] This protein avidly binds fatty acids (preferentially unsaturated long-chain fatty acids) and appears to function as an intracellular transport protein for long-chain fatty acids. This protein is closely related or identical to the Z protein for which a role as a cytoplasmic binding protein for organic anions and dyes was proposed.[96]

Medium-chain triglycerides (MCT, carbon chain 6–10) can be absorbed intact (up to 30% of an oral dose). They are acted upon avidly by pancreatic lipase, are more stable in water than long-chain fatty acids, and form micelles more readily with the bile acids. In the intestinal cell they are not reesterified, but exit as fatty acids directly to the capillary venous system and portal vein (Figure 15-8). This greater efficiency of handling of MCT at several stages of digestion/absorption is the reason for their use in patients with malabsorption.[94]

Pancreatic insufficiency Pancreatic secretion may be reduced to 10% of normal without azatorrhea or steatorrhea; when between 2 and 10% of normal output, mild to moderate steatorrhea (less than 25 g/day) ensues; and when between 0 and 2% of normal capacity to secrete enzymes, steatorrhea is profound (25–80 g/day).[97] Theoretically, in the patient with pancreatic insufficiency steatorrhea should be abolished, if oral pancreatin could assure the arrival of exogenous lipase in the duodenum in amounts equivalent to 10% of normal. In practice, restoration of normal fat balance is not easily achieved by oral enzyme therapy.[98]

Fat malabsorption in CF *Pancreatic function* Numerous studies in CF have documented the gross steatorrhea in 85% of patients with pancreatic insufficiency.[9,38,75,76,85] Prospective studies on the loss of pancreatic function in CF are limited as the methods for documenting this decrease in function were cumbersome (fecal fat estimation, secretin-pancreozymin stimulation test).

A noninvasive method of assessing pancreatic function indirectly by administering a synthetic peptide that requires chymotrypsin for cleavage and measuring the *p*-aminobenzoic acid in the urine may offer a methodology to follow patients with CF and document more accurately the percentage of remaining pancreatic function.[99,100] Plasma immunoreactive trypsin is elevated in infants with CF and below normal in older children and adults. Prospective measurements of circulating immunoreactive trypsin could be a useful measure of pancreatic function.[101] Current methods for calculating the dosage of pancreatic enzymes for replacement are largely clinical, consisting of observations of number and type of bowel movements and weight gain.

Fecal fat The range of fecal fat excretion in 190 untreated CF patients showed that up to 80% of the ingested fat may be excreted.[80] An enormous range of steatorrhea was found, with 72% of patients having a fecal fat greater than 30% of intake. The mean fecal fat excretion as percentage of intake was 38.5%. The excretory rate of fat was 18.3 times the rate for excretion in the normal subject. With pancreatic supplements, the amount of fat excreted per unit of fat intake was still 12–13 times normal. The average improvement in fat excretion with

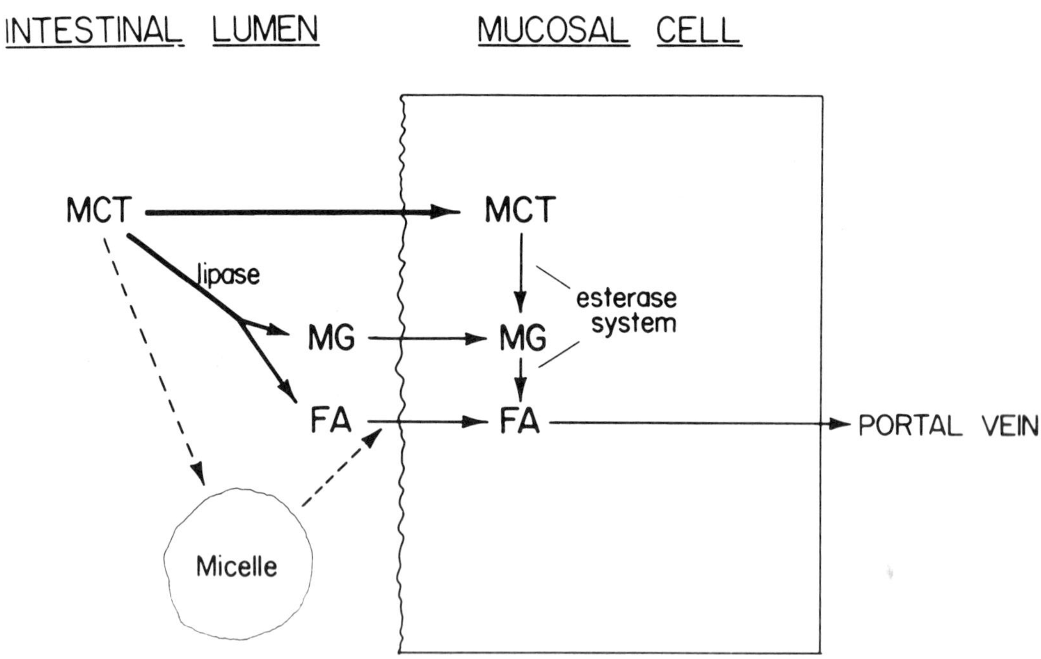

Figure 15-8 Fate of medium-chain triglyceride (MCT) in the intestine. Comparison with Figure 15-7 reveals that MCT has advantages over dietary fat (LCT) at each stage of digestion and absorption. Reproduced from Gray GM: In Sleisinger MH, Fordtran JS (eds): *Gastrointestinal Disease, Pathophysiology, Diagnosis, Management,* Philadelphia, WB Saunders, 1973, p 252 (reference 94), with permission.

supplements of cimetidine, sodium bicarbonate, and the combination of cimetidine and sodium bicarbonate for each routine was 33%. Durie et al[102] showed that at fat intakes under 120 g/day, fat excretion was more affected by cimetidine and bicarbonate than at higher intakes. They concluded that the amount of pancreatic enzyme required by a patient appears to be directly influenced by the amount of substrate in the diet.

Another important therapeutic observation concerns the digestion of medium-chain triglycerides (MCTs) which are contained in the formula Pregestimil, the formula of choice in infants with cystic fibrosis. Durie et al[103] showed that fat excretion was greatly improved by the addition of pancreatic enzymes to the MCT-containing formula, falling from a mean of 26% of intake to 8.6% of intake. These findings fit in with what is known of the normal digestion of MCTs as described earlier in this section.

Absorption of fatty acids The intestinal absorption of saturated and unsaturated long-chain fatty acids has been compared experimentally in rats.[104] Although intraluminal solubility of palmitate (a saturated fatty acid) is less than linoleate (an unsaturated fatty acid), initial uptake of the two lipids by intestinal mucosa was similar. However, significant differences in rate of entry into the cell and/or rate of microsomal metabolism result, for the saturated fatty acid, in a significantly less rapid reesterification and therefore overall absorption. These findings were thought to account for the greater absorption of unsaturated fatty acids reported in patients with steatorrhea.

Fernandes et al[105] found that fatty acid absorption in children with steatorrhea was determined by three factors: (1) chain length—the absorption was found to decrease as the chain length rises; (2) degree of saturation—fatty acids with one or more double bonds are absorbed to a greater degree than are their saturated counterparts, and the C_{18} polyunsaturated acids were absorbed more completely than is oleic acid; and (3) the composition of the dietary fats—the degree of absorption of any given fatty acid was greater if it was fed with less-well-absorbed fatty acids. They recommended that patients with steatorrhea should be fed unsaturated fats.

Limited studies of radioactively labeled fatty acids in CF have shown that oleic acid and palmitic acid are poorly absorbed.[106,107] On theoretical grounds, the fatty acid absorption would have been expected to be normal if pancreatic achylia was the only lesion. Kuo and Huang[108] studied the effects of medium-chain triglycerides upon fat absorption, plasma lipids, and depot fat in children with cystic fibrosis. Despite the abnormally depressed plasma and tissue polyunsaturated fatty acid levels encountered in these children, further decreases in the relative proportions of linoleic and arachidonic acids after medium-chain triglyceride feeding for a period of 5–9 months were noted. Surprisingly, clinical manifestations of essential fatty acid deficiency did not appear and, moreover, the feeding actually helped to promote growth and development in these patients. In another study by Lloyd-Still et al[109] a high linoleic acid supplement in the diet of 11 CF patients did not correct the essential fatty acid deficiency.

These observations show that there are a variety of abnormalities in fatty acid absorption in CF, and there is some evidence that the interconversion of the various fatty acids may be abnormal and possibly related to changes in desaturase activity. Further studies are required to try and delineate the defects in fatty acid metabolism, if we are to understand how to approach the problem of dietary supplementation in these patients.

Vitamins, trace metals, and fatty acids For detailed discussion of this subject, see Chapter 16.

Bile acid abnormalities Abnormalities in bile salt kinetics, serum levels, and fecal losses of bile acids are discussed in Chapter 18. Bile acid pool size is low in untreated infants and children with CF and returns to normal with pancreatic enzyme replacement.[110] Total bile acid synthesis changes little with therapy. Bile acid malabsorption has been demonstrated by several investigators, and the fecal bile acid losses vary between 24 and 57 mg/kg/day in most studies.[110-114] The bile acid losses are best explained by the binding of bile acid to undigested protein, fiber, or carbohydrate,[110,113] although Harries et al[115] disagree and hypothesize that there may be a defect in the primary mucosal phase of bile salt absorption similar to that seen with amino acids in cystic fibrosis. Fecal bile acid loss is normal in CF children without steatorrhea.

Smalley et al[114] studied 16 CF children with steatorrhea and compared three regimens of diet and therapy: a normal diet with pancreatic supplement, a diet of reduced long-chain triglycerides with added medium-chain triglycerides, and the same diet with added pancreatic supplements. On each of these three regimens steatorrhea and fecal bile acid loss were significantly less than on no treatment, with the lowest excretion occurring on the diet of reduced long-chain triglycerides with added medium-chain triglycerides and pancreatic enzyme supplements.

Roy et al[116] studied fecal fat, bile acid, and rectal microflora in 7 control children and in three groups of CF children: 7 off antibiotics, 10 on oral cloxacillin, and 6 on intravenous cloxacillin, gentamicin, and carbenicillin for at least two weeks. Antibiotics had little or no effect on fat excretion, but led to a significant decrease ($P < 0.01$) of fecal bile acid on the triple-antibiotic therapy. Reduced deconjugation of bile acids and formation of secondary bile acids was associated with a marked reduction of the anaerobic flora in the children on triple therapy compared to controls. They suggested that the reduction of the anaerobic flora by antibiotics in CF decreases the adsorption of bile acids to dietary residues and microbes, thus favoring bile acid absorption and leading to decreased fecal loss of bile acids. These observations are compatible with the improvement in growth noted in CF infants treated with antibiotics.

Studies on duodenal bile acids in CF[115] showed changes in total bile acid concentration, glycine–taurine conjugate ratios, and percentage of dihydroxy bile acids that contribute to lowering of the critical micellar concentration. Furthermore, biliary lipid is lithogenic in untreated CF and responds to pancreatic enzymes.[117] Serum bile acids did not increase significantly in untreated CF patients following meals compared to controls,[118] but they returned to normal with pancreatic enzyme supplementation. Addition of cimetidine to pancreatic enzymes significantly decreased the postprandial serum bile acid concentration compared to the response seen with enzymes alone.[113] The authors were unable to interpret whether decreased gallbladder contractility, decreased intestinal transit, or increased hepatic extraction of bile acids from portal blood was responsible for these abnormalities.

Summary Children with CF excrete large amounts of bile acids in their stools. This leads to decreased duodenal concentration, a contracted pool size, and a biliary lipid composition with a high lithogenic index. This disorder of bile acid metabolism is not present in CF without pancreatic insufficiency, and responds to some extent to pancreatic enzyme supplementation. It can be further reduced by a diet low in long-chain fatty acids with added medium-chain triglycerides. Antibiotics that reduce the anaerobic fecal flora also reduce fecal bile acid loss. The pathogenesis of the bile acid malabsorption in CF remains obscure, but is consistent with a broken enterohepatic circulation. Intraluminal factors such as increased adsorption of bile acids to dietary residues have been postulated, but other factors may be involved.

Gastrointestinal Hormones in CF

Knowledge of the gastrointestinal hormones has resulted from the ability to measure minute amounts of these substances by radioimmunoassay. The polypeptides located in the "gut" endocrine organ are also found in the central nervous system where they exert neurotransmitter function. They are classified as follows[119]: (1) the gastrin family, which consists of gastrin, cholecystokinin (CCK), and related peptides; (2) the secretin family, consisting of secretin, pancreatic glucagon, gastric inhibitory polypeptide (GIP), and vasoactive intestinal polypeptide (VIP); and (3) other hormones and polypeptides, enteroglucagon, somatostatin, motilin, pancreatic polypeptide, neurotensin, substance P, and bombesin.

Insulin and pancreatic glucagon belong to the gastrointestinal hormones in a broader sense and these are discussed in Chapter 19.

Adrian et al[73] studied the pancreatic and gut hormone response to a milk drink in 10 children with cystic fibrosis. Plasma insulin and gastric inhibitory polypeptide were significantly reduced in CF compared to controls ($P < 0.05$ and $P < 0.005$, respectively). Fasting levels of pancreatic polypeptide were significantly lower in CF ($P < 0.01$), and fasting enteroglucagon levels were significantly elevated in CF ($P < 0.001$). No significant differences were seen in basal or postmilk responses of plasma glucagon, gastrin, secretin, vasoactive intestinal peptide, or motilin in cystic fibrosis. The authors concluded that in CF the pancreatic polypeptide cell is more susceptible to the effects of the disease process than the beta or alpha cell. Some aspects of the abnormalities in the gastrointestinal endocrine system were similar to those seen in celiac disease and in tropical sprue. These abnormalities in hormonal response may contribute to the failure to restore the steatorrhea to normal in CF despite adequate pancreatic enzyme supplementation.

GASTROINTESTINAL MANIFESTATIONS OF CF

Table 15-3 summarizes the clinical complications affecting the gastrointestinal tract in CF and is adapted from several papers.[120-122] Pancreatic complications are discussed in Chapter 17, and the endocrine abnormalities are reviewed in Chapter 19. Vitamin deficiencies are included in Chapter 16. All the clinical complications of liver disease are discussed in Chapter 18. Meconium ileus and associated disorders are discussed in Chapter 11 and 21. Hypoproteinemia is discussed in this chapter under protein absorption.

Table 15-3
Gastrointestinal Manifestations of Cystic Fibrosis

	Approximate Incidence (%)
Pancreas	
Total achylia	80–90
Partial or normal function	10–20
Growth retardation	variable
Glucose intolerance	30–42
Diabetes	2–5
Pancreatitis	<1
Pancreatic calcification	<1
Vitamin deficiencies (A, E, K)	variable
Liver	
Focal biliary fibrosis	14–19
Cirrhosis/portal hypertension	4–5
Neonatal cholestasis	3
Gallstones	7
Obstructive jaundice (postneonatal)	<1
Fatty infiltration	30–66
Intestine	
Meconium ileus, atresia, volvulus	10–15
Rectal prolapse	10–22
Meconium ileus equivalent	10–35
Intussusception	1
Hypoproteinemia	5
Duodenal ulcer	<1
Pneumatosis intestinalis	<1
Appendicitis	<1

Intussusception

Intussusception (Figure 15-9) is a well-recognized complication of CF, occurring in approximately 1% of patients, with an average age of presentation of 9½ years (range 4–16 years).[123] All patients had pancreatic insufficiency. The etiology is similar to meconium ileus equivalent resulting from the thick putty-like inspissated stool in the cecum. In the Holsclaw et al[123] series of 19 patients, an operation was performed in 19 of the 22 episodes. However, since the advent of Gastrografin enema therapy,[124] an operation is rarely required if the diagnosis is recognized early. For further discussion of this complication see Chapter 21.

Rectal Prolapse

Rectal prolapse was reported to occur in 22.6% of 386 patients.[125] Rectal prolapse in CF is related to a combination of steatorrhea, poor musculature secondary to malnutrition, and increased abdominal pressure from chronic coughing. It occurs most frequently between 6 months and 3 years of age and is rarely encountered after 5 years of age. In 16 patients rectal prolapse was the presenting complaint of cystic fibrosis. In three patients the diagnosis of CF was made 7, 8, and 10 years after the initial complaint. Sometimes direct questioning is required to elicit this complication which may have been forgotten by the parents.

In 48 patients rectal prolapse lasted longer than six months. The condition usually responds to dietary therapy and pancreatic supplements. The earlier the diagnosis of CF, the less the likelihood of rectal prolapse. Surgical correction is rarely required. Cystic fibrosis is the commonest cause of rectal prolapse in the pediatric age group in the United States. Rectal prolapse in a child is an indication for a sweat test, irrespective of whether there are symptoms suggestive of cystic fibrosis.

Pneumatosis Intestinalis

This is a rare complication of CF (Figure 15-10) with only two case reports,[126,127] although personal communication has elicited several other unreported cases. Most of these patients are over 18 years of age and have severe pulmonary insufficiency. The patient may be symptom-free and the pneumatosis found as an incidental finding on the chest x-ray; at other times it may cause abdominal pain.

No active treatment is required unless a complication, such as intestinal obstruction, volvulus, perforation, pneumoperitoneum, or hemorrhage, ensues. Pneumatosis intestinalis has been reported in association with rectal prolapse,[127] and we have seen it with diabetes. Few of these patients have survived long after the diagnosis was made; their death is usually from cor pulmonale and unrelated to the pneumatosis. Chronic pulmonary diseases, such as asthma, may be complicated by pneumatosis intestinalis, and it has been postulated that air dissects from the alveoli to the gut via the mediastinum and retroperitoneal space. The pneumatosis in CF usually involves the colon and the origin of the gas in the large intestine is more difficult to explain.

Duodenal Ulcer

In the autopsy study of Oppenheimer and Esterly[19] there were 12 (8%) instances of peptic ulceration involving the stomach and duodenum in 146 patients. One patient had a perforation and another a serious hemorrhage. Most of these findings were considered terminal and the result of stress ulceration. The incidence of duodenal ulcer during life in CF is rare, and the few case reports are poorly documented.[128] This is surprising in view of the deficient pancreatic bicarbonate secretion present in over 80% of these patients together with evidence of gastric hyperacidity.[62] Barium studies in CF are frequently misinterpreted as showing evidence of duodenitis, whereas these abnormalities are the result of the excessive mucus present in the duodenum and not from ulceration. (Figure 15-11) We have personal experience of one 8-year-old CF patient with a duodenal ulcer complicated by hematemesis. Endoscopically documented ulcers in CF have not yet been reported. There are no data at present to substantiate any increased incidence of peptic ulcer in living patients with cystic fibrosis. The treatment of these ulcers is no different from other non-CF patients and could include therapy with cimetidine and antacids.

APPROACH TO NUTRITIONAL THERAPY

The data discussed in this chapter have demonstrated the complexity of factors in-

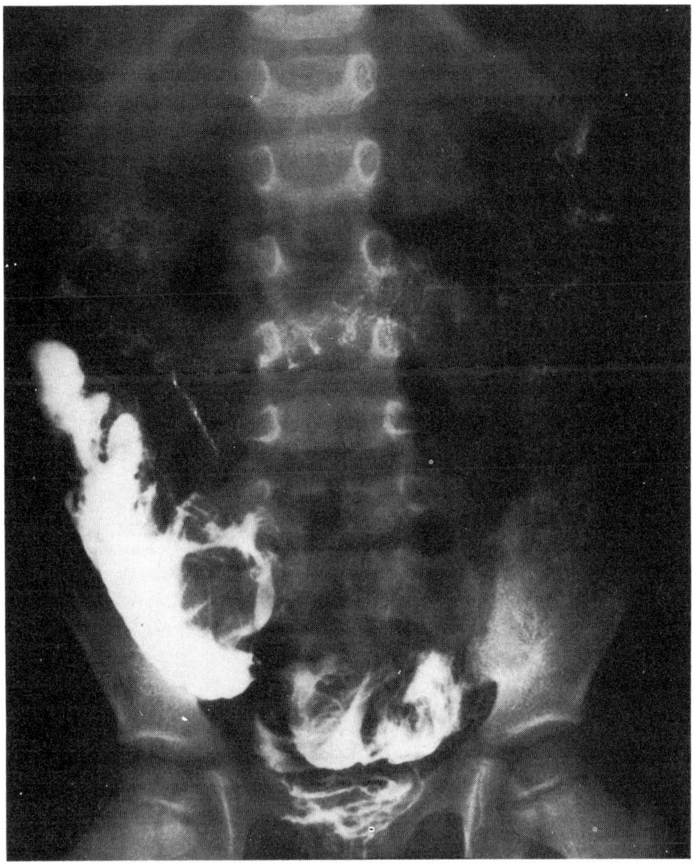

Figure 15-9 Seven-year-old male. The well-defined rounded filling defect is the intussusceptum formed by the small bowel. Its presence on the postevacuation radiographs indicates that the intussuception was not successfully reduced by the barium enema. (Courtesy Dr. Sandra Fernbach.)

volved in our approach to growth failure and nutritional supplementation in these patients. Table 15-4 has been modified from Hubbard[9] to show some of the considerations for individualizing dietary recommendations for patients with cystic fibrosis.

Caloric Intake

Caloric intake has been shown to be deficient in a significant proportion of CF patients. Reduced caloric intake is especially prominent in infants with the severe bronchiolitis syndrome and in older children and adults with cor pulmonale. Adeniyi-Jones et al,[7] in their metabolic balance studies, measured basal oxygen consumption and found that CF patients had a 30% higher basal energy expenditure expressed as basal metabolic rate or as oxygen consumption

Table 15-4
Factors Modifying Our Approach to Dietary Supplementation in Cystic Fibrosis

Factor
Caloric intake/nutritional assessment
Age and activity
Severity of illness/effects of infection
Psychological effects
Degree of pancreatic insufficiency
Fat
Protein
Carbohydrate
Hormonal imbalance, ie, diabetes
Drug interactions

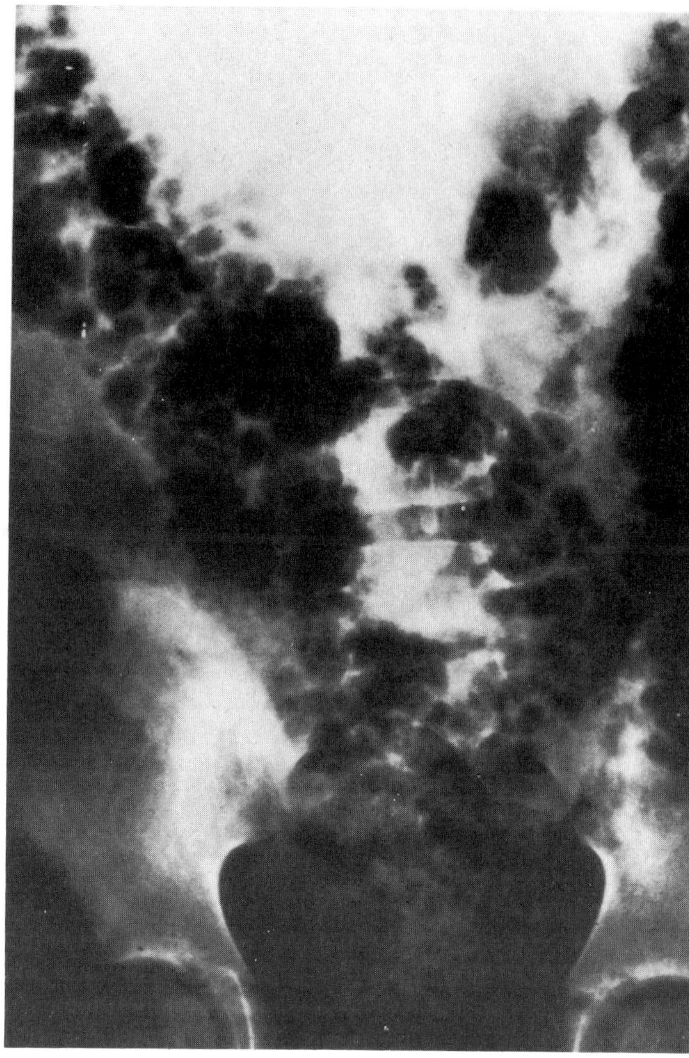

Figure 15-10 The bubbly appearance of the abdomen is due to air in bowel wall—pneumatosis cystoides intestinalis. When pneumatosis occurs in shorter lengths of bowel, it may be difficult to differentiate from meconium ileus equivalent. (Courtesy Dr. William Tooley.)

compared to controls. Similar findings were reported by Cropp and Rosenberg,[129] who showed that as lung function deteriorated and lung disease worsened in CF, total basal oxygen consumption and caloric requirements of the body increased.

When pulmonary dysfunction is marked, basal oxygen consumption may rise to 60–90% above predicted values. When caloric intakes cannot be increased in proportion to the high energy cost of breathing, CF patients will lose weight regardless of the effectiveness of their gastrointestinal absorption (see Figures 15-3 and 15-4).

Detailed nutritional assessment by a skilled nutritionist is a valuable resource and may elicit deficiencies in the family diet that can be corrected. Supplements of snacks, medium-chain triglyceride oil, Polycose, and powdered skim milk are examples of caloric supplementation that are easily available. The replacement of soda by milk or similar nutritious liquids is advised. The best caloric supplement in these patients is still not defined, and it is important not to recommend a diet that is unpalatable or expensive as cooperation will be poor. If we apply principles learned in the care of patients with inflammatory bowel disease, it is more important to try to increase the total caloric intake with foods that the patients enjoy, rather than to be too rigid in what we or the family believe the children should eat. A high-protein diet should be encouraged, and the fat intake should be kept below 100–120 g/day in the older patient.

Effects of Age and Activity

The infant with CF will be benefited by a formula containing medium-chain triglycerides (MCTs), and Pregestimil is recommended. Pancreatic supplements will further significantly decrease the steatorrhea in

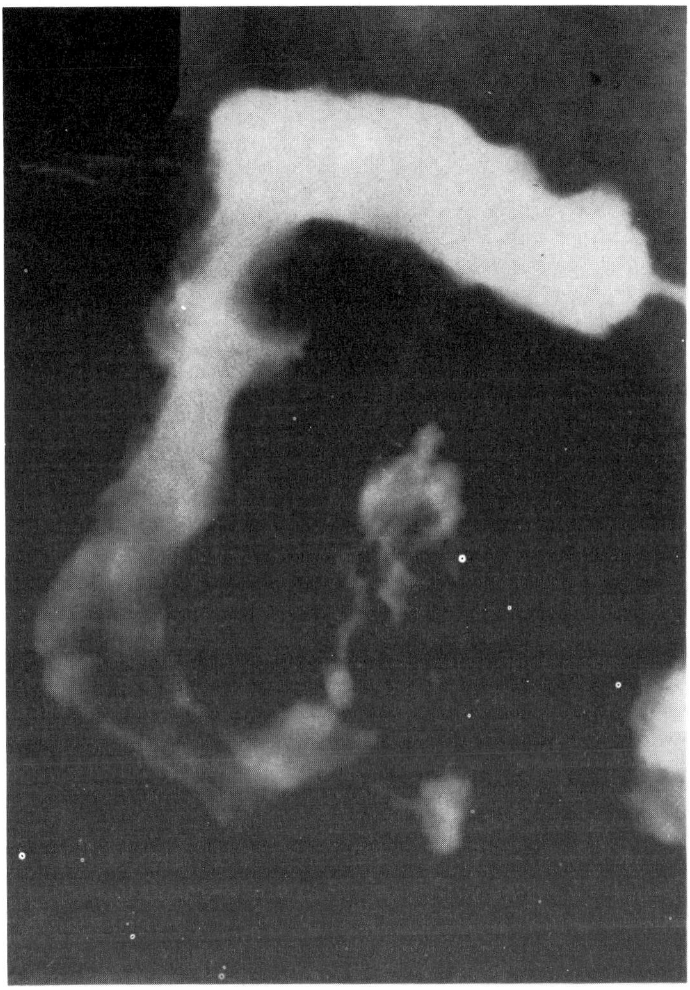

Figure 15-11 Eleven-year-old female. Smudged mucosa and multiple indentation of the barium-filled duodenal loop due to inspissated secretions within Brunner's glands. This appearance may be mistaken for areas of ulceration. Varices which develop in the presence of hepatic fibrosis have a similar appearance. (Courtesy Dr. Sandra Fernbach.)

children on Pregestimil.[103] In older children the addition of MCT oil is beneficial, but unfortunately many patients find it unpalatable.

Increased activity usually increases appetite and can affect caloric intake. Gurwitz et al[6] suggested that this factor is responsible for the increased survival of males with CF compared to females. Data to prove whether increased activity leads to increased coughing and improved pulmonary function, or whether it is the effect on caloric intake that is important, are lacking to test this hypothesis.

Severity of Illness and Effects of Infection

The effects of infection on nutritional parameters have been described. In principle, increased caloric intake and vitamins are required, but it is rarely possible to achieve these goals. Data on the effects of intravenous hyperalimentation to CF patients under these conditions are scanty except for patients with meconium ileus recovering from surgery. The benefits of this form of therapy need to be evaluated in terms of tolerance, acceptability, complications, and expense. Constant infusion of elemental diets through a silicone-lined nasogastric catheter (which can remain in situ for weeks) has been used for children with other diseases (eg, inflammatory bowel disease). Unfortunately, an indwelling nasogastric tube poses problems for the patient with CF by interfering with pulmonary drainage. Isolated reports of this form of therapy have been published,[130] but in our experience this form of therapy is rarely tolerated.

Psychological Factors

The importance of psychological factors aggravating anorexia and decreasing caloric intake cannot be overemphasized. Active intervention is required not only for the individual patient, but for the family that may be functioning poorly owing to depression. This area has a special relevance in the adolescent and older patient who may show marked deterioration in clinical status because of rapid weight loss, leading to decreased pulmonary drainage and exacerbation of pulmonary infection.

Degree of Pancreatic Insufficiency

Pancreatic insufficiency with resultant fat malabsorption is the major cause of the growth failure in cystic fibrosis. Table 15-5 summarizes the conditions in CF associated with impaired lipolysis. In attempting to restore fat malabsorption in CF to normal, numerous variables require consideration, including the efficacy of the various pancreatic preparations, the dosage, dosage schedule, effects of gastric acid, size and composition of meals, and the varying degrees of pancreatic insufficiency in the individual subject. Several of these variables have been studied in CF, such as the effects of enteric-coated pancreatic enzyme preparations, bicarbonate, cimetidine, and long- and medium-chain fatty acid supplementation. Unfortunately, none of these changes restores the steatorrhea in CF to normal, and it is likely there are several other factors involved in CF that are different from other causes of pancreatic insufficiency seen in the adult.

There is a critical intake of fat between 100 and 120 g/day in older patients, over which increased amounts of pancreatic enzymes cease to affect the steatorrhea. At present the role of fatty acid supplementation in CF is difficult to define. Protein malabsorption can be improved with casein hydrolyzates, and the deleterious effects of soy protein in these infants has been mentioned.

Effects of Hormonal Imbalance

Abnormalities in hormone status, such as diabetes, will affect growth failure. The role of anabolic steroids and other hormone abnormalities are discussed in Chapter 19.

Drug Interactions

These can result in positive or negative effects on caloric intake and should always be considered.

Table 15-5
Conditions in CF Associated with Impaired Lipolysis

Altered duodenal pH
  Gastric acid hypersecretion?
Pancreatic insufficiency
  Loss of lipase and bicarbonate secretion
Decreased luminal bile salts
  Decreased hepatic synthesis of bile salts?
  Decreased delivery of bile salts to intestinal lumen
  Decreased effective concentration of conjugated bile salts
  Increased intestinal loss of bile salts
Physical barriers to absorption
  Viscous mucus?
Defects in intestinal mucosal cell function
  Impaired fatty acid absorption
  Defects in fatty acid binding protein?
  Defects in lipoprotein transport?
  Anatomical defects in intestinal structure?
Hormonal imbalance
  Gastrointestinal hormone abnormalities

Summary

The role of dietary supplementation in CF requires carefully controlled trials of individual therapics before specific recommendations can be given. These studies have not yet been performed. It is important to avoid pitfalls in this sensitive area in view of our past history of uncontrolled supplementations such as the Allan diet[131] and claims for supplementation with selenium. Supplements of trace minerals have been recommended by some authorities,[8] but the basis for these recommendations is not at present well documented. Recommendations for vitamin and mineral supplements in CF are discussed in Chapter 16.

ADDENDUM

Since this chapter was written, an excellent comprehensive review of the gastrointestinal manifestations of cystic fibrosis was published by Park and Grand,[132] containing 274 references.

REFERENCES

1. Shwachman H: Cystic fibrosis. *Curr Probl Pediatr* 1978;8:5–72.
2. Sproul A, Huang NN: Growth patterns in children with cystic fibrosis. *J Pediatr* 1964;65:664–676.
3. Kraemer R, Rudeberg A, Hadorn B, et al: Relative underweight in cystic fibrosis and its prognostic value. *Act Paediatr Scand* 1978; 67:33–37.
4. Gaskin K, Gurwitz D, Corey M, et al: Improved pulmonary function in cystic fibrosis patients without pancreatic insufficiency. In *Proceedings Eighth International Congress of Cystic Fibrosis.* Toronto, Canadian Cystic Fibrosis Foundation, 1980, pp 226–230.
5. Corey ML: Longitudinal studies in cystic fibrosis. In *Proceedings Eighth International Congress of Cystic Fibrosis.* Toronto, Canadian Cystic Fibrosis Foundation, 1980, pp 246–255.
6. Gurwitz D, Corey M, Francis PWJ, et al: Perspectives in cystic fibrosis. *Pediatr Clin North Am* 1979;26:603–615.
7. Adeniyi-Jones SK, Suskind R, Kean B, et al: Growth, energy metabolism and T_3 levels in malnutrition in cystic fibrosis. *Cystic Fibrosis Club Abstr* 1979;20:22.
8. Chase HP, Long MA, Lavin MH: Cystic fibrosis and malnutrition. *J Pediatr* 1979;95: 337–347.
9. Hubbard VS: Nutrient requirements of patients with cystic fibrosis. In *Proceedings Eighth International Congress of Cystic Fibrosis.* Toronto, Canadian Cystic Fibrosis Foundation, 1980, pp 149–160.
10. Kirschner BS, Voinchet O, Rosenberg IH: Growth retardation in inflammatory bowel disease. *Gastroenterology* 1978;75:504–511.
11. Kelts DG, Grand RJ, Shen G, et al: Nutritional basis of growth failure in children and adolescents with Crohn's disease. *Gastroenterology* 1979;76:720–727.
12. Rosenberg IH: Nutritional support in inflammatory bowel disease. *Gastroenterology* 1979;77:393–396.
13. Grand RJ, Watkins JB, Torti FM: Development of the human gastrointestinal tract: A review. *Gastroenterology* 1976;70: 790–810.
14. Hanosh M: A review: Fat digestion in the newborn: Role of lingual lipase and preduodenal digestion. *Pediatr Res* 1979;13: 615–622.
15. Hsia DYV: Birth weight in cystic fibrosis of the pancreas. *Ann Hum Genet* 1959;23: 289–299.
16. Imrie JR, Fagan DG, Sturgess JM: Quantitative evaluation of the development of the

exocrine pancreas in cystic fibrosis and control infants. *Am J Pathol* 1979;95:697–707.

17. Lloyd-Still JD: Clinical studies on the effects of malnutrition during infancy on subsequent physical and intellectual development, in Lloyd-Still JD (ed): *Malnutrition and Intellectual Development.* Lancaster, MTP Press Ltd, 1976, pp 103–159.
18. Lloyd-Still JD, Hurwitz I, Wolff PH, et al: Intellectual development after severe malnutrition in infancy. *Pediatrics* 1974;54: 306–311.
19. Oppenheimer EH, Esterly JR: Pathology of cystic fibrosis. Review of literature and comparison with 146 autopsied cases. *Perspect Pediatr Pathol* 1975;2:241–278.
20. Farber S: Pancreatic function and disease in early life. V pathologic changes associated with pancreatic insufficiency in early life. *Arch Pathol* 1944;37:238–250.
21. Bodian M: *Fibrocystic Disease of the Pancreas. A Congenital Disorder of Mucus Production—Mucosis.* London, William Heineman Medical Books Ltd, 1952.
22. Thomaidis TS, Arey JB: The intestinal lesions in cystic fibrosis of the pancreas. *J Pediatr* 1963;63:444–453.
23. Freye HB, Kurtz SM, Spock A, et al: Light and electron microscopic examination of the small bowel of children with cystic fibrosis. *J Pediatr* 1964;64:575–579.
24. Dische Z, di Sant'Agnese PA, Pallavicini C, et al: Composition of mucoprotein fractions from duodenal fluid of patients with cystic fibrosis of the pancreas and from controls. *Pediatrics* 1959;24:74–91.
25. Morin CL, Roy CC, Lasalle R, et al: Small bowel mucosal dysfunction in patients with cystic fibrosis. *J Pediatr* 1976;88:213–216.
26. Neutra MR, Trier JS: Rectal mucosa in cystic fibrosis. Morphological features before and after short-term organ culture. *Gastroenterology* 1978;75:701–710.
27. Specian RD, Neutra MR: Regulation of intestinal mucus secretion: The role of parasympathetic stimulation. In *Proceedings Eighth International Congress of Cystic Fibrosis.* Toronto, Canadian Cystic Fibrosis Foundation, 1980, p 36a.
28. Monthly Vital Statistics Report, National Center for Health Statistics, HRA 76-1120, Vol. 25, 3, Supplement. June 22, 1976. DHEW, Public Health Service, Health Resources Administration, 5600 Fishers Lane, Rockville, Maryland 20852.
29. Greulich WW, Pyle SI: *Radiographic Atlas of Skeletal Development of the Hand and Wrist, 2nd Ed.* Stanford, Stanford University Press, 1959.
30. Green M, Richmond JB: *Pediatric Diagnosis.* Philadelphia, WB Saunders, 1980.
31. Sills RH: Failure to thrive. The role of clinical and laboratory evaluation. *Am J Dis Child* 1978;132:967–969.
32. Whitten CF, Pettit MG, Fischoff J: Evidence that growth failure from maternal deprivation is secondary to undereating. *JAMA* 1969;209:1675–1682.
33. Horner JM, Thorsson AV, Hintz RL: Growth deceleration patterns in children with constitutional short stature: Aid to diagnosis. *Pediatrics* 1978;62:529–534.
34. Food and Nutrition Board, National Research Council: *Recommended Dietary Allowances, 9th ed.* Washington, DC, National Academy of Sciences, 1980, pp 1–185.
35. Owen GM, Kram KM, Garry PJ, et al: A study of nutritional status of pre-school children in the United States 1968–1970. *Pediatrics* 1974;53(suppl):597–646.
36. Committee Report. Assessment of protein nutritional status. *Am J Clin Nutr* 1970;23: 807–819.
37. Berry HK, Kellogg FW, Hunt MM, et al: Dietary supplement and nutrition in children with cystic fibrosis. *Am J Dis Child* 1975;129:165–171.
38. Dodge JA, Yassa JG: Food intake and supplementary feeding programmes. In *Proceedings Eighth International Congress of Cystic Fibrosis.* Toronto, Canadian Cystic Fibrosis Foundation, 1980, pp 125–136.
39. Joint FAO/WHO Expert Committee on Nutrition: Food Fortification, Protein–Calorie Malnutrition. Geneva, WHO Technical Report Series No. 477, 1971.
40. Seone N, Latham MC: Nutritional anthropometry in the identification of malnutrition in childhood. *J Trop Pediatr Environ Child Health* 1971;41:106–120.
41. Brasel JA: Endocrine adaptation to malnutrition. *Pediatr Res* 1980;14:1299–1303.
42. Grant DB, Hambley J, Becker D, et al: Reduced serum sulphation factor activity in patients with protein–calorie malnutrition. *Arch Dis Child* 1973;48:596–600.
43. Green OC, Fefferman R, Nair S: Plasma growth hormone levels in children with cystic fibrosis and short stature. Unresponsiveness to hypoglycemia. *J Clin Endocrinol Metab* 1967;27:1059–1061.
44. Barbezat GO, Hansen JDL: The exocrine pancreas and protein–calorie malnutrition. *Pediatrics* 1968;42:77–92.
45. Samuel AM, Kadivel GV, Pagel BD, et al: Adrenocorticoids and corticoid binding globulins in protein-calorie malnutrition. *Am J Clin Nutr* 1976;29:889–894.

46. Scrimshaw NS: Effect of infection on nutrient requirements. *Am J Clin Nutr* 1977; 30:1536–1544.
47. Beisel WR: Magnitude of the host nutritional responses to infection. *Am J Clin Nutr* 1977;30:1236–1247.
48. Beisel WR: The influence of infection or injury on nutritional requirements during adolescence, in McKigney JI, Munro HN (eds): *Nutrient Requirements in Adolescence.* Cambridge, MA, The MIT Press, 1976, p 257.
49. Beisel WR: Interrelated changes in host metabolism during generalized infectious illness. *Am J Clin Nutr* 1972;25:1254–1260.
50. Beisel WR: Infectious diseases, in Schneider HA, Anderson CE, Coursin DB (eds): *Nutritional Support of Medical Practice.* New York, Harper and Row, 1977, pp 350–366.
51. Beisel WR: Effect of infection on human protein metabolism. *Fed Proc* 1966;25: 1682–1687.
52. Matthews WJ, Williams M, Oliphant B, et al: Hypogammaglobulinemia in patients with cystic fibrosis. *N Engl J Med* 1980; 302:245–249.
53. Powanda MC, Wannemacher RW, Cockerell GL: Nitrogen metabolism and protein synthesis during pneumococcal sepsis in rats. *Infect Immun* 1972;6:266–272.
54. Vitale JJ: The impact of infection on vitamin metabolism: An unexplored area. *Am J Clin Nutr* 1977;30:1473–1477.
55. Pollack H, Bookman JJ: Riboflavin excretion as a function of protein metabolism in the normal, catabolic and diabetic human being. *J Lab Clin Med* 1951;38:561–572.
56. Rivlin RS: Riboflavin metabolism. *N Engl J Med* 1970;283:463–472.
57. Felig P, Marliss E, Pozefsky T, et al: Amino acid metabolism in the regulation of gluconeogenesis in man. *Am J Clin Nutr* 1970; 23:986–992.
58. Blackburn GL: Lipid metabolism in infection. *Am J Clin Nutr* 1977;30:1321–1332.
59. Beisel WR, Edelman R, Nauss K, et al: Single-nutrient effects on immunologic functions. *JAMA* 1981;245:53–58.
60. Walsh JH: Control of gastric secretion, in Sleisenger MH, Fordtran JS (eds): *Gastrointestinal Disease.* Philadelphia, WB Saunders, 1973.
61. Roulet M, Weber AM, Paradis Y, et al: Gastric emptying and lingual lipase activity in cystic fibrosis. *Pediatr Res* 1980;14:1360–1362.
62. Cox KL, Isenberg JN, Ament ME: Gastric acid hypersecretion in cystic fibrosis. *Clin Res* 1980;28:96A.
63. Gray GM, Cooper HL: Protein digestion and absorption. *Gastroenterology* 1971;61:535–544.
64. Silk DBA, Chung YC, Berger KL, et al: Comparison of oral feeding of peptide and amino acid meals to normal subjects. *Gut* 1979;20:291–299.
65. Koretz RL, Meyer JH: Elemental diets—facts and fantasies. *Gastroenterology* 1980;78:393–410.
66. Shahidi NT, Diamond LK, Shwachman H: Anemia associated with protein deficiency: A study of 2 cases with cystic fibrosis. *J Pediatr* 1961;59:533–542.
67. Fleisher DS, Digeorge AM, Barness LA, et al: Hypoproteinemia and edema in infants with cystic fibrosis of the pancreas. *J Pediatr* 1964;64:341–348.
68. Fleisher DS, Digeorge AM, Auerbach VH, et al: Protein metabolism in cystic fibrosis of the pancreas. *J Pediatr* 1964;64:349–356.
69. Dolan TF: Hemolytic anemia and edema as the initial signs in infants with cystic fibrosis. *Clin Pediatr* 1976;15:597–600.
70. Strober W, Peter G, Schwartz RH: Albumin metabolism in cystic fibrosis. *Pediatrics* 1969;43:416–426.
71. West CD, Wilson JL, Eyles R: Blood amino nitrogen levels: Changes in blood amino nitrogen levels following ingestion of proteins and a protein hydrolysate in infants with normal and with deficient pancreatic function. *Am J Dis Child* 1946;72:251–273.
72. Milla PJ, Rassam UB, Kilby A, et al: Small intestinal absorption of amino acids and dipeptide in pancreatic insufficiency. In *Proceedings Eighth International Congress of Cystic Fibrosis.* Toronto, Canadian Cystic Fibrosis Foundation, 1980, p 177.
73. Adrian TE, McKiernan J, Johnstone DI, et al: Hormonal abnormalities of the pancreas and gut in cystic fibrosis. *Gastroenterology* 1980;79:460–465.
74. Vaughan WJ, Lindgren FT, Whalen JB, et al: Serum lipoprotein concentrations in cystic fibrosis. *Science* 1978;199:783–786.
75. Shmerling DH, Forrer JCW, Prader A: Fecal fat and nitrogen in healthy children and in children with malabsorption or maldigestion. *Pediatrics* 1970;46:690–695.
76. Lapey A, Kattwinkel J, di Sant'Agnese PA, et al: Steatorrhea and azotorrhea and their relation to growth and nutrition in adolescents and young adults with cystic fibrosis. *J Pediatr* 1974;84:328–334.
77. Gibbons ISE, Seakins JWT, Ersser RS: Tyrosine metabolism and fecal amino acids in cystic fibrosis of the pancreas. *Lancet* 1967;1:877–878.
78. Seakins JWT, Ersser RS, Gibbons ISE: Protein

malabsorption and faecal amino acids in cystic fibrosis. In *Fifth International Cystic Fibrosis Conference*. Cambridge, Cystic Fibrosis Research Trust, 1969, p 275.

79. Seakins JWT, Ersser RS, Gibbons ISE: Studies on the origin of fecal amino acids in cystic fibrosis. *Gut* 1970;11:600–609.
80. Forstner G, Gall G, Corey M, et al: Digestion and absorption of nutrients in cystic fibrosis. In *Proceedings Eighth International Congress of Cystic Fibrosis*. Toronto, Canadian Cystic Fibrosis Foundation, 1980, p 137.
81. Anderson TA, Meeuwisse GW, Fomon SJ: Carbohydrate, in Fomon SJ (ed): *Infant Nutrition*. Philadelphia, WB Saunders, 1974.
82. Greaves JP, Hollingsworth DF: Changes in the pattern of carbohydrate consumption in Britain. *Proc Nutr Soc* 1964;23:136–142.
83. Burke V, Anderson CM: Normal digestive and absorptive functions of the small intestine, in Anderson CM, Burke V (eds): *Pediatric Gastroenterology*. Oxford, Blackwell Scientific Publications, 1975.
84. Buts JP, Morin CL, Roy CC, et al: One-hour blood xylose test: A reliable index of small bowel function. *J Pediatr* 1978; 90:729–733.
85. Shwachman H, Leubner H, Catzel P: Mucoviscidosis. *Adv Pediatr* 1955;7:249–323.
86. Shwachman H, Dooley RR, Guilmette F, et al: Cystic fibrosis of the pancreas with varying degrees of pancreatic insufficiency. *Am J Dis Child* 1956;92:347–368.
87. Hadorn B, Zoppi G, Shmerling DH, et al: Quantitative assessment of exocrine pancreatic function in infants and children. *J Pediatr* 1968;73:39–50.
88. Davidson GP, Koheil A, Forstner GG: Salivary amylase in cystic fibrosis: A marker of disordered autonomic function. *Pediatr Res* 1978;12:967–970.
89. Handwerger S, Roth J, Gorden P, et al: Glucose intolerance in cystic fibrosis. *N Engl J Med* 1969;281:451–461.
90. Gibbons ISE: Disaccharides and cystic fibrosis of the pancreas. *Arch Dis Child* 1969;44:63–68.
91. Antonowicz I, Lebenthal E, Shwachman H: Disaccharidase activities in small intestinal mucosa in patients with cystic fibrosis. *J Pediatr* 1978;92:214–219.
92. Schaad U, Kraemer R, Gaze H, et al: One-hour blood-xylose in cystic fibrosis. *Arch Dis Child* 1978;53:756–757.
93. Fomon SJ: Fat, in Fomon SJ (ed): *Infant Nutrition*. Philadelphia, WB Saunders, 1974.
94. Gray GM: Mechanisms of digestion and absorption of food, in Sleisenger MH, Fordtran JS (eds): *Gastrointestinal Disease*. Philadelphia, WB Saunders, 1973.
95. Ockner RK, Manning JA: Fatty acid binding ing protein in small intestine. Identification, isolation, and evidence for its role in cellular fatty acid transport. *J Clin Invest* 1974; 54:326–338.
96. Levi AJ, Gatmaitan Z, Arias IM: Two hepatic cytoplasmic protein fractions, Y and Z, and their possible role in the hepatic uptake of bilirubin, sulfobromophthalein and other anions. *J Clin Invest* 1969;48: 2156–2167.
97. DiMagno EP, Go VLW, Summerskill WHJ: Relations between pancreatic enzyme outputs and malabsorption in severe pancreatic insufficiency. *N Engl J Med* 1973;288:813–815.
98. Meyer JH: The ins and outs of oral pancreatic enzymes. *N Engl J Med* 1977;296: 1347–1348.
99. Nousia-Arvanitakis S, Arvanitakis C, Desai N, et al: Diagnosis of exocrine pancreatic insufficiency in cystic fibrosis by the synthetic peptide N-benzoyl-L-tyrosyl-*p*-aminobenzoic acid. *J Pediatr* 1978;92:734–737.
100. Arvanitakis C, Cooke AR: Diagnostic tests of exocrine pancreatic function and disease. *Gastroenterology* 1978;74:932–948.
101. Durie PR, Largman C, Brodrick JW, et al: Plasma immunoreactive pancreatic cationic trypsinogen in cystic fibrosis: A sensitive indicator of exocrine pancreatic dysfunction. *Pediatr Res* 1981;15:1351–1355.
102. Durie PR, Bell L, Linton W, et al: Effect of cimetidine and sodium bicarbonate on pancreatic replacement therapy in cystic fibrosis. *Gut* 1980;21:778–786.
103. Durie PR, Newth CJ, Forstner GG, et al: Malabsorption of medium chain triglycerides in infants with cystic fibrosis: Correction with pancreatic enzyme supplements. *J Pediatr* 1980;96:862–864.
104. Ockner RK, Pittman JP, Yager JL: Differences in the intestinal absorption of saturated and unsaturated long chain fatty acids. *Gastroenterology* 1972;62:981–992.
105. Fernandes J, Van de Kamer JH, Weijers HA: Differences in absorption of the various fatty acids studied in children with steatorrhea. *J Clin Invest* 1962;41:488–494.
106. Blomstrand R, Lindquist B, Paabo K: The intestinal absorption of carbon-labelled oleic and palmitic acid in the normal infant and in cystic fibrosis of the pancreas. *Helv Paediatr Acta* 1955;6:640–648.
107. Reemtsma K, di Sant'Agnese PA, Malm JR, et al: Cystic fibrosis of the pancreas: Intestinal absorption of fat and fatty acid labelled with I^{131}. *Pediatrics* 1958;22:525–532.
108. Kuo PT, Huang NN: The effect of medium chain triglyceride upon fat absorption and plasma lipid and depot fat of children with cystic fibrosis of the pancreas. *J Clin Invest*

1965;44:1924–1933.

109. Lloyd-Still JD, Johnson SB, Holman RT: Essential fatty acid status in cystic fibrosis and the effects of safflower oil supplementation. *Am J Clin Nutr* 1981;34:1–7.
110. Watkins JB, Tercyak AM, Szczepanik P, et al: Bile salt kinetics in cystic fibrosis: Influence of pancreatic enzyme replacement. *Gastroenterology* 1977;73:1023–1028.
111. Weber AM, Roy CC, Morin CL, et al: Malabsorption of bile acids in children with cystic fibrosis. *N Engl J Med* 1973;289: 1001–1005.
112. Goodchild MC, Murphy GM, Howell AM, et al: Aspects of bile acid metabolism in cystic fibrosis. *Arch Dis Child* 1975;50: 769–778.
113. Boyle BJ, Long WB, Balistreri WF, et al: Effect of cimetidine and pancreatic enzymes on serum and fecal bile acids and fat absorption in cystic fibrosis. *Gastroenterology* 1980;78:950–953.
114. Smalley CA, Brown GA, Parkes MET, et al: Reduction of bile acid loss in cystic fibrosis by dietary means. *Arch Dis Child* 1978;53:477–482.
115. Harries JT, Muller DPR, McCollum JPK, et al: Intestinal bile salts in cystic fibrosis: Studies in the patient and experimental animal. *Arch Dis Child* 1979;54:19–24.
116. Roy CC, Delage G, Fontaine A, et al: The fecal microflora and bile acids in children with cystic fibrosis. *Am J Clin Nutr* 1979; 32:2404–2409.
117. Roy CC, Weber AM, Morin CL, et al: Abnormal biliary lipid composition in cystic fibrosis. *N Engl J Med* 1977;297:1301–1305.
118. Balistreri WF, Suchy FJ, Heubi JE: Serum bile acid response to a test meal stimulus: A sensitive test of ileal function. *J Pediatr* 1980;96:582–589.
119. Henrichs I, Teller WM: Pathophysiology of gastrointestinal hormones: Implications for pediatrics. *Eur J Pediatr* 1980;135:3–11.
120. Grand RJ: Changing patterns of gastrointestinal manifestations of cystic fibrosis. *Clin Pediatr* 1970;9:588–593.
121. Shwachman H: Gastrointestinal manifestations of cystic fibrosis. *Pediatr Clin North Am* 1975;22:787–805.
122. Barbero GJ, Shwachman H, Grand R, et al: Gastrointestinal and nutritional manifestations of cystic fibrosis, in Mangos JA, Talamo RC (eds): *Cystic Fibrosis: Projections into the Future.* Miami, Symposia Specialists, 1976.
123. Holsclaw DS, Rocmans C, Shwachman H: Intussusception in patients with cystic fibrosis. *Pediatrics* 1971;48:51–58.
124. Noblett HR: Treatment of uncomplicated meconium ileus by gastrografin enema: A preliminary report. *J Pediatr Surg* 1969;4: 190–197.
125. Kulczycki LL, Shwachman H: Studies in cystic fibrosis of the pancreas: Occurrence of rectal prolapse. *N Engl J Med* 1958;259: 409–412.
126. White H, Rowley WF: Cystic fibrosis of the pancreas: Clinical and roentgenographic manifestations. *Radiol Clin North Am* 1963;1:539–556.
127. Wood RE, Herman CJ, Johnson KW, et al: Pneumatosis coli in cystic fibrosis: Clinical, radiological and pathological features. *Am J Dis Child* 1975;129:246–248.
128. Aterman K: Duodenal ulceration and fibrocystic pancreas disease. *Am J Dis Child* 1961;101:102–107.
129. Cropp GJA, Rosenberg PN: Energy costs of breathing in cystic fibrosis: Relation between severity of pulmonary disease and basal oxygen consumption. *Cystic Fibrosis Club Abstr* 1981;22:15.
130. Bradley JA, Axon, ATR, Hill GL: Nocturnal elemental diet for retarded growth in a patient with cystic fibrosis. *Br Med J* 1979;1:167.
131. Allan JD, Mason A, Moss AD: Nutritional supplementation in treatment of cystic fibrosis of the pancreas. *Am J Dis Child* 1973;126:22–26.
132. Park RW, Grand RJ: Gastrointestinal manifestations of cystic fibrosis: A review. *Gastroenterology* 1981;81:1143–1161.

16

Nutrition in Cystic Fibrosis: Vitamins, Fatty Acids, and Minerals

Philip M. Farrell

Van S. Hubbard

Because of the pancreatic and gastrointestinal disturbances described in the previous chapter, the majority of patients with cystic fibrosis (CF) are susceptible to malnutrition. Not surprisingly, nutrient deficiencies are most likely to occur, especially in a clinically obvious fashion, during the first few years of life when growth rates are greatest. Nevertheless, considerable variation in nutritional status is evident among CF patients at the time of diagnosis or during the early childhood years. This may be attributed to the numerous variables which influence nutrition and growth in a given CF patient including: (1) the degree of steatorrhea and azotorrhea; (2) the occurrence of intestinal resection, in association with meconium ileus or subsequent bowel obstructions, causing increasing malabsorption; (3) growth rate; (4) the presence and severity of chronic respiratory disease and infection; (5) various dietary considerations such as the quantity and quality of food consumed; (6) the relative efficiency of macronutrient utilization; and (7) the magnitude of nutrient stores which is determined by numerous factors including digestive/absorptive function, the size of the individual, and previous dietary history. The quantity of nutrients consumed varies widely[1,2] and is related to appetite, availability of desirable foods, and the ability to eat. Occasionally, the tachypnea and dyspnea associated with lung disease in children with CF may become a major factor by decreasing the appetite and ability to feed. Although the quality of food consumed in developed countries is generally satisfactory, this is not always true. In addition, there is very little margin of safety afforded by typical American and European diets for some of the fat-soluble vitamins, such that a deficiency state can readily occur as a consequence of steatorrhea.

Before proceeding to a discussion of nutrient deficiencies, it would be worthwhile to mention the well-recognized concept that the degree of malnutrition may vary in nutrient-deficiency states. At the mild end of the spectrum, one finds patients with either depleted stores or low circulating concentrations of a given nutrient, but with no associated signs or symptoms. More pronounced or prolonged deficiency will lead to metabolic abnormalities, structural changes, and functional disturbances, including a progression to overt pathophysiologic disturbances. Therefore, it should be emphasized that many CF patients described in the literature have not necessarily shown clinical malnutrition, but rather a state of biochemical malnutrition.

Another issue that will arise in the minds of readers pertains to whether or not nutritional status can significantly influence the overall course of cystic fibrosis. This important question remains to be answered with definitive evidence. Although severe malnutrition undoubtedly can aggravate the disease, milder degrees of nutrient deficiencies (eg, low blood levels of vitamins A and E) may or may not be clinically detrimental. However, there is some evidence suggesting that biochemical malnutrition can subtly affect CF patients in an adverse fashion. For instance, patients with intact pancreatic function appear to have a milder course of disease.[3] In addition, aggressive nutritional management, including supplementation protocols involving malnourished patients with CF, has revealed overall benefit and improved pulmonary status.[4,5] Furthermore, CF centers of North America that practice intensive nutritional management (admittedly with similar attention to respiratory care) can legitimately boast of increased patient longevity. Nevertheless, convincing data are needed on the importance of good nutrition in order to support the routine institution of vigorous nutritional intervention programs. Furthermore, improved methods must be developed to assess nutritional status in a comprehensive but convenient and minimally invasive fashion.

OVERVIEW OF NUTRIENT DEFICIENCIES IN CYSTIC FIBROSIS

The major nutritional concerns in cystic fibrosis are summarized in Table 16-1. Macronutrients deserving attention include energy, protein, and fat. Caloric requirements are generally increased in CF because of malabsorption, respiratory disease, infection, or other problems such as glucose intolerance leading to glucosuria. In contrast to the usual textbook description of the voracious appetite of children with CF, dietary surveys reviewed by Chase et al[6] indicate that ingestion of calories averaged only about 80% of the recommended daily allowance (RDA) for energy. Although the RDA values are established for active, healthy populations, it is of great concern that low total food consumption apparently occurs in a substantial proportion of patients with CF. As a guideline, it has been suggested[7] that energy intake be increased at least 50% in children with CF. Because of the heterogeneity of these patients, however, no precise general recommendations for caloric intake can be offered. Occasionally, a CF patient can grow in a normal fashion and avoid nutrient deficiencies by consuming no more than the RDA. On the other hand, patients with advanced pulmonary disease may need as much as twice the normal intake of calories. Detailed discussion of

Table 16-1
Major Nutritional Concerns in Cystic Fibrosis

Energy (calories)	Increased requirement because of malabsorption, respiratory disease and other complications
Protein	Appropriate quantity and quality are needed especially during infancy
Fat	Provides an important source of calories, as well as essential fatty acids
Fat-soluble Vitamins A, D, E, and K	All may be deficient in CF patients
Miscellaneous minerals	Sodium, calcium, iron, zinc, and selenium

the energy needs of CF patients may be found in a recent article by Hubbard and Mangrum.[2]

Protein intake by children with CF must be increased to compensate for azotorrhea and to support the accretion of amino acids in growing tissue. Thus, the major risk of protein deficiency occurs during the first year of life when the average consumption is more than 1.5 g/kg body weight/day, in contrast to a minimum requirement of approximately 0.6 g/kg body weight/day in adults.[8] Human breast milk, which is relatively low in protein (7% of calories), and soy-based formula (formerly deficient in methionine) have been particularly associated with hypoproteinemic edema and growth retardation.[9,10]

Fat nutrition in cystic fibrosis has received a great deal of attention during recent years. Although some restriction of lipid intake has often been recommended for CF patients in an attempt to reduce the abdominal symptoms of malabsorption, dietary fat is recognized as important for providing an excellent source of energy and for enhancing the palatability of a child's diet. In addition, certain polyunsaturated fatty acids such as linoleate cannot be adequately synthesized in mammalian tissues and thus are nutritionally essential. Because low levels of linoleate have been observed repeatedly in CF patients with pancreatic insufficiency, a section has been included in this chapter on the essential fatty acids.

In regard to the micronutrients, most of the clinical concern and research have focused on vitamins, particularly the fat-soluble vitamins, and certain trace minerals. Deficiencies of vitamins A, E, and K have been described repeatedly in CF patients. In fact, more investigation has been carried out on these vitamins than any class of nutrients potentially abnormal in cystic fibrosis. Accordingly, this chapter focuses on the fat-soluble vitamins and provides a separate section for each, reviewing their chemistry, biology, and the status of these compounds in cystic fibrosis. In addition, discussions of research needs and recommendations for treatment are included for each nutrient. It should be pointed out, however, that nutrient-metabolite interaction is an important concept in nutrition. Thus, various vitamins, minerals, and even macronutrients such as essential fatty acids should ideally be considered in relationship to one another. Table 16-2 summarizes some of the nutrient interrelationships that are pertinent to cystic fibrosis. Further details as well as background information in general may be found in other references.[11,12]

Because water-soluble vitamins have received meager attention in cystic fibrosis, only the following brief summary is warranted. Usually, CF patients are urged to take one or two multivitamin pills per day because of the expectation that increased metabolism and excretion of the water-soluble vitamins will occur in conjunction with chronic infection; however, increased turnover of the B group and vitamin C has not been demonstrated in CF patients. Recent investigations[13-15] have found that the average values for vitamin B_1 (thiamine), vitamin B_2 (riboflavin), vitamin B_6 (pyridoxine), folate, and vitamin C (ascorbic acid) were similar in the CF and control populations. In each study, an occasional patient

Table 16-2
Nutrient Interactions Relevant to Cystic Fibrosis

Vitamin A	Zinc (via RBP) Vitamin E (antioxidant protection)
Vitamin D	Protein (via RBP and β-carotene-15,15′-dioxygenase) Calcium and phosphorus (bone mineralization) Vitamin K (via osteocalcin)
Vitamin E	Essential fatty acids (membrane antioxidant) Iron (inactivation of tocopherol) Selenium (glutathione peroxidase)
Vitamin K	Vitamin E (excess appears to promote K deficiency)
Zinc	Essential fatty acids (unknown mechanism) Protein (synthesis)

had a subnormal value, but none demonstrated clinical evidence of deficiency. Adequacy of levels did not correlate with the amount of vitamin supplement being taken. Random screening of 28 patients with CF at the National Institutes of Health (Hubbard, unpublished data) demonstrated normal circulating concentrations of folate and ascorbic acid. Vitamin B_{12} malabsorption has been associated with untreated pancreatic insufficiency;[16,17] however, pancreatic enzyme therapy and/or bicarbonate ingestion will correct this abnormality. Furthermore, it has been determined that pancreatin preparations provide approximately 1 mg of vitamin B_{12} per gram dry weight.[16] Although there have been reports of macrocytic anemia responsive to parenteral B_{12} administration in CF patients, usually no evidence for depletion of this vitamin is found.[16,18,19] Clearly, there is a need for more research on the B vitamins and ascorbate.

In view of the limited data available on water-soluble vitamins, it is not possible to offer a recommendation for supplements based on experimental evidence. Thus, until adequate research is carried out, it seems prudent for CF patients to consume approximately twice the RDA of the B group and vitamin C by ingesting a multivitamin preparation in addition to a normal diet. To our knowledge, there appears to be no benefit from taking larger doses of these vitamins, especially in the individual who has been evaluated biochemically and found to have normal levels.

VITAMIN A

General Background[20,21]

Although night blindness of nutritional etiology has been known for thousands of years, it was not until the early part of the 20th century that vitamin A was identified. The active factor was initially isolated from animal fats and fish oils, but in 1922 was shown to be associated with the yellow carotenes of plants. This subsequently led to the discovery that β-carotene was a "provitamin" and could be converted to the functional vitamin by enzymes of the intestinal mucosa.

The chemistry of vitamin A is somewhat complex in that there are several biologically active compounds including retinol (vitamin A_1), 3-dehydroretinol (vitamin A_2), retinal (the aldehyde derivative and functional form of vitamin A in vision), retinoic acid, and the provitamin carotenoids (the most important of which is β-carotene). Although vitamin A alcohols exist in several isomeric forms, all-*trans*-retinol (shown in Figure 16-1) is the major naturally occurring form in the diet. As discussed subsequently, when preformed vitamin A is consumed, it is actually retinal esters which serve as the chemical form of the nutrient. Examination of the structure of β-carotene (Figure 16-1) indicates that this symmetrical molecule can readily be oxidized to produce two molecules of retinol. Analysis of vitamin A in biological fluids and tissues has been carried out most commonly using physical or chemical methods. The trifluoroacetic acid method has been popular, but the use of high-pressure liquid chromatography[22] offers major advantages and is now the preferred analytical technique. As discussed subsequently, this

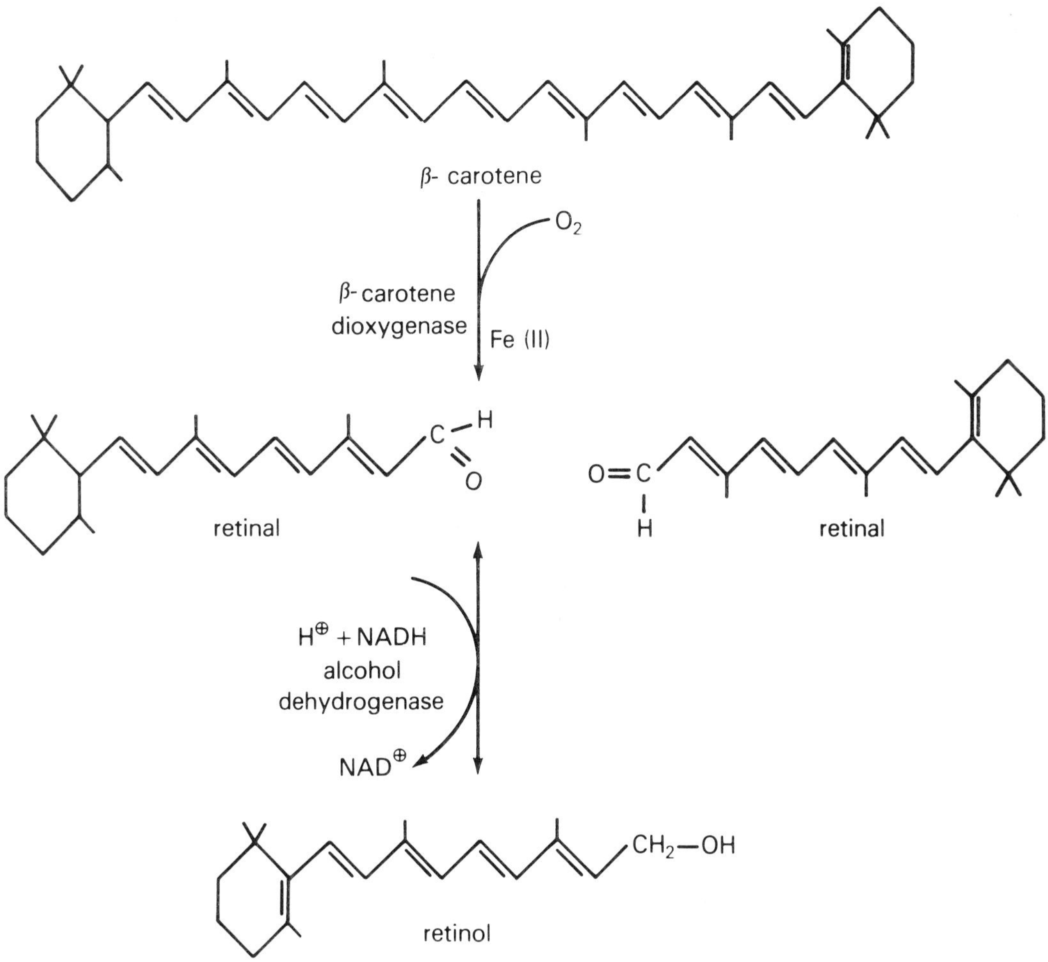

Figure 16-1 Metabolism of β-carotene. Each molecule of β-carotene can theoretically yield two molecules of retinol; however, 100% efficiency of absorption and conversion of β-carotene to retinol does not occur and functionally about one molecule of retinol is formed for each molecule of carotene ingested.

method for simultaneously determining retinol and retinyl esters on 0.1 ml plasma samples should be accompanied by measurement of retinol binding protein (RBP). Although bioassays for vitamin A activity are rarely used at the present time in nutrition research, use of techniques such as rat growth test and vaginal smear assay have indicated that 0.6 μg of β-carotene and 0.3 μg of retinol correspond to one international unit of vitamin A.

The dietary intake of vitamin A varies from day to day, suggesting that the hepatic stores and plasma transport system are potentially of major importance. Two categories of foods can serve as a source of vitamin A. Various plants, particularly brightly colored vegetables like carrots, but not fruits, can provide the carotenoid pigments for oxidation into vitamin A. The small intestine plays an important role in vitamin A metabolism by first converting β-carotene to retinal by the action of β-carotene-15,15-dioxygenase and then reducing the product to retinol via a nonspecific aldehyde reductase system. Liver, milk products, and eggs serve as the source of retinyl esters from which retinol is released in the proximal small intestine by the action of pancreatic retinyl ester hydrolase and a second hydrolase associated with the intestinal brush border. Free retinol is then absorbed into the intestinal mucosal cells in a micellar form where it may be reesterified and incorporated into chylomicrons. It should be noted that the efficiency of absorption and metabolism is less than 50% as determined with low doses in small animals such as rats.[23] Furthermore, absorption of retinol is significantly hampered when the diet is unusually low in fat or when steatorrhea is present. Not only are the pancreas and intestinal mucosa important in the "digestion," uptake, and chemical transformation of vitamin A, but bile salts are also essential in the normal absorption process.

Retinyl esters derived from either carotene or preformed vitamin A are transported in chylomicrons through the lymphatic system and into the blood stream for deposition in the liver and storage (as retinyl esters). Release into the blood stream takes place after hydrolysis to free retinol. The plasma transport of secreted retinol occurs in association with a specific complex consisting of the retinol binding protein (RBP) and prealbumin; zinc is also required for the secretory process to operate normally. Generally, plasma levels of both vitamin A and prealbumin are proportionate to the level of RBP.[24] In the fasting state, only approximately 10% of circulating vitamin A is esterified; however, in the postabsorptive period, the percentage of retinyl esters increases markedly. The concentration of circulating retinol is maintained relatively constant until hepatic stores are depleted of vitamin A, and then the blood level may fall rapidly. Thus, hepatic storage of vitamin A, principally as retinyl palmitate, protects against day-to-day variations in dietary consumption and short-term malabsorption. Excretion of vitamin A takes place after conjugation in the liver to retinyl glucuronides. A major degree of enterohepatic circulation occurs and leads to significant reabsorption of vitamin A. This offers another protection against sudden depletion.

The functional role of vitamin A in the retina was established by a series of investigations which elucidated the interaction of retinal with a protein (opsin), thus creating the light-sensitive rhodopsin complex. Vitamin A performs other important metabolic functions involving cellular membranes and epithelial surfaces; however, the biochemical nature of these activities requires further study. It is also known that vitamin A functions in the synthesis of glycopeptides. This might explain the occurrence of conjunctival keratomalacia and the squamous metaplasia with keratinization that occurs along the respiratory epithelium in vitamin A deficiency (see Chapter 12).

Status in Cystic Fibrosis

The vitamin A nutriture of patients with cystic fibrosis has been studied in some detail. Shortly after CF was recognized as a distinct syndrome, Andersen[25] reported evidence of vitamin A deficiency in 10 of 49 patients. Because marked keratinizing metaplasia of the bronchial epithelium was present, Anderson felt that vitamin A deficiency might be contributing to the pathophysiology of the pulmonary disease. Coincidentally, she also found that 7 of 12 vitamin A-deficient infants described in the literature had pancreatic fibrosis lesions typical of CF. Subsequently, many case reports of low vitamin A levels in CF patients have been documented.[26–29] The clinical features described include xerophthalmia and night blindness, although increased intracranial pressure may also be found[29] at the time CF is diagnosed.

Surveys of vitamin A status in CF patients have been carried out with attention to both retinol and, in limited work thus far, retinol binding protein (RBP). These studies (Table 16-3) have often revealed low plasma vitamin A concentrations, even in patients supplemented with 10,000 units/day, but significantly increased levels in liver.[30,31] According to Smith et al[32] and Jacobs et al,[33] RBP levels are also significantly decreased. Based on these observations, one might suspect that a defect exists in the mobilization/ transport system in patients with CF and that supplementation doses of vitamin A used routinely may be too high. Although it was originally proposed that decreased RBP

Table 16-3
Plasma and Liver Vitamin A in Patients with Cystic Fibrosis and in Control Subjects*

Patient	Sex	Age (yr)	Plasma		Liver	
			Albumin (g/100 ml)	*Vitamin A (μg/100 ml)*	*Lipid (g/100 g)*	*Vitamin A (μg/g)*
1	M	17	4.4	77	3.8	482
2	F	14	2.7	14	8.2	127
3	F	14	3.1	18	6.4	68
4	F	9	2.3	10	24.7	23
5	M	17	3.2	6	5.6	197
6	F	23	2.9	13	4.5	379
7	M	17	1.8	16	4.5	85
8	M	11	3.0	30	7.1	995
9	M	9	3.7	17	5.2	156
10	F	12	2.8	15	2.9	230
11	F	19	2.1	8	4.4	862
CF patients, mean ± SD			2.9 ± 0.7	20 ± 19	5.2 ± 1.5*	317 ± 300†
Control subjects, mean ± SD			3.4 ± 0.5‡	38 ± 11‡	4.2 ± 0.5§	126 ± 164§

*From Underwood and Denning.[31]
†Concentration of vitamin A in liver was significantly higher in the children with CF than in the control subjects ($P < 0.05$).
‡Mean of 9 subjects.
§Mean of 18 subjects.

levels could be attributed to liver disease in cystic fibrosis, there have been patients with no evidence of liver disease who also have low RBP. Zinc deficiency can impair the vitamin A transport system,[33] but this was not found to be the cause in a study by Palin et al[34] involving measurement of RBP after zinc supplementation. Subclinical protein malnutrition can also lower the circulating concentration of this rapidly metabolized protein[35] and needs to be studied in CF patients concurrent with vitamin A and RBP assessment. The hepatic retinyl ester hydrolase has not been evaluated in CF patients, nor have any measurements been made of vitamin A in target organs such as the eye and lungs.

Although there is appropriate rationale for placing patients with CF on supplements of vitamin A, the issues described above make it difficult to recommend a dose, particularly since more research is needed on evaluation of retinol status. Guidelines in the literature[6,36] suggest from 5000 units (the RDA) to 25,000 units per day in addition to dietary sources. On the basis of the data available at present, as well as the concerns raised about toxicity, it seems reasonable to supplement CF patients having malabsorption with 5000–10,000 units/day. It has been demonstrated that the water-soluble emulsified form of vitamin A is better absorbed than the natural fat-soluble form.[37] Nevertheless, our experience indicates that circulating retinol levels can often be maintained by utilizing vitamin A supplements commonly found in multivitamin preparations, thus eliminating the need for a separate medication.

VITAMIN D

General Background[38,39]

Signs of vitamin D deficiency, particularly rickets, have been documented since ancient times as a result of reduced sunlight exposure from northern migration, clothing, and urbanization. In the 19th century, the therapeutic use of cod liver oil and the benefits of sunlight exposure for osteomalacia were recognized. Then, in 1922, the term vitamin D was proposed for the antirachitic factor of cod liver oil. This was followed by the important discovery of Steenbock[40] that compounds with antirachitic activity could be produced in food by ultraviolet irradiation. Steenbock's experiments led to the fortification of foods with vitamin D and the virtual elimination of nutritional rickets in developed countries. Because vitamin D can potentially be synthesized in adequate amounts from 7-dehydrocholesterol by ultraviolet exposure (an uncontrolled, chemical reaction), it is not necessarily an essential dietary component but can be considered a hormone. Nevertheless, ingestion of vitamin D is required by urban populations who have chosen to limit their exposure to sunlight. Thus, for practical purposes, vitamin D should be regarded as an essential nutrient, particularly since storage of vitamin D is limited and because patients with CF who have advanced lung disease may not obtain adequate sunlight exposure.

The chemistry and metabolism of the D vitamins have been extensively studied in recent years. As presented in Figure 16-2, vitamins D_2 and D_3, the most prevalent antirachitic compounds, are derived from ergosterol and 7-dehydrocholesterol, respectively, and are often referred to as ergocalciferol and cholecalciferol. The further metabolism of these steroid compounds has been elucidated in the laboratory of DeLuca[38,39] and is summarized in Figure 16-3. A series of hydroxylation reactions, the first occurring predominantly in the liver and the second exclusively in the kidney, lead to the synthesis of 25-OH-cholecalciferol and 1,25-$(OH)_2$-cholecalciferol, as well as other, minor metabolites. The most potent natural form of vitamin D known, which is ten times more active than cholecalciferol, is the 1,25-$(OH)_2$-D_3 compound.

Analysis of vitamin D and the hydroxylated derivatives is currently performed using high-pressure liquid chromatography. This approach separates all the metabolites which can then be analyzed on the basis of their absorbance in the ultraviolet region. Radioimmunoassays can also be utilized, but

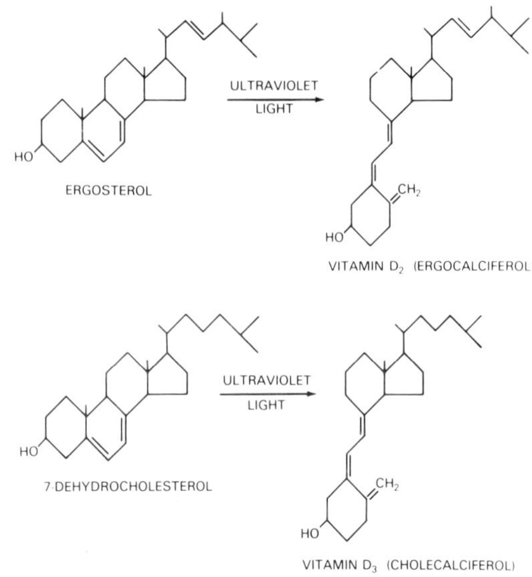

Figure 16-2 Vitamin D metabolism. Exposure to sunlight is important in the biochemistry of vitamin D. This is indicated by the reaction in which ultraviolet light promotes conversion of the provitamins, ergosterol and 7-dehydrocholesterol to vitamin D_2 and vitamin D_3, respectively.

are no longer the preferred methods. Bioassays of vitamin D activity (using the classical rat-line tests with silver nitrate staining of sectioned bone or using isolated intestinal loop techniques) are also helpful for some purposes.[41]

Foods fortified with vitamin D represent a major dietary source in developed countries. In children, processed milk which contains 400 IU/quart of vitamin D (formerly D_2 exclusively, now D_3 in some instances) contributes most of the ingested vitamin. It should be recognized that adequate ingestion of calcium and phosphorus must also occur in order to maintain bone mineralization. Vitamin D is absorbed in the jejunum and/or ileum along with dietary fat. Bile salts are essential for the absorption process;[42] this leads to the transport of vitamin D in the chylomicrons of the lymphatic system and eventual delivery to the venous circulation. Cholecalciferols are then taken to the liver for the first hydroxylation reaction. Only limited stores of vitamin D are present in liver. Transport of hydroxylated cholecalciferols occurs by interaction with a protein serving as the carrier of vitamin D in the bloodstream.

The function of vitamin D in supporting mineralization of bone has been well established.[39] Vitamin D is essential for calcium absorption across the intestinal mucosa and also is capable of playing a permissive role in stimulating the mobilization of calcium from bone. When deficiency occurs in a growing child, rickets may be expected; however, osteomalacia due to bone demineralization will take place in adults or children whose bones are no longer growing. In addition, pathologic fractures may appear. The molecular mechanism of action for vitamin D has not been fully elucidated, but appears to involve interaction with nuclear receptors and induction of calcium–phosphorus transport proteins. It should be noted that vitamin D interacts with parathyroid hormone, which is capable of stimulating the synthesis of 1,25-$(OH)_2$-cholecalciferol for enhancing intestinal calcium absorption in states of calcium deficiency.

Status in Cystic Fibrosis

Although reports of osteoporosis and pathologic fractures in CF patients have appeared in the literature,[43,44] rickets has rarely been diagnosed,[45,46] in contrast to the situation in other malabsorption syndromes such as biliary atresia. Studies of vitamin D absorption in patients with CF have not been published to our knowledge, but a few reports have appeared on blood vitamin D metabolites. Mean serum levels of 25-OH-D (the major circulating metabolite of vitamin D) in 17 patients with CF were reported by Hubbard et al[47] to fall generally within the normal range; however, three subjects were below 15 ng/ml, and one had no detectable hydroxycholecalciferol. Hahn et al[48] found that 16 of 21 patients had serum 25-OH-D values below 15 ng/ml and that the mean level in cystic fibrosis (12 ng/ml) was significantly less than that of controls (19 ng/ml). Neither of these studies was adequately controlled for sunlight exposure. Although CF patients from each study did have "deficient" levels of 25-OH-D, none had clinical or roentgenographic evidence of rickets. In general, the patients had been receiving daily supplements of at least 800 units of vitamin D, such that their intake was generally three times that of the healthy controls. Two unsupplemented CF patients without steatorrhea were reported[47] as having above-normal serum 25-OH-D levels, which would suggest that the lower serum levels of 25-OH-D seen in the supplemented patients with steatorrhea provide circumstantial evidence for malabsorption of this vitamin. It must be kept in mind, however, that the majority of circulating 25-OH-D may be derived from vitamin D_3 via endogenous production with

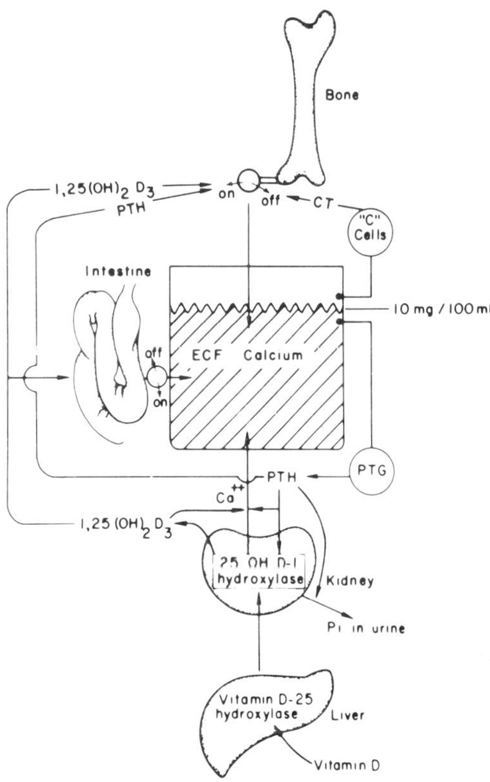

Figure 16-3 Vitamin D metabolism and the regulation of plasma (ECF) calcium concentration. Low circulating calcium is detected by the parathyroid gland and leads to PTH secretion which, in turn, stimulates production of 1,25-$(OH)_2D_3$ to mobilize calcium. Reproduced with permission from DeLuca (1982).

exposure to sunlight, according to a study of normal adults by Haddad and Hahn.[49]

In the above surveys, circulating calcium concentrations were generally within the normal range, although in the study by Hahn et al[48] mean serum calcium in patients with CF was significantly reduced (normal = 9.69 mg/dl; CF = 9.33 mg/dl). A positive correlation of circulating 25-OH-D levels with both serum calcium concentration and radiologic evidence of decreased bone mineralization was also observed in this study. Mischler et al[50] reported bone demineralization in 44% of patients with CF evaluated by direct photon absorptiometry. The incidence of demineralization was much greater in females than in males, particularly among adolescents; however, all patients under 10 years had normal bone mineral content. Solomons et al[13] did not observe decreased bone density, but their population had a mean age of 11 years compared to nearly 21 years in the study of Hahn et al[48] and greater than 15 years in the study of Mischler et al[50]. None of these investigations included evaluation of calcium balance or measurement of transport protein.

Several questions arise from these limited observations on vitamin D metabolites and calcium in blood and bone. Perhaps some of the subtle differences reported for calcium and 25-OH-D indicate that the interpretation of the normal range must be reconsidered for these populations. It would be useful to have more comprehensive assessment of vitamin D, parathormone, calcium, phosphorus, and bone mineralization in CF patients, as well as data on all vitamin D metabolites and a better evaluation of endogenous synthesis. As far as treatment is concerned, further research is needed before recommendations can be made beyond taking 1–2 multivitamins per day containing 400 IU of vitamin D.

VITAMIN E

General Background[51,52]

Vitamin E was discovered in 1922 as a fat-soluble factor that prevented fetal death in animals fed a diet containing rancid lard. Subsequently, the term "tocopherol" was suggested from the Greek words "tos" (meaning childbirth) and "phero" (meaning to bring forth) and "ol" (for the alcohol portion of the molecule). Lipids with vitamin E activity were isolated from wheat germ oil and their chemical synthesis achieved in the 1930s. The chemistry of vitamin E is more complex than the other fat-soluble vitamins because there are eight naturally occurring compounds with the characterisitc biologic activity.[53] The most abundant and active isomer is α-tocopherol, the structure of which is shown in Figure 16-4 as both the alcohol and the quinone produced after oxidation. There are three other tocols, differing from α-tocopherol with respect to methyl group substitutions on the ring, and four tocotrienols. From a practical point of view, the vitamers of importance to human nutrition are β-tocopherol, with methyl groups in the carbon 5 and 8 positions, and γ-tocopherol with methyl groups in the carbon 7 and 8 positions. β-Tocopherol is approximately one third as active as the α-isomer, while γ-tocopherol has a biologic activity equal to about 10% of α-tcopherol based on in vivo comparisons of activity. The standard vitamin E compound is *dl*-α-tocopheryl acetate, 1 mg being designated as having 1 international unit (IU) of activity. The natural occurring compound, *d*-α-tocopherol, has 1.49 units of vitamin E activity per milligram.

Several methods have been used to assess vitamin E status. Traditionally, the Emmerie-Engel reaction has been utilized for colorimetric determinations of plasma or serum tocopherol concentrations. This involves reaction of a lipid extract with ferric chloride which, after conversion to ferrous iron, can be measured colorimetrically by production of complexes such as ferrous bathophenathroline. The colorimetric methods can also be used in conjunction with thin-layer chromatography in order to separate α-tocopherol from the β- and γ-isomers, which generally contribute approximately 20% to the total tocopherol content of plasma. In recent years, Bieri et al[22] have

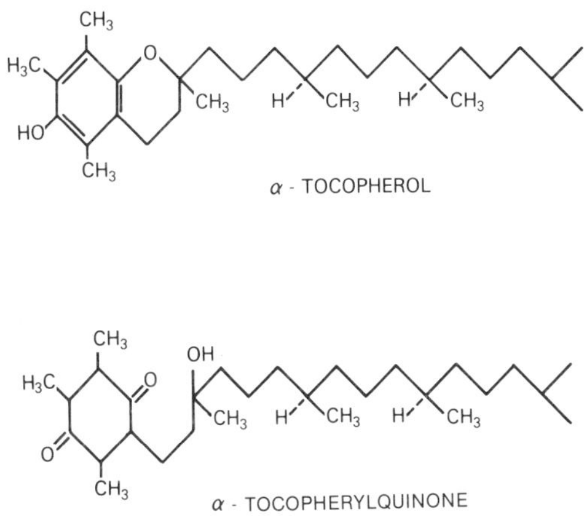

Figure 16-4 Vitamin E. The various tocopherol isomers have the same ring structure, but differ in the methyl substitutions as discussed in the text. α-Tocopherol is the most abundant and biologically active form. α-Tocopherol quinone is the oxidative product of α-tocopherol.

developed a method of analysis based on high-pressure liquid chromatography which separates the various tocopherol isomers and is now considered the ideal analytical method for tocopherol isomers. In addition to plasma tocopherol determinations, vitamin E status can also be assessed with the peroxide hemolysis test,[54,55] which provides an index of the tocopherol concentration of erythrocytes incubated in dilute hydrogen peroxide. Although the test is not entirely specific, hemolysis of greater than 5% during a 3-hr incubation strongly suggests vitamin E deficiency. Most of the reports on the vitamin E status of patients with cystic fibrosis, as reviewed by Farrell,[56] have presented tocopherol concentrations per unit volume of plasma. It has been demonstrated, however, that vitamin E levels in blood can vary depending on the concentration of total lipids.[57] Therefore, Horwitt et al[57] have proposed that tocopherol concentrations be expressed relative to total plasma lipids, a recommendation supported by the work of Farrell et al.[58,59]

The major sources of vitamin E consumed by Americans and Europeans are the vegetable and seed oils such as corn oil, soybean oil, and safflower oil. The concentration of tocopherols in these oils depends to some extent on the amount of polyunsaturated fatty acid (PUFA) present. Also, the isomers of vitamin E found in a given source show considerable variation. For instance, lipid extracts of soybeans contain predominantly γ-tocopherol rather than the α-vitamer which is the predominant form in animal-based dietary sources such as liver and lard.

The absorption of tocopherols depends upon factors generally involved in lipid digestion and intestinal uptake. This includes bile salts and pancreatic enzymes. In general, the degree of tocopherol absorption will vary in association with lipid absorption, as reviewed by Bieri and Farrell;[60] however, the efficiency of absorption decreases as large amounts of tocopherol are consumed. Once absorbed, tocopherols are transported via lymphatics to the venous system and then taken up by several tissues including liver, lung, heart, and adipose tissue. Although it has been suggested that adipocytes "store" vitamin E, since the majority of tocopherol in the body is found there, it should be recognized that the tocopherol present in adipose tissue is not readily available to other tissues.[61] Thus, plasma tocopherol levels fall promptly when vitamin E is excluded from the diet.

Vitamin E is known to function as a biological antioxidant, protecting the PUFA of membrane phospholipids from oxidation.[62] The vitamin carries out this function by becoming oxidized itself and stopping the chain reaction of fatty acid peroxidation. Other functions have been proposed for vitamin E[63,64] but have not been established. Although animals develop a wide variety of pathologic changes as listed in Table 16-4, tocopherol-deficient humans have only been shown to develop hemolytic disease, which is usually mild, and possibly neuromuscular degeneration in association with long-term severe tocopherol deficiency.[56,65]

Status in Cystic Fibrosis

The earliest report of possible pathologic effects of vitamin E deficiency in cystic fibrosis[45] involved an infant who showed

Table 16-4
Pathology of Vitamin E Deficiency in Animals

Lesions of the Reproductive System
Embryopathy
Testicular atrophy
Myopathy
Lesions of the central nervous system
Nutritional encephalomalacia
Localized axonal dystrophy
Lesions of the cardiovascular system
Exudative diathesis
Necrotizing arteritis
Myocardial necrosis
Hematopoietic disorders
Hemolysis
Anemia
Hepatic necrosis
Lipopigment accumulation

necrotic changes in skeletal muscle resembling the lesions associated with tocopherol deficiency in various animal species (Table 16-4). Subsequently, several reviews[56,60,66] have been published on the vitamin E-deficient state of patients with CF. Study of the possible consequences of vitamin E deficiency in cystic fibrosis has focused on erythrocyte stability, the neuromuscular system, and the morphology of the intestinal tract.

Dolan[67] reported five infants with CF who developed hemolytic anemia associated with low vitamin E levels. The effects of vitamin E deficiency and repletion on various hematological indices have been studied in older CF patients by Farrell et al.[55,59] Unsupplemented CF patients with pancreatic insufficiency had significant reduction in their plasma levels of α-tocopherol and α-tocopherol/triglyceride and α-tocopherol/total lipid ratios. Also, erythrocytes from these vitamin E-deficient patients demonstrated increased susceptibility to oxidation as assessed by the in vitro peroxide hemolysis test. Despite the observation of normal hemoglobin and hematocrit values, RBC counts, and reticulocyte counts, determination of [^{51}Cr]RBC survival indicated a decreased mean half-life of 22 days compared to 28 days in control subjects. Supplementation with 200 IU/day α-tocopheryl acetate resulted in normalization of plasma α-tocopherol levels, improvement in values for peroxide-induced hemolysis, and correction of [^{51}Cr]RBC survival times. Farrell et al[55] also determined fatty acid composition of erythrocytes in their study, showing increased palmitoleic and oleic acids and decreased linoleic acid, but no statistical difference in the peroxidizable indices of the fatty acids of the CF erythrocyte compared to normal controls. Hubbard and Dunn[68] subsequently determined the erythrocyte fatty acid composition from vitamin E-supplemented patients with cystic fibrosis and reported similar results. Data from other studies suggest that vitamin E supplementation does not appear to affect the fatty acid composition of plasma or erythrocyte lipids.[69,70]

The neuromuscular system has been investigated in CF because of the recognition of myopathy associated with vitamin E deficiency in animals. These studies have been limited to evaluation of plasma enzymes such as creatine kinase which originate from muscle, assessment of creatinuria, and a small number of histologic examinations of striated muscle. Nitowsky et al[71] observed increased creatine excretion in tocopherol-deficient CF patients, a disturbance generally found in muscular dystrophy. Although the abnormal creatinuria was responsive in 12 of 14 patients to vitamin E supplementation, this change is not specific for muscle necrosis and can be partially attributed to muscle wasting.[56] Enzymes which are characteristic of skeletal muscle damage and are strikingly elevated in muscular dystrophy have only rarely been elevated in cystic fibrosis or in patients with other gastrointestinal disorders accompanied by low vitamin E levels. Histological studies have also been generally unrevealing and have only shown rare or mild abnormalities.[56] Evaluation of muscle performance in CF patients before and after vitamin E supplementation resulted in no differences within the patients themselves or from a normal control group.[72,73]

According to Sung,[74] patients with CF have a neuroaxonal dystrophy that affects primarily the gracile nucleus and resembles lesions observed in animals with vitamin E deficiency. These lesions are not specific for cystic fibrosis since they appeared frequently in routine autopsies of adults beyond 30 years old; however, they were recognized at a much earlier age, ie, 6–22 years.[74] The association with vitamin E has been substantiated in a more recent study in which autopsies of 47 CF patients were reviewed by Sung et al.[75] Axonal dystrophy in the gracile nucleus occurred, particularly in patients older than 10 years. Comparison of the overall incidence in patients autopsied between 1952 and 1969 and those investigated between 1970 and 1980 revealed a decrease in axonal dystrophy from 79% (15/19) to 36% (10/28), respectively. The decreased incidence of neurologic lesions was associated with a greater number of patients receiving vitamin E supplementation, an increase in the length of time on vitamin E supplementation, and initiating such treatment at an earlier age. Sung et al[75] also reported the invariable occurrence of more severe axonal dystrophy in patients with congenital biliary atresia over one year of age; these patients usually have more severe vitamin E deficiency that is unresponsive to oral supplementation.[56,76] In contrast to Sung's conclusions, Cavalier and Gambetti[77] reported that although direct correlation between severity of neuroaxonal dystrophy and duration of disease was observed, the incidence and severity of the abnormalities did not decrease in association with prescribed vitamin E supplements. A major weakness of all the neuropathological studies involving material from patients with CF is that actual assessment of the vitamin E status of the patients was not performed. Other neuropathologic lesions described by Geller et al[78] include microscopically visible degeneration in the posterior funiculi of spinal cord sections in 17 of 106 autopsy specimens from patients with CF. The degeneration was predominantly limited to the fasciculus gracilus, occurred bilaterally, and was found only in sections from the cervical and thoracic segments. Although the posterior column abnormality was not clinically evident, five of seven patients with the diagnosis of peripheral polyneuropathy also had degeneration present. Again, no discussion of vitamin E status was included in this report; however, posterior column degeneration is among the earliest changes described in animals on vitamin E-deficient diets.[78] Other clinical case reports[79,80] have also described posterior column dysfunction occurring concurrent with vitamin E deficiency in patients without cystic fibrosis. (See Chapter 22 for further discussion of this topic.)

Ceroid pigment, also referred to as lipofuscin, accumulates in the smooth muscle of vitamin E-deficient animals, presumably as a result of the intracellular accummulation of peroxidized, unsaturated lipids. This pigment has been invariably present upon examination of necropsy tissue from vitamin E-deficient CF patients more than 2 years old. In fact, Kerner and Goldbloom[81] found ceroid pigment in tissue at all levels of the intestinal tract, liver, urinary bladder, trachea, and lungs. At the present time, no functional disturbance has been attributed to the presence of this material.

Thus, considerable research has already been conducted on tocopherol deficiency in cystic fibrosis, but there is a need to elucidate the cellular functions of vitamin E, its possible role in the nonrespiratory functions of the lung, and to establish the dose required by patients with CF (especially those with the combination of pancreatic insufficiency and significant liver disease). It would also be useful to study vitamin E requirements of patients receiving PUFA supplements and to define further the neuromuscular consequences of human tocopherol deficiency.

Supplementation with vitamin E, ideally using a water-miscible preparation,[82,83] is required to prevent tocopherol deficiency. In contrast to vitamin A, blood levels of vitamin E do reflect tissue concentrations, for no abnormality in tocopherol transport is apparent.[31] The supplement usually prescribed ranges from 50 IU for infants to 200 IU for adults; however, recent data[59] suggest that these doses are excessive, based on tocopherol–lipid ratio values obtained during assessment of nutritional status in supplemented patients.

VITAMIN K

General Background

Vitamin K was discovered in 1929 during a series of investigations with chicks who developed hemorrhages when fed a diet extracted of lipid. Thus, the term vitamin K was coined for this "koagulation" vitamin. The vitamin was subsequently isolated from alfalfa and its structure identified in 1939.[84,85] The chemistry of vitamin K has been well established ever since Doisy and associates identified vitamin K_1 (phylloquinone) as 2-methyl-3-phytyl-1,4-naphthoquinone. This compound, whose structure is shown in Figure 16-5, is synthesized by various plants and is the only coagulation factor produced in plants. Vitamin K_2 was originally isolated from fish meal, differs from phylloquinone in the isoprene side chain, and is known as menaquinone-7. Other menaquinone derivatives with variable length side chains can be synthesized in animals and birds and are considered vitamin K_2 homologs. Because the concentrations of vitamin K in biological fluids and tissues are very low, chemical determinations are extremely difficult. In addition, vitamin K homologs are labile to alkali and light. When extracts are highly concentrated, vitamin K compounds can be identified by their distinctive absorbance spectrum. Another method of analysis involves bioassay using chicks fed a vitamin K-deficient diet and then given the test substance such as a tissue extract or plasma; measurement of the blood prothrombin level is utilized as the measure of response to vitamin K. It would be highly advantageous, however, to have a chemical method available for routine analysis of vitamin K.

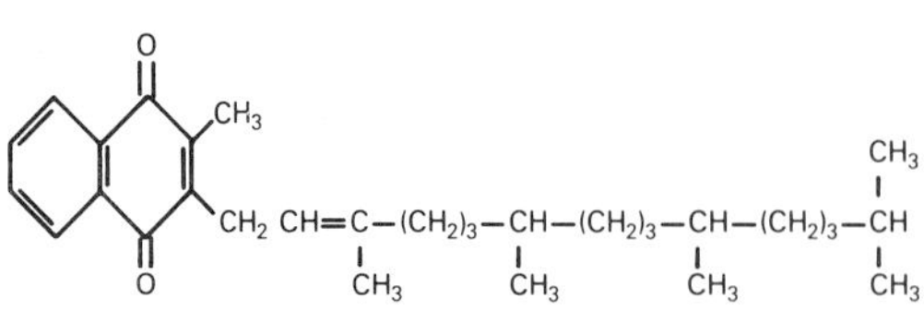

PHYLLOQUINONE (VITAMIN K_1)

Figure 16-5 Vitamin K. Phylloquinone (vitamin K_1) is a product synthesized by plants. It differs from the other vitamin K analogs as a result of its isoprene side chain.

Good dietary sources of vitamin K are green leafy vegetables such as lettuce, cabbage, broccoli, and asparagus. Cheese, butter, and beef liver also provide moderate amounts of vitamin K. Study of the intestinal absorption of vitamin K indicates that 30–70% uptake occurs, depending upon the source and other factors. Vitamin K compounds, like other fat-soluble vitamins, are incorporated into chylomicrons and transported via lymphatics to the venous circulation. It is generally assumed that absorption of vitamin K will be decreased in patients with steatorrhea and in individuals given nonabsorbable lipids such as mineral oil. Vitamin K_1 is rapidly deposited in the liver, with approximately 50% of a parenterally administered dose appearing within 1 hr and 20% of an oral dose being found in the liver in 2 hr. Approximately half the liver content of vitamin K is phylloquinone from the diet and the remainder is accounted for by menaquinones. Several metabolites of phylloquinone and the menaquinones have been recovered from the urine, particularly sulfate and glucocuronide derivatives. In humans and omnivorous animals, intestinal synthesis of higher-molecular-weight menaquinones (menaquinone-7 to menaquinone-13) occurs as a result of bacterial flora. Although these compounds derived from intestinal flora are found in the liver, the magnitude of in vivo vitamin K synthesis and the turnover of these compounds have not been determined precisely; as discussed subsequently, this raises issues about supplementation of CF patients with vitamin K.

The function of vitamin K with respect to blood coagulation has been closely related to prothrombin (factor II) and three other coagulation proteins (factors VII, IX, and X). In vitamin K-deficient subjects, the administration of phylloquinone or menaquinone leads to a prompt response such that prothrombin levels will return toward normal in 4–6 hr. It has been suspected for many years that the mechanism of vitamin K action involves regulation of the production of these proteins by the liver. Although some data suggested interaction with genetic material to stimulate specific mRNA synthesis,[84] recent evidence strongly indicates that the site of action of vitamin K involves posttranslational carboxylation of glutamate residues in prothrombin precursors.[85] This generates γ-carboxyglutamate residues which are necessary components of the active protein. Vitamin K is also active in the production of the newly discovered bone matrix protein "osteocalcin" which contains γ-carboxyglutamate.[86]

Status in Cystic Fibrosis

Deficiency of vitamin K has been observed in some patients with cystic fibrosis. Because methods for determination of circulating vitamin K are not available, assessment of vitamin K status has depended upon measurement of prothrombin time. Several reports have appeared describing hypoprothrombinemia and bleeding in patients with CF.[87–90] In all cases, the patients were less than 4 months of age. Thus, infants with a hemorrhagic tendency should be evaluated for cystic fibrosis when they have a prolonged prothrombin time. According to a report by Torstenson et al,[87] all the vitamin K-dependent coagulation proteins were low, while the non-vitamin K-dependent factors were normal in two infants with CF studied extensively. Normalization of hypoprothrombinemia occurred with vitamin K therapy in these subjects.

Occurrence of hypoprothrombinemia could potentially be attributable to several factors in CF patients. Malabsorption of vitamin K might occur and is likely to be more of a problem in the previously undiagnosed patient with steatorrhea and in the infant with inadequately developed bowel flora. Secondly, CF patients with chronic respiratory tract infections are frequently taking antibiotics which, although absorbed, could conceivably alter the bacterial flora of the intestinal tract and possibly decrease synthesis of vitamin K. To the authors' knowledge, the magnitude of this effect has not been determined in patients on chronic antibiotic therapy other than neomycin or in those with malabsorption; however, it may be estimated[84] that as much as half the vitamin K arises in the gastrointestinal tract, based on the observation that germfree rats require about twice as much in their diet as conventional rats.[91] Another factor in the production of vitamin K deficiency in cystic fibrosis relates to dietary sources. Special food supplements and formulas consumed by CF patients may provide inadequate vitamin K.[92]

Because of concern that vitamin K deficiency might develop in patients with cystic fibrosis, it has been recommended that supplementation take place with either 50–100 μg of vitamin K daily or 2.5–5 mg weekly.[6,36] This dose would appear to be high in view of the 1 μg/kg estimated daily requirement for dietary vitamin K; however, the degree of absorption is uncertain when large amounts of fat-soluble vitamins are consumed. Most CF centers have routinely supplemented infants up to 1 year of age and some children on antibiotic therapy, even though 4 weeks or longer of neomycin ingestion is needed to lower prothrombin levels. Although there is no well-established basis for vitamin K supplementation of patients with hemoptysis, this practice has often been followed. Regardless of the practices followed by CF centers, it should be recognized that almost all children, adolescents, and adults with chronic lung disease and malabsorption (including those with hemoptysis) have maintained normal prothrombin times without vitamin K supplements even while taking daily antibiotics. Only infants and CF patients with extensive biliary cirrhosis are expected to have prolonged prothrombin times.[93] These children should be treated with vitamin K supplements in order to improve their blood coagulation.

Because new biochemical and immunologic methods are being developed for measurement of vitamin K and K-dependent coagulation proteins, it will become more feasible to carry out research in this area. Certainly, there is a pressing need to assess vitamin K status of CF patients under various conditions to determine if a subclinical coagulopathy can occur in CF patients who do not receive supplements. In addition, this might allow the complete assessment of vitamin K synthesis by intestinal bacteria. As these methods improve, development of sound guidelines for vitamin K supplementation may become possible.

ESSENTIAL FATTY ACIDS

General Background[94,95]

Dietary fat is important as a high-density source of calories, for improving the palatability of food, and for providing essential fatty acids (EFA). Therefore, the traditional tendency to restrict fat consumption by CF patients might be expected to cause adverse nutritional consequences. Of particular concern, relative to the nutritional deficiencies, is the potential lack of adequate amounts of essential fatty acids such as linoleate. EFA are those polyunsaturated fatty acids that cannot be adequately synthesized de novo to support growth, production of biological membranes, and functioning of certain metabolic processes. Three fatty acids are recognized as being essential, namely linoleate, linolenate, and arachidonate, although the latter can be synthesized if adequate linoleate is ingested. The structures of these fatty acids are shown in Figure 16-6. As described subsequently, linoleic acid is especially important because it can be converted to arachidonic acid which can in turn be metabolized into prostaglandins.

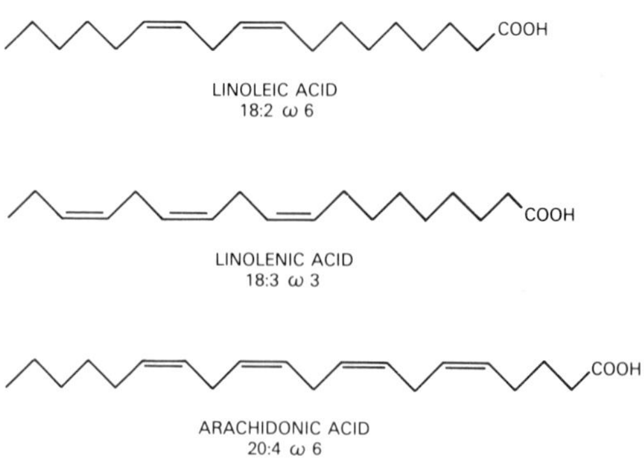

Figure 16-6 Essential fatty acids. These fatty acids cannot be synthesized de novo in humans. The structures shown are identified by the "ω" shorthand nomenclature system, in which the number following the "ω" indicates the position of the first double bond counting from the methyl terminus.

Before discussing EFA deficiency, it would be helpful to review the nomenclature and metabolism of relevant fatty acids.[96] Because fatty acids are carboxylic acids containing a long hydrocarbon chain, they can be designated according to the general rules of organic nomenclature. The hydrocarbon chain may be straight or branched, saturated or unsaturated, and may contain ring structures. Table 16-5 lists the common saturated and unsaturated fatty acids up to 24 carbons in length with their systematic and generic or trivial names. Because of their long names, it is convenient to designate fatty acids by a shorthand notation. A numerical notation consisting of the number of carbon atoms followed by the number of double bonds is often employed, eg, palmitic acid is 16:0 and palmitoleic acid is 16:1. When using such a shorthand notation, there are several methods of signifying the location of the double bonds in unsaturated fatty acids. For example, linoleic acid may be represented as: $18{:}2\Delta^{9,12}$, as 18:2(9,12), as $18{:}2^{9,12}$, or as $18{:}2\omega6,9$. Note that the last system, employing "ω" to signify the location of the double bonds, entails numbering of the molecule from the methyl end rather than from the carboxyl end. This system recognizes the metabolic relationships among polyunsaturated fatty acids, as determined by their terminal structures. The ω nomenclature for double-bond locations has become popular among nutritionists in recent years and is often shortened further to indicate only the first double bond counting from the methyl terminus. Thus, for linoleic acid, 18:2ω6 is used to designate an 18-carbon fatty acid with two double bonds, the terminal one of which is formed at the sixth carbon from the methyl group; since the double bonds are all methylene interrupted, it is not necessary to use the designation 18:2ω6,9. The ω system has been used in this chapter and is recommended because of its relevance to cellular metabolism and the widespread acceptance it enjoys.

Mammalian species can produce most of the common fatty acids completely de novo from carbohydrate or protein. To make palmitic acid (16:0), for instance, acetyl-CoA and malonyl-CoA are the only precursors necessary. Palmitate is therefore classified as a nonessential fatty acid. Two other abundant fatty acids, stearic acid (18:0) and oleic acid (18:1Δ^9 or 18:1ω9), are synthesized in the liver by either simple elongation of palmitoyl-CoA or by elongation and subsequent desaturation. In contrast to the ω9 family of fatty acids, linoleate (18:2ω6) and higher PUFAs of the ω6 family cannot be formed de novo because of an inability to introduce a second double bond into oleic acid, ie, between the double bond in the C-9 position and the methyl end of the hydrocarbon chain. This is the basis for linoleate being an essential fatty acid which must be supplied in the diet. Once absorbed, linoleate undergoes a series of desaturations and elongations to produce the polyunsaturated fatty acids characteristic of an organism. Thus, 18:2ω6 serves the important function of being a precursor for fatty acids such as arachidonate (20:4ω6).

Fatty acids are measured in plasma and tissues after extraction with organic solvents, production of volatile methyl ester derivatives, and gas chromatographic separation. It is important that complete separation of fatty acids be achieved, especially the PUFAs of 18 and 20 carbon chain lengths. In states of essential fatty acid deficiency, one finds decreased linoleate, usually decreased arachidonate (depending upon the severity of EFA deficiency), and also the appearance of an unusual fatty acid synthesized from oleate (18:1ω9). As illustrated in Figure 16-7, this "pathologic" fatty acid is a 20-carbon compound with three double bonds—hence a triene. It is referred to as 5,8,11-eicosatrienoic acid or 20:3ω9.

Table 16-5
Fatty Acids in Human Tissues

Number of Carbons	Systematic Name	Common Name
Saturated straight-chain fatty acids		
14	Tetradecanoic	Myristic
16	Hexadecanoic	Palmitic
18	Octadecanoic	Stearic
20	Eicosanoic	Arachidic
22	Docosanoic	Behenic
24	Tetracosanoic	Lignoceric
Unsaturated straight-chain fatty acids		
16:1Δ^9	9-Hexadecenoic	Palmitoleic
18:1Δ^9	9-Octadecenoic	Oleic
18:2$\Delta^{9,12}$	9,12-Octadecadienoic	Linoleic
18:3$\Delta^{9,12,15}$	9,12,15-Octadecatrienoic	Linolenic
18:3$\Delta^{6,9,12}$	6,9,12-Octadecatrienoic	γ-Linolenic
20:3$\Delta^{8,11,14}$	8,11,14-Eicosatrienoic	Homo-γ-linolenic
20:3$\Delta^{5,8,11}$	5,8,11-Eicosatrienoic	Triene
20:4$\Delta^{5,8,11,14}$	5,8,11,14-Eicosatetraenoic	Arachidonic

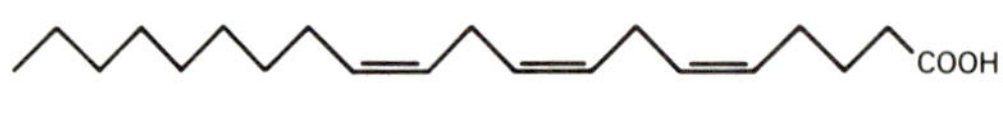

EICOSATRIENOIC ACID
20:3 ω 9

Figure 16-7 Eicosatrienoic acid. This fatty acid is the chain elongation product of oleic acid (18:1ω9) and increases in amount in association with essential fatty acid deficiency. Eicosatrienoic acid is the 20:3 isomer used in calculating triene/tetraene ratio (20:3ω9/20:4ω6).

Because of the presence of this triene and the customary decrease in the tetraenoic acid, arachidonate, measurement of the "triene–tetraene ratio" can be used for diagnosis of EFA deficiency. In studies of animals, a ratio above 0.4 is considered diagnostic of EFA deficiency; however, a value of 0.2 has been used recently for humans.

In general, practically any common source of dietary fat will provide linoleic acid as a component of triglycerides. Bile salts and lipases (including pancreatic juice) are, therefore, necessary for absorption. The minimum amount of linoleic acid consumption required to prevent EFA deficiency, as identified in studies with rats, is 1–2% of total caloric intake. Humans might require a greater amount of linoleic acid, especially during periods of rapid growth.

In regard to metabolic functions, it should be pointed out that all fatty acids longer than eight carbons in chain length cross biological membranes slowly and must be converted to acylcarnitine intermediates for entry into the mitochondria. Evidence from study of lower animals indicates that essential fatty acids may be important in the efficient transport of cholesterol and for the stabilization of biologic membranes (as components of phospholipids). Because essential fatty acids are necessary in the formation of prostaglandins, all functions of prostaglandins could potentially be altered in EFA deficiency. The signs of EFA deficiency in animals include growth retardation, scaly dermatitis, increased susceptibility to respiratory tract infections, and loss of hair. In humans, most of the same abnormalities have been observed, especially in patients on long-term, fatfree parenteral alimentation.

Status in Cystic Fibrosis

The first study of fatty acids in blood and tissue lipids of patients with CF was published by Kuo et al.[97] They compared the fatty acid composition of serum chylomicrons and adipose tissue from 15 patients with CF, who had variable degrees of steatorrhea, with data obtained in a control group consisting of 12 children who had no evidence of malabsorption. Decreased linoleic acid (18:2ω6) and increased palmitoleic (16:ω9) and oleic (18:1ω9) acids were the predominant alterations of fatty acid composition observed. Ever since their recognition of an abnormality of fatty acid composition, various explanations for the etiology of this biochemical disturbance in cystic fibrosis have been proposed. The possible influence of concomitant hepatic disease was studied by Caren and Corbo,[98] who determined the fatty acid composition of the four major plasma lipid fractions in 8 normal children, 20 normal adults, 23 patients with CF, 7 patients with advanced cirrhosis, and 9 patients with hepatitis. The results indicated that the patients with primary liver disease had alterations of their fatty acid profiles similar to those seen in cystic fibrosis, including decreased 18:2ω6 and increased 16:1ω9 and 18:1ω9. Changes were observed in all lipid fractions (free fatty acids, triglycerides, phospholipids, and cholesterol esters). Thus, these authors concluded that the fatty acid changes were a reflection of underlying liver disease in cystic fibrosis.

Other investigators have proposed that the altered fatty acid composition may be related to the basic defect in cystic fibrosis, which could be potentiated by the maldigestion and malabsorption of fats. Rivers and Hassam[99] suggested that an enzymatic defect in fatty acid desaturation was responsible for the fatty acid changes observed in CF. They further proposed that the occurrence of this defect coupled with decreased absorption of

EFA would account for the course of the disease. Although their hypothesis would provide a theoretical explanation for some observations in cystic fibrosis, no direct enzyme measurements were reported. Press[100] and Watts et al[101] concluded that the changes of fatty acid composition observed in patients with CF were similar to alterations seen in other patients as a consequence of either malabsorption or dietary deficiency of essential fatty acids; thus, there was no need to postulate a metabolic defect specific to CF to explain the findings.

Several groups have attempted to answer the question regarding the cause of the altered fatty acid composition in cystic fibrosis by comparing results obtained in patients with and without malabsorption.[68–70,102,103] The status of the exocrine pancreas has been based on stool fat and nitrogen, pancreatic enzyme activity in duodenal fluid, serum amylase isozymes, serum carotene, and/or results of the benzoyl-tyrosyl-*p*-aminobenzoic acid absorption test of pancreatic function. These studies have shown that patients with CF having clinically normal exocrine pancreatic functions show fatty acid profiles in blood lipids which do not differ from controls. These observations indicate that the abnormalities of fatty acid composition in patients with CF are a secondary consequence of inadequate linoleate absorption due to maldigestion and/or insufficient dietary fat, although the data of Caren and Corbo[98] suggest that the abnormal fatty acid profiles were not simply a consequence of dietary factors. Results of dietary surveys by Caren and Corbo,[98] Hubbard and di Sant'Agnese (unpublished data), and Mischler, Farrell, and Lemen (unpublished data) have shown that many CF patients consume linoleic acid at greater than 2% of total calories. Furthermore, the alterations of fatty acid composition are found in patients receiving pancreatic enzyme supplements, even though steatorrhea is significantly reduced.

Although there have been several attempts to provide fatty acid supplementation for patients with CF, with the objective of augmenting caloric intake and/or normalizing the fatty acid profiles,[104–106] the outcome of such studies has been variable. Kuo and Huang[107] reported accentuation of the already abnormal fatty acid profiles of plasma lipids and adipose tissue when medium-chain triglycerides were substituted in the diet for the longer-chain triglycerides. Elliott and co-workers published several reports[108–110] leading to the association of normalized sweat electrolyte concentrations and improved clinical status of patients following parenteral administration of fat emulsions approximately every other week. These workers made the assumption that fat infusions would at least partially correct the fatty acid profiles (no fatty acid determinations were performed) and suggested that treating cystic fibrosis with linoleate-containing fat might influence the course of disease. Subsequent studies[104,111] have not substantiated the claims regarding improvement of clinical and laboratory evaluations as a result of fat infusions. Additionally, it has now been determined that intravenous fat emulsions would have to be given more frequently than every two weeks in order to maintain improvement in the fatty acid profiles.[104] In fact, the therapy would probably be needed at least two to three times per week when given as 10% Intralipid in a dose approximating 10–20 ml/kg/infusion (Hubbard and Dunn, unpublished data).

Using the oral linoleic acid supplementation approach, Rosenlund et al[105] treated patients with CF for one year with corn oil (1 g/kg/day) given with meals. They observed variable improvement in their patients, including a decreased sweat sodium and a normalization of the serum fatty acid profiles; however, clinical status was not significantly affected. Lloyd-Still et al[112] subsequently carried out dietary supplementation with safflower oil (1 g/kg/day) for one year and observed no significant change in sweat chloride concentrations. The fatty acid profiles of their group of subjects were not described in this report; however, in a subsequent paper[106] it was reported that correction of the fatty acid disturbances did not occur.

Although both corn oil and safflower oil are good sources of linoleic acid and are readily available, inadequate patient compliance with the recommended supplement must be considered as one explanation for the variable results observed during long-term evaluations of oral fatty acid treatment. In a more recent dietary supplementation study with Microlipid (triglyceride emulsion containing 54% linoleate and given daily in a volume that supplied 7% of calories as EFA), Mischler et al[113] found that compliant patients normalized their plasma 18:2ω6 levels, whereas those who admitted irregular consumption of the supplement did not achieve correction. These data further suggested that more than 7% of calories as linoleate may be needed for prompt correction of the diminished EFA stores.

Although the alteration of fatty acids in cystic fibrosis does not appear to be caused by a defect in linoleic acid metabolism and thus is not related to the basic defect in the disease, it remains a biochemical abnormality which is present in the majority of CF patients, ie, those with pancreatic insufficiency. Based on animal studies, it would be expected to adversely influence some of the manifestations of the disease. Of interest in this connection is the recent observation[114,115] that CF patients with normal fat absorption, and thus normal fatty acid profiles, have lower mean sweat electrolyte concentrations than patients with pancreatic insufficiency. Such observations do not necessarily imply that the high sweat electrolyte concentrations in CF patients are the result of abnormal fatty acid composition of the membranes; however, it is conceivable that the altered fatty acid composition may potentiate the underlying defect. Therefore, in further studies regarding the relationship of linoleate supplementation to sweat electrolyte composition, it is imperative that both fatty acid profiles and sweat electrolyte concentrations be determined concurrently. It would also be helpful to assess more of the possible metabolic effects of correcting linoleate deficiency, for instance, evaluation of prostaglandins.

MINERALS

The nutritional status of CF patients with respect to macrominerals and trace minerals has been of considerable interest, but in general has not been studied in sufficient depth. Furthermore, the techniques used for assessing trace minerals have often been unsatisfactory. This is not surprising in view of the fact that even in healthy adults there is controversy over methods used to evaluate some of these dietary elements such as zinc and sodium.

Macrominerals of concern in cystic fibrosis include calcium, phosphorus, and sodium. The factorial approach and metabolic balance techniques are often used in normal subjects to evaluate these elements in conjunction with assessment of growth, other relevant dietary components such as protein, and the impact of the environment. Calcium and phosphorus are discussed briefly in the section on vitamin D. Unfortunately, comprehensive studies of calcium and phosphorus balance in relationship to bone mineralization have not yet been carried out in CF patients. As discussed previously, however, there is evidence[21] that bone demineralization occurs frequently in cystic fibrosis, particularly in the older patients, and that this can lead to pathologic fractures. As the longevity of patients with CF continues to increase, there will be even greater concern for the state of calcium and phosphorus nutrition.

Sodium is of concern in cystic fibrosis because of the high salinity of sweat. There is a major requirement for sodium during growth, primarily to support expansion of the extracellular fluid volume. The requirement is particularly high during the first 6 months of life when as much as 0.5 mEq/kg/day are needed for the increases in this compartment. Sodium requirements can be estimated from information on the salinity and expected daily volume of sweat under a variety of environmental conditions. The consequences of sodium or salt depletion in patients with cystic fibrosis can be catastrophic in hot climates and lead to severe hyponatremic dehydration and shock. Indeed, it was the clinical observation of this phenomenon that led to discovery of the sweat electrolyte defect and diagnostic test for cystic fibrosis by di Sant'Agnese et al.[116] Under conditions of moderate ambient temperature and humidity, insensible water loss in the adult averages 500–800 ml/day. Because as much as 75% of the cutaneous insensible water loss results from diffusion rather than sweat gland secretion, a substantial portion of the water is essentially electrolyte-free. Assuming a sweat sodium concentration of 30 mEq/liter, it may be calculated that a maximum sodium loss of 4 mEq/day will occur under such conditions. This corresponds to 92 mg of elemental sodium or 234 mg of sodium chloride since 1 mEq of sodium is 23 mg, and this corresponds to 58.5 mg of salt. In a hot climate, particularly under conditions of strenuous physical activity, adults may readily lose up to 3 liters of additional water per day from sweating and will require at least 2 g/day of extra salt per liter of additional insensible water loss.

Most of the sodium in the diet is consumed as salt (NaCl) with the major sources being cheese, milk, meat, poultry, eggs, and fish. A substantial amount is also added from the salt shaker and from convenience foods. It should be noted that cereals, fruits, and vegetables are naturally low in sodium, but that modern processing techniques have led to higher salt contents. Thus, it can be calculated that American adults consume 10–20 times the amount of sodium required. Indeed, the renal conservation of sodium is efficient enough that the healthy adult can maintain sodium balance with an intake of little more than the minimal requirement of infants.

In patients with cystic fibrosis, it is clear that salt supplements may be required in hot environments when exposure and/or physical exertion causes increased sweating. The extra salt required for adolescent and adult patients can be assumed to be two- to fourfold greater than the estimate given previously for healthy adults. One would expect, therefore, that a supplement of 4–8 g NaCl/day would be needed per liter of extra insensible water loss. Because the American diet usually contains excessive sodium, however, it is unlikely that patients with CF would require that level of supplementation. Furthermore, most patients are not continuously exposed to hot environments, where sweating is profuse over a long period of time.

From a practical point of view, physicians caring for patients with CF should recognize that the problem of salt loss is only of major concern in hot climates or during heat-wave conditions. Even then, the need for additional salt is limited to those patients who are generating increased sweat, ie, those with extra sweat electrolyte losses. Thus, there is no good rationale for the traditional practice of recommending routine consumption of salty foods and aggresive use of the salt shaker, particularly in view of the rising sodium content of the American diet. In fact, as the longevity of patients with CF continues to increase and cor pulmonale becomes an increasing problem, a lifelong habit of ingesting salty food becomes an obstacle to effective management of heart failure by sodium restriction. We would, therefore, recommend that patients not be encouraged to salt their food aggressively, but rather should consume a regular diet in which the meat and milk food groups will provide adequate sodium chloride. If patients are consistently exposed to hot environments with enough physical activity to increase their sweat volume, salt tablets should be consumed in a dose of 250 mg to 2 g two or three times daily (depending upon the size of the patient, the degree of exposure, and the level of physical activity). Measurement of serum electrolytes in conditions of high ambient temperatures is obviously important, just as monitoring fluid and electrolyte status is important in patients with gastroenteritis. (See Chapter 4 for further discussion of these problems.)

The microminerals or trace elements that have attracted the greatest attention in cystic fibrosis are copper, selenium, iron, and zinc. There has been controversy over the question as to how one can best evaluate micromineral status of the general population as well as patients with diseases that can lead to malnutrition. In general, minerals such as copper, zinc, and selenium function at the cellular level as cofactors for enzymes of intermediary metabolism. Thus, plasma and urine concentrations of these minerals may vary from day to day and thus not provide a good indication of nutritional status. Measurement of the activity of the metalloenzyme, on the other hand, can provide a more reliable index of nutritional status. There have been limited studies on copper status in cystic fibrosis. Kopito and Shwachman[117] reported values for two sera samples and six urine specimens that were considered normal. Solomons et al[13] measured plasma copper and its transport protein (ceruloplasmin) and found that the mean concentrations of each were significantly increased in patients with cystic fibrosis; of 16 patients studied, 15 showed copper levels above the control mean value of 103 mg/dl. Hubbard (unpublished data) also found copper and ceruloplasmin concentrations to be generally increased in cystic fibrosis. In addition, van Stekelenberg et al[118] reported that the copper content in fingernail clippings was significantly elevated in cystic fibrosis. Although elevations in ceruloplasmin might be attributable to the fact that this protein is an acute-phase reactant in patients with infection, the explanation for high copper levels is not readily apparent. It should be pointed out, however, that copper is largely excreted in bile and that patients with biliary stasis conceivably have defective copper excretion. Further research will be needed to evaluate this possibility.

Selenium is an essential cofactor for the enzyme glutathione peroxidase and, therefore, is closely associated with vitamin E as part of the cellular antioxidant system. The nutritional interrelationships between selenium and vitamin E are well established and reviewed extensively by Hoekstra[119] and Draper.[120] Because selenium deficiency in animals can be associated with abnormalities seen in cystic fibrosis such as pancreatic degeneration with scarring and growth retardation, there have been claims that this trace element plays an important role in cystic fibrosis. Normally, dietary protein provides considerable selenium such that protein malnutrition can be associated with selenium deficiency. Thus, meats and seafoods are good sources, whereas grains are variable, and fruits and vegetables contain very little selenium. There are regions of the world, such as Tibet and New Zealand, where the selenium content of the soil is low enough to cause low circulating levels of selenium and even a myocardiopathy which may be fatal (Keshan disease). Evaluation of selenium status has involved measurement of either plasma or red blood cell concentrations, along with determinations of glutathione peroxidase activity. Plasma levels vary from day to day and can be misleading, but erythrocyte selenium is more stable. Investigation of patients with CF has been carried out in recent years to determine if a deficiency developed in association with this disease. Heinrich et al[121] reported that intestinal absorption of protein-bound selenomethionine was decreased in two patients with cystic fibrosis. Underwood, et al[122] found that mean plasma levels of selenium were mildly reduced in 23 patients with CF to a mean value of 13.1 mg/dl compared to a control value of 20.6 mg/dl; however, there was considerable overlap in data between the CF population and the controls. Castillo et al[123] and Lloyd-Still and Ganther[124] have also found that serum and whole-blood selenium levels in CF patients are lower than age-matched controls, but not as low as circulating concentrations in the population of New Zealand. Furthermore, the activity of glutathione peroxidase in erythrocytes, which provides a reliable index of deficiency, was the same in cystic fibrosis as in control subjects. This occurred despite the reduced selenium concentrations and provides a good indication that these patients with CF have adequate selenium nutriture. Thus, there is no basis at the present time for recommending selenium supplementation, particularly because of the possibility of toxic side effects.

Iron is an essential component of hemoglobin, myoglobin, various cytochromes, and many important enzymes. In addition to being found in functional forms, iron is bound to a storage protein (ferritin) and a transport protein (transferrin). Nutritional deficiency is first evident in the storage sites, and anemia is a relatively late sign of iron depletion. Regulation of iron nutriture occurs largely at the level of the intestinal mucosa where major adjustments are made in percentage absorption, depending on the magnitude of iron stores. Dietary sources include meats, beans, eggs and iron-fortified foods, but the bioavailability of the nutrient in these foods is quite variable.

The iron status of patients with cystic fibrosis has been of concern ever since Andersen[43] reported that hemosiderosis of the liver was evident in 13 of 49 autopsies. This pathology was confined almost exclusively to infants less than 7 months old, an observation supported by Stein et al.[125] Normally, iron stores present at birth are being used actively by 7 months of age for expansion of the red cell mass; however, this may not occur in growth-retarded infants such as those with untreated cystic fibrosis. In another autopsy series of patients who died at 1 month to 38 years of age, Longnecker[126] found that hepatic iron stores were similar in magnitude to controls during the first year. Minimal levels of stainable hepatic iron were observed by Stein et al[125] and by Longnecker[126] after 1 year of age. Gilly et al[127] subsequently examined bone marrow iron microscopically in 38 patients with CF, aged 3 months to 10 years, and found normal stores in 9, while 13 had depleted iron stores; 16 patients had excessive iron stores including 10 who were older than 6 months and generally had been on pancreatic enzyme therapy for 2 years.

The issue of whether or not pancreatic enzyme therapy increases iron absorption has been controversial, largely because of studies which have not been sufficiently comprehensive or controlled. Heme iron absorption was studied by Smith[128] in 15 patients with CF who generally had been on pancreatic enzymes for more than one year, had hemoglobin levels of less than 12 g/dl, and low plasma iron concentrations. All subjects receiving enzyme replacement therapy absorbed less iron than previously untreated infants and also absorbed less than controls. Furthermore, serial studies in two patients showed that when pancreatin was added, reduction of iron absorption occurred. Heinrich et al[121,129] have investigated absorption in relationship to iron stores using both inorganic forms and heme iron. Their methodology involved whole-body counting on the 14th day after giving a test dose of the ferrous salt to assess absorption. Although the ranges were wide for both CF and normal children, there was no significant difference in iron absorption between the two groups when matched for stores as assessed by bone marrow examination. Three CF patients with normal iron stores and four with depleted iron stores were examined with and without concurrent pancreatic enzyme administration. The average absorption was not reduced to a statistically significant level in either subgroup of patients with CF. Absorption of heme iron was also observed to be no different than in adult controls when matched for iron status.

From our interpretation of the studies related to iron nutrition, we conclude that the development of hemosiderosis in cystic fibrosis (if it occurs at all) is a pathologic phenomenon limited to infants, particularly those not receiving pancreatic enzymes. Whether the increased tissue iron in infants is a result of the untreated state or a reflection of residual fetal iron stores is not known; however, the pathological accumulation of iron is certainly not a problem in the older patient. Also, the issue of the effect of pancreatic disease on iron absorption has not been fully resolved. It might be expected that increased absorption of iron salts would take place in association with pancreatic insufficiency because there is a lower intestinal pH which favors the solubility and reduction of iron to the ferrous form which is better absorbed.[130] On the other hand, what role pancreatic enzyme supplements play in the absorption of iron remains unclear since a direct effect on the transport of iron from the intestinal lumen has not been established, although one might expect that enzymes would favor the absorption of heme iron.[17,131] Iron status should, therefore, be evaluated periodically in patients with CF, ideally by comprehensive assessment including ferritin levels. Supplementation should be provided before anemia or low plasma iron levels are detected. In patients who are unresponsive, other causes of anemia should be explored.

Zinc has been of interest in cystic fibrosis for many reasons, including the association of zinc deficiency with growth retardation and altered immunologic status.[132,133] Zinc is an essential constituent of numerous enzymes involved in most mammalian metabolic pathways. Although there is no single zinc-containing enzyme that can explain the biochemical and clinical changes occurring in zinc deficiency, there is reason to believe that enzymes involved in nucleic acid synthesis and degradation are critically dependent upon zinc for maintaining cellular functions.[134] Because evidence of zinc deficiency develops rapidly in experimental animals when intake is restricted, it is felt that a limited pool of biologically available zinc is present to support these metalloenzymes. Sources of dietary zinc include meat, liver, eggs, and seafood. Although whole-grain products such as wheat or rye bread contain zinc, it is not readily bioavailable; thus, grain products and vegetables do not provide sufficient zinc in an absorbable form. There are areas within the United States and in other parts of the world (eg, New Zealand and the Middle East) where the soil is deficient in zinc, resulting in the spontaneous appearance of zinc deficiency in animals raised for their dietary contribution of meat. The most prominent signs of zinc deficiency in animals and man are loss of appetite, failure to grow normally, skin alterations, impaired regeneration of wounds, and decreased taste acuity. Zinc deficiency influences other nutrients and is associated with decreased retinol-binding protein levels. Also, signs of essential fatty acid deficiency are more pronounced when zinc is low. In recent years, it has become appreciated that marginal states of zinc nutrition exist in segments of the population.[135] This has been shown both in elderly individuals and in children. These patients may rapidly develop decreased taste acuity, loss of appetite, evidence of altered immunocompetence, and loss of weight.

Methods for assessment of zinc nutritional status are somewhat controversial. Although many studies have involved measurement of plasma zinc levels, this may change rapidly from day to day and is unlikely to reflect total body stores of the mineral. Also, circulating zinc concentrations can be decreased when albumin levels are low or when inflammation develops. Erythrocyte zinc is also of questionable value. Measurement of the zinc concentration of hair is satisfactory when severe deficiency occurs, but may not be helpful to diagnose a rapidly developing state of deficiency. Urinary zinc values are also difficult to interpret. The test for taste acuity has been useful, but is subjective and used primarily for research. Some evidence suggests that saliva or sweat might also be useful, but this has not been established. Because of the problems with assessment of zinc status, the best approach is to use multiple indices such as plasma zinc, hair zinc, and measurement of proteins which depend upon zinc such as alkaline phosphatase and/or retinol-binding protein. It must be recognized, however, that these proteins are influenced by other nutritional and metabolic abnormalities.

In cystic fibrosis, plasma levels of zinc have been reported as decreased in association with growth retardation.[33,136] In particular, 18 patients with poor growth studied by Halstead and Smith[136] had a mean zinc concentration of 75 mg/dl, a value lower than 10 patients with normal growth (plasma zinc = 90 mg/dl; normal mean = 89 mg/dl). The children with growth retardation also had pulmonary infection which might explain the results. Nevertheless, there have been some patients identified with low plasma zinc concentrations when no acute infection was evident. Jacob et al[33] reported that 7 of 18 such patients had plasma zinc levels below 70 mg/dl. Other studies have not generally revealed a difference in plasma zinc concentrations when patients with CF have been compared to age-matched controls or siblings, even when growth retardation was present.[13,34,137] Hair concentrations of zinc, as well as plasma levels, were measured by Palin et al[34] and were not found to differ when 36 patients with CF were compared to 17 siblings. In addition, they found no association between growth and zinc levels. During a brief zinc supplementation trial with these patients, the authors found that zinc levels increased in the patients with CF, but the same change was found in control siblings and there were no measurable differences in processes known to be dependent upon zinc. Thus, further studies will be necessary before final conclusions can be reached regarding the zinc status of patients on a day-to-day basis. Because the intake of food can be reduced during times of severe infection, especially when appetite is decreased and vomiting occurs, this micromineral deserves further study.

SUMMARY AND DIETARY GUIDELINES

This chapter has reviewed available data concerning selected nutrients which are potentially altered in cystic fibrosis. One of the important messages learned from reviewing the literature is that much of the research in this area has been superficial or has involved inadequate methods of nutritional assessment. Furthermore, relatively small populations of patients with CF have been utilized for most investigations; this is of particular concern because of the marked heterogeneity of the disease. Because of the limitations in research thus far, it is difficult to reach conclusions that can be applied to the CF population as a whole. Nevertheless, there is sufficient information in the literature to recognize that deficiencies can occur in caloric intake, fat-soluble vitamins, essential fatty acids, and possibly protein and some of the minerals.

Guidelines for the caloric requirements of patients with CF have been summarized by Hubbard and Mangrum.[2] In general, initial intake of approximately 150% of the RDA for energy and macronutrients has been recommended for the "average" child with cystic fibrosis. The source of calories should be distributed such that at least 15–20% is derived from protein and 35–40% from fat. If an attempt is made to place patients on a regular diet, protein and fat requirements will be thus met because of the high consumption of these energy sources. The practice of taking one or two multivitamins per day provides patients with at least twice the RDA for most micronutrients, assuming a well-balanced diet. Particular attention must be given to the fat-soluble vitamins A, E, and K. It is ideal to have methods available for assessing a given patient's nutritional status relative to these micronutrients, as well as several other essential dietary components. Until further research has been carried out, however, final recommendations of methods for assessing certain nutrients such as vitamin A and zinc will have to be deferred.

Guidelines for an adequate diet have been discussed by Harper[138] and by Goodhart[139] and include the following elements. Variety in food selection should be the first basic principle; this can be achieved by choosing from the four major food groups (dairy, meat, fruit/vegetable, grain/cereal). An excessive intake of any one nutrient or food should be avoided. Fiber may be included in moderate amounts. A regular program of physical activity should be incorporated into the dietary planning.

The goal of each CF center should be to support normal growth and development in their patients, even if they have pancreatic insufficiency. Although this objective cannot always be achieved, it should nevertheless be given the highest priority possible. By optimizing nutritional habits, using pancreatic enzyme supplements effectively, and treating patients with micronutrients as required, physicians should be able to prevent malnutrition and thereby enhance the health of patients with cystic fibrosis. Hopefully, this will have a beneficial impact on both the quality and the quantity of life.

ACKNOWLEDGMENTS

We thank Paul A. di Sant'Agnese, MD, ScD (Med), for his contribution on issues relating to malnutrition in cystic fibrosis; Janet L. Greger, PhD, and Howard E. Ganther, PhD, for suggestions concerning reliable assessment of micromineral status; Elaine H. Mischler, MD, for sharing data on linoleate deficiency; and Kathleen E. McMahon, MS, for information on dietary guidelines. Dr. Farrell's relevant support includes grants from the Cystic Fibrosis Foundation and the National Institutes of Health (1-P50-HL-27358).

REFERENCES

1. Hubbard VS: Nutrient requirements of patients with cystic fibrosis, in Sturgess JM (ed): *Perspectives in Cystic Fibrosis, Proceedings of the 8th International Cystic Fibrosis Congress.* Toronto, Imperial Press, 1980, pp 149–160.
2. Hubbard VS, Mangrum PJ: Energy intake and nutritional counseling in cystic fibrosis. *J Am Diet Assoc* 1982;80:127–131.
3. Gaskin K, Gurwitz D, Durey P, et al: Improved respiratory prognosis in patients with cystic fibrosis with normal fat absorption. *J Pediatr* 1982;100:857–862.
4. Shepherd R, Cooksley WGE, Cooke WDD: Improved growth and clinical, nutritional, and respiratory changes in response to nutritional therapy in cystic fibrosis. *J Pediatr* 1980;97:351–357.
5. Corey ML: Longitudinal studies in cystic fibrosis, in Sturgess JM (ed): *Perspectives in Cystic Fibrosis, Proceedings of the 8th International Cystic Fibrosis Congress.* Toronto, Imperial Press, 1980, pp 246–255.
6. Chase HP, Long MA, Lavin MH: Cystic fibrosis and malnutrition. *J Pediatr* 1979;95: 337–347.
7. Huang NN, Holsclaw D, Hilman BC, et al: Dietary care, in Huang NN (ed): *Guide to Drug Therapy in Patients with Cystic Fibrosis.* Atlanta, The National Cystic Fibrosis Research Foundation, 1972.
8. Munro HN, Crim MC: The proteins and amino acids, in Goodhart RS, Shils ME (eds): *Modern Nutrition in Health and Disease.* Philadelphia, Lea & Febiger, 1980.
9. Dolan TF, Rowe DS, Gibson LE, Edema and hypoproteinemia in infants with cystic fibrosis. *Clin Pediatr* 1970;9:295–297.
10. Lee PA, Roloff DW, Howatt WF: Hypoproteinemia and anemia in infants with cystic fibrosis. *JAMA* 1974;228:585–588.
11. Goodhart RS, Shils ME. *Modern Nutrition in Health and Disease.* Philadelphia, Lea & Febiger, 1980.
12. di Sant'Agnese PA, Hubbard VS: The pancreas, in Taussig LM (ed): *Cystic Fibrosis.* New York, Brian C. Decker, in press.
13. Solomons NW, Wagonfeld JB, Rieger C, et al: Some biochemical indices of nutrition in treated cystic fibrosis patients. *Am J Clin Nutr* 1981;34:462–474.
14. Littlewood JM, Congdon PJ, Bruce G, et al: Vitamin status in treated cystic fibrosis patients, in Sturgess JM (ed): *Perspectives in Cystic Fibrosis, Proceedings of the 8th International Cystic Fibrosis Congress.* Toronto, Imperial Press, 1980, pp 166–171.
15. Congden PJ, Bruce G, Rothburn MM, et al: Vitamin status in treated patients with cystic fibrosis. *Arch Dis Child* 1981;56:708–714.
16. Deren JJ, Arora B, Toskes PP, et al: Malabsorption of crystalline vitamin B_{12} in cystic fibrosis. *N Engl J Med* 1973;288:949–950.
17. Bernstein L, Herbert V: The role of pancreatic exocrine secretions in the absorption of vitamin B_{12} and iron. *Am J Clin Nutr* 1973; 26:340–346.
18. Rucker R, Harrison G: Vitamin B_{12} deficiency in cystic fibrosis. *N Engl J Med* 1973; 289:329.
19. Barness LA: Vitamin B_{12} absorption in cystic fibrosis. *N Engl J Med* 1973;289:45.
20. Lui NS, Roels OA: Vitamin A and carotene, in Goodhart RS, Shils ME (eds): *Modern Nutrition in Health and Disease.* Philadelphia, Lea & Febiger, 1980.
21. Sauberlich HE, Hodges RE, Wallace DL, et al: Vitamin A metabolism and requirements in the human studied with the use of labelled retinol. *Vitam Horm* 1974;32:252–275.
22. Bieri JG, Tolliver TLJ, Catignani GL: Simultaneous determination of alpha tocopherol and retinol in plasma or red cells by high pressure liquid chromatography. *Am J Clin Nutr* 1979;32:2143–2149.
23. Bieri JG, McKenna MC: Expressing dietary values for fat-soluble vitamins: Changes in concepts and terminology. *Am J Clin Nutr* 1981;34:289–295.
24. Smith FA, Raz A, Goodman DW: Radioim-

munoassay of human plasma retinol-binding protein. *J Clin Invest* 1970;49:1754–1761.
25. Andersen DH: Cystic fibrosis of the pancreas, vitamin A deficiency and bronchiectasis. *J Pediatr* 1939;15:763–771.
26. Petersen RA, Petersen VS, Robb RM: Vitamin A deficiency with xerophthalmia and night blindness in cystic fibrosis. *Am J Dis Child* 1968;116:662–665.
27. Keating JP, Feigin RD: Increased intracranial pressure associated with probable vitamin A deficiency in cystic fibrosis. *Pediatrics* 1970;46:41–46.
28. Kulczycki LL: Malabsorption with vitamin A deficiency in a college girl treated for cystic fibrosis. *Acta Paediatr Scand* 1971;60:371–372.
29. Abernathy RS: Bulging fontanelle as presenting sign in cystic fibrosis: Vitamin A metabolism and effect on cerebrospinal fluid pressures. *Am J Dis Child* 1976;130:1360–1362.
30. Underwood BA, Denning CR: Correlations between plasma and liver concentrations of vitamins A and E in children with cystic fibrosis. *Bull NY Acad Med* 1971;47:34–50.
31. Underwood BA, Denning CR: Blood and liver concentrations of vitamins A and E in children with cystic fibrosis of the pancreas. *Pediatr Res* 1972;6:26–31.
32. Smith FR, Underwood BA, Denning CR, et al: Depressed plasma retinol-binding protein levels in cystic fibrosis. *J Lab Clin Med* 1972;80:423–433.
33. Jacob RA, Sandstead HH, Solomons NW, et al: Zinc status and vitamin A transport in cystic fibrosis. *Am J Clin Nutr* 1978; 31:638–644.
34. Palin D, Underwood BA, Denning CR: The effect of oral zinc supplementation on plasma levels of vitamin A and retinol-binding protein in cystic fibrosis. *Am J Clin Nutr* 1979;32:1253–1259.
35. Shetty PS, Jung RT, Watrasiewicz KE, et al: Rapid-turnover transport proteins: An index of subclinical protein–energy malnutrition. *Lancet* 1979;2:230–232.
36. Warwick WJ: Vitamin administration, in Huang NN (ed): *Guide to Drug Therapy in Patients with Cystic Fibrosis.* Atlanta, The National Cystic Fibrosis Research Foundation, 1972.
37. Warwick WJ, Hansen LG, Sharp H: Absorption of vitamin A in patients with cystic fibrosis. *Clin Pediatr* 1976;15:807–810.
38. DeLuca HF: Some new concepts emanating from a study of the metabolism and function of vitamin D. *Nutr Rev* 1980;38:169–180.
39. DeLuca HF: New developments in the vitamin D endocrine system. *J Am Diet Assoc* 1982;80:231–235.
40. Steenbock H: The induction of growth promoting and calcifying properties in a ration by exposure to light. *Science* 1924;60: 224–225.
41. DeLuca HF. Vitamin D, in Goodhart RS, Shils ME (eds): *Modern Nutrition in Health and Disease.* Philadelphia, Lea & Febiger, 1980.
42. Blomstrand R, Forsgren L: Intestinal absorption and esterification of vitamin D_3-1,2-^{3}H in man. *Acta Chem Scand* 1967;21:1662.
43. Andersen DH: Cystic fibrosis of the pancreas and its relation to celiac disease: Clinical and pathological study. *Am J Dis Child* 1938;56: 344–399.
44. Lowe CU, May CD, Reed SC: Fibrosis of the pancreas in infants and children. A statistical study of clinical and hereditary features. *Am J Dis Child* 1949;78:349–374.
45. Oppenheimer EH: Focal necrosis of striated muscle in an infant with cystic fibrosis of the pancreas and evidence of lack of absorption of fat-soluble vitamins. *Bull Johns Hopkins Hosp* 1956;98:353–358.
46. Parfitt MA, Nassim JR, Collins J, et al: Metabolic studies in a case of fibrocystic disease of the pancreas with reference to treatment and to the incidence of bone disease. *Arch Dis Child* 1962;37:25–33.
47. Hubbard VS, Farrell PM, di Sant'Agnese PA: 25-Hydroxycholcalciferol levels in patients with cystic fibrosis. *J Pediatr* 1979;94:84–86.
48. Hahn TJ, Squires AE, Halstead LR, et al: Reduced serum 25-hydroxyvitamin D concentration and disordered mineral metabolism in patients with cystic fibrosis. *J Pediatr* 1979;94:38–42.
49. Haddad JG, Hahn TJ: Natural and synthetic sources of circulating 25-hydroxyvitamin D in man. *Nature* 1973:244:515–517.
50. Mischler EH, Chesney PJ, Chesney RW, et al: Demineralization in cystic fibrosis detected by direct photon absorptiometry. *Am J Dis Child* 1979;133:632–635.
51. Horwitt MK: Vitamin E, in Goodhart RS (ed): *Modern Nutrition in Health and Disease.* Philadelphia, Lea & Febiger, 1980.
52. Machlin LJ: *Vitamin E: A Comprehensive Treatise.* New York, Marcel Dekker, 1980.
53. Kasparek S: Chemistry of tocopherols and tocotrienols, in Machlin LJ (ed): *Vitamin E: A Comprehensive Treatise.* New York, Marcel Dekker, 1980.
54. Horwitt MK, Harvey CC, Duncan GD, et al: Effects of limited tocopherol intake in man with relationships to erythrocyte hemolysis and lipid oxidations. *Am J Clin Nutr* 1956;4:408–419.
55. Farrell PM, Bieri JG, Fratantoni JF, et al:

The occurrence and effects of human vitamin E deficiency: A study in patients with cystic fibrosis. *J Clin Invest* 1977;60:233–241.

56. Farrell PM: Deficiency states, pharmacological effects, and nutrient requirements, in Machlin LJ (ed): *Vitamin E: A Comprehensive Treatise.* New York, Marcel Dekker, 1980.
57. Horwitt MK, Harvey CC, Dahm CH, et al: Relationships between tocopherol and serum lipid levels for determination of nutritional adequacy. *Ann NY Acad Sci* 1972;203: 233–236.
58. Farrell PM, Levine S, Murphey LL, et al: Plasma tocopherol levels and tocopherol-lipid relationships in a normal population of children as compared to healthy adults. *Am J Clin Nutr* 1978;31:1720–1726.
59. Farrell PM, Mischler EH, Gutcher GR: Evaluation of vitamin E deficiency in children with lung disease. *Ann NY Acad Sci* 1982;393:96–106.
60. Bieri JG, Farrell PM: Vitamin E. *Vitam Horm* 1976;34:31–75.
61. Bieri JG, Evarts RP: Effects of plasma lipid level on tissue deposition of alpha tocopherol, abstracted. *Fed Proc* 1975;34:913.
62. McKay PB, King MM: Vitamin E: Its role as a biologic free radical scavenger and its relationship to the microsomal mixed-function oxidase system, in Machlin LJ (ed): *Vitamin E: A Comprehensive Treatise.* New York, Marcel Dekker, 1980.
63. Catignani GL: Role in nucleic acid and protein metabolism, in Machlin LJ (ed): *Vitamin E: A Comprehensive Treatise.* New York, Marcel Dekker, 1980.
64. Corwin LM: The role of vitamin E in mitochondrial metabolism, in Machlin LJ (ed): *Vitamin E: A Comprehensive Treatise.* New York, Marcel Dekker, 1980.
65. Nelson JS: Pathology of vitamin E deficiency, in Machlin LJ (ed): *Vitamin E: A Comprehensive Treatise.* New York, Marcel Dekker, 1980.
66. Park RW, Grand RJ: Gastrointestinal manifestations of cystic fibrosis: A review. *Gastroenterology* 1981;81:1143–1161.
67. Dolan TF: Hemolytic anemia and edema as initial signs in infants with cystic fibrosis. *Clin Pediatr* 1976;15:597–600.
68. Hubbard VS, Dunn GD: Fatty acid composition of erythrocyte phospholipids from patients with cystic fibrosis. *Clin Chim Acta* 1980;102:115–118.
69. Hubbard VS, Dunn GD, di Sant'Agnese PA: Abnormal fatty-acid composition of plasma-lipids in cystic fibrosis: A primary or secondary defect? *Lancet* 1977;2:1302–1304.
70. Mischler EH, Farrell PM, Brown DJ, et al: Plasma fatty acid alternations in cystic fibrosis as related to pancreatic and vitamin E status. *Cystic Fibrosis Club Abstr* 1979; 20:65.
71. Nitowsky HM, Gordon HH, Tildon JT: Studies of tocopherol deficiency in infants and children. IV. The effect of alpha tocopherol on creatinuria in patients with cystic fibrosis of the pancreas and biliary atresia. *Bull Johns Hopkins Hosp* 1956;98:361–371.
72. Levin S: Muscular performance and vitamin E in cystic fibrosis, abstracted. *Arch Dis Child* 1974;49:247.
73. Darby CW, Davidson AGF, Desai ID: Muscular performance in cystic fibrosis patients and its relationship to vitamin E. *Arch Dis Child* 1973;48:72–75.
74. Sung JH: Neuroaxonal dystrophy in mucoviscidosis. *J Neuropathol Exp Neurol* 1964; 23:567–583.
75. Sung JH, Park SH, Mastri AR, et al: Axonal dystrophy in the gracile nucleus in congenital biliary atresia and cystic fibrosis (mucoviscidosis): Beneficial effects of vitamin E therapy. *J Neuropathol Exp Neurol* 1980;39: 584–597.
76. Guggenheim MA, Ringerl SP, Silverman A, et al: Progressive neuromuscular disease in children with chronic cholestasis and vitamin E deficiency: Diagnosis and treatment with alpha tocopherol. *J Pediatr* 1982;100:51–58.
77. Cavalier SJ, Gambetti P: Dystrophic axons and spinal cord demyelination in cystic fibrosis. *Neurology* 1981;31:714–718.
78. Geller A, Gilles F, Shwachman H: Degeneration of fasciculus gracilis in cystic fibrosis. *Neurology* 1977;27:185–187.
79. Swaiman KF, Halverson D, Sharp HL: Sea-blue histiocyte associated with posterior column dysfunction in childhood. *Neurology* 1973;23:474.
80. Swaiman KF, Garg BP, Lockman LA: Sea-blue histiocyte and posterior column dysfunction: A familial disorder. *Neurology* 1975;25:1084–1087.
81. Kerner F, Goldbloom RB: Investigations of tocopherol deficiency in infancy and childhood. *AMA J Dis Child* 1960;99:597–603.
82. Harries JT, Muller DPE: Absorption of different doses of fat soluble and water miscible preparations of vitamin E in children with cystic fibrosis. *Arch Dis Child* 1971;46: 341–344.
83. Hubbard VS, Adams AJ, Farrell PM, et al: Vitamin E absorption in cystic fibrosis. *Cystic Fibrosis Club Abstr* 1977;18:55.
84. Olson RE: Vitamin K, in Goodhart RS (ed): *Modern Nutrition in Health and Disease.* Philadelphia, Lea & Febiger, 1980.
85. Suttie J: Vitamin K, in Machlin LP (ed):

Handbook of Vitamins. New York, Marcel Dekker, in press.

86. Hauschka PV, Lian JB, Gallop PM: Direct identification of the calcium-binding amino acid, gamma-carboxyglutamate, in mineralized tissue. *Proc Natl Acad Sci USA* 1975; 72:3925–3929.
87. Torstenson OL, Humphrey GB, Edson JR, et al: Cystic fibrosis presenting with severe hemorrhage due to vitamin K malabsorption: A report of three cases. *Pediatrics* 1970;45:857–861.
88. Dolan TF, Gibson LE: Possibility of cystic fibrosis in infants with vitamin K deficiency. *J Pediatr* 1970;77:515.
89. Walters TR, Koch HLF: Hemorrhagic diathesis and cystic fibrosis in infancy. *Am J Dis Child* 1972;124:641–642.
90. Carpentieri U, Gustavson LP, Haggard ME: Misdiagnosis of neglect in a child with bleeding disorder and cystic fibrosis. *South Med J* 1978;71:854–855.
91. Gustafsson BE, Daft FS, McDaniel EG, et al: Effects of vitamin K-active compounds and intestinal microorganisms in vitamin K-deficiency germfree rats. *J Nutr* 1962;78: 461–468.
92. Committee on Nutrition, American Academy of Pediatrics: Vitamin K supplementation for infants receiving milk substitute infant formulas and for those with fat malabsorption. *Pediatrics* 1971;48:483–487.
93. Corrigan JJ, Taussig LM, Beckerman R, et al: Factor II (prothrombin) coagulant activity and immunoreactive protein: Detection of vitamin K deficiency and liver disease in patients with cystic fibrosis. *J Pediatr* 1981;99:254–257.
94. Holman R: Essential fatty acid deficiency. *Prog Chem Fats Other Lipids* 1968;9:275–348.
95. Alfin-Slater RB, Aftergood L: Lipids, in Goodhart RS (ed): *Modern Nutrition in Health and Disease.* Philadelphia, Lea & Febiger, 1980.
96. Sanders RL: Introduction to lipid biochemistry, in Farrell PM (ed): *Lung Development: Biological and Clinical Perspectives.* New York, Academic Press, 1982, vol 1.
97. Kuo PT, Huang NN, Bassett DR: The fatty acid composition of the serum chylomicrons and adipose tissue of children with cystic fibrosis of the pancreas. *J Pediatr* 1962;60:394–403.
98. Caren R, Corbo L: Plasma fatty acids in pancreatic cystic fibrosis and liver disease. *J Clin Endocrinol* 1966;26:470–477.
99. Rivers JPW, Hassam AG: Defective essential-fatty-acid metabolism in cystic fibrosis. *Lancet* 1975;2:642–643.
100. Press M: Essential-fatty-acid metabolism in cystic fibrosis. *Lancet* 1975;2:871–872.
101. Watts R, Taylor S, Postuma R, et al: Essential-fatty-acid metabolism in cystic fibrosis. *Lancet* 1975;2:983.
102. Galabert C, Filliat M, Chazalette JP: Fatty-acid composition of serum-lecithins in cystic fibrosis patients without steatorrhea. *Lancet* 1978;2:903.
103. Rogiers V, Crokaert R, Vix H: Altered phospholipid composition and changed fatty acid pattern of the various phospholipid fractions of red cell membranes of cystic fibrosis children with pancreatic insufficiency. *Clin Chim Acta* 1980;105:105–115.
104. Chase HP, Cotton EK, Elliott RB: Intravenous linoleic acid supplementation in children with cystic fibrosis. *Pediatrics* 1979;64:207–213.
105. Rosenlund ML, Selekman JA, Kim HK, et al: Dietary essential fatty acids in cystic fibrosis. *Pediatrics* 1977;59:428–432.
106. Lloyd-Still JD, Johnson SB, Holman RT: Essential fatty acid status in cystic fibrosis and the effects of safflower oil supplementation. *Am J Clin Nutr* 1981;34:1–7.
107. Kuo PT, Huang NN: The effect of medium-chain triglycerides upon fat absorption and plasma lipids and depot fat of children with cystic fibrosis of the pancreas. *J Clin Invest* 1965;44:1924–1933.
108. Elliott RB: The effect of essential fatty acid on sweat sodium concentrations in cystic fibrosis, abstracted. *Aust Paediatr J* 1972;8: 217.
109. Elliott RB, Robinson PG: Unusual clinical course in a child with cystic fibrosis treated with fat emulsion. *Arch Dis Child* 1975;50: 76–78.
110. Elliott RB: A therapeutic trial of fatty acid supplementation in cystic fibrosis. *Pediatrics* 1976;57:474–479.
111. Davidson GP, Phelan PD, Townley RRW: A controlled trial using intravenous infusion of Soya oil emulsion in the treatment of children with cystic fibrosis. *Aust Paediatr J* 1978;14:80–82.
112. Lloyd-Still JD, Simon SH, Wessel HLU, et al: Negative effects of oral fatty acid supplementation on sweat chloride in cystic fibrosis. *Pediatrics* 1979;64:50–52.
113. Mischler EH, Farrell PM, Parrell SW, et al: Correction of essential fatty acid deficiency in cystic fibrosis. *Cystic Fibrosis Club Abstr* 1982;23:133.
114. Stern RC, Boat TF, Abramowsky CR, et al: Intermediate range sweat chloride concentration and pseudomonas bronchitis. *JAMA* 1978;239:2676–2680.
115. Davis PB, Hubbard VS, di Sant'Agnese PA:

Low sweat electrolytes in a patient with cystic fibrosis. *Am J Med* 1980;69:643-646.
116. di Sant'Agnese PA, Darling PA, Perera GA, et al: Abnormal electrolyte composition of sweat in cystic fibrosis of the pancreas: Clinical significance and relationship to disease. *Pediatrics* 1953;12:549-563.
117. Kopito L, Shwachman H: Spectroscopic analysis of tissues from patients with cystic fibrosis and controls. *Nature* 1964;202:501-502.
118. van Stekelenburg GJ, van de Laar AJB, van Der Laag J: Copper analysis of nail clippings: An attempt to differentiate between normal children and patients suffering from cystic fibrosis. *Clin Chim Acta* 1975; 59:233-240.
119. Hoekstra WG: Biochemical function of selenium and its relation to vitamin E. *Fed Proc* 1970;34:2083-2089.
120. Draper HH: Nutrient interrelationships, in Machlin LJ (ed): *Vitamin E: A Comprehensive Treatise.* New York, Marcel Dekker, 1980.
121. Heinrich HC, Gabbe EE, Bartels H, et al: Bioavailability of food iron-(^{59}Fe), vitamin B_{12}-(^{60}Co) and protein bound selenomethionine-(^{75}Se) in pancreatic exocrine insufficiency due to cystic fibrosis. *Klin Wochenschr* 1977;55:595-601.
122. Underwood BA, Denning CR, Navab M: Polyunsaturated fatty acids and tocopherol levels in patients with cystic fibrosis. *Ann NY Acad Sci* 1972;203:237-247.
123. Castillo R, Landon C, Eckhardt MW, et al: Selenium and vitamin E status in cystic fibrosis. *J Pediatr* 1981;99:583-585.
124. Lloyd-Still JD, Ganther HE: Selenium and glutathione peroxidase levels in cystic fibrosis. *Pediatrics* 1980;65:1010-1012.
125. Stein AA, Porta E, Powers S, et al: Studies on surgical biopsies of pancreas and liver in four cases of cystic fibrosis. *Ann Surg* 1963; 157:516-524.
126. Longnecker DS: Hepatic iron stores in patients with cystic fibrosis. *Arch Pathol* 1965;80:148-152.
127. Gilly R, Mouriguand C, Bachelot C: Bone marrow iron in cystic fibrosis. *Mod Probl Pediatr* 1967;10:263-268.
128. Smith RS: Iron absorption in cystic fibrosis. *Br Med J* 1964;1:608-609.
129. Heinrich HC, Bender-Gotze Ch, Gabbe EE, et al: Absorption of inorganic iron-($^{59}Fe^{2+}$) in relation to iron stores in pancreatic exocrine insufficiency due to cystic fibrosis. *Klin Wochenschr* 1977;55:587-593.
130. Davis AE, Badenoch J: Iron absorption in pancreatic disease. *Lancet* 1962;2:6-8.
131. Conrad ME, Benjamin BI, Williams HL, et al: Human absorption of hemoglobin-iron. *Gastroenterology* 1967;53:5-10.
132. Fraker PF, Zwickl CM, Luecke RW: Delayed type hypersensitivity in zinc deficiency adult mice: Impairment and restoration of responsivity to nitrofluorobenzene. *J Nutr* 1982;112:309-313.
133. Pekarek RS, Sandstead HH, Jacob RA, et al: Abnormal cellular immune responses during acquired zinc deficiency. *Am J Clin Nutr* 1979;32:1466-1471.
134. Li TK, Vallee BL: The biochemical and nutritional roles of other trace elements, in Goodhart RS, Shils ME (eds): *Modern Nutrition in Health and Disease.* Philadelphia, Lea & Febiger, 1980.
135. Greger JL, Geissler AH: Effects of zinc supplementation on taste acuity of the aged. *Am J Clin Nutr* 1978;31:633-637.
136. Halstead JA, Smith JC: Plasma-zinc in health and disease. *Lancet* 1970;1:322-324.
137. Solomons NW, Rieger CHL, Jacob RA, et al: Zinc nutriture and taste acuity in patients with cystic fibrosis. *Nutr Res* 1981;1:13-24.
138. Harper AE: What are appropriate dietary guidelines? *Food Technol* 1978;32:48-53.
139. Goodhart RS: Criteria of an adequate diet, in Goodhart RS (ed): *Modern Nutrition in Health and Disease.* Philadelphia, Lea & Febiger, 1980.

17

The Pancreas in Cystic Fibrosis

Emanuel Lebenthal

David Baswell

The terms cystic fibrosis of the pancreas,[1] fibrocystic disease of the pancreas,[2] and mucoviscidosis of the pancreas[3] have been utilized to describe the pathologic appearance of the pancreas in cystic fibrosis (CF). Historically, the malabsorption and pancreatic lesions were recognized[1] prior to the associated chronic lung disease. The gastrointestinal symptoms due to pancreatic insufficiency were used to establish the diagnosis before the description of elevated electrolytes in apocrine glands and the routine use of pilocarpine iontophoresis for sweat electrolytes became available.[4] Clinical symptoms and laboratory data suggestive of pancreatic insufficiency are seen in 85–90% of CF patients during the first year of life; the remaining 10–15% of patients have sufficient pancreatic reserve to avoid symptoms of maldigestion and malabsorption. It has been estimated that more than 90% of pancreatic function must be absent for symptoms of pancreatic insufficiency to be apparent. The few patients without clinical evidence of malabsorption may still have a partial pancreatic exocrine lesion; the extent of possible morphologic alterations of their pancreases has not been established.

Physiologic pancreatic insufficiency in the first months of life is well known (absent to low amylase and low lipase). This transient low pancreatic output in early postnatal life should not be confused with the pancreatic insufficiency of CF.

The relationship of the disruption of normal pancreatic development to the natural progression of pancreatic lesions in CF is poorly understood, and only scarce data are available. An understanding of the evolution of pancreatic insufficiency in CF will assist in the clinical evaluation and the treatment of the CF patient and possibly in understanding the pathophysiology of the pancreatic lesion.

Despite the relative paucity of data, the aims of this chapter are to evaluate the alterations of pancreatic structure and function during development and in later life, to correlate those changes with the clinical manifestations in patients who suffer from CF, and to contrast different diagnostic techniques in the differential diagnosis of pancreatic insufficiency and steatorrhea. The treatment and the difficulties which may be encountered with dietary manipulation, oral pancreatic enzyme replacement, and the use of new therapeutic modalities, such as bile salts, cimetidine, and bicarbonate, will be discussed.

ANATOMY AND EMBRYOLOGY

The structural and functional modifications in the pancreas in cystic fibrosis have led to the hypothesis that the structural changes seen may occur as an abnormal event during development in utero.[5] In order to better appreciate this hypothesis, an understanding of the normal anatomical and physiological development of the pancreas becomes mandatory.

The normal pancreas develops in two parts, the dorsal and ventral pancreatic anlage. During the fourth week of gestation the dorsal anlage arises as a diverticulum from the endoderm of the primitive duodenum. By the seventh week part of the head and the entire body and tail of the pancreas have been formed. The ventral anlage arises as a diverticulum from the primitive bile duct; this portion rotates above the duodenum and, by the sixth to seventh week, fuses with the dorsal anlage to complete the formation of the head of the pancreas.[6,7] The duct of the dorsal portion (accessory pancreatic duct) opens into the duodenum and remains patent in up to 70% of adults.[8] The ventral duct opens with the common bile duct at the ampulla of Vater. Following fusion of the two anlage, communication is established between the two ducts. The dorsal duct has little or no further enlargement; the ventral duct continues to increase in size and becomes the major duct of the exocrine pancreas.[7]

Tubules appear at about 7 weeks, and zymogen granules, the Golgi apparatus, and the rough endoplasmic reticulum appear at 12 weeks (Figure 17-1).[9] Crescent- and spindle-shaped zymogen granules, unique to this period, are not seen later in life. From 14 to 20 weeks (Figure 17-2), acinar lobules bud from the tubules and become lined with centroacinar cells. At this stage these cells are less differentiated than acinar cells and have a less elaborate mitochondrial structure, Golgi apparatus, and endoplasmic reticulum; the microvilli show a greater degree of irregularity.[9] Further development of the pancreas consists of additional elaboration of these organelles (Figure 17-3 and 17-4).

The pancreas of the adult is a flattened triangular gland about 10–15 cm in length and weighing 60–110 g.[7,10] It is a compound racemose gland which is nodular in appearance; the lobules may be visualized easily with the naked eye.[11] The pancreatic ductules are surrounded by centroacinar cells; the ductules drain into intralobular ducts which anastomose to become the main pancreatic ducts. The intralobular ducts and main ducts are lined with low columnar and columnar epithelium, respectively.

The exocrine acini are round or short tubular structures which, in groups, make up the lobules. The acini are made up of single rows of pyramidal epithelial cells with the apices converging on a central lumen which drains into the small pancreatic ductules.[12] The acinar cell has unique organelles that include condensing vacuoles and zymogen granules. The nucleus of the acinar cell is towards the base of the cell. The Golgi apparatus appears in the midportion of the

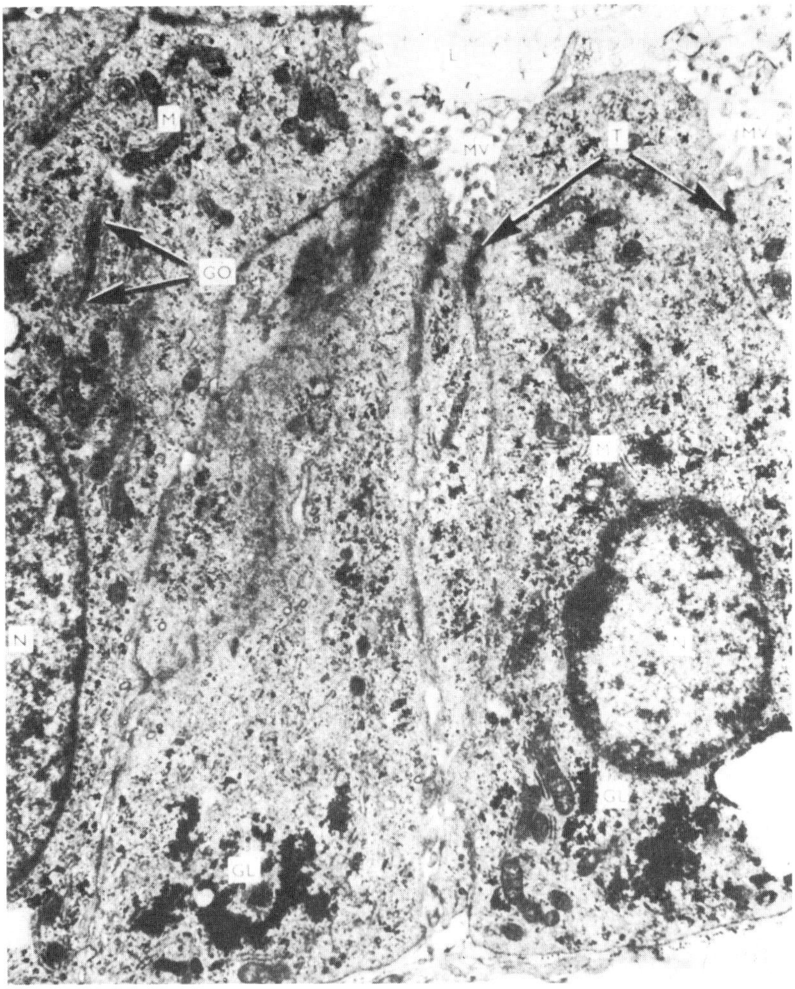

Figure 17-1 Human fetal pancreas at approximately 9 weeks gestion. A primitive ductular pattern is seen as are tubules (T), Golgi appratus (GO), mitochrondria (M), glycogen (GL).

cell; the size and exact location depend upon the state of cellular activity.

Enzymes are synthesized in the rough endoplasmic reticulum;[13–15] the completed protein is sequestered in the rough endoplasmic reticular cisternae and transferred to the Golgi apparatus from which condensing vacuoles containing secretory proteins are elaborated. With the elimination of water, the secretory proteins are further concentrated in the condensing vacuoles which eventually mature into the zymogen granules. These zymogen granules migrate towards the apical region and act as storage depots until stimulated to discharge their contents. Exocytosis occurs after the zymogen membrane fuses with the cellular membrane at the apex of the cell; this fused membrane ruptures, and the contents of the zymogen granule are released into the ductule.[16] Controversy exists as to the mechanism of enzyme secretion. Parallel secretion (concentrations of enzymes remain constant at varying rates of secretion) of pancreatic enzymes is accepted by most[17–19] as the actual representation of enzyme secretion by the acinar cell. Nonparallel transport and secretion have been suggested as well.[20–22]

HORMONAL CONTROL OF PANCREATIC SECRETION

There appears to be a basal release of enzymes from the acinar cell,[23,24] but secretion is predominantly caused by the stimulation of a meal or secretagogue. Pancreatic secretagogues are classified into two groups, peptide hormones and cholinergic agents. Two mechanisms of stimulus-secretion coupling have been proposed. Vasoactive intestinal peptide (VIP) and secretin are believed to act through an increase in adenylcyclase,[25] with resultant accumulation of cyclic AMP within acinar cells.[26] Pancreozymin-cholecystokinin (PZ-CCK) and cholinergic agents, on the other hand, cause an increased efflux of calcium from acinar cells[27] with a corresponding increase in intracellular concentration of cyclic GMP.[28] Two classic intestinal peptide hormones that are responsible for controlling pancreatic secretion are secretin and PZ-CCK. Secretin predominantly affects ductular and centroacinar cells, causing an increase in the secretion of HCO_3^- and water. An initial increase of protein secretion is usually noted but is felt to be a "wash-out" phenomenon caused by the sudden increase in fluid in the ducts. A slight but sustained increase in enzyme over the basal secretion has been noted, suggesting that secretin is also a stimulant of enzyme release.[16] In contrast, PZ-CCK stimulates the pancreas to produce secretions high in enzyme concentration and low in HCO_3^- and in volume. Secretin and PZ-CCK potentiate

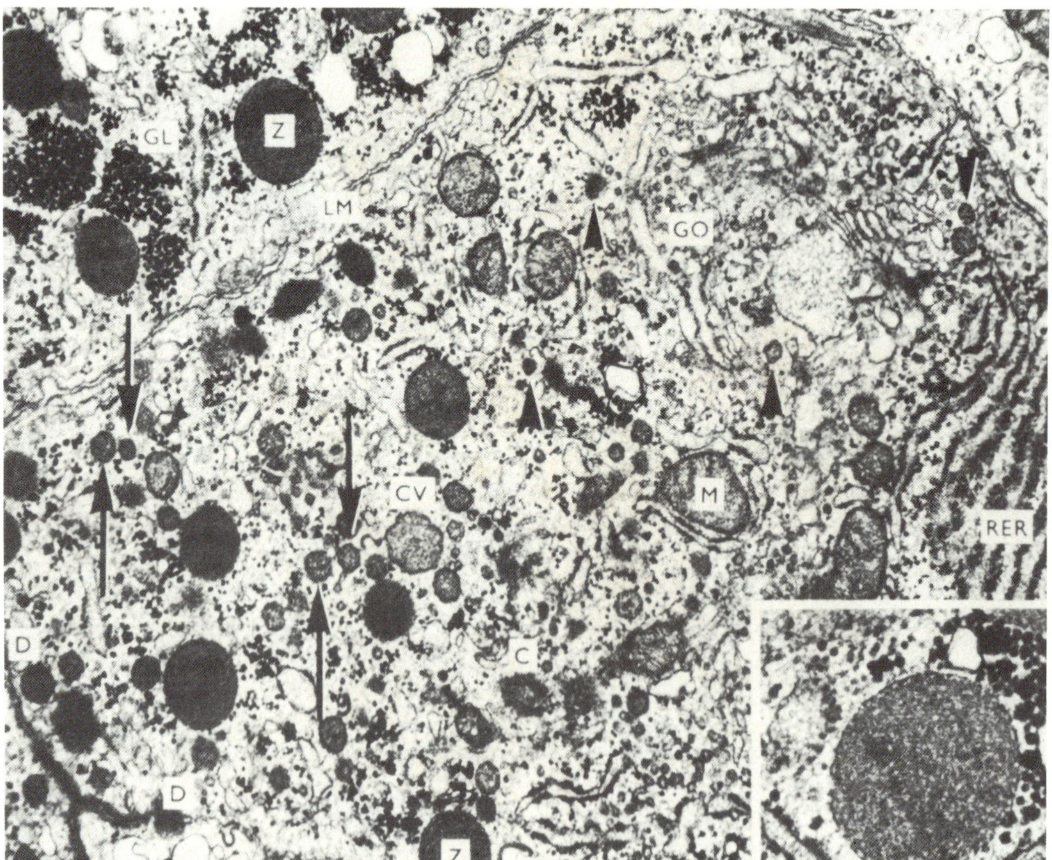

Figure 17-2 Human fetal pancreas at 16 weeks. Seen are prominent Golgi (GO), rough endoplasmic reticulum (RER), condensing vacuole (CV), zymogen granule (Z).

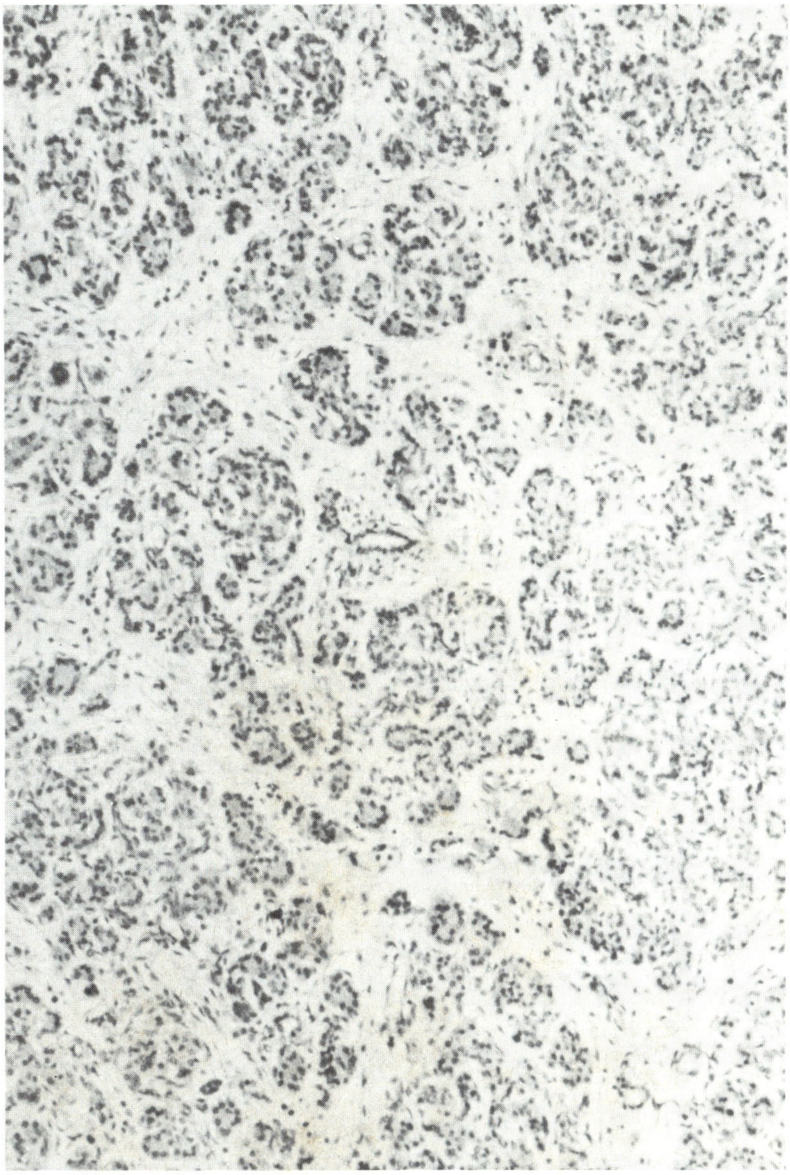

Figure 17-3 Human fetal pancreas at 21 weeks.

each other when given in combination; the response in both water and electrolyte secretion and enzyme production following stimulation with the two secretagogues together is greater than that seen when each stimulant is given alone.[29,30]

In contrast to the pancreas in adults, PZ-CCK has no effect on the secretion of enzymes in newborns, minimal effect at 1 month, and normal response at 2 years, suggesting the possibility of immature stimulus–secretion mechanisms early in life.[31]

SECRETION OF ENZYMES

In order to correctly interpret the secretory response of enzymes in CF at various ages, one must know the normal sequential appearance of enzymes in zymogen granules and then in duodenal fluid during different periods of development.

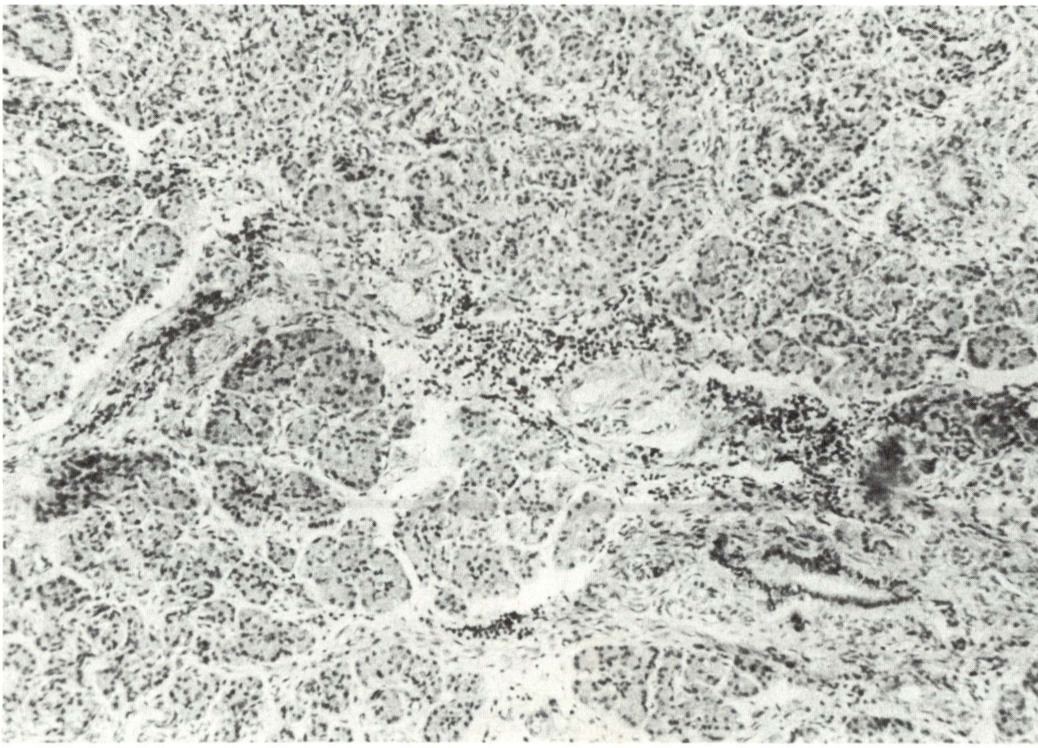

Figure 17-4 Pancreas of full-term infant. Shows well-developed acini and minimal fibrous tissue.

Trypsinogen is found in homogenates of fetal pancreas in normal amounts very early in gestation, followed by chymotrypsinogen, procarboxypeptidases A and B, lipase, and amylase. Trypsinogen appears in the fetal pancreas at 16 weeks and lipase at 32 weeks.[9] Amylase is virtually absent in the fetal and newborn pancreas and is not detected in autopsy specimens until about 2–4 months of age.[32] Enterokinase, found in the proximal small intestine as early as the 26th week of gestation,[33] activates trypsinogen into trypsin, which in turn activates the other proteolytic proenzymes.

Duodenal secretions from premature and full-term infants in the neonatal period have revealed virtually no amylase, markedly diminished lipase, and low carboxypeptidase B as compared to 2-year-old controls. Chymotrypsin and trypsin in the unstimulated duodenal fluids were 50% and nearly 100% of the control values, respectively.[31] Thus, in the normal newborn, there is a transient physiologic pancreatic insufficiency for lipase and amylase.

SECRETION OF ELECTROLYTES AND WATER

Normal human pancreatic fluid obtained at various rates of secretion is isotonic to the extracellular fluid. This suggests that water enters into the pancreatic ductules with the solutes. The predominant cations, Na^+ and K^+, are secreted at fixed concentrations. The anions, Cl^- and HCO_3^-, vary with the rate of secretion. At high flow rates, HCO_3^- concentration is high, reaching 150 mEq/liter, while at lower flow rates, Cl^- is the predominant anion. Studies[34] suggest that the acinar cell secretes Cl^- and that centroacinar and ductular cells secrete HCO_3^-. It would appear that centroacinar and ductular cells, after stimulation, contribute most of the water and HCO_3^- to the pancreatic fluid.

The pancreas of the premature or term

newborn seems to lack the ability to respond to PZ-CCK or secretin. A similar low secretory response of fluid and electrolytes is observed following stimulation with either hormone. The ability to differentiate between PZ-CCK develops by one week of life; by that time, stimulation with secretin results in low secretion of fluid and electrolytes qualitatively similar to, but quantitatively less than, older infants or children.[35]

The effect of CF on the response of the pancreas after PZ-CCK and secretin has been studied.[36] Marked alterations were noted in CF patients compared to normal controls. Volume of secretion was 20% that of controls, protein was found to be 63%, HCO_3^- 9%, Na^+ 18%, K^+ 25%, Ca^{2+} 33%, and Mg^{2+} 60% of control values. Secretion of Na^+, K^+, and Mg^{2+} was more reduced following secretin stimulation. Fluid volume and HCO_3^- secretion were both reduced after stimulation with either hormone.

PATHOLOGY OF THE PANCREAS IN CF

The pathological findings in the pancreas depend on the age of the patient and the severity of the disease.[37] Although infants and children with CF have been reported in whom the pancreas was histologically normal at autopsy,[38] histometric studies have suggested that the ratio of acinar to connective tissue may already be altered before the expected pathological changes are seen.[5] In patients with long-standing disease, the pancreas grossly appears small, hard, and nodular with an increase in fat; multiple cystic structures may be present. Stenosis or obstruction of large pancreatic ducts is occasionally seen,[39] but in general the pancreatic ductular lesions are those of small duct obstruction by secretions and cellular debris.[37]

Four histological grades of abnormality of the pancreas have been described;[40] the lesions are focal and not uniform throughout the pancreas. Grade I is characterized by intraluminal eosinophilic concretions. Grade II is more advanced with exocrine atrophy, intra- and interlobular fibrosis with ductal ectasia, and microcysts may also be present. Grade III includes the findings of acinar atrophy and liposclerosis. In grade IV, scar tissue with scattered islets of Langerhans are seen with total loss of acinar cells and ductal obliteration.[41] Type IV lesions are more commonly found in the tail of the pancreas, type III in the body and types I and II in the head of the pancreas; all four types may coexist in the same specimen. The series of Vawter et al[41] reports 6.8% of pancreases as predominantly type I, 17.2% as type II, 55% as type III, and 17.2% as type IV. In a larger study a grading system of 0 to 4+ is used.[37] The pancreatic abnormalities are reported to progress as the patient grows older; 25% of patients less than 6 weeks old are reported to have no detectable lesion, but when all ages are included, this figure drops to 8.9%. In the older patients studied, 85% have grade 4+ lesions. The islets of Langerhans are spared in most cases until late in the disease.

The earliest lesions seen in CF are the appearance of eosinophilic concretions in acini and ductules.[37] It has been suggested that as pancreatic ductules become obstructed by precipitated secretions and cellular debris, acinar and ductular distention occurs. These abnormalities may lead to acinar disruption, followed by release of proteolytic enzymes and resulting in autodigestion of the pancreas. Replacement of degenerate acini by small cysts, fibrous tissue, and fat subsequently occurs[37,42] (Figures 17-5, 17-6, 17-7).

In a study of autopsy material, acini from minimally involved pancreases have been found to be reduced by 33% of controls; in more severely involved specimens, acini were reduced to 5% of controls. Acinar and ductular volumes were increased by up to 1700%, suggesting distention of these structures. Elevated calcium concentrations, greater than ten times control levels, were noted in the obstructed ductal structures.[42] The early ductular enlargement, and subsequent accumulation of calcium-rich material, was suggested as responsible for the eventual obstructive process.

The early decrease in acinar cell number and increase in volume has been confirmed

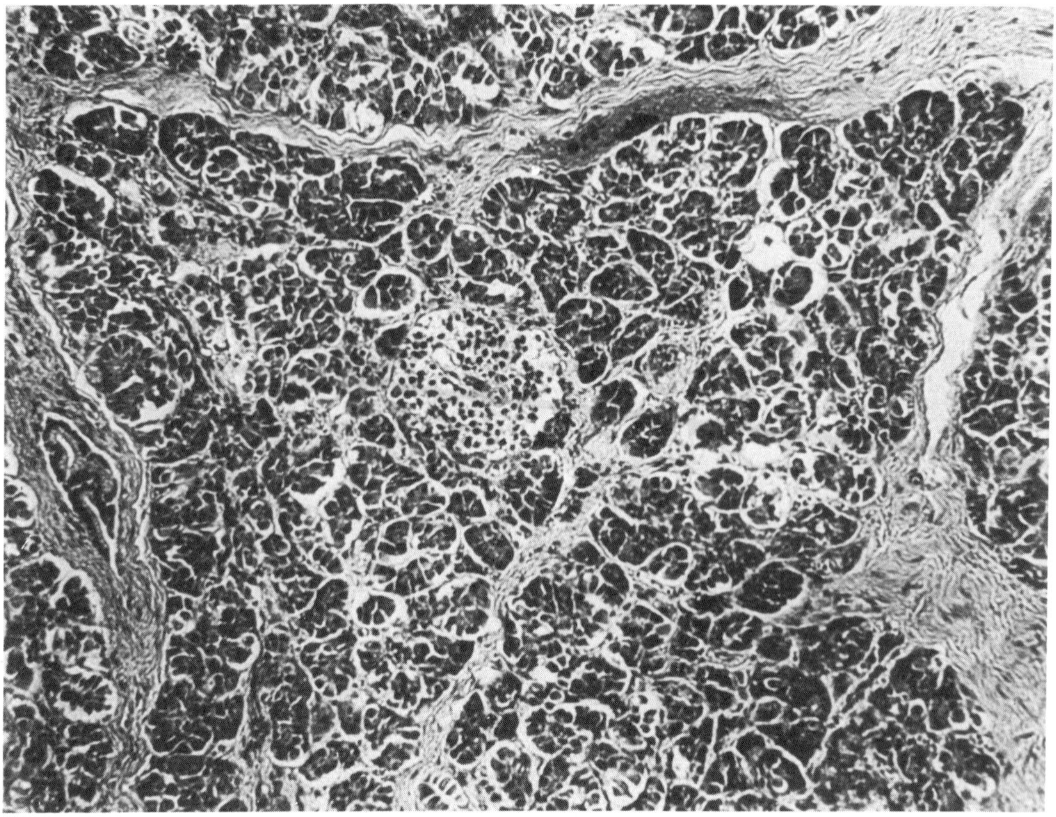

Figure 17-5 Cystic fibrosis. Pancreas shows early degrees of fibrous changes.

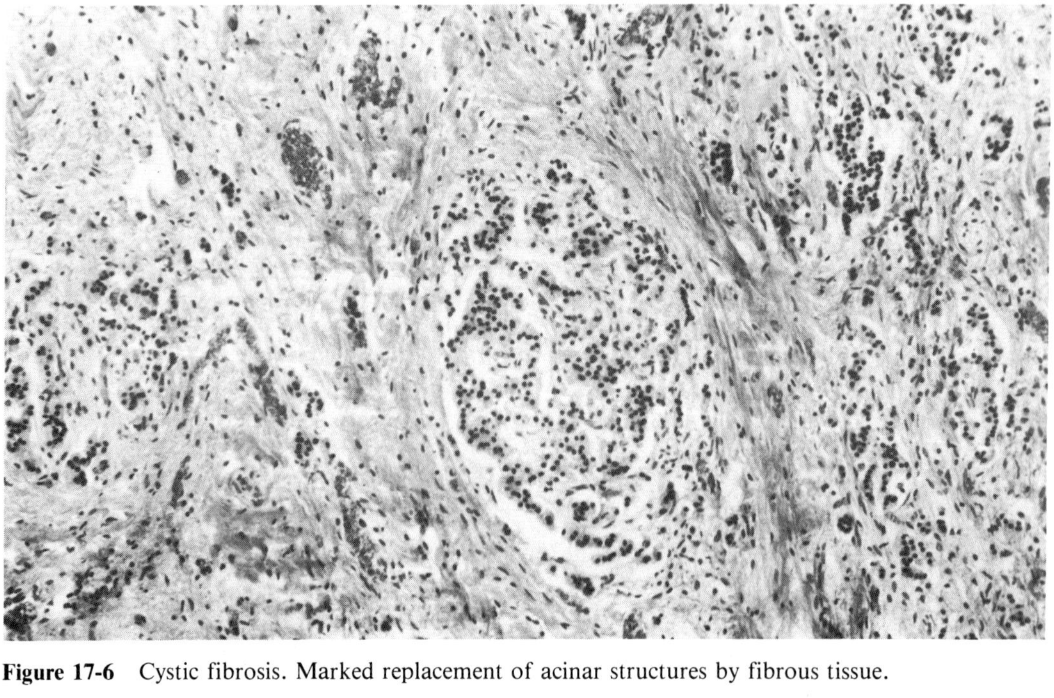

Figure 17-6 Cystic fibrosis. Marked replacement of acinar structures by fibrous tissue.

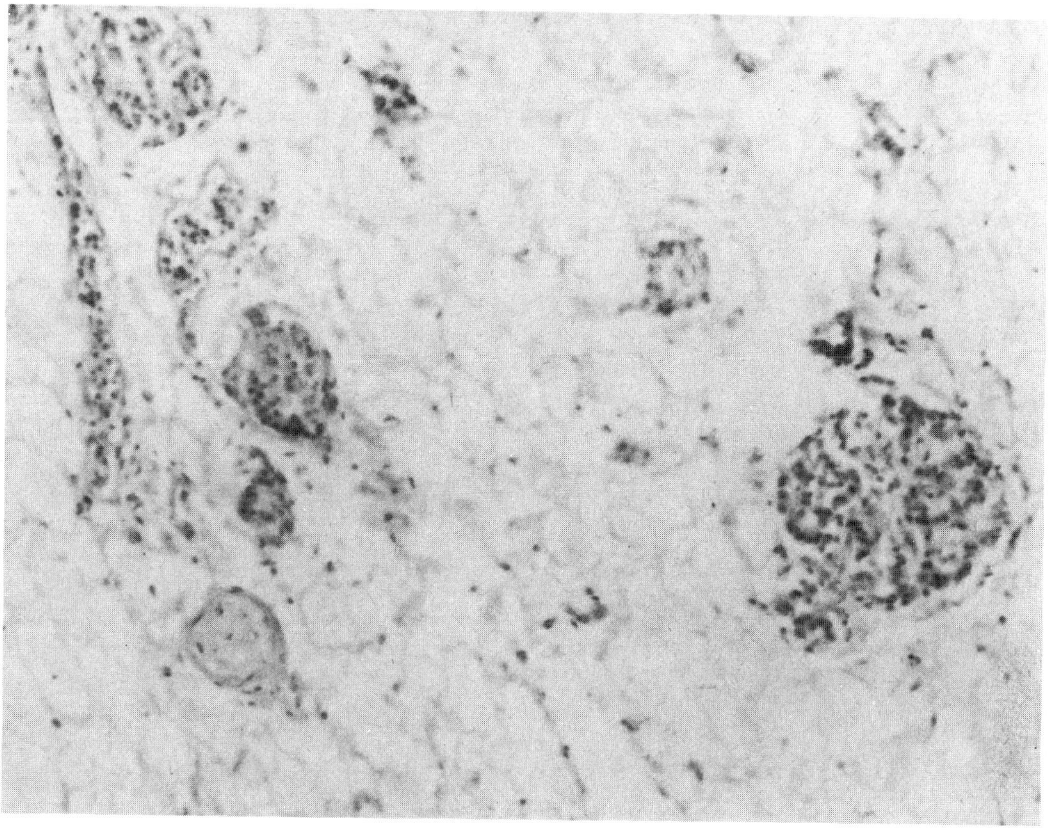

Figure 17-7 Pancreas from 24-year-old cystic fibrosis patient, showing replacement of pancreatic tissue with fat. Only rare islets of Langerhans are seen.

in subsequent histometric studies.[5] A comparison of the ratio of acinar to connective tissue, and of the volume of acinar and duct lumens in autopsy specimens from patients with CF to age-matched controls was made. The ratio of acinar to connective tissue in CF pancreases decreased from 35 weeks postconception to 52 weeks. During the same time period, the volume of acinar and duct lumens increased when compared to controls. There was found to be a lack of exocrine tissue before and at birth. These findings suggest that in CF, changes in the pancreas are evolving during gestation, that early normal maturation of the pancreas is not taking place, and further degeneration may supervene after birth (see Chapter 3).

CLINICAL MANIFESTATIONS OF PANCREATIC INVOLVEMENT

Despite the early thoughts that cystic fibrosis was primarily a pancreatic disease, it has become clear that multiple organ systems are involved, as described in other chapters. Many of the gastrointestinal manifestations can be attributed either directly or indirectly to the pancreatic lesion.

Meconium Ileus

This is the earliest clinical manifestation of cystic fibrosis. Small intestinal obstruction, usually of the distal ileum, may be seen in up to 15% of infants born with cystic fibrosis[43] and is felt to be related to the highly viscous meconium. The etiology of the high shear value of this meconium is unknown, but may be related to the decrease in pancreatic enzymes, the decrease in water, the increase in protein, or to the altered secretions of small intestinal mucus (elevated levels of glycoproteins). Signs and symptoms of distal small-bowel obstruction are present by 48–72 hr; there is a history of lack of meconium passage, emesis which is frequently bilious, and abdominal distention. Abdominal palpation will reveal dilated bowel loops and may reveal a mass in the right lower quadrant and pelvis. Radiologic evaluation demonstrates distended bowel loops without air fluid levels; barium enema frequently reveals a microcolon of disuse.

The diagnosis of meconium ileus must be suspected in any infant presenting with small-bowel obstruction, and a sweat test is mandatory. Other etiologies of obstruction to be considered include small-intestinal atresia, Hirschsprung's disease, malrotation, volvulus, congenital bands, and meconium plug syndrome. Treatment may be surgical, but in uncomplicated cases, a carefully performed Gastrografin® enema may relieve the obstruction.[44,45] Volume depletion may occur due to fluid and electrolyte shifts when hypertonic enemas are used. A similar, but less severe, situation may be seen with delayed passage of meconium without obstruction (see Chapters 11 and 12).

Pancreatic Insufficiency

The most common clinical features referrable to the gastrointestinal tract are secondary to pancreatic insufficiency. The patient may present with a large protuberant abdomen, wasted buttocks, malnutrition, and failure to thrive in spite of ingesting prodigious quantities of food. Stools tend to be frequent, bulky, oily, light-colored, and malodorous. The steatorrhea is secondary to deficiency of pancreatic lipase; a low bile acid pool, increased viscosity of the duodenal fluid, low bicarbonate secretion, and possibly other abnormalities of digestion and absorption may contribute to the picture of malabsorption. Undiagnosed infants with pancreatic insufficiency may have severe failure to thrive which may be complicated by hypoproteinemia (and edema) secondary to the inability to adequately digest and absorb dietary protein. Deficiency of fat-soluble vitamins (A, D, E, and K) is secondary to fat malabsorption. The vitamin deficiency states are more thoroughly discussed in Chapter 16.

Rectal prolapse may be seen in up to 20% of untreated patients by 3 years of age. It is felt that the prolapse is caused by the frequent passing of large and bulky stools and to the increase in intraabdominal pressure due to persistent coughing. Treatment mainly consists of replacement with pancreatic enzymes and adequate diet.

Intestinal obstruction from inspissated and impacted stool in infants and older patients has been inappropriately called "meconium ileus equivalent." Viscous intestinal secretions mixed with only partially digested food in the absence of normal pancreatic enzyme secretion may lead to constipation and partial or complete bowel obstruction in as many as 10% of patients with CF.[46] This complication is more common in patients who initially presented with meconium ileus.[47] Recurrent bouts of abdominal pain and an abdominal mass in a patient known to have cystic fibrosis is strongly suggestive of this syndrome. Treatment with oral and rectal administration of *N*-acetylcysteine and/or Gastrografin enema will usually dissolve the inspissated mass of stool and abnormal mucopolysaccharide secreted by bowel mucous glands. In rare cases when conservative management of the acute episode is unsuccessful, surgical intervention may be necessary. Chronic treatment requires increased pancreatic enzyme replacement and the ongoing use of cathartics like mineral oil or Colace.

Intussusception[48] or volvulus[44] may lead to acute or recurrent complications similar to bowel obstruction as discussed above. When intussusception occurs in children ages 2 or older, a sweat test should be performed to rule out CF. Intussusception in early stages could be relieved by barium enema.

Diabetes mellitus is 25 times more common in CF than in the general population, occurring in 1–2% of the pediatric age group and increasing to 13% of patients more than 25 years old.[49] Abnormal glucose tolerance tests may be seen in a greater number of patients. Although pancreatic alpha and beta cells appear to be normal until late in the course of disease,[37,41] abnormally low insulin responses to glucose loads or to diet may be noted.[50,51] It is presumed that the diabetes and insulinopenia is secondary to ongoing pancreatic autodisruption, the replacement of normal pancreatic tissue with fat and fibrous tissue, and the eventual disruption of normal Langerhan's islets (see Chapter 19).

Recurrent pancreatitis[52] is a complication seen in a group of cystic fibrosis patients without clinical signs of pancreatic insufficiency. Their pancreatic secretions are more viscous than normal, presumably leading to partial ongoing obstruction of pancreatic ducts and recurrent episodes of autodigestion of the pancreas by active pancreatic enzymes. Some of these patients may have episodes of acute pancreatitis precipitated by fatty meals, alcohol ingestion, cholecystectomy, or tetracycline usage. Pancreozymin-secretin stimulation revealed essentially normal enzymes but deficient HCO_3^- in their duodenal fluid. Selenomethionine (^{75}Se) uptake scanning revealed activity only in the head of the pancreas,[52] a finding consistent with pathology reports.[41] Treatment of this form of pancreatitis is by supplementation with pancreatic enzymes and the usual management for acute pancreatitis.

Differential Diagnosis of Malabsorption Seen in CF

Intestinal malabsorption secondary to pancreatic insufficiency is one of the usual hallmarks of cystic fibrosis (Table 17-1). Most patients will fail to gain weight normally during infancy and childhood. They frequently will have loose, bulky, greasy, and foul-smelling stools, but this may be difficult to appreciate in infancy. When a patient presents with failure to thrive and diarrheal stools suggestive of malabsorption, cystic fibrosis must be suspected. Included in the differential diagnosis are celiac disease, chronic nonspecific diarrhea, small-intestinal mucosal injury of any etiology, chronic parasitic infestation, and other causes of pancreatic insufficiency, ie, Shwachman-Diamond syndrome, isolated deficiencies in lipase, amylase, trypsinogen, and enterokinase. The presence of a positive sweat test would rule out all of the diseases under consideration except cystic fibrosis. Conversely, normal pancreatic function may rarely be present in cystic fibrosis and a normal secretin test will rule out cystic fibrosis.

Table 17-1
Causes of Malabsorption

Intestinal
Lymphangiectasia
Bacterial overgrowth
Mucosal injury
Parasitism
Celiac disease
Acrodermatitis enteropathica
Milk and/or soy protein allergy
Crohn's disease
Pancreatic
Cystic fibrosis
Shwachman-Diamond syndrome
Isolated enzyme deficiencies
Lipase
Trypsinogen
Enterokinase

LABORATORY ASSESSMENT OF PANCREATIC FUNCTION

Meconium

Screening of newborn infants by testing meconium for increased albumin content has been attempted as a means of establishing the early diagnosis of CF. The theoretical application is based on the increased albumin in stool and meconium seen in pancreatic insufficiency.[53,54] Initial results obtained following introduction of test strips[55] were encouraging; subsequent evaluations revealed high numbers of false-positive and false-negative results, thus making this form of screening unacceptable[56,57] (see Chapter 2).

Stool

Examination of stools can give an impression as to whether or not pancreatic insufficiency exists. A history of failure to thrive in association with stools that are bulky, voluminous, malodorous, frothy, and difficult to flush is strongly suggestive of steatorrhea. The presence of undigested meat fibers and/or an oily appearance of the stool further supports the existence of pancreatic insufficiency. Microscopic examination of stool during the first 6 months of life will reveal the presence of fat globules in most normal individuals as in those with cystic fibrosis;[58] after that time the presence of undigested meat fibers and/or fat globules suggests pancreatic disease and the need for more extensive evaluation.

The diagnosis of steatorrhea, which may be suggestive of insufficient pancreatic lipase, is perhaps best made by evaluating the excretion of fat in stool during a 72-hr collection. The patient must be on a diet adequate in fat, otherwise false-negative results may be obtained. Infants will require 3 g/kg body weight; older children should receive 50–100 g/day.

The quantitative measurement of trypsin and/or chymotrypsin in stool can yield valuable information regarding the presence of these proteolytic enzymes. The activity of the enzymes hydrolyzing the arginine and lysine peptide bonds of known substrates can be estimated.[59–61] A qualitative estimate of activity may also be made by incubating stool with x-ray film or gelatin.[49]

Blood

Amylase may be measured in the serum and may be from two primary sources: the salivary glands and the pancreas. These isoamylases may be separated electrophoretically in polyacrylamide gels. Patients with cystic fibrosis (or other forms of pancreatic insufficiency) will be lacking in, or have low levels of, pancreatic amylase and tend to have elevated levels of salivary amylase such that the total serum amylase may be normal. It was suggested that this noninvasive test of pancreatic amylase activity can be useful in the diagnosis of pancreatic insufficiency.[62–68]

Serum lipase may also be measured. Most of the lipase measurable in serum is of pancreatic origin, although pharyngeal lipase may be detected.[69,70] A decrease in serum lipase is therefore suggestive of a deficiency in pancreatic lipase.

Radioimmunoassay of pancreatic enzymes[71] has been done to establish ranges for patients with and without pancreatic disease. Immunoreactive trypsin is produced only by the pancreas and is the most thoroughly evaluated marker.[72,73] It correlates well with duodenal fluid trypsin activity and has been advocated for neonatal screening for the presence of pancreatic involvement in CF.[74]

Chymotrypsin activity in duodenal fluids may be measured indirectly. A synthetic tripeptide, *N*-benzoyl-L-tyrosyl-*p*-aminobenzoic acid (PABA), is given orally. Chymotrypsin splits *p*-aminobenzoic acid from the peptide. PABA is subsequently absorbed by the gut, conjugated in the liver and excreted in the urine. The amount of PABA measured in the urine or blood may serve as an indicator of pancreatic chymotrypsin.[75–78] Serum PABA can be measured in a similar manner in order to avoid timed collection of urine specimens.[79]

Radiology

Radiologic evaluation of the pancreas in patients with cystic fibrosis is rarely needed for diagnosis; however, ultrasonography, computerized axial tomographic (CAT) scanning, and endoscopic retrograde cholangiopancreatography may be of help in the evaluation. Ultrasound examination will usually reveal the pancreas to be smaller than usual and to have increased echogenecity;[80] the echogenecity increases with age as the pancreas becomes smaller in size.[81] If pancreatitis is present, a large, anechoic pancreatic head may be noted.

CAT scanning adds no useful information beyond that already available through ultrasonography; a small fibrous pancreas is seen.

Endoscopic retrograde cholangiopancreatography (ERCP) has been performed on cystic fibrosis patients with normal pancreatic function;[52] findings included a beaded pattern with narrowing of ducts and normal-appearing pancreatic ducts.

Measurement of Pancreatic Enzymes

The laboratory evaluation (including pancreozymin and secretin stimulation, if available) of the patient with suspected CF may be laborious but is essential in order to establish the degree of pancreatic dysfunction which may be used to assess ongoing changes in the pancreas. The most direct method of establishing pancreatic function in patients suspected of having pancreatic insufficiency is through the collection and evaluation of pancreatic secretions following stimulation with the above secretagogues (Figure 17-8). The duodenum is intubated under fluoroscopic visualization using a double-lumen Dreiling tube. Resting duodenal fluid is collected and tested for pH and yellow color in order to assure tube placement. Baseline collection of duodenal fluid is carried out over two 10-min periods. Pancreozymin–cholecystokinin, 2 units/kg, is then administered intravenously, and three 10-min collections are made. Secretin, 2 units/kg, is injected, and three additional 10-min collections are carried out. The fluids obtained are assayed for amylase, lipase, trypsin, chymotrypsin; volume of collection, pH of fluid, viscosity, and electrolyte content (especially bicarbonate) are also determined.

All of the tests described above, with the exception of the pancreozymin–secretin stimulation, reveal only indirect, qualitative information regarding pancreatic insufficiency. No accurate information can be gained regarding the availability of individual enzymes present in duodenal secretions.

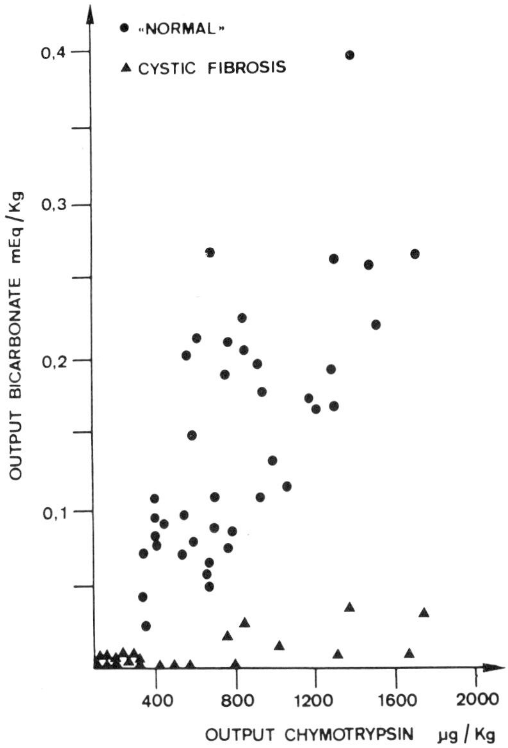

Figure 17-8 Pancreozymin–secretin test in cystic fibrosis. Outputs of bicarbonate (*y* axis) and chymotrypsin (*x* axis) in 40 children without gastrointestinal disease, 12 children with cystic fibrosis with steatorrhea, and 10 children with cystic fibrosis without steatorrhea. In all cases of cystic fibrosis bicarbonate output is abnormally low, but those children without steatorrhea have low normal to normal chymotrypsin outputs. Reproduced from Hadorn B: The exocrine pancreas, in Anderson CM, Burke V (eds): *Pediatric Gastroenterology*. Oxford, Blackwell Scientific Publications, 1975, with permission.

Only by measurement of pancreatic enzymes present in the basal and poststimulation pancreatic secretions can a reliable interpretation of the secretory status of the pancreas be made.

Evaluation of Pancreatic Function in CF

Pancreatic functions in CF patients are usually abnormal. The duodenal fluid from these patients demonstrates increased viscosity, and markedly reduced secretion of bicarbonate, water, and electrolytes; in 85–90% of affected patients, enzymes are markedly decreased or absent.[36,52,82–86] Increased stool fat and protein will usually be noted, depending on the severity of the pancreatic lesion. Stool trypsin and chymotrypsin activity will be low or absent. Serum amylase may be normal, but isoamylase evaluation will reveal that the salivary form is predominant; in a like manner serum lipase will be predominantly of the pharyngeal type. An elevated enterokinase[87] has also been noted in duodenal fluids for CF patients. This may be secondary to a reduced or zero level of pancreatic proteases, especially trypsinogen.

Most patients with cystic fibrosis exhibit complete pancreatic insufficiency. Approximately 10–15% of patients will not have symptoms suggestive of deficiency of pancreatic enzymes,[36,84,88] but will show normal or near-normal secretion of these enzymes in response to pancreozymin. Further evaluation with secretin reveals a markedly diminished secretion of HCO_3^- and of total volume.[36,84] Most of the patients in this group have the other clinical and laboratory manifestations of cystic fibrosis, but a smaller subgroup has been described with borderline or normal sweat tests, familial pulmonary disease (including sibs with classical cystic fibrosis), and normal pancreatic function and histology but with an abnormal bicarbonate response to secretin.[52,89,90]

THERAPY OF PANCREATIC INSUFFICIENCY

The replacement of pancreatic acinar tissue with fibrous and fatty tissue occurs in the majority of patients with cystic fibrosis and leads to partial or total absence of pancreatic enzymes in the duodenum. The end result is maldigestion and malabsorption of carbohydrates, fats, and proteins. The deficiency in pancreatic enzymes may be circumvented by dietary modifications and the use of enzyme preparations from bovine or porcine pancreatic tissue as substitutes for deficiencies in endogenous pancreatic enzymes.

Dietary alterations include low-fat diets and medium-chain triglycerides (MCT) and unsaturated fatty acid substitution for long-chain fats. In this manner, the steatorrhea may be lessened as is the frequency and bulk of stools. Patients with CF have been fed diets of beef serum hydrolysates, MCT, and glucose polymers[91,92] in an attempt to bypass the digestive abnormalities; these patients show gains in weight, clinical scores, and serum albumin measurements. Such diets are rarely accepted by patients and therefore compliance is a major difficulty. In the very young patients semielemental formulas such as Pregestimil and Portagen are helpful; at times hyperalimentation is needed when marasmus prevails. During the first year of life, the provision of approximately 150 kcal/kg will usually allow adequate growth. We recommend replacement of fat-soluble vitamins using twice normal dosages. A more complete discussion of the vitamin and dietary needs of CF patients may be found in Chapters 15 and 16.

The use of pancreatic supplements is universal, and they are usually given with meals. Taken orally, these preparations theoretically will provide enough pancreatic enzyme to prevent the maldigestion and malabsorption of CF. Different preparations vary in enzyme content, formulation, and bioavailability (Table 17-2). In addition, individual variation in residual enzyme secretion will cause variation in dosage requirements. Appropriate doses result in a decrease in the number of stools and a decrease in the bulk and odor of stools. Normal digestion and absorption is rarely achieved, although normalization of growth may occur.

The difficulties of administration of enzyme replacement therapy are due to many factors. Acid and peptic inactivation of lipase occurs below pH 4.5 and of trypsin below pH 3.5. Oral pancreatin dosages in adults have been found to provide less than 22% of ingested trypsin and less than 8% of ingested lipase at the ligament of Treitz.[93,94] It is suspected that the increased gastric acidity[95] and lowered duodenal pH secondary to depressed HCO_3^- secretion[36] are responsible for the measured decrease in enzyme activity. Enteric coating to protect against acid denaturation has been attempted,

Table 17-2
Pancreatic Supplements

Name	Product	Dose	Lipase USP units	Protease USP units	Amylase USP units	Other
Viokase (Viobin)	Pancreatin tablets or powder	Tablet or ⅓ packet	6,500	32,000	48,000	
Pancreatin-High Lipase (Vitaline)	Pancreatin tablet	Tablet	12,000	60,000	60,000	
Cotazym (Organon)	Pancrelipase	Capsule	8,000	30,000	30,000	
		25-mg packet	16,000	60,000	60,000	
		50-mg packet	40,000	150,000	150,000	
Cotazym-65B		Capsule	8,000	30,000	30,000	65 mg conjugated bile salts
Cotazym S		Capsule, enteric-coated microspheres	5,000	20,000	20,000	
Ilozyme (Warren-Teed)	Pancrelipase	Tablet	11,000	30,000	30,000	
Pancrease Johnson & Johnson)	Pancrelipase	Capsule-enteric	4,000	25,000	20,000	

but the absence of a duodenal environment with sufficient alkalinity may interfere with dissolution of the microspheres or tablets. Other efforts to overcome the acid-pepsin inactivation included the concomitant administration of pancreatic enzyme with either antacids or cimetidine;[96–98] either regimen improves fat digestion and decreases steatorrhea, but high doses of HCO_3^- are unpalatable and generally unacceptable in a pediatric population. The long-term effects of cimetidine in childhood are unknown, and therefore it cannot be recommended for lifelong usage.

It has been suggested[99] that some patients with cystic fibrosis have increased fecal losses of bile salts and therefore a decrease in their intestinal availability. The interruption in the enterohepatic circulation of bile salts and their loss in stool and low concentration in the duodenum may disrupt the intraluminal interaction of lipase, bile salts, and triglycerides, resulting in an inability to form micelles and a worsening of already present steatorrhea. Bile salt malabsorption is more pronounced in untreated patients and may still be seen after pancreatic supplements are used. A preparation of pancrelipase with supplemental bile salts (Cotazym 65-B, Organon) is specifically designed for this group of patients.

There is controversy as to what is the best time to administer the pancreatic supplements; we prefer to give the supplement after the meals. The formulation of the pancreatic supplement may play a role in enzyme availability. Dispersion of enzymes into the meal for more even distribution may delay their passage into the duodenum and increase their exposure to the acidic environment.[100] Enteric coating to circumvent the gastric acidity may hinder their even dissolution[94] or at a time consistent with arrival of food particles in the duodenum.[101]

Wide variation in individual enzyme deficiencies also leads to other difficulties since the various preparations have enzymes present in fixed quantities. To our knowledge, differential requirements of individual enzymes have not been evaluated.

Three preparations of pancreatic replacement are commonly used. Pancreatin is extracted from the pancreas of the swine, beef, or ox; each milligram contains at least 25 USP units of amylase, 25 USP units of protease, and 2 USP units of lipase.[102] The most commonly used form of pancreatin, Viokase (Viobin), has a much higher ratio of lipase to amylase than other commercially available formulations. The recommended pancreatin dosage is from 1 to 6 tablets taken orally after each meal, the maximum daily dosage not to exceed 6 g/day; this would provide adequate amylase, protease, and lipase to digest 150 g of starch, 150 g protein, and 12 g of fat under optimal conditions in vitro.[103]

Pancrelipase is a concentrate of porcine pancreatic enzymes containing at least 24 USP units of lipase, 100 USP units of amylase, and 100 USP units of protease per milligram. Compared to pancreatin, the lipase activity is increased 12-fold and the amylase and protease activity fourfold.

Both pancreatin and pancrelipase tablets may be enteric-coated to resist acid inactivation. The associated problems have been alluded to previously. A newer pancrelipase preparation, enteric-coated microspheres (ECMS) (Pancrease, Johnson & Johnson, and Cotazym S, Organon), has become available which purports to overcome many of the problems previously seen. The enzyme activity is higher (4000 NF units lipase, 20,000–25,000 NF units each of amylase and protease, respectively), per capsule, yet fewer capsules need be used because the microspheres are more evenly dispersed in the stomach, and the pH-dependent polymer coating is resistant to acid pHs but dissolves in alkaline pHs, making more enzyme available in the duodenum. The therapeutic effects of lower doses compared to standard pancreatin and pancrelipase have been noted;[104–107] one fifth to one half the number of capsules are needed to attain the same clinical effectiveness. Recent studies[96] have shown only little additional effectiveness with antacid or cimetidine when used with ECMS, suggesting that the duodenal pH is effective in disruption of the enteric coatings.

Complications of pancreatic replacement therapy include: (1) the persistence of an inadequate digestive process, especially of fats; (2) the presence of perianal irritation and excoriations felt to be secondary to excess proteases; and (3) hyperuricemia and uricosuria,[108,109] which is thought to be caused by excessive intake of purines in the pancreatic extract preparation. Treatment of uricosuria and the excretion of uric acid crystals consists of lowering the dosage of pancreatic extracts to the minimum dose which prevents significant steatorrhea, decreasing oral intake of fats, supplementing with MCT oil, and increasing nitrogen and carbohydrate caloric intake[110] (see Chapter 23).

CONCLUSION

Pancreatic involvement and insufficiency in patients with CF contributes to the mortality and poor nutritional status of the disease.

In early infancy, physiologic low lipase and absent amylase can be confused with pancreatic insufficiency. The unique feature of exocrine pancreatic function in cystic fibrosis is that the bicarbonate output and fluid volume in response to secretin is always diminished. The earliest lesions seen in CF are the appearance of eosinophilic concretions in acini and ductules. Not all patients with CF have pancreatic insufficiency from birth; about 10–15% of patients have sufficient pancreatic function in infancy to avoid symptoms.

Many of the gastrointestinal manifestations of CF can be attributed directly or indirectly to the pancreatic lesion; in other words, malabsorption, meconium ileus, intussusception, volvulus, intestinal obstruction, rectal prolapse, fecal impaction, and growth failure can be the result of pancreatic insufficiency. Recurrent pancreatitis can occur in patients with CF and normal pancreatic function. The incidence of diabetes mellitus and insulinopenia increase with age.

It is important to establish the degree of pancreatic dysfunction, preferably with a pancreozymin–secretin test. The replacement of pancreatic enzymes is difficult, and normal digestion and absorption is rarely achieved. New therapeutic modalities such as bile salts, cimetidine, bicarbonate, or acid lipase and amylase should be tested more carefully. More thorough investigation of the pancreatic lesion and the pathophysiology of the pancreatic insufficiency might be helpful in elucidating the cellular defect in cystic fibrosis.

REFERENCES

1. Andersen DH: Cystic fibrosis of the pancreas and its relation to celiac disease. *Am J Dis Child* 1938;56:344–399.
2. Bodian ML: *Fibrocystic Disease of the Pancreas. A Congenital Disorder of Mucus Production (Mucosis).* London, Wm. Heinemann Medical Books, 1952.
3. Shwachman H, Leubner H, Catzel P: Mucoviscidosis, in Levine SZ (ed): *Advances in Pediatrics.* Chicago, Year Book Medical Publishers, 1955.
4. di Sant'Agnese P, Darling R, Perera G, et al: Abnormal electrolyte composition of sweat in cystic fibrosis of the pancreas. *Pediatrics* 1953;12:549–563.
5. Imrie JR, Fagan DG, Sturgess JM: Quantitative evaluation of the development of the exocrine pancreas in cystic fibrosis and control infants. *Am J Pathol* 1979;95: 697–707.
6. Patten BM: *Human Embryology, 3rd ed.* New York, McGraw-Hill, 1968.
7. Gray H: The pancreas, in Gross CM (ed): *Anatomy of the Human Body.* Philadelphia, Lea & Febiger, 1966.
8. Kleitsch WP: Anatomy of the pancreas. A study with special reference to the duct system. *Arch Surg* 1955;71:795–802.
9. Laitio M, Lev R, Orlic D: The developing human fetal pancreas: An ultrastructural and histochemical study with special reference to exocrine cells. *J Anat* 1974;117: 619- 634.
10. Grant JCB: *A Method of Anatomy, Descriptive and Deductive, 4th ed.* Baltimore, Williams & Wilkins, 1948.
11. Brandberg LL: The pancreas, in Sleisenger MH, Fordtran JS (eds): *Gastrointestinal Disease.* Philadelphia, WB Saunders, 1978.
12. Bloom W, Fawcett DW: *A Textbook of Histology, 10th ed.* Philadelphia, WB Saunders, 1975.
13. Palade GE, Siekevitz P: Intracisternal granules in exocrine cells of pancreas. *J Biophys Biochem Cytol* 1956;2:417–422.
14. Palade GE, Siekevitz P, Caro LG: The exocrine pancreas, in De Reuck AVS, Cameron MP (eds): *Ciba Foundation Symposium.* London, Churchill, 1962.
15. Siekevitz P, Palade GE: A cytochemical study of the pancreas of the guinea pig. *J Biophys Biochem Cytol* 1960;7:619–630.
16. Meyer JH: Pancreatic physiology, in Sleisenger MH, Fordtran JS (eds): *Gastrointestinal Disease.* Philadelphia, WB Saunders, 1978.
17. Steer MI, Glazer G: Parallel secretion of digestive enzymes by the in vitro rabbit pancreas. *Am J Physiol* 1976;231:1860–1865.
18. Tartakoff AM, Jamieson JD, Scheele GA, et al: Studies on the pancreas of the guinea pig. Parallel processing and discharge of exocrine proteins. *J Biol Chem* 1975;250: 2671–2677.
19. Scheele GA, Palade GE: Studies on the guinea pig pancreas. Parallel discharge of exocrine enzyme activities. *J Biol Chem* 1975;250:2660–2670.
20. Rothman SS: Protein transport by the pancreas. *Science* 1975;190:747–753.
21. Dagorn JC, Sahel J, Sarles H: Nonparallel secretion of enzymes in human duodenal juice collected by endoscopic retrograde catheterization of the papilla. *Gastroenterology* 1977;73:42–45.
22. Dagorn JC, Estival A: Nonparallel secretion from rat pancreas in vivo studies. *J Physiol* 1979;290:51–58.
23. Jamieson JD, Palade GE: Synthesis, intracellular transport, and discharge of secretory proteins in stimulated pancreas exocrine cells. *J Cell Biol* 1971;50:135–138.
24. Kramer MF, Poert C: Unstimulated secretion of protein from rat exocrine pancreas cells. *J Cell Biol* 1972;52:147–158.
25. Klaeveman HC, Conlon TP, Gardener JD: Effects of gastrointestinal hormones on adenylcyclase activity on pancreatic exocrine cells, in Thompson JC (ed): *Symposium on Gastrointestinal Hormones.* Austin, University of Texas Press, 1975.
26. Gardner JD, Conlon TP, Adams TD: Cyclic AMP in pancreatic acinar cells: Effects of gastrointestinal hormones. *Gastroenterology* 1976;70:29–35.
27. Shelby HT, Gross LP, Lichty P, et al: Action of cholecystokinin and cholinergic agents on membrane-bound calcium in dispersed pancreatic acinar cells. *J Clin Invest* 1976;58: 1482–1493.
28. Gardner JD, Jackson MJ: Regulation of amylase release from dispersed pancreatic acinar cells. *J Physiol* 1977;270:439–454.
29. Meyer JH, Spingola LJ, Grossman MI: Endogenous cholecystokinin potentiates exogenous secretion on pancreas of dog. *Am J Physiol* 1971;221:742–747.
30. Wormsley KJ: Response to secretin and pancreozymin in man. *Scand J Gastroenterol* 1971;6:342–350.

31. Lebenthal E, Lee PC: Development of functional response in human exocrine pancreas. *Pediatrics* 1980;66:556–560.
32. Lebenthal E, Lev R, Lee PC: Perinatal development of the exocrine pancreas, in Lebenthal E (ed): *Textbook of Gastroenterology and Nutrition in Infancy.* New York, Raven Press, 1981.
33. Antonowicz I, Lebenthal E: Developmental pattern of small intestinal enterokinase and disaccharidase activities in the human fetus. *Gastroenterology* 1977;72:1299–1303.
34. Lightwood R, Reber HA: Micropuncture study of pancreatic secretion in the cat. *Gastroenterology* 1979;72:61–66.
35. Zoppi G, Andreotti G, Pajno-Ferrarra F, et al: The development of specific responses of the exocrine pancreas to pancreozymin and secretin stimulation in newborn infants. *Pediatr Res* 1973;7:198–203.
36. Zoppi G, Shmerling H, Gaburro D, et al: The electrolyte and protein contents and outputs in duodenal juice after pancreozymin and secretin stimulation in normal children and in patients with cystic fibrosis. *Acta Pediatr Scand* 1970;59:692–696.
37. Oppenheimer EH, Esterly JR: Pathology of cystic fibrosis: Review of the literature and comparison with one hundred and forty-six autopsied cases. *Perspect Pediatr Pathol* 1975;2:241–278.
38. Oppenheimer E, Esterly J: Cystic fibrosis of the pancreas. Morphologic findings in infants with and without diagnostic pancreatic lesions. *Arch Pathol* 1973;96:149–154.
39. Allen RA, Baggenstoss AH: The pathogenesis of fibrocystic disease of the pancreas. Study of the ducts by serial section. *Am J Pathol* 1955;31:337–351.
40. Danks DM, Allen J, Andersen CM: A genetic study of fibrocystic disease of the pancreas. *Ann Hum Genet* 1965;28:323– 356.
41. Vawter GF, Shwachman H: Cystic fibrosis in adults: An autopsy study. *Pathol Ann* 1979; 14:357–382.
42. Kopito LE, Shwachman H, Vawter GF, et al: The pancreas in cystic fibrosis: Chemical composition and comparative morphology. *Pediatr Res* 1976;10:742–749.
43. McPartin J, Dickson J, Swair V: Meconium ileus, immediate and long term survival. *Arch Dis Child* 1972;47:207–210.
44. Shwachman H: Cystic fibrosis. *Curr Probl Pediatr* 1978;8:1–72.
45. Waggett H, Bishop H, Koop E: Experience with Gastrografin enema in the treatment of meconium ileus. *J Pediatr Surg* 1970;5: 649–654.
46. Matseshe J, Go V, DiMagno E: Meconium ileus equivalent complicating cystic fibrosis in post neonatal children and young adults. *Gastroenterology* 1977;72:732–736.
47. Jaffe B, Graham W, Goldman L: Post infancy intestinal obstruction in children with cystic fibrosis. *Arch Surg* 1966;92:337–343.
48. Holsclaw DS, Rocmans C, Shwachman H: Intussusception in patients with cystic fibrosis. *Pediatrics* 1971;48:51.
49. Shwachman H, Grand RJ: Cystic fibrosis, in Sleisenger MH, Fordtran JS (eds): *Gastrointestinal Disease.* Philadelphia, WB Saunders, 1978.
50. Adrian T, McKiernan J, Johnstone D, et al: Hormonal abnormalities of the pancreas and gut in cystic fibrosis. *Gastroenterology* 1980; 79:460–465.
51. Kjellman N, Larsson Y: Insulin release in cystic fibrosis. *Arch Dis Child* 1975;50: 205–209.
52. Shwachman H, Lebenthal E, Khaw KT: Recurrent acute pancreatitis in patients with normal pancreatic enzymes. *Pediatrics* 1975; 55:86–95.
53. Green MN, Clarke J, Shwachman H: Studies in cystic fibrosis of the pancreas: Protein pattern meconium ileus. *Pediatrics* 1958; 21: 635–639.
54. Ryley H, Neal L, Brogan T, et al: Plasma proteins in meconium from normal infants and from babies with cystic fibrosis. *Arch Dis Child* 1974;49:901–904.
55. Stephan U, Busch E, Kollberg H, et al: Cystic fibrosis detection by means of a test strip. *Pediatrics* 1975;55:35–38.
56. Ryley H, Neale L, Bray P: False negative meconium tests for cystic fibrosis. *Lancet* 1976; 2:365–366.
57. Berger H, Reynolds S, Lee K: False-positive meconium screen. *Lancet* 1977;2:458.
58. Zoppi G, Andreotti G, Pajno-Ferrara F, et al: Exocrine pancreas function in premature and full term neonates. *Pediatrics* 1972;6: 880–886.
59. Haverback BL, Dyce BJ, Gutentag RJ, et al: Measurement of trypsin and chymotrypsin in stool: A diagnostic test for pancreatic insufficiency. *Gastroenterology* 1963;44:588– 597.
60. Barbero GJ, Sibinga MS, Marino JM, et al: Stool trypsin and chymotrypsin value in the diagnosis of pancreatic insufficiency in cystic fibrosis. *Am J Dis Child* 1966;112:536–540.
61. Bonin A, Roy CC, LaSalle R, et al: Fecal chymotrypsin: A reliable index of exocrine pancreatic function in children. *J Pediatr* 1973;83:594–600.
62. Wolf RO, Taylor LL: Isoenzyme demonstration technique. *Am J Clin Pathol* 1968;49: 871–876.
63. Taussig LM, Wolf RO, Wood RE, et al: Use of serum amylase isoenzymes in evaluation of

pancreatic function. *Pediatrics* 1974;54: 229-235.

64. Skude G, Kollberg H: Serum isoamylases in cystic fibrosis. *Acta Pediatr Scand* 1976;65: 145-149.
65. Wolf RO, Taussig LM, Ross ME, et al: Quantitative evaluation of serum pancreatic isoamylases in cystic fibrosis. *J Lab Clin Med* 1976;87:164-168.
66. Takacs O, Sohar I, Laszlo A, et al: Distribution of serum amylase isoenzymes in cystic fibrosis homozygotes and heterozygotes. *Acta Paediatr Acad Sci Hung* 1977;18: 21-26.
67. Kenny D, Cooke A, Tempany E, et al: Activity of serum alpha amylases in cystic fibrosis. *Clin Chim Acta* 1978;89:429-433.
68. Gillard BK, Simbala JA, Feig SA: Serum amylase isoenzymes in cystic fibrosis patients. Evidence for a generalized defect in exocrine gland secretory regulation. *Pediatr Res* 1980;14:1168-1172.
69. Hamosh M, Klaeveman HL, Wolf RO, et al: Pharyngeal lipase and digestion of dietary triglyceride in man. *J Clin Invest* 1975;55: 908-913.
70. Berk JE: Serum amylase and lipase. New perspectives. *JAMA* 1967;199:98-102.
71. Temler RS, Felber JP: Radioimmunoassay of enzymes of the exocrine pancreas (trypsin, chymotrypsin, chymotrypsinogen). *Biochem Biophys Acta* 1971;236:72-83.
72. Heinrich HC, Gabbe EE, l'Uagic F: Immunoreactive serum trypsin in diseases of the pancreas. *Klin Wochenschr* 1979;57: 1237-1238.
73. Stagg BH, Wood TP: Radioimmunoassay of trypsin. *Ann Clin Biochem* 1979;16: 147-151.
74. Burlina A, Rizzotti P, Tonon M, et al: Serum immunoreactive trypsin in cystic fibrosis. *Scand J Gastroenterol Suppl* 1980;15(Suppl 62):35-43.
75. Imondi AR, Stradley RP, Wohlgemuth RL: Synthetic peptides in the diagnosis of exocrine pancreatic insufficiency in animals. *Gut* 1972;13:726-731.
76. Gyr K, Stalder GA, Schiffman I, et al: Oral administration of a chymotrypsin-labile-peptide. A new test of exocrine pancreatic function in man. *Gut* 1976;17:27-32.
77. Arvanitakis C, Greenberger NJ: Diagnosis of pancreatic disease by a synthetic peptide. *Lancet* 1976;1:663-666.
78. Sacher M, Kobsa A, Shmerling DH: PABA screening test for exocrine pancreatic function in infants and children. *Arch Dis Child* 1978;53:639-641.
79. Dockter G, Nacu I, Kohlberger E: Determination of protease-cleaved *p*-aminobenzoic acid (PABA) in serum after oral administration of *N*-benzoyl-L-tyrosyl-*p*-aminobenzoic acid (PABA-peptide) in children. *Eur J Pediatr* 1981;135:277-279.
80. Willi UV, Reddish JM, Teele RL: Cystic fibrosis: Its characteristic appearance on abdominal sonography. *Am J Roentgenol* 1980; 134:1005-1010.
81. Spehl-Robberecht M, Baran D, Dab I, et al: Ultrasonic study of pancreas in cystic fibrosis. *Ann Radiol* 1981;24:49-52.
82. Brooks F: Testing pancreatic function. *N Engl J Med* 1972;286:300-303.
83. Dreiling DA, Janowitz HD: The measurement of pancreatic secretory function, in *Ciba Foundation Symposium on the Exocrine Pancreas.* London, J&A Churchill, 1962.
84. Hadorn B, Zoppi G, Shmerling DH, et al: Quantitative assessment of exocrine pancreatic function in infants and children. *J Pediatr* 1968;73:39-50.
85. Howat HT, Braganza JM: Assessment of pancreatic dysfunction in man, in Howat HT, Sarles H (eds): *The Exocrine Pancreas.* Philadelphia, WB Saunders, 1979.
86. Lebenthal E: Pancreatic function and assessment, in Lebenthal E. (ed): *Digestive Diseases in Children.* New York, Grune & Stratton, 1978.
87. Lebenthal E, Lee PC: Effect of pancreozymin and secretin on intraluminal enterokinase, trypsin, and chymotrypsin activities of cystic fibrosis and control children. *Digestion* 1982;23:39-47.
88. Shwachman H, Gahm N: Studies in cystic fibrosis of the pancreas; a simple test for the detection of excessive chloride in the skin. *N Engl J Med* 1956;255:999-1001.
89. Sarsfield JK, Davies JM: Negative sweat tests and cystic fibrosis. *Arch Dis Child* 1975;50: 463-466.
90. Huff DS, Huang NN, Arey JB: Atypical cystic fibrosis of the pancreas with normal levels of sweat chloride and minimal pancreatic lesions. *J Pediatr* 1979;94:237-239.
91. Allan JD, Milner J, Moss D: Therapeutic use of an artificial diet. *Lancet* 1970;1:785-786.
92. Berry HK, Kellogg FW, Hunt MM, et al: Dietary supplement and nutrition in children with cystic fibrosis. *Am J Dis Child* 1975; 129:165-171.
93. DiMagno EP, Malagelada JM, Go VLW, et al: Fate of orally ingested enzymes in pancreatic insufficiency. Comparison of two dosage schedules. *N Engl J Med* 1977;296: 1318-1322.
94. Graham DY: Enzyme replacement therapy of exocrine pancreatic insufficiency in man. *N Engl J Med* 1977;296:1314-1318.
95. Cox K, Isenberg J: Hypersecretion of gastric acid in patients with pancreatic exocrine

insufficiency due to cystic fibrosis, abstracted. *Gastroenterology* 1975;74:1022.

96. Gow R, Bradbear R, Francis P, et al: Comparative study of varying regimens to improve steatorrhea and creatorrhea in cystic fibrosis: Effectiveness of an enteric-coated preparation with and without antacids and cimetidine. *Lancet* 1981;2:1071–1074.
97. Nassif EG, Younoszai MK, Weinberger MM, et al: Comparative effects of antacids, enteric coating, and bile salts on the efficacy of oral pancreatic enzyme therapy in cystic fibrosis. *J Pediatr* 1981;98:320–323.
98. Cox K, Isenberg J, Osher A, et al: The effect of cimetidine in maldigestion in cystic fibrosis. *J Pediatr* 1979;94:488–492.
99. Weber A, Roy C, Morin C, et al: Malabsorption of bile acids in children with cystic fibrosis. *N Engl J Med* 1973;289:1001–1005.
100. Meyer J: The ins and outs of oral pancreatic enzymes. *N Engl J Med* 1977;296:1347–1348.
101. Meyer J, Mandiola S, Shadcheur A, et al: Dispersion of solid food by the canine stomach. *Gastroenterology* 1977;72:A79, 1102.
102. United States Pharmacopoeial Convention: *The United States Pharmacopocia XX and The National Formulary XV*. Rockville, Maryland, 1980, pp 580–584.
103. Cho Y, Aviado D: Clinical pharmacology for pediatricians. Pancreatic enzyme preparations with special reference to enterically coated microspheres of pancrelipase. *J Clin Pharmacol* 1981;21:224–237.
104. Holsclaw PS, Fohl JC, Keith HH: Enhancement of enzyme replacement therapy in cystic fibrosis. *Cystic Fibrosis Club Abstr* 1979;20: 19.
105. Holsclaw PS: Long term benefits of pH-sensitive enteric coated enzymes in CF. In *Proceedings of the Eighth International Congress on Cystic Fibrosis.* Toronto, Canadian Cystic Fibrosis Foundation, 1980, p 19a.
106. Khaw KT, Adeniyi-Jones S, Gorden D, et al: Comparative effectiveness of Viokase, Cotazym and Pancrease in children with cystic fibrosis. *Cystic Fibrosis Club Abstr* 1977;18: 57.
107. Weber AM, Caheldere B, Roy CC, et al: Effectiveness of enteric coated pancrease in cystic fibrosis children under 4 years old. *Cystic Fibrosis Club Abstr* 1979;20:18.
108. Stapleton FB, Kennedy J, Nousia-Arvanitakis S, et al: Hyperuricosuria due to high dose pancreatic extract therapy in cystic fibrosis. *N Engl J Med* 1976;295:246–248.
109. Davidson GP, Hassel FM, Crozier D, et al: Iatrogenic hyperuricemia in children with cystic fibrosis. *J Pediatr* 1978;93:976–978.
110. Nousia-Arvanitakis S, Stapleton FB, Liushaw MA, et al: Therapeutic approach to pancreatic extract-induced hyperuricosuria in cystic fibrosis. *J Pediatr* 1977;90: 302–305.

18

The Liver in Cystic Fibrosis

John D. Lloyd-Still

INCIDENCE

Hepatic disease detected by clinical examination developed in 2.2% (15 of 693) patients seen over an 18-year period at the CF center in Cleveland.[1] di Sant'Agnese and Davis[2] reviewed the literature and found cirrhosis present in 5% (10 of 221) CF patients more than 12 years old. In CF patients over 25 years, Shwachman et al[3] reported liver involvement in 5.7% (4 of 70); two of these patients had portal hypertension and two had intermittent jaundice.

The incidence of hepatic involvement in CF from pathological studies varies from necropsy figures for focal biliary cirrhosis between 9% (18 of 198 patients)[4] and 19% (28 of 164 patients)[5] to the incidence of multilobular biliary cirrhosis with nodular scarring of 2.4% (4 of 164 patients).[5] Among newborns who died with CF, 33% (11 of 36) had diffuse cholestasis and an additional eight showed periportal changes, proliferation of bile ductules, and/or periportal fibrosis and inflammation.[5] Pathologic studies during life by means of liver biopsy showed abnormalities in 17.8% (15 of 84 patients)[6] to 40% (20 of 50 patients)[7] by light microscopy.

One may attempt to define the incidence of liver involvement in CF by evaluating abnormalities in tests of liver function. These vary from 37.5% (15 of 40 patients)[8] to 42.5% (31 of 146 patients)[9] for alkaline phosphatase, to 36% (15 of 42 patients) with raised serum bile acids[10] and 78% with abnormal liver scans.[11]

Thus when defining the incidence of hepatic involvement in CF, one needs to clarify whether one is defining the clinical, pathological, or biochemical parameters of involvement.

PATHOLOGY AND PATHOGENESIS

The pathologic changes in CF are discussed in detail in Chapter 3. Since the basic defect in the disease remains unknown, we cannot completely explain the pathogenesis of the hepatic lesions. Bodian[12] proposed the name "focal biliary fibrosis" as a specific hepatic lesion in CF. He postulated that granular eosinophilic secretions lodge in bile ducts, resulting in ductular dilatation, hyperplasia, proliferation, and finally periductal inflammation and fibrosis. In simple terms, the bile in CF is considered to be too "sticky." Confirmation of this abnormality can be demonstrated in newborn CF infants with cholestasis,[5] and excessive mucoid material is often noted in extra- and intrahepatic bile ducts.[13] Rarely this mucoid material produces obstructive jaundice later in life.

Children with CF associated with pancreatic insufficiency have increased fecal losses of bile acids,[14,15] with a resultant reduced bile salt pool size[16] which is responsive to the administration of pancreatic enzymes. Biliary lipid composition was found to be lithogenic in untreated CF and to respond to pancreatic enzymes.[17] This abnormality presumably accounts for the increased incidence of gallstones in these patients.[18]

A number of factors that may be involved in worsening the underlying liver problems are detailed in Table 18-1. Fatty infiltration of the liver is found in starvation, prolonged undernutrition, and is a characteristic feature of kwashiorkor. Fatty liver is a frequent finding in newly diagnosed infants with CF, but whether CF infants presenting with hypoalbuminemia are especially prone to develop hepatic complications is unknown. Fatty changes in the liver are also frequently present at autopsy in older children whose course is characterized by prolonged periods of malnutrition prior to death. The low levels of lipoproteins reported in CF[19] could result in impaired removal of hepatic triglycerides. Analysis of liver lipid content from patients with kwashiorkor shows an increased concentration of palmitic acid and a decrease in the concentration of linoleic acid,[20] findings that are similar to those found in the serum of CF patients.[21]

Table 18-1
Possible Factors Involved In Liver Pathology in CF

Focal biliary fibrosis → cirrhosis
Bile stasis, granular eosinophilic secretions
Lithogenic bile
Decreased lipoproteins → impaired removal triglycerides
Fatty infiltration, hypoproteinemia, malnutrition
Hemosiderosis
Neonatal Cholestasis, obstructive jaundice
Endotoxemia secondary to meconium ileus
Cholangiolitis, microgallbladder
Viruses—cytomegalovirus, hepatitis A, B, others
Ischemia secondary to cor pulmonale
Abnormal immune responses
Iatrogenic: intravenous hyperalimentation; anabolic steroids; other drugs

Other possible damaging agents include intravenous hyperalimentation, and drugs such as antibiotics and anabolic steroids which may cause cholestasis or hepatocellular damage. Excessive iron absorption secondary to pancreatic insufficiency can lead to hemosiderosis,[4] which was present in 17% (33 of 198 autopsies) and is more common in infants.[5] The liver performs an important function in protection from the effects of toxins absorbed from the intestine, and in situations such as meconium ileus, endotoxins may be absorbed in increased amounts and damage the liver. Gallstones may lead to obstructive jaundice and ascending cholangitis. Patients with CF may acquire infection from hepatotoxic viruses such as hepatitis B, hepatitis A, non-A non-B hepatitis, the cytomegalovirus, and others, but there is no evidence that these viruses pursue an unusual course in these patients. Anoxia may be an important factor leading to hepatic ischemia in the terminal stages, and in theory cardiac cirrhosis may ensue. Inhibition of leukocyte migration by purified liver-specific lipoprotein derived from hepatocyte plasma membrane was found in 9 of 11 children with liver disease and in 5 of 14 with CF without overt liver disease ($P < 0.025$). This suggested that sensitization against liver membrane antigens, either primary or secondary, may contribute to the progression of liver damage in CF.[22]

Shwachman[23] found a familial tendency to cirrhosis associated with CF; in the Boston series three families with a total of seven patients were affected, a familial incidence of 15%.[36] There is marked individual variation in the progression of the hepatic lesion in CF. This is especially true of infants who may recover completely from an episode of prolonged neonatal cholestasis or alternatively may succumb from the effects of cirrhosis within a few months. In the older child with hepatosplenomegaly, the liver involvement usually slowly progresses to cirrhosis and portal hypertension.

CLINICAL SYNDROMES

Neonatal Cholestasis

Cystic fibrosis is an important cause of prolonged obstructive jaundice in the neonatal period, and a sweat test is mandatory in the work-up of these infants in order to prevent unnecessary laparotomy. Although neonatal cholestasis caused by CF is considered rare (in Mowat's[24] experience CF accounted for only 2 of 126 infants referred with this problem), Table 18-2 summarizes 23 reported CF infants with this clinical presentation.[24-32] Roy[26] found that 5 of 24 newly diagnosed CF patients had obstructive jaundice and meconium ileus, while four others were malnourished with hepatomegaly, variable degrees of steatosis, and transient elevations of transaminases. We have seen three infants with meconium ileus and prolonged cholestatic jaundice (average duration 4 months) in the last four years. This apparently increasing incidence may be related either to improved diagnosis (every infant with intestinal obstruction in our institution now receives a sweat test) or to changes in therapy (intravenous hyperalimentation may cause cholestasis, especially after the first 14 days).

Fourteen (61%) of the 23 infants (Table 18-2) had meconium ileus associated with jaundice. Hepatosplenomegaly was usually present. The serum bilirubin was elevated up to 20 mg/dl and was predominantly direct-reacting. The transaminase levels were in the range of 200–300 international units (IU), and the alkaline phosphatase was between 25–48 King Armstrong units. The duration of jaundice varied from 1 to 9 months and was longer in those infants with meconium ileus. Two infants had documented cytomegalovirus infection. Nine (39%) of the infants died, but at autopsy cirrhosis was present in only one of these infants. In children who died later, liver histology showed mild changes consisting of mucus plugging, bile plugs, and fibrosis.

The management of these infants may be extremely difficult. The majority are severely malnourished, necessitating intravenous hyperalimentation which may further aggravate the cholestasis. We have observed a syndrome analogous to the "inspissated bile syndrome" with the bilirubin reaching up to 40 mg/dl. Many of these infants develop pulmonary complications which increase the nutritional deficits. Some authorities have advocated a direct approach by exploration and insertion of a T tube into the gallbladder or common bile duct with attempts made to flush out the "sticky" bile. One of the more important factors in outcome is the ability to correct the negative caloric balance. Despite the persistence of jaundice for up to 9 months, these infants can make an almost complete recovery (Figure 18-1). However, this complication of CF carries a high mortality (39%).

Hepatic Complications in the Older Patient

Fatty infiltration of the liver Fatty infiltration of the liver is a common finding at autopsy in CF patients, being present in 66% (131 of 198 patients).[4] When liver biopsies

Table 18-2
Relevant Clinical Details of Reported CF Infants with Obstructive Jaundice

Reference	Patients	Onset	Durations	Outcome	Meconium ileus	Autopsy liver	Biopsy liver	Associated findings
22	1							
	2							
23	1	Birth		1 wk.*	Yes			
24	1				Yes			
	2				Yes			
	3				Yes			
	4				Yes			
	5				Yes			
25	1	3 wk	4 mo	4 mo*	Yes	Cirrhosis		CMV†
	2	3 wk	5 mo	Recovered	—			
	3	1 mo	3 mo	8 yr*	Yes	Normal		
	4	1 wk	4 mo	Recovered	—			
26	1	1 wk		Recovered	—		Fibrosis	
27	1	Birth		3 days*	Yes	CMV inclusions		CMV
28	1	1 wk		20 days*	Yes	Bile plugs		
	2	6 mo		6 mo*	—	Fibrosis		
	3	9 mo		14 mo*	—	Fibrosis		
	4	2 mo		4 mo*	—	Fibrosis		
29	1	3 wk	1 mo	Recovered	—			
30	1		1 mo	Recovered	Yes		Bile stasis	
Personal series	1	1 wk	8 mo	Recovered	Yes		Fibrosis	
	2	1 wk	8 mo	Recovered	Yes		Fibrosis	
	3	1 wk	9 mo	6 mo*	Yes			
Totals	23	4 wk	4 mo	9*	14			

*Died.
†CMV = Cytomegalovirus.

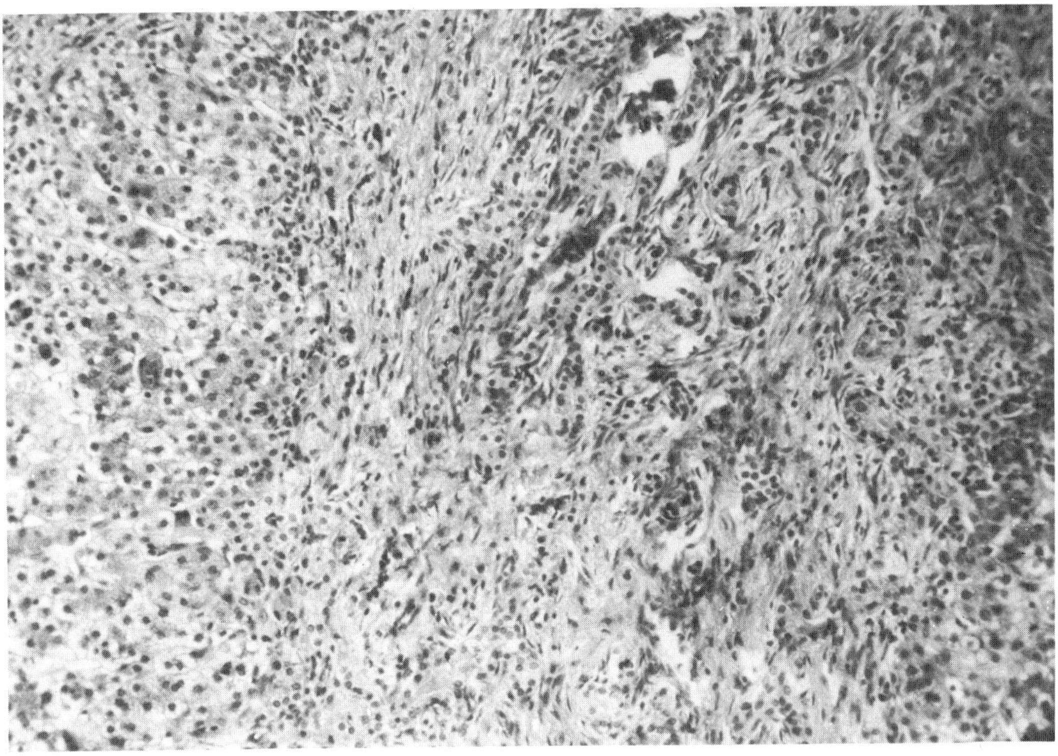

Figure 18-1 Liver biopsy on a 3-month-old infant with CF operated on for meconium ileus. His course was complicated by malnutrition and prolonged cholestasis. Liver function showed bilirubin total 8.5 mg/dl, direct 5.0 mg/dl, SGOT 189 IU/liter, SGPT 232 IU/liter, alkaline phosphatase 75 Bodansky units. He made a complete recovery, and at 5 years of age his weight and height are at the 25th percentile, with normal liver function. The biopsy (hematoxylin-eosin, magnification × 250) shows extensive focal biliary fibrosis between normal hepatocytes. Note the eosinophilic granular secretions. Bile duct proliferation is present.

were performed during life, fatty changes were found in 30% (15 of 50 patients).[6] Fatty infiltration of the liver is a characteristic feature of protein–calorie malnutrition (kwashiorkor) which is frequently present in infants newly diagnosed with CF. The follow-up of surviving cases of severe kwashiorkor has failed to demonstrate cirrhosis.[33] Apart from alcoholic liver disease, macrovesicular fatty infiltration of the liver is usually considered a harmless manifestation of disturbed lipid metabolism and of little importance. The clinical significance of fatty liver in CF is unknown; rare cases have been reported which presented with massive hepatomegaly, edema, hypoalbuminemia, and fatty infiltration.[34]

Cirrhosis This presentation is one of the more common hepatic complications of CF, with an incidence of focal biliary cirrhosis of 9–19%,[4,5] whereas multilobular cirrhosis was found in 2.4%.[5] Fifteen (2.2%) of 693 patients with CF seen over an 18-year period developed clinical hepatic disease,[1] and in 13 of these patients all symptoms were secondary to portal hypertension. Liver biopsies were performed in eight of these patients, and all showed evidence of biliary cirrhosis. di Sant'Agnese and Davis[2] reviewed the literature and quoted an incidence of cirrhosis of 5% in 221 adolescents and adults with CF. Thus, it seems likely that cirrhosis will become an increasing problem as the life expectancy for patients with CF improves.

The early stages of development of cirrhosis in CF are usually asymptomatic, and this complication is suspected when abdominal examination reveals hepatomegaly or splenomegaly. The liver is usually hard and nodular (Figures 18-2–18-6). Other signs of portal hypertension, including a prominent collateral venous pattern, abdominal distention, and ascites, appear later. The degree of pulmonary involvement is variable. Gradually the liver diminishes in size while the spleen becomes enlarged, resulting in signs of hypersplenism with granulocytopenia, anemia, and thrombocytopenia. Progressive evidence of liver decompensation with lowered albumin, hypoprothrombinemia, ascites, jaundice, and hepatic failure may ensue. In other patients the first sign of hepatic involvement may be bleeding from esophageal varices. In the pediatric age group CF accounts for one third of patients with cirrhosis from all causes and for 50% of children with symptoms of portal hypertension.[35] It is mandatory to perform a sweat test in all children presenting with portal hypertension of unknown cause.

Portal hypertension The largest series of CF patients with portal hypertension (48 in a total clinic population of 2500) was reported by Schuster et al.[36] Unfortunately, documentation of liver pathology was not given, but one can assume from the data of Stern et al[1] that these patients probably had evidence of biliary cirrhosis. The management of portal hypertension in CF is controversial. Contraindications to shunting procedures include extensive pulmonary involvement or hepatic decompensation. It is difficult to assign a specific figure to pulmonary contraindications, but the results in patients with a clinical score[37] of less than 60 were very poor.[36]

Portosystemic shunting procedures are effective in reducing the risk of esophageal bleeding. Schuster et al[36] state that a shunting procedure should be performed prior to respiratory deterioration because of the progressive nature of the pulmonary disease. The major argument against shunting procedures in cirrhosis is the high incidence of postshunt hepatic encephalopathy. Advocates of shunting procedures in CF claim that hepatic encephalopathy does not occur if the patients are correctly selected (ie, good

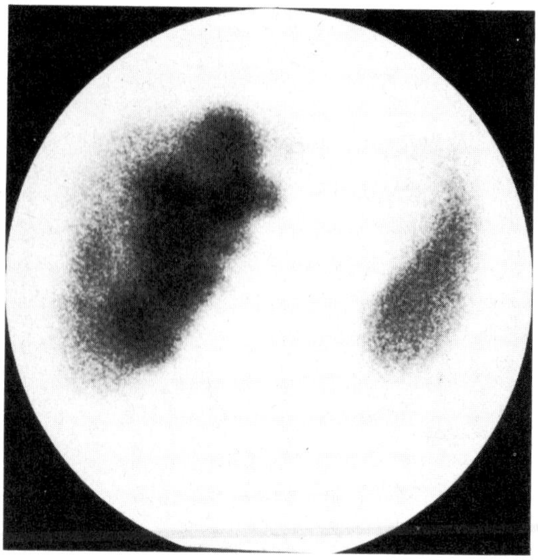

Figure 18-2 Technetium pertechnate scan on an 11-year-old CF patient with hepatosplenomegaly. The isotope in the liver is unevenly distributed, corresponding to the macronodular cirrhosis. The spleen is markedly enlarged. Liver function shows normal bilirubin, SGOT 56 IU/liter, SGPT 85 IU/liter, alkaline phosphatase 56 Bodansky units. Esophageal varices were present. She had one hemetemesis secondary to aspirin gastritis treated conservatively. Three years later she developed uncontrollable hemetemesis requiring over 16 units of blood and underwent a successful splenorenal shunt with preservation of the spleen. Pulmonary function is 75% of predicted.

pulmonary status and no evidence of hepatic decompensation). The limited data on the seven patients shunted and reported by Stern et al[1] support this statement, but the larger series of Schuster et al[36] does not, in that 25% (9 of 36 patients) died from postoperative complications shortly after the shunting procedure. Isolated case reports confirm that hepatic encephalopathy can occur following shunt surgery in CF.[38] Schuster et al[36] have argued that such patients were operated on too late as an emergency procedure, and should have had a prophylactic shunt performed earlier.

Several other factors further complicate this problem. First, some children with portal hypertension can spontaneously develop their own shunts.[36,39] Second, hematemesis may arise from gastric erosions secondary to

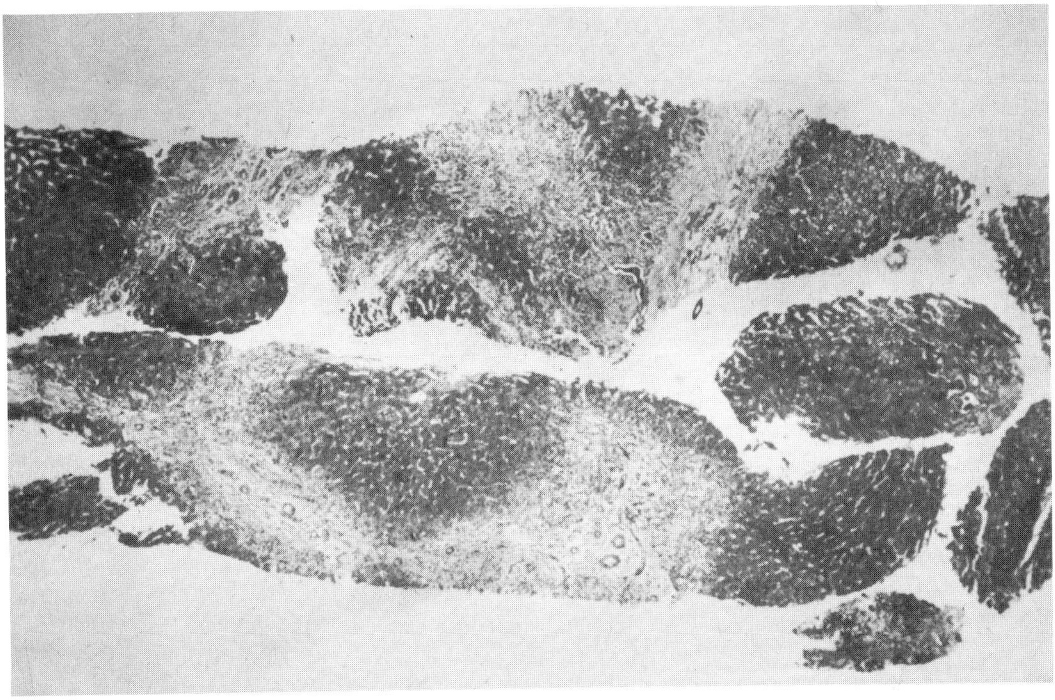

Figure 18-3 Liver biopsy (hematoxylin-eosin, magnification × 40) on the same patient. Note the fragmentation caused by the extensive fibrosis. Nodules characteristic of cirrhosis are present.

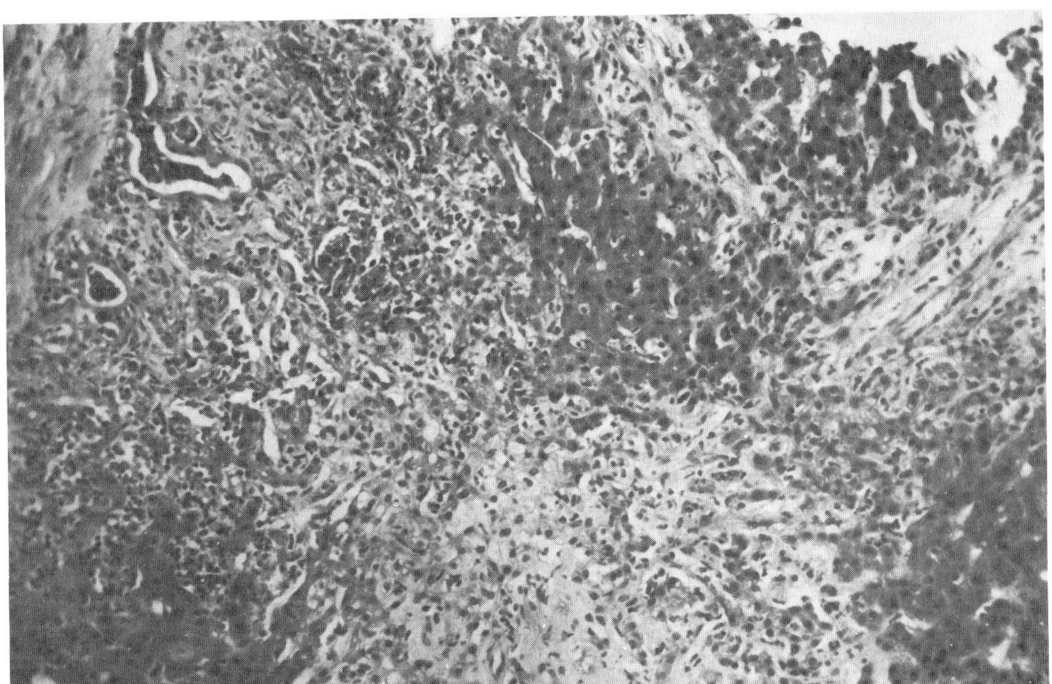

Figure 18-4 Hematoxylin-eosin, magnification × 250 of the same biopsy. Marked fibrous infiltrate is present, and eosinophilic granular secretions are visible.

aspirin rather than from bleeding esophageal varices. Thus, it is essential to perform endoscopy to confirm the diagnosis, and all these patients should be advised to avoid salicylates. Last, the natural history of portal hypertension in CF is unclear. Most will ultimately die from progressive pulmonary involvement, and it is uncertain whether esophageal bleeding will hasten demise. Limited data[36] and personal communication have revealed a number of CF patients with portal hypertension who have survived up to 10 years following a variceal bleed without hepatic decompensation.

How then can we sort out this dilemma? Mowat[24] has agreed with the criteria of Schuster et al[36] and recommends surgery in patients with demonstrable varices, portal pressure greater than 27 cm of water, and adequate pulmonary status, providing that the alimentary bleeding was not provoked by aspirin. If hypersplenism is present, splenectomy should be combined with portal decompression. We suggest another criterion, and do not recommend surgery until the patient has had at least one significant bleeding episode (sufficient to drop the hematocrit at least 5% and/or to require transfusion). Further data on long-term follow-up of these patients may help to clarify the indications for surgery.

The work-up of these patients is described in detail in textbooks of pediatric liver disease[24,39] and may include hematological evaluation including clotting factors, endoscopy, barium esophagram, splenic venography, superior mesenteric arteriography and ultrasonography.

Once having decided to recommend surgery, there is controversy concerning preoperative care and the specific shunt procedure to be utilized. In Boston, all patients have an elective tracheostomy performed 5–7 days prior to the definitive procedure to prevent postoperative pulmonary complications. However, Stern et al[1] have not found tracheostomy necessary. The type of shunt seems to make little difference as long as the accepted criteria of vessel size and accessibility are followed.[36] Since hypersplenism is almost always present, splenectomy has been performed routinely with a splenorenal shunt and, in most instances, with a portocaval shunt. Other surgeons perform a splenorenal shunt by a posterior approach below the transverse colon and thus retain the spleen. If the portal pressure is reduced, the spleen shrinks, and other evidence of hypersplenism returns to normal. The portocaval shunt may be technically difficult because of a characteristic retroperitoneal fibrosis which is sometimes present in CF patients. Postsplenectomy sepsis was not documented in the Boston series, but this is a potential problem[40] and pneumococcal vaccine and continuous penicillin prophylaxis should be administered.

The impressive results with shunt surgery reported by Stern et al[1] are probably related to a highly selected patient group with excellent liver function and pulmonary status (87–100% of predicted normal values). Unfortunately, data on liver function were not given by Schuster et al,[36] and it may be that their high mortality (9 early deaths and 11 late deaths following surgery in 36 patients) was related to less selective criteria.

Hypersplenism This complication of CF is usually associated with portal hypertension, and the previous discussion noted that most surgeons removed the spleen at the time of a shunt procedure. These patients may have symptomatic thrombocytopenia, anemia, and granulocytopenia. Postoperatively the platelet count may rise to values greater than 800,000/mm^3, a concentration associated with an increased risk of thrombosis in major blood vessels. Schuster et al[36] have argued that it is better to perform one definitive procedure in order to avoid the complication of deteriorating pulmonary status. Stern et al[1] reported seven patients with hypersplenism without variceal bleeding. One underwent a shunt procedure and is alive 3 years later. One of the other six patients died. Generally, the associated symptoms with the portal hypertension will determine the timing of surgery.

Gallstones, cholangitis and obstructive jaundice Abnormality of the contents and/

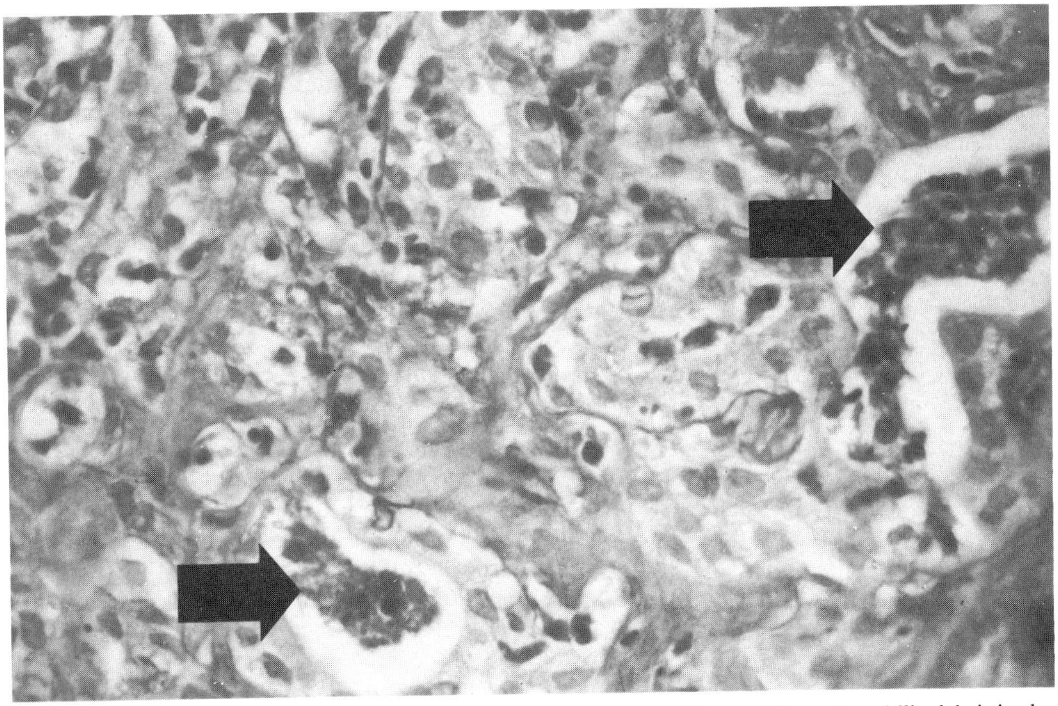

Figure 18-5 Hematoxylin-eosin, magnification × 350 of the same biopsy. The eosinophilic debris in the bile canaliculi is shown by the arrows. Note the irregular appearance of the hepatocytes.

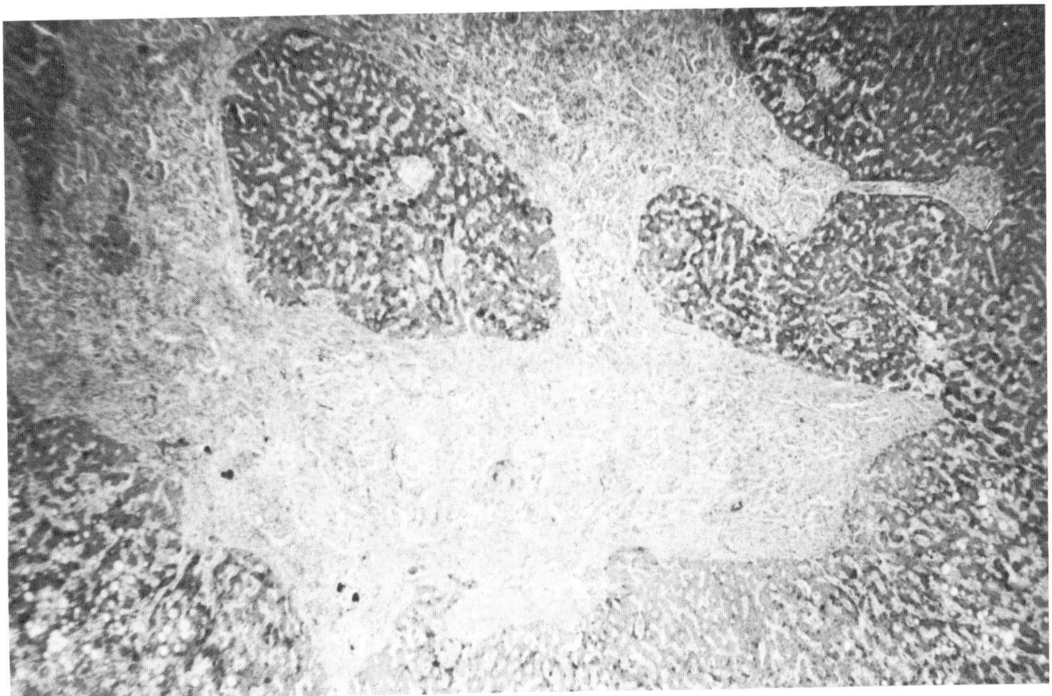

Figure 18-6 Liver at autopsy (trichrome, magnification × 250) on a 16-year-old CF patient showing a far advanced cirrhotic nodule surrounded by extensive fibrous tissue. The surrounding hepatocytes are normal. Slight fatty infiltration is present in the right upper quadrant. No symptoms were present during life referable to her liver disease.

or the mucosa of the gallbladder (Figure 18-7) were noted in 33% (24 of 72) autopsied cases of CF.[41] The lesions consisted of mucoid material in the lumen (white bile) and numerous multiloculated mucus-containing cysts in the epithelium and submucosa. These lesions were not associated with age, focal biliary cirrhosis, or meconium ileus. Isenberg et al[42] performed oral cholecystograms on 66 patients with CF. Thirty (45%) were judged abnormal (22 nonvisualized, 4 microgallbladder, 1 structural abnormality, and 3 with calculi). Intravenous cholangiograms were performed in the 22 nonvisualized gallbladders; a further 6 were considered normal while abnormalities included 8 nonvisualizing, 5 microgallbladder, 2 structural abnormalities, and 1 calculi.

The authors speculated that these results might be related to poor absorption of the lipophilic oral contrast material. They stressed that nonopacification of the gallbladder was not an indication for surgery in CF patients and found no association between abdominal pain and gallbladder abnormalities. Irregularities of the gallbladder outline were

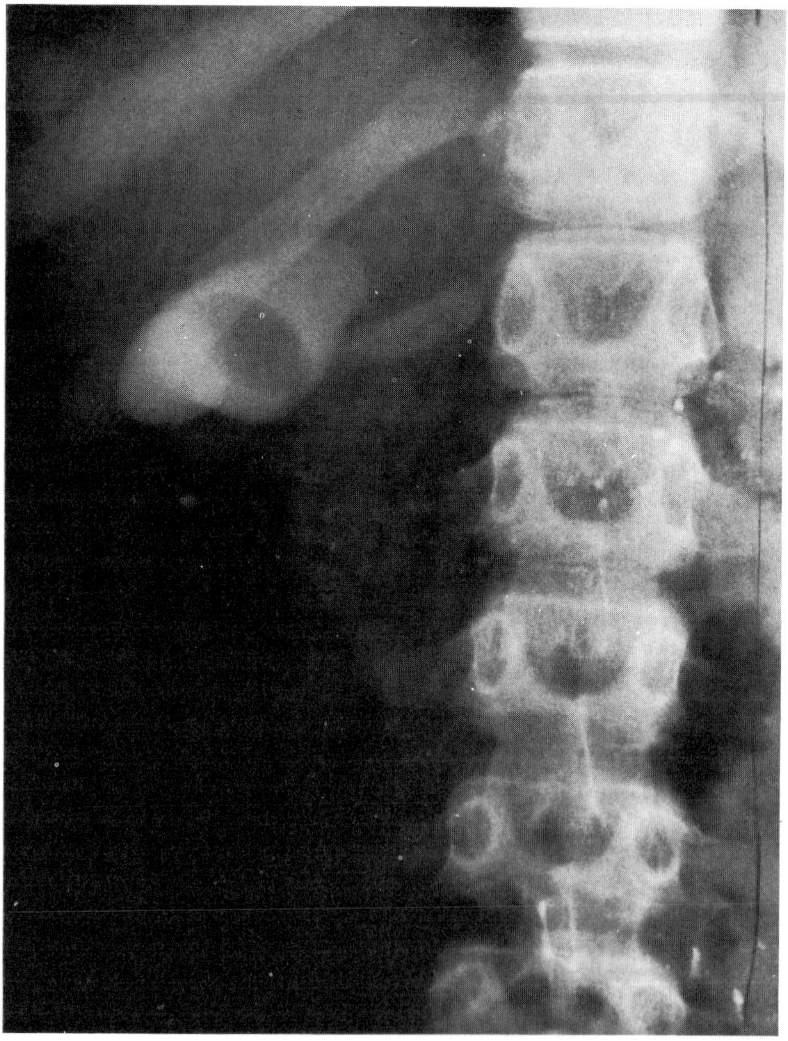

Figure 18-7 12-year-old female. A single nonopaque calculus is identified within the contrast-filled gallbladder. Multiple small densities within the abdomen are the undissolved portions of the tablets given to produced gallbladder opacification. (Courtesy of Dr. Sandra Fernbach.)

considered to be due to submucosal cysts as shown at autopsy.[41] Similar findings from France[43] and Denmark[18] showed abnormal gallbladders in over 40% of patients. Isenberg et al[42] noted no correlation between external biliary tree abnormalities and multifocal biliary cirrhosis which was present in 40% of their patients. These findings are surprising as one might expect that the potential for bile stasis would increase the risk of cholangitis and play a role in producing cirrhosis.

Warwick et al[44] studied the association of gallstones in CF and found calculi present in 8.6% of patients (6 of 70) investigated by oral and intravenous cholangiography. Two patients had symptoms of cholecystitis. They found that the incidence of gallbladder abnormalities increased with age, and speculated that their treatment program with drugs known to cause cholestasis (sulfonamides, anabolic steroids, and oral contraceptives) may have contributed to their high incidence of abnormalities.

Ultrasound of the hepatobiliary tract[45] demonstrated calculi in 5% (2 of 37 CF patients); 47% less than 10 years and 37% over 10 years had microgallbladders, and hepatic fibrosis was present in 76%. Recently, intrapancreatic bile duct compression causing obstructive jaundice in a 29-year-old patient with CF was reported.[46] It seems likely that as survival improves, an increasing number of older CF patients with complications secondary to gallbladder abnormalities, calculi, and cholecystitis will be encountered.

LABORATORY ABNORMALITIES

Abnormal liver function tests in CF are common (Table 18-3), but pathologic correlations with these abnormalities have only been reported by three groups.[6,42,44] Isenberg et al[42] noted that only 65% (13 of 20) biopsy-proven patients with multifocal biliary cirrhosis had elevations of serum gammaglutamyl transpeptidase (γGT). Similar poor correlations between clinical, biochemical, and biopsy findings were noted by Dietzsch et al.[6] Therefore, caution is necessary before assuming a direct correlation between the serum abnormalities and liver pathology.

Kattwinkel et al[8] examined sera from 91 normal individuals (ages 4–30 years) and 49 patients with CF (ages 3–41 years) for total alkaline phosphatase and its isoenzymes, transaminases, 5-nucleotidase, and γGT. They found that in normal children levels of SGOT, γGT, total alkaline phosphatase, and its bone isoenzyme are age dependent, whereas SGPT, 5-nucleotidase, and intestinal and liver fractions of alkaline phosphatase are independent of age up to 30 years. One third of CF patients had biochemical evidence of hepatobiliary disease before clinical signs were evident, and γGT,

Table 18-3
Incidence of Reported Abnormalities Related to the Liver in Cystic Fibrosis

Investigation	Incidence (%)	Reference
Gammaglutamyltranspeptidase	29–40	8, 42
Liver alkaline phosphatase	38–50	8, 9
Serum glutamic-oxaloacetic transaminase (SGOT)	38	8
Serum glutamic-pyruvic transaminase (SGPT)	30	8
5-Nucleotidase	12	8
Sulfobromophthalein (BSP)	26	43
Serum bile acids ↑	21–33	10
Fecal bile acids ↑	88	48
Duodenal bile acids ↓	61	53
Liver biopsies	18–40	6, 42
Liver scans	78–88	11, 54
Ultrasound gallbladder/liver	84	45
Cholecystogram and cholangiogram	43–45	42, 43

the transaminases, and the hepatic isoenzyme of alkaline phosphatase were the most reliable indicators of this complication. Specifically, of 40 CF patients investigated the following were abnormally elevated: γGT (40%), liver alkaline phosphatase (38%), SGOT (38%), SGPT (30%), and 5-nucleotidase (12%).

Similar findings were reported by Boat et al,[9] who found the total alkaline phosphatase was elevated in nearly 25% of all hospitalized patients with CF and that this figure rose to 50% for patients 16 years and older. Several identifiable causes of high liver alkaline phosphatase levels in CF patients include chronic hepatic congestion, drug hepatotoxicity, overt biliary cirrhosis, and, most commonly, subclinical focal biliary cirrhosis. Isenberg et al[42] noted elevations of γGT in 29% (19 of 66 patients). Bilirubin levels were in the normal range,[8] except in the rare patient with neonatal cholestasis or other obstructive or viral hepatitis syndromes.

Bromsulfophthalein (BSP) Kinetics

Grand et al[47] performed BSP kinetic studies in CF and made the following observations:

1. In normal children or in CF children with normal livers, BSP kinetics are described by a single exponential curve with hepatic removal significantly higher than in normal adults.
2. Minimal hepatic disease in children with CF may be detected by analysis of BSP kinetics which show a biexponential phase disappearance curve.
3. All children with CF and cirrhosis demonstrated significant impairment in biliary secretory function and increased hepatic to plasma reflux which differentiated them from other patients with cirrhosis.
4. The lower hepatic to plasma reflux after portosystemic shunting may reflect improved sinusoidal flow.
5. Compartmental analysis of BSP kinetics has significant predictive value for the presence and progression of liver disease in CF, but does not identify a primary characteristic transport defect.

Further documentation of these abnormalities is unlikely as BSP administration is no longer approved by the Food and Drug Administration in the United States.

Bile Acids

A number of abnormalities have been reported in bile salt kinetics, fecal bile acids, duodenal, and serum bile acids in CF.

Bile salt kinetics Watkins et al[16] investigated bile acid kinetics by stable isotope techniques in six untreated CF patients (ages 3½ months to 4½ years). Before administration of pancreatic enzyme replacement, fat excretion equaled 50 ± 4% of intake and was reduced to 20 ± 10% of intake after therapy. Total bile acid pool size nearly doubled during enzyme replacement from 379 ± 32 μmol/kg to 620 ± 36 μmol/kg. Total bile acid synthesis changed little with therapy.

These data indicate that both primary and secondary bile acids are conserved within the enterohepatic circulation during enzyme therapy and that the mechanism for the regulation of bile acid synthesis is intact in CF. Watkins et al[16] found that large amounts of bile acids continued to be excreted in the feces during therapy and suggested that interruption of the enterohepatic circulation continues and deficiencies of the intraluminal phase may persist during enzyme therapy. They postulated that the excess bile acid loss in CF might be binding within the intraluminal phase, either to unhydrolyzed lipid or to maldigested protein or carbohydrate.

Fecal bile acids Weber et al[14] found that quantitative fecal bile acids (mg/24 hr/m^2 of body surface area) in 24 children with untreated pancreatic insufficiency secondary to CF were increased (743.2 ± 53.3) compared to 18 controls (110 ± 11.0). Bile acid loss in CF was comparable to that of six infants after ileal resection (957.7 ± 195.1). In six CF children without pancreatic disease the bile acid loss was 133.4 ± 15.9 and did not differ from controls.[48]

Goodchild et al[15] confirmed these findings but found no correlation between fecal bile acid and fecal fat excretion. They noted an inverse relation between fecal bile acid values and age. Those patients with overt liver disease tended to have the lowest fecal bile acid values. Roller and Kern[49] found a much lower excretion of fecal bile acids and normal [^{14}C]cholylglycine breath tests in their CF patients (age range 11–24 years, mean 18 years) and considered bile acid malabsorption to be of minimal clinical significance. The discrepancy between these findings and others[14,16] are probably explained by the older age of the patients.

Roy et al[50] studied fecal fat, bile acid, and rectal microflora in 7 control children and in three groups of CF children: 7 off antibiotics, 10 on oral cloxacillin, and 6 on intravenous cloxacillin, gentamicin, and carbenicillin for at least two weeks. Antibiotics had little or no effect on fat excretion, but led to a significant decrease ($P < 0.01$) of fecal bile acid on the triple antibiotic therapy. Reduced deconjugation of bile acids and formation of secondary bile acids was associated with a marked reduction of the anaerobic flora in the children on triple therapy compared to controls. They suggested that the reduction of the anaerobic flora by antibiotics decreases the adsorption of bile acids to dietary residues and microbes and favors bile acid absorption, thus leading to decreased fecal loss of bile acids in CF.

Serum bile acids Lloyd-Still and Demers[10] measured the concentrations of four fasting serum bile acids by radioimmunoassay in 42 CF patients ranging in age from 1 month to 16 years. The concentrations of cholylglycine (0.96 ± 2.25 μmol/liter, N = 0.15 ± 0.08) and chenodeoxycholylglycine (0.93 ± 1.15 μmol/liter, N = 0.13 ± 0.14) were slightly above normal. Increased concentrations of bile acids were detected in 6/39 with cholylglycine, 13/39 with chenodeoxycholylglycine, and 4/19 with sulfolithocholylglycine. Similar findings were found in infants with prolonged cholestasis and CF. Goodchild et al[15] reported that 3 of 6 children with CF had elevated serum bile acids; 2 of the 3 with raised serum bile acid levels had evidence of hepatic disease.

When the levels of serum cholylglycine were studied in response to a meal in 8 CF patients[51] not receiving pancreatic supplementation, the mean increase in serum cholylglycine concentration was significantly smaller ($P < 0.01$) than in controls. However, when these same patients were studied during the administration of pancreatic supplements, the response approximated that seen in normal adults. Balistreri et al[51] interpreted these findings as indicating intact ileal transport processes in CF, thus adding support to the hypothesis that intraluminal factors are responsible for the increased fecal bile acid loss in CF. Addition of cimetidine to pancreatic enzymes significantly decreased the postprandial serum bile acid concentration compared to the response seen with enzymes alone.[52] The authors were unable to interpret whether decreased gallbladder contractility, decreased intestinal transit, or increased hepatic extraction of bile acids from portal blood was responsible for these abnormalities.

BILIARY ABNORMALITIES

Bile Salts

Harries et al[53] found that the total bile salt concentration, glycine–taurine conjugate ratios, and percentage of dihydroxy bile acids in 13 patients with CF and pancreatic insufficiency of pancreatic enzymes were 3.5 (1.3–6.6) mmol/liter, 8.6 (10–3.1), and 37 (10–60) compared with control values of 7.4 (3.0–16.0) mmol/liter, 3.0 (1.3–4.5), and 61 (52–70), respectively. The differences between the control and CF values were statistically significant ($P < 0.01$–$P < 0.001$). In two patients with normal pancreatic function, duodenal bile salts were both quantitatively and qualitatively normal.

They interpreted these results as consistent with an interrupted enterohepatic circulation. However, they failed to find evidence that unhydrolyzed dietary substrates play a role in the interrupted enterohepatic circulation. They hypothesized that there may be a defect in the primary mucosal phase of bile salt absorption similar to that found with amino acids in CF. Other possibilities include a progressive reduction in the bile salt pool secondary to inadequate compensatory synthesis of bile salts by the liver. Alternatively, more proximal regions of the small intestine may develop the mucosal capacity to absorb bile salts.

Biliary Lipid Composition

Roy et al[17] compared biliary lipid composition in 26 patients with CF, 7 children with cholelithiasis without CF, and 13 controls. In 14 patients with CF who had stopped taking pancreatic enzymes for one week, molar percentage of lipid concentration accounted for by cholesterol (16.3 ± 2.9) and saturation index (2.0 ± 0.3) were comparable to values of the cholelithiasis group and higher ($P < 0.01$) than the controls. In 12 patients with CF receiving pancreatic enzymes, the molar percentage of cholesterol (8.6 ± 1.7) and the saturation index (1.0 ± 0.1) did not differ from controls. In CF there was a preponderance of cholic over chenodeoxycholic, both off (1.7 ± 0.2) and on (1.9 ± 0.3) therapy, as compared to the cholelithiasis (0.7 ± 0.1) and control (0.8 ± 0.0) groups. The glycine–taurine ratio of conjugated bile acids was lower in enzyme-treated patients with CF (3.7 ± 0.0) than in patients off treatment (6.4 ± 1.0), but was higher ($P < 0.01$) than in controls (1.8 ± 0.2). They concluded that bile is lithogenic in untreated CF and responds to pancreatic enzymes. The high molar percentage of cholesterol provides a physicochemical explanation for the increased incidence of gallstones in CF.

Liver Scans

Colloidal indium and technetium pertechnetate injected intravenously are taken up by the reticuloendothelial cells of the liver. Distortion of hepatic architecture by fibrosis leads to impairment of hepatic uptake, and with portal hypertension there is an increased uptake by the spleen and bone marrow. Feigelson et al[54] reported 22 abnormal scans among 25 CF patients. Goodchild et al[11] confirmed this finding with 13 of 16 scans being abnormal. Nine of the 13 CF patients with abnormal scans had no convincing evidence of hepatic abnormality on clinical examination or serological tests. No correlation was noted between the degree of abnormality on scan, age of the patient, or their clinical score. They concluded that liver scanning in CF is unlikely to make a significant contribution to an assessment of prognosis.

SUMMARY

Serious complications from liver involvement in CF occur in a small minority (2%) of patients. These patients may become candidates for a variety of shunt operations to relieve the portal hypertension which is secondary to the biliary cirrhosis. These procedures need to be performed before there is significant deterioration of pulmonary function. It is unlikely that surgery will prolong life, as prognosis is usually dependent on the severity of pulmonary disease. In some patients the liver disease predominates and will result in liver failure.

At least one third of CF patients develop evidence of liver involvement as evidenced by abnormal biochemical indices, changes on liver biopsy, or abnormal liver scans. The significance of these abnormal findings in terms of survival, nutrition, and general well-being is poorly understood. The changes in the liver pathology are thought to result from a similar process to that occurring in other organs, such as the lungs and pancreas, and the bile in CF is known to be abnormal in both constituents and flow rate.

The abnormal bile constituents have been documented to result in the formation of lithogenic bile, calculi, cholecystitis, submucus cysts of the gallbladder, and obstructive jaundice. The incidence of these abnormalities increases with the age of the patients. Thus, as survival for CF patients improves, the incidence of hepatic involvement will likely increase.

REFERENCES

1. Stern RC, Stevens DP, Boat TF, et al: Symptomatic hepatic disease in cystic fibrosis: Incidence, course, and outcome of portal systemic shunting. *Gastroenterology* 1976;70:645-649.
2. di Sant'Agnese PA, Davis PB: Cystic fibrosis in adults: 75 cases and a review of 232 cases in the literature. *Am J Med* 1979;66:121-132.
3. Shwachman H, Kowalski M, Khaw KT: Cystic fibrosis: A new outlook. 70 patients above 25 years of age. *Medicine* 1977;56:129-149.
4. Craig JM, Haddad H, Shwachman H: The pathological changes in the liver in cystic fibrosis of the pancreas. *Am J Dis Child* 1957; 93:357-369.
5. Oppenheimer EH, Esterly JR: Pathology of cystic fibrosis. Review of the literature and comparison with 146 autopsied cases. *Perspect Pediatr Pathol* 1975;2:241-278.
6. Dietzsch HJ, Gottschalk B, Hinkel GK, et al: The value of bioptic follow-up examinations for controlling the course of liver involvement in cystic fibrosis. In *Proceedings Eighth International Congress Cystic Fibrosis* Toronto, Canadian Cystic Fibrosis Foundation, 1980, p 220.
7. Sharp HL, Warwick WJ: Hepatic function and structure in cystic fibrosis. *Cystic Fibrosis Club Abstr* 1968;9:4-5.
8. Kattwinkel J, Taussig LM, Statland BE, et al: The effects of age on alkaline phosphatase and other serologic liver function tests in normal subjects and patients with cystic fibrosis. *J Pediatr* 1973;82:234-242.
9. Boat TF, Doershuk CF, Stern RC, et al: Serum alkaline phosphatase in cystic fibrosis. *Clin Pediatr* 1974;13:505-512.
10. Lloyd-Still JD, Demers LM: Serum glycine-conjugated bile acids in pediatric hepatobiliary disorders. *Am J Clin Pathol* 1979; 71:444-451.
11. Goodchild MC, Banks AJ, Drolc Z, et al: Liver scans in cystic fibrosis. *Arch Dis Child* 1975;50:813-815.
12. Bodian M: *Fibrocystic Disease of the Pancreas. A Congenital Disorder of Mucus Production—Mucosis.* London, William Heinemann, 1952.
13. Oppenheimer EH, Esterly JR: Hepatic changes in young infants with cystic fibrosis: Possible relation to focal biliary cirrhosis. *Pediatrics* 1975;86:683-689.
14. Weber AM, Roy CC, Morin CL, et al: Malabsorption of bile acids in children with cystic fibrosis. *N Engl J Med* 1973;289:1001-1005.
15. Goodchild MC, Murphy GM, Howell AM, et al: Aspects of bile acid metabolism in cystic fibrosis. *Arch Dis Child* 1975;50:769-778.
16. Watkins JB, Tercyak AM, Szczepanik P, et al: Bile salt kinetics in cystic fibrosis: Influence of pancreatic enzyme replacement. *Gastroenterology* 1977;73:1023-1028.
17. Roy CC, Weber AM, Morin CL, et al: Abnormal biliary lipid composition in cystic fibrosis. *N Engl J Med* 1977;297:1301-1305.
18. Rovsing H, Sloth K: Microgallbladder and biliary calculi in mucoviscidosis. *Acta Radiol* 1973;14:588-592.
19. Vaughan WJ, Lindgren FT, Whalen JB, et al: Serum lipoprotein concentrations in cystic fibrosis. *Science* 1978;199:783-786.
20. MacDonald I, Hansen JDL, Bronte-Stewart B: Liver depot and serum lipids during early recovery from kwashiorkor. *Clin Sci* 1963; 24:55-61.
21. Hubbard VS, Dunn GD, di Sant'Agnese PA: Abnormal fatty-acid composition of plasma-lipids in cystic fibrosis: A primary or a secondary defect? *Lancet* 1977;2:1302-1304.
22. Mieli-Vergani G, Psacharopoulos HT, Nicholson AM, et al: Immune responses to liver membrane antigens in patients with cystic fibrosis and liver disease. *Arch Dis Child* 1980;55:696-701.
23. Shwachman H: Gastrointestinal manifestations of cystic fibrosis. *Pediatr Clin North Am* 1975;22:787-805.
24. Mowat A: Hepato-biliary lesions in cystic fibrosis, in Mowat A (ed): *Liver Disorders in Childhood.* London, Butterworths, 1979, pp 269-279.
25. Schwarz HP, Kraemer R, Thurnheer U, et al: Liver involvement in cystic fibrosis. *Helv Paediatr Acta* 1978;33:351-364.
26. Roy CC: Gastrointestinal and hepatobiliary complications: Changing pattern with age. In *Proceedings Eighth International Congress Cystic Fibrosis.* Toronto, Canadian Cystic Fibrosis Foundation, 1980, p 190.
27. Valman HB, France NE, Wallis PG: Prolonged neonatal jaundice in cystic fibrosis. *Arch Dis Child* 1971;46:805-809.
28. Rosenstein BJ, Oppenheimer EH: Prolonged

obstructive jaundice and giant cell hepatitis in an infant with cystic fibrosis. *J Pediatr* 1977;91:1022–1023.

29. Oppenheimer EH, Esterly JR: Congenital cytomegalovirus infection and bileduct obstruction in newborn infant with cystic fibrosis of pancreas. *Lancet* 1973;2:1031–1032.
30. Gatzimos CD, Jowitt RH: Jaundice in mucoviscidosis (fibrocystic disease of pancreas). *Am J Dis Child* 1955;89:182–186.
31. Taylor WF, Qaqundah BY: Neonatal jaundice associated with cystic fibrosis. *Am J Dis Child* 1972;123:161–162.
32. Talamo RC, Hendren WH: Prolonged obstructive jaundice. Report of a case in a neonate with meconium ileus and jejunal atresia. *Am J Dis Child* 1968;115:74–79.
33. Thaler H: Relation of steatosis to cirrhosis. *Clin Gastroenterol* 1975;4:273–280.
34. Wilroy RS, Crawford SE, Johnson WW: Cystic fibrosis with extensive fat replacement of the liver. *J Pediatr* 1966;68:67–73.
35. di Sant'Agnese PA, Blanc WA: A distinctive type of biliary cirrhosis of the liver associated with cystic fibrosis of the pancreas. *J Pediatr* 1956;18:387–409.
36. Schuster SR, Shwachman H, Toyama WM, et al: The management of portal hypertension in cystic fibrosis. *J Pediatr Surg* 1977;12: 201–206.
37. Shwachman H, Kulczycki LL: Long term study of one hundred and five patients with cystic fibrosis: Studies made over a five to fourteen year period. *Am J Dis Child* 1958; 96:6–15.
38. Case report. Clinico-pathological conference. *N Engl J Med* 1979;300:420–427.
39. Alagille D, Odievre M: Portal hypertension, in Alagille D, Odievre M (eds): *Liver and Biliary Tract Disease in Children*. New York, John Wiley, 1979, pp 262–295.
40. Balfanz JR, Nesbit ME, Jarvis C, et al: Overwhelming sepsis following splenectomy for trauma. *J Pediatr* 1976;88:459–460.
41. Esterly JR, Oppenheimer EH: Observations in cystic fibrosis of the pancreas. I. The gallbladder. *Bull Johns Hopkins Hosp*. 1962; 110:247–255.
42. Isenberg JN, L'Heureux PR, Warwick WJ, et al: Clinical observations on the biliary system in cystic fibrosis. *Am J Gastroenterol* 1976;65:134–141.
43. Feigelson J, Pecau Y, Sauvegrain J: Liver function studies and biliary tract investigations in mucoviscidosis. *Acta Pediatr Scand* 1970;59:539–544.
44. Warwick WJ, L'Heureux PR, Sharp HL, et al: Gallstones and cystic fibrosis, In *Proceedings Seventh International Congress Cystic Fibrosis*. Paris, Jouve, 1976, p 484.
45. Fenstersheib MD, Werlin SL, Bruns WT, et al: Ultrasound evaluation of the hepatobiliary tract in cystic fibrosis. *Pediatr Res* 1979; 13:398.
46. Lambert JR, Cole M, Crozier DN, et al: Intrapancreatic common bile duct compression causing jaundice in an adult with cystic fibrosis. *Gastroenterology* 1981;80:169–172.
47. Grand RJ, Lebenthal E, Jacobson M, et al: Predictive value of BSP kinetics for early liver involvement in cystic fibrosis. In *Proceedings Seventh International Congress Cystic Fibrosis*. Paris, Jouve, 1976, p 463.
48. Weber AM, Roy CC, Chartrand L, et al: Relationship between bile acid malabsorption and pancreatic insufficiency in cystic fibrosis. *Gut* 1976;17:295–299.
49. Roller RJ, Kern F: Minimal bile acid malabsorption and normal bile acid breath tests in cystic fibrosis and acquired pancreatic insufficiency. *Gastroenterology* 1977;72:661–665.
50. Roy CC, Delage G, Fontaine A, et al: The fecal microflora and bile acids in children with cystic fibrosis. *Am J Clin Nutr* 1979;32: 2404–2409.
51. Balistreri WF, Suchy FJ, Heubi JE: Serum bile acid response to a test meal stimulus: A sensitive test of ileal function. *J Pediatr* 1980; 96:582–589.
52. Boyle BJ, Long WB, Balistreri WF, et al: Effect of cimetidine and pancreatic enzymes on serum and fecal bile acids and fat absorption in cystic fibrosis. *Gastroenterology* 1980;78: 950–953.
53. Harries JT, Muller DPR, McCollum JPK, et al: Intestinal bile salts in cystic fibrosis. *Arch Dis Child* 1979;54:19–24.
54. Feigelson J, Pecau Y, Perez R: Liver scanning and liver function in cystic fibrosis. *Acta Paediatr Scand* 1972;61:337–342.

19

Endocrinological Complications Associated with Cystic Fibrosis

Orville C. Green

Chronic disease and malnutrition affect the functions of the endocrine system to variable degrees in different individuals. As a general rule, such disorders are found to be secondary, with restoration toward normal when the disease is ameliorated or when adequate nutritive status is restored. Children with cystic fibrosis seldom have their basic disorder restored completely to normal, but they do represent a population in whom the degrees of severity of disease and basic nutritional supplies are highly variable. Therefore, it is not surprising that secondary dysfunction of the endocrine glands will vary between patients when specific hormonal functions are assayed. In this review, data are obtained from the studies of groups of children with cystic fibrosis; unfortunately few published studies have correlated the endocrinologic findings with scales of severity of disease. Such a correlation might clarify much of the present conflicting evidence as to the presence or absence and degree of hormonal dysfunction in this group of patients.

The endocrine system traditionally has been thought of as a cybernetic system with negative-feedback loops from a target organ whose product (humoral hormone) acts upon a detector system (hypothalamic or pituitary) which controls production of the tropic stimulator. These may involve "long loops," between hypothalamus and target gland, or "short loops" within the hypothalamic-pituitary axis or within target cells. Inhibitory hormones may also function in these loops to switch off stimulators. The humoral hormonal messengers produced by target glands not only control these cybernetic loops, but also exert their effects upon peripheral tissues through a variety of membrane and cytoplasmic receptor systems. The peptide hormones usually act through the membrane receptor-adenylate cyclase ("second messenger") system, while the steroid hormones act through cytoplasmic receptors. Clinical experience suggests to us that most of the hormonal dysfunctions seen in children with cystic fibrosis appear to involve abnormal cell membrane mechanisms rather than cytoplasmic systems, although very little basic research into these endocrine mechanisms has occurred. We shall consider each of these systems and its function in children with cystic fibrosis and, in addition, review the present knowledge of disordered carbohydrate metabolism and the hormonal systems involved.

GROWTH

General Concepts

The endocrine system of the child appears to be primarily concerned with growth and, at adolescence, the emphasis changes to focus upon adult reproduction. Human growth in length may be divided into four major phases, each with different controlling factors: fetal growth, neonatal growth, childhood growth, and adolescent growth. Each phase has different metabolic modulators but requires a basic nutrient fuel supply. Variations in weight gain in these four phases may reflect alterations in growth in length (skeletal growth), but generally are more directly related to nutritional supply and caloric expenditure. Therefore, in the following discussion the term "growth" will reflect primarily increments in length, not weight. Weight will be reflected by nutritional status and is reviewed in Chapter 15.

Fetal Growth

Human fetal growth appears to be relatively independent of the endocrine system as we know it. The rate of growth in a normal gestation of 10 lunar months exceeds that of most malignancies. A wide variety of transplacental insults (infections, maternal smoking, maternal use of alcohol, etc) as well as genetic influences may stunt fetal growth. Of interest, children who are later found to have congenital deficiencies of pituitary secretions and thyroid hormone function are usually of normal length at birth.[1] There are only two publications mentioning birth size of babies later diagnosed as afflicted with cystic fibrosis.[2,3] Both refer only to weight, and each series found similar average birth weights of 2.9 kg, in contrast to expected average birth weights of 3.3 kg for full-term infants. It is possible that the decreased birth weight of children later diagnosed as afflicted with cystic fibrosis is due to decreased fat content.

The only clearly defined growth stimulus in human fetal life is insulin. The hyperglycemia and hyperinsulinism of infants of diabetic mothers produces macrosomia in the infant. Fetal pancreatic deficiency results in severe intrauterine growth retardation and emaciation.[4] Infants born with diabetes mellitus, which is usually transient, also suffer from growth retardation and emaciation.[5] Insulin therapy restores growth in these children. Other known growth factors which appear to be important in extrauterine life, such as somatomedin-C and pituitary growth hormone, have not been demonstrated to be important in fetal growth. There is no evidence that prolactin or placental lactogen play any role in fetal growth.

Evidence for pancreatic beta-cell abnormalities in cystic fibrosis will be reviewed later in this chapter, but it is tempting to postulate that mild insulin lack in newborn cystic fibrosis infants is reflected in these lower birth weights. The primary fuels of fetal life are glucose and amino acids; the fat depots of normal neonates are primarily glucose-derived.[6] No data on the composition of neonatal fat depots in children with cystic fibrosis are available, but if this depot fat were found to differ from that of normal infants, there may be some support for a speculation on altered fetal fuels during gestation in cystic fibrosis.

There are undoubtedly many yet undiscovered factors involved in fetal growth, and these may be related to the small size of newborns with cystic fibrosis. Of particular interest would be studies of vitamin D and metabolites in these infants, since bone growth is dependent upon the conversion of vitamin D_3 to 1,25-dihydroxy-D_3 and the liver is important in this function.

Neonatal Growth

This growth phase reflects a change from rapid rates of fetal growth to a gradual deceleration toward the childhood phase of diagnosis and treatment thereafter result in growth. The known conventional hormonal mechanisms controlling growth become important (growth hormone, somatomedins, thyroid hormone, and vitamin D metabolites). In the only large study of infants with cystic fibrosis, Sproul and Huang[7] have demonstrated that both boys and girls with cystic fibrosis, evaluated as a group, actually show a "catch-up" from below the third percentile of normal for both mean height and mean weight at 3 months of age, to reach the third to 10th percentiles of normal by 24 months of age. Ranges are wide, as shown in Figure 19-1. Figure 19-2 shows their data for children in the childhood and adolescent ages. The data collected at age 3 months suggest either that these children were below the third percentile of normal for length at birth, or that the first 3 months of life are associated with marked failure to thrive and that diag-

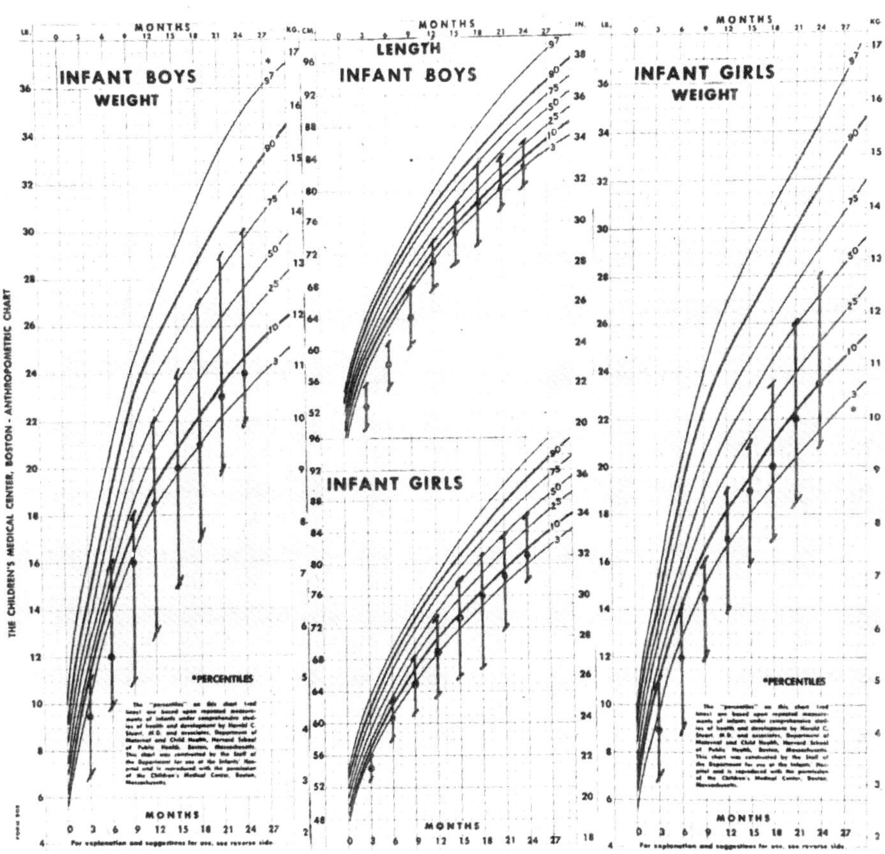

Figure 19-1 Ranges and medians for height and weight of infants with cystic fibrosis from ages 3 months to 2 years. From Sproul A, Huang N (reference 7) reproduced with permission.

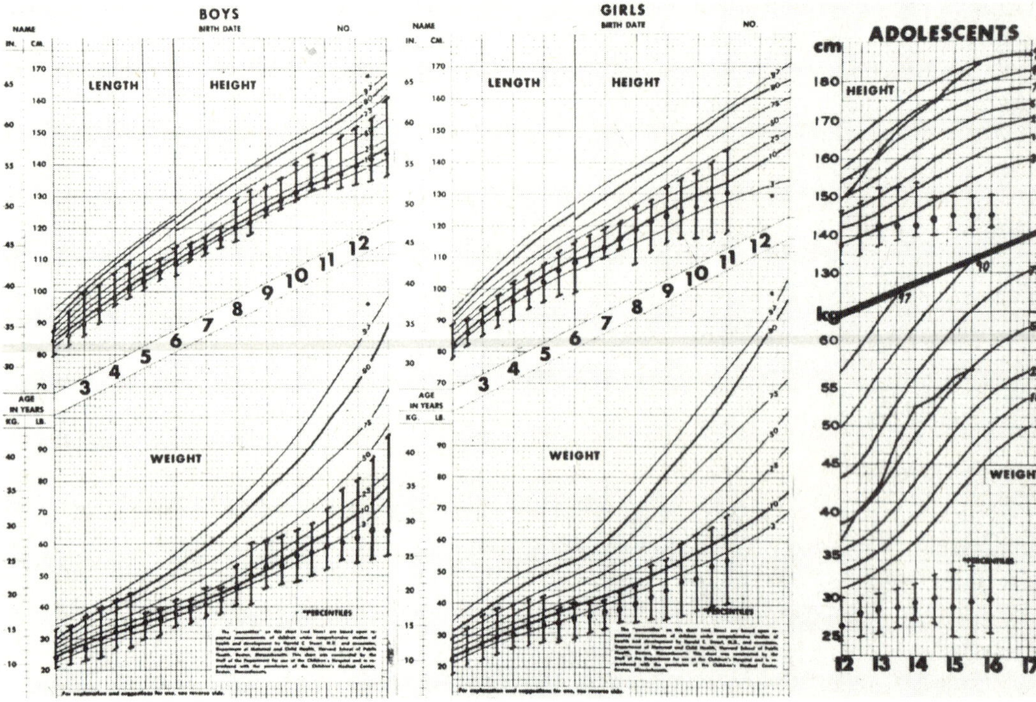

Figure 19-2 Ranges and medians for height and weight of children with cystic fibrosis from ages 2 years to 16 years. From Sproul A, Huang N (reference 7) reproduced with permission.

nosis and treatment result in marked improvement. No specific studies of hormonal mechanisms controlling growth at this time of life have been published for infants with cystic fibrosis.

Childhood Growth

This growth phase (from about age 2 years to adolescence) is the period of life most thoroughly studied and reported in the literature, in both normal children and disease states. Traditional views of mechanisms concerning growth during this phase have concerned pituitary function (growth hormone, thyrotropic hormone), thyroid hormone secretion, and study of the various somatomedins controlling cartilagenous bone growth. The past decade has seen a rapidly increasing store of information concerning growth-hormone-dependent stimuli to bone growth—the somatomedins. Originally defined as "sulfation factor" by Salmon and Daughaday[8] because of an effect of serum on stimulation of sulfate uptake into immature cartilage, it is now known that several factors can be demonstrated in normal serum which can stimulate sulfate uptake or can stimulate protein uptake in an insulin-like fashion.[9] Insulin itself has been considered a somatomedin by some workers. Most reports in the available literature have utilized the bioassay cartilage technique, but assays using other methods, specifically a radioimmunoassay for somatomedin-C and a more specific receptor assay, are now used increasingly in clinical studies. Because of nonspecific plasma factors, these techniques do not always give the same findings in patients with disease conditions other than growth-hormone deficiency and may even give discrepant results when studying those children.[10]

Figure 19-3 outlines the present concept of pituitary growth hormone secretion stimulating production of the somatomedins (presumably primarily from the liver) which then cause bone and tissue growth. It can be seen that a number of factors can affect somatomedin synthesis and activity in spite of normal pituitary growth hormone secretion.

Inhibitors include steroid hormones (glucocorticoids and estrogens), various sytemic illnesses, and especially malnutrition. Other ill-defined circulating inhibitors seem to be present in some studies.[11]

It is now accepted that a traditional feedback long loop exists between serum somatomedin levels and hypothalamic–pituitary growth hormone release.[12] This mechanism is thought to result from somatomedin stimulation of somatostatin at the hypothalamic–pituitary level. The concept of long-loop feedback explains the findings of elevated growth hormone levels in certain conditions of illness and malnutrition. Children with protein–calorie malnutrition have some of the highest resting levels of growth hormone in the literature[13] but are found to be deficient in somatomedin.[14] Other conditions documented to have low levels of somatomedins associated with high levels of growth hormone include the Laron type of dwarfism,[15] liver disease,[16] and newborn infants.[17]

Sproul and Huang published the first reports of serial measurements of height and weight in 50 children with cystic fibrosis, correlating severity of pulmonary involvement with degree of growth retardation (Figure 19-2). There was significant retardation of physical growth when compared to normal standards at all age periods. The initial "catch-up" rate of growth previously mentioned during infancy raised the mean measurements to between the 3rd and 10th percentiles of normal by age 2 years; rates of growth were then maintained in those percentiles until approximately 9 years of age when a deceleration in growth rate appeared. After age 9 years, a deceleration in growth rate was accompanied by a slowing of skeletal maturation. A significant correlation was demonstrated between growth retardation and severity of pulmonary involvement, but no correlation was found between retardation of growth and degree of pancreatic insufficiency.

The correlation of growth retardation in this childhood phase of growth with degree of pulmonary involvement suggests that nutrition plays a minimal role in the failing growth rates in these children. However, most clinics have observed improvement in rates of growth with improvement in nutritional status.[18] Specific diets have been recommended to improve nutrition with claims that weight and height gains result.[19] Therapies such as anabolic agents, aimed at improvement of nutritional status, have been recommended and have produced significant short-term increments in appetite and weight gain as well as growth.[20,21]

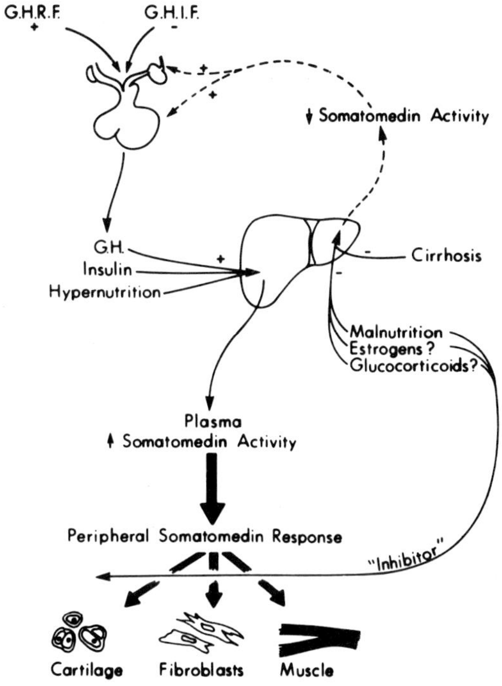

Figure 19-3 The somatomedin hypothesis. Growth hormone (GH), insulin, and hypernutrition will stimulate production of somatomedins which in turn will stimulate growth of cartilage, fibroblasts, and muscle. Estrogen, glucocorticoids, cirrhosis, and malnutrition will decrease somatomedin production, which in turn results in growth-hormone release as a compensatory response. Inhibitors to the peripheral action of somatomedins may be present in certain conditions such as malnutrition. GHRF = growth-hormone releasing factor (from hypothalamus); GHIF = growth hormone inhibitory factor (somatostatin). From Chochinov RH, Daughaday WH: Current concepts of somatomedin and other biologically related growth factors. *Diabetes* 1976;25:994–1004, reproduced with permission from the American Diabetes Association, Inc.

Studies of hormonal mechanisms in children with cystic fibrosis have included reports of growth hormone secretion, somatomedin activity, thyroid function, and vitamin D metabolism. The first report of growth hormone levels in children with cystic fibrosis[22] indicated an elevation in mean fasting levels with relatively poor response to a standard pituitary secretory challenge of induced hypoglycemia. These results were similar to those found in severe conditions of malnutrition such as kwashiorkor but were of lesser magnitude. The children studied in that report were all below the third percentile of normal for height and had severe involvement with pulmonary cystic fibrosis. Later reports suggested that many children with cystic fibrosis have normal fasting growth hormone levels and normal prolactin levels.[23] A normal response of growth hormone to hypoglycemia in three of four patients with mild to excellent clinical scores was reported by Handwerger et al.[24] Elevated growth hormone levels were confirmed in 15 studies reported by Milunski et al.[25]

None of these studies specifically correlated individual patient responses with a specific clinical score of severity. The implication of the finding of elevated growth hormone levels in some patients with cystic fibrosis who are not growing well suggests that somatomedin responses are abnormal. This speculation was confirmed by a report of decreased bioassayable somatomedin levels in cystic fibrosis[26] but was contradicted by a later report measuring somatomedin activity with the placental radioreceptor assay and the finding that somatomedin levels in this procedure were normal, as were fasting growth hormone levels.[27]

The usual relationship found in patients with chronic malnutrition has been a low somatomedin level in the presence of normal or elevated growth hormone levels. Thus present reports of studies concerning growth hormone and somatomedin in children with cystic fibrosis do not provide a specific answer for the progressive deceleration in growth rates seen as the children reach age 9 years and older. They also fail to provide an answer to the question as to whether or not growth deceleration is secondary to pulmonary dysfunction or malnutrition. The primary problem with the studies has been a failure to correlate the laboratory results with specific scoring systems of either pulmonary dysfunction or states of malnutrition in the study population.

There is general agreement in the literature that the deceleration in the growth rates observed in this population is accompanied by a progressive retardation in skeletal maturity[7,21] and that in spite of this delay, normal adult height may be achieved in children who survive.[28] One must assume that the children with the most severe pulmonary disease leading to death prior to achievement of full maturity contributes a bias to growth measurements after adult heights have been achieved and that severe pulmonary involvement has eliminated possible severe growth failure from the final data.

Adolescent Growth

As the human child advances in childhood growth, there are progressive changes in body maturity which may be evaluated by skeletal radiographs. This type of maturational change from growing cartilage to bone requires normal thyroid function and normal vitamin D metabolism, but is under other as yet ill-defined controls which may be affected by nutritional status, emotional status, stress, and chronic illness. An accepted concept among workers in the field of human growth is the assumption that some change occurs in the human organism when the skeletal maturity reaches a specific age, generally between 10 and 12 years.

At this time, changes occur also in the central nervous system with respect to hormonal activity and hypothalamic gonadotropin-releasing hormone. The low level of activity during childhood now changes into a specific pulsatile pattern with an amplitude and frequency which causes the anterior pituitary gland to secrete the gonadal-stimulating hormones: follicle-stimulating hormone (FSH), and luteinizing hormone (LH). Disorders of amplitude and frequency of gonadotropin-releasing-hormone (GnRH) pulses will result in disorders of gonadal function, and some abnormalities of pituitary–gonadal function can be treated by pulsatile administration of GnRh (hypothalamic amenorrhea) or by the continuous administration of large doses of GnRH analogs causing the pituitary to become refractory to normal pulsatile patterns (children with sexual precocity). In response to the proper frequency and amplitude of GnRH pulses, the pituitary releases FSH and LH to stimulate the target gonad.[29] The target may be thought of as an "endocrine gonad" which produces sex hormones in response to FSH and LH, and as an "exocrine gonad" which produces sperm in the testis and ova in the ovary.

The hormonal secretions of the endocrine gonad of the adolescent human cause a second growth spurt that appears to be unique in primates. Cartilaginous and bone growth is stimulated by sex hormones superimposed upon and independent of the somatomedins of childhood. Sex hormonal administration may cause these growth spurts even in children without pituitary–growth hormone–somatomedin activity.

Steroidal stimulated growth, however, results in the slowly progressive closure of the epiphyseal growth plates, heralding fusion and cessation of growth. Androgens are more potent growth stimulators than estrogens, which cause a more rapid fusion of epiphyses. Thus, the iatrogenic administration of androgens and estrogens, or other causes of sexual precocity before the skeleton has reached a level of 10–11 years, will result in growth acceleration but will imply an ultimate stature which has been reduced by too early fusion.[30]

Long clinical experience with abnormalities of these mechanisms has led to the concept that adolescent changes will occur in otherwise normal children when their skeletal maturity reaches 11–12 years irrespective of the chronological age. The diagnosis of "delay of maturity" accounts for 55% of all complaints of short stature in pediatric endocrine clinics.[31] This concept has been expanded to include certain chronic illnesses, and cystic fibrosis is one of those. Sproul and Huang[7] have shown that a delay in skeletal maturity occurs with the slowing of growth after age 9 years; this delay in skeletal maturity is then associated with a delay in the timing of adolescence. Clinical studies in adolescent children and adults with cystic fibrosis have confirmed that the hormonal changes of puberty do occur, but are generally delayed in association with the retardation in progress of skeletal maturity.[28,32]

Ultimate stature is eventually achieved in a relatively normal height range in those patients who survive. It must be recognized, however, that patients with cystic fibrosis who survive to pass through adolescence and achieve adulthood are those with the least severe manifestations of the disease and the best medical care. The study by Mitchell-Heggs et al[32] could not correlate slow growth rate with severe lung infection or malabsorption, although the childhood study of Sproul and Huang[7] did correlate slow growth with more severe lung disease.

SEXUAL DEVELOPMENT

In addition to causing the height growth spurt of adolescence, the sex hormones cause the growth of the reproductive organs in the body. Patients with cystic fibrosis will show the growth responses of those organs (penis, breasts, uterus), but the function of these organs may be seriously impaired by the generalized disturbance of secretory activity. In males with cystic fibrosis, penile and prostatic growth and sexual function are not impaired. Secondary sexual characteristics develop normally with time, although later than in normal boys.[33] The hormonal status of pituitary FSH and LH as well as gonadal testosterone has been evaluated in only 3 patients with cystic fibrosis.[34] Even though sperm production from the exocrine testis was deficient, these levels of FSH and LH and testosterone were reported to be normal. This report has apparently been accepted in the literature without additional confirming studies. Although not impotent, most males are infertile, with aspermia[35] due to epididymal abnormalities, absent or defective vasa deferentia, and dilated or absent seminal vesicles.[36] Spermatogenesis occurs in the testis, but the ejaculate is aspermic, although a survey of treatment centers has revealed that 2–3% of affected males may be fertile.[37]

Females will achieve full development of sexual maturation unless severe disease is present. In normal females, menarche is dependent upon achieving a critical body weight[38] which may be affected by nutritional status and degree of athletic endeavor. These factors obviously will vary considerably from patient to patient and irregular menses would be expected. Menarchal age is delayed in relation to severity of illness.[39] Abnormalities of the cervical mucous-secreting glands have been described,[40] but these abnormalities have not seemed to affect child-bearing capability. Impaired fertility is common in the female but pregnancies have occurred; by 1966, ten births to women with cystic fibrosis had been reported[41] with five mothers showing no adverse effects, but five showing deterioration of pulmonary function with the pregnancy. A national survey in 1980 revealed 129 pregnancies in 100 women with CF, with 87 live births.[42] One infant had CF. An additional concern of pregnancy in these women is the effect upon the developing fetus of the varieties of medication administered to the mother.

The varying degrees of impairment of fertility in both men and women with cystic fibrosis reflects the variable involvement of different organ systems so common in this disorder. As more children reach adolescence and maturity, there will be more concern with marriage, reproductive capacity, and the effects of gestation on maternal lung pathology. Additional studies and improved methods of management will be needed, both to assist the mother through the pregnancy which may be harmful to her and to protect the fetus against harm from transplacental toxic substances which may be administered to the mother.

ADRENAL FUNCTION

Adrenal function has been investigated for both androgenic secretion and glucocorticoid secretion as well as aldosterone activity. Urinary 17-ketosteroid excretion has been found to be normal in terms of total ketosteroids and ketosteroid fractions (androsterone, etiocholanolone, dehydroepiandrosterone, and 11-ketoandrosterone).[35,43,44] The latter publications also indicated normal urinary glucocorticoid excretion. In unpublished studies from our own laboratory, urinary 17-ketosteroids, 17-hydroxycorticosteroids, and serum cortisol levels have all been found to be within normal ranges when adjusted for body size and skeletal maturity. Although considerable interest has revolved around the control of salt loss through the sweat glands and possible aldosterone abnormalities (see Chapters 4 and 5), no primary abnormalities of aldosterone have been reported.

Children with cystic fibrosis may have normal or slightly elevated aldosterone urinary excretion rates and secretion rates have been calculated in 6 children.[45] This study reported normal aldosterone secretion rates, metabolic clearance rates, plasma concentrations, and volumes of distribution for aldosterone in parents of cystic fibrosis children and in 5 of the 6 children with cystic fibrosis studied. One child had an abnormally high secretion rate which was attributed to relative salt depletion. Urinary 17-hydroxycorticosteroids were normal in all patients also.

Some children with cystic fibrosis have been prone to severe salt depletion and develop severe metabolic alkalosis with hypochloremia and hypokalemia as well as hyponatremia. Three such patients have been reported with detailed studies of the renin-aldosterone system.[46] All three infants were found to have marked hyperreninemia, hyperaldosteronemia, and hyperaldosteronuria. Repletion with adequate salt and water restored the abnormalities to normal. Studies of urinary 17-ketosteroids and

17-hydroxycorticosteroids were normal in these patients.

These data all support the conclusion that adrenal function responds in a secondary fashion to the salt and water depletion that may be found in patients with cystic fibrosis. No evidence exists to incriminate adrenal disorders as a primary cause of the loss of electrolytes through the sweat. (See Chapter 5 for further discussion of the role of aldosterone in CF.)

In addition, studies have been carried out concerning the administration of androgens to patients with cystic fibrosis. The administration of testosterone, dehydroepiandrosterone, and anabolic agents to patients with cystic fibrosis have shown no effects upon sweat secretory activity.[47] Treatment of patients with delay of growth and retarded skeletal maturity utilizing androgens modified as "anabolic agents" has produced temporary beneficial results in terms of growth, increased weight gain, and improved pulmonary function.[20,21] Anabolic therapy is now utilized in many clinics. These agents must be metabolized in the liver and use of these drugs even in normal children has resulted in varying degrees of cholestasis.[48] A rare complication is the risk of liver tumor.[49] Therefore when these drugs are utilized in this patient population, liver function must be monitored. Treatment with these agents provides temporary improvement with an increase in height but most patients will show an advance in skeletal maturity greater than the height achieved. This undesirable effect may be outweighed by the subjective improvement, weight gain, and increased physical performance as a result of therapy.

CALCIUM METABOLISM

A few studies have appeared concerning calcium metabolism and relationships to parathyroid hormone activity and vitamin D metabolism. Overt rickets is now a vary rare occurrence in patients with cystic fibrosis. Although fat-soluble forms of vitamin D may be poorly absorbed through the gut, and liver metabolism of vitamin D may be defective, rickets is unusual. One recent case of vitamin D-deficiency rickets with abnormal liver function tests and myopathy has been reported with these manifestations leading to the diagnosis of cystic fibrosis.[50] Decreased levels of the hormone 1,25-dihydroxy-vitamin D_3 with elevated parathyroid hormone levels were found. Treatment with vitamin D and pancreatic enzymes led to full recovery of the rickets and the myopathy. Most patients demonstrate normal gastrointestinal calcium absorption with normal serum calcium and phosphorus responses to administered exogenous parathyroid hormone even though endogenous parathyroid hormone assays may sometimes be found to be elevated and to suppress subnormally in response to calcium infusion.[51]

THYROID FUNCTION

Goiter and hypothyroidism secondary to iodide therapy in children with cystic fibrosis has been reported as a secondary complication.[52,53] The administration of iodide solutions to normal individuals is not a cause of hypothyroidism or goiter. In one prospective study of patients with cystic fibrosis, 15 of 18 patients studied developed goiter or hypothyroidism or both while receiving 540 mg of iodide daily as a saturated solution of potassium iodide.[54]

This finding led to a detailed study of 25 patients with cystic fibrosis between ages 2 and 24 years in an effort to determine whether an intrathyroidal abnormality was present in cystic fibrosis. The study group had Shwachman scores of over 70. Studies included the perchlorate discharge test; the thyroid-releasing-hormone (TRH) test; and peripheral analyses for thyroid-stimulating hormone (TSH), serum thyroxine, and serum triiodothyronine.[55] No evidence of an intrathyroidal defect was found. Serum TSH responses to TRH were not abnormal. Serum thyroxine concentration was normal but serum triiodothyronine concentration was decreased in these patients with cystic fibrosis. The suggestion was made that decreased peripheral conversion of thyroxine to triiodothyronine was associated with illness and did not constitute a specific thyroidal abnormality in cystic fibrosis. The mechanism whereby patients with cystic fibrosis develop hypothyroidism when given iodides could not be clarified. Of interest, patients with hypothyroidism may have sweat chloride analyses indistinguishable from patients with cystic fibrosis.[56,57] An additional report suggests that TRH may inhibit pancreatic enzyme secretion in normal humans.[58] TRH is not a significant circulating hormone but is involved primarily in the short-loop release of TSH through the hypothalamic–anterior pituitary–portal system. These studies were carried out by administration of large quantities of TRH and the physiologic significance remains obscure.

The conclusion of studies of thyroid function in patients with cystic fibrosis suggests that patients given iodide solutions are at risk for the development of goiter and/or hypothyroidism and should receive physiologic replacement thyroid hormone therapy if either condition develops.

CARBOHYDRATE INTOLERANCE IN PATIENTS WITH CF

Diabetes mellitus is defined as a symptom complex of glucosuria with hyperglycemia and comprises an heterogeneous group of diseases rather than a single disorder. Many of these diseases have a genetic component. The two most common forms of diabetes mellitus have been classified as type I (also called insulin-dependent diabetes mellitus, IDDM; juvenile onset diabetes, JOD) and type II (insulin independent diabetes mellitus, IIDM; maturity onset diabetes, MOD). JOD has been found to be positively correlated with certain tissue typing antigens (HLA-B8, HLA-BW15, mixed lymphocyte types DR-3, DR-4), but even within this subgroup, heterogeneity is found. MOD characteristically arises in older persons and is frequently associated with obesity and decreased peripheral insulin receptors. Pancreatic insulin secretion in MOD is not totally impaired but may be decreased relative to hyperglycemia. In contrast to JOD, MOD does not require insulin therapy. Undefined genetic patterns appear to be present in MOD but also suggest heterogeneity. Type II diabetes (MOD) may infrequently occur in the child and adolescent and is then called maturity onset diabetes of the young (MODY).

A variety of genetic syndromes have also been associated with the development of diabetes and the type may be type I, type II, or MODY. In these genetic syndromes, type II may sometimes progress to type I and require insulin therapy. The genetic association may be strong and unaccompanied by pancreatic destruction, as in the Prader-Willi syndrome, or the association may be considered secondary to progressive pancreatic disease, as is seen in cystic fibrosis. Because the genetics of type I and type II disease are still not clearly defined, the question remains as to whether these other genetic diseases and secondary conditions are truly causative, or whether these patients actually have a genetic predisposition to diabetes. In childhood populations, JOD occurs in approximately 2 per 1000 children and MODY is considerably rarer.

The unusually high incidence (10%) of glucose intolerance in the cystic fibrosis population was first mentioned in 1938.[59] Table 19-1 summarizes reports of glucose intolerance from selected studies in a variety of clinics. The percentage of glucose intolerance varies from 8% to 75%, with an overall figure of 43%. Insulin dependence appears to occur in about 1% of patients. These figures far exceed the expected incidence in an otherwise normal childhood population. Three authors suggested a genetic predisposition from family studies,[25,60,61] but other studies, including our own, have found no familial incidence. A genetic linkage to type I or type II diabetes mellitus is unlikely since cystic fibrosis does not occur in families with these forms of diabetes in a higher proportion than in the general population; it is only the reverse association of diabetes occurring in patients with cystic fibrosis that is seen. No tissue typing studies have been published

Table 19-1
Glucose Intolerance to Testing*

Author	Year	Number Studied	Number Glucose Intolerant	Percentage
Lowe et al[62]	1949	35	3	8%
Rosan et al[61]	1962	30	12	40%
Handwerger et al[24]	1969	31	13	42%
Milner[65]	1969	61	16	26%
Milunski et al[25]	1971	15	2	13%
Wang et al[60]	1973	58	43	75%
Wilmshurst et al[68]	1975	8	6	75%
Selden et al[70]	1976	38	19	50%
Lippe et al[71]	1977	13	7	54%
Green (unpublished data)		16	10	62%
Totals		305	131	43%

*Summary of published reports of incidence of glucose intolerance discovered in study groups of patients with cystic fibrosis reported from 10 clinics. Our own unpublished data are included. Regulation of carbohydrate metabolism is disordered in almost half of all patients studied.

in cystic fibrosis patients with diabetes mellitus, but a genetic linkage might be postulated if the tissue types of type I diabetes were found to be present in those children who have become insulin dependent.

Failure of the Endocrine Pancreas and Diabetes Mellitus in Patients with Cystic Fibrosis

Initial reports of glucose intolerance, glycosuria, and insulin dependence in patients with cystic fibrosis were interpreted as showing coincidental development of two disorders in the same patient.[62,63] Experimental studies in rabbits with ligation of the pancreatic duct appeared to support the concept that the acinar cells could suffer severe damage while the islet cells remained intact.[64] This concept gradually changed, with additional studies demonstrating direct association between the presence of cystic fibrosis and diabetes mellitus.

In 1962, Rosan et al[61] reported their observations on 10 patients with cystic fibrosis known to have diabetes (8 of whom required insulin therapy) and an additional 30 patients not previously known to be diabetic. Although they stated that only 5 of these 30 were found to be diabetic by their criteria, 12 were found to be abnormally intolerant to glucose loading with peak glucose levels of 190 mg/dl. Only 18 of the 30 patients could be considered to have normal responses. They concluded that "subclinical" diabetes must exist in a high proportion of patients with cystic fibrosis but that diabetes did not appear to shorten survival. This subclinical diabetic condition was found to coexist for many years, and they suggested that it may progress to complete insulin dependence. When insulin-dependent diabetes did develop, it was indistinguishable from JOD (type I), except for the infrequent occurrence of ketosis. Only 23% of their patients had a family history of any form of diabetes. Insulin requirements were variable, in the range of 0.3–1.5 units/lb/day (0.6–3.3 units/kg/day).

Subsequently, with the advent of radioimmunoassay methods for insulin analysis, it was found that, when compared to normals, all patients with cystic fibrosis had lowered levels of endogenous insulin for all levels of blood glucose; detailed studies in 31 patients led to the present concept that a large percentage of patients have moderate to severe glucose intolerance due to anatomic disorganization and fibrosis of the endocrine pancreas and that these abnormalities are a complication of the basic pancreatic disease rather than a concomitant association with the genetic disorder of type I or type II diabetes mellitus.[24] Twenty-three of the 31 patients had mild to excellent clinical CF scores. Four of these patients were studied over an 18-month period with apparent deterioration in insulin secretion.

Studies in 61 additional children from England[65] reported blood glucose and serum insulin levels after oral and intravenous glucose, and also after intravenous glucagon and tolbutamide in a few patients. Two patients in this series were already known to be diabetic, and 16 additional patients were found to be glucose intolerant to oral testing. Of the 8 children tested with intravenous glucose, all were abnormal, but the insulin response to intravenous loading was greater than to oral loading. Milner[65] concluded that insulin release was defective but that these patients may also show a defective release of the gut hormones which augment insulin release in response to oral glucose loading in normal patients.

Additional publications studying glucose tolerance in children with cystic fibrosis have appeared.[25,66–71] All studies agree that insulin secretion in response to hyperglycemia is defective. There was general agreement that the defective release is secondary to disorganization and fibrosis of the islet cells, although the suggestion by Milner that some gut factor was deficient was supported by the studies of Clodi.[66] The differences in intravenous and oral glucose loading with respect to insulin response is consistent enough to warrant further investigation.

Our own studies of beta-cell responsiveness are shown in Table 19-2 and Figure 19-4. Oral glucose loading followed by intravenous glucagon stimulation has been shown to be a maximal stimulus to insulin production, and the data have been reported in children.[72] We have concluded from our studies that the beta cell in cystic fibrosis patients not only shows defective insulin secretion but has a very poor insulin reserve when

Table 19-2
Glucose and Insulin Responses in Children with Cystic Fibrosis Compared to Normal Children

	Cystic fibrosis		Normal*	
Time (min)	*Glucose (mg/dl)*	*Insulin (μU/ml)*	*Glucose (mg/dl)*	*Insulin (μU/ml)*
0	70.9 ± 4.7	6.1 ± 1.3	84.7 ± 2.8	11.7 ± 1.8
30	136.9 ± 8.3	19.3 ± 4.2	124.9 ± 5.1	
60	162.6 ± 11.7	31.0 ± 6.1		
90	156.5 ± 13.8	33.6 ± 6.7		
120	129.4 ± 12.2	23.1 ± 3.8		58.1 ± 6.6
150	102.5 ± 13.0	16.3 ± 5.2		
180	66.1 ± 6.4	8.1 ± 2.0	86.7 ± 2.9	24.5 ± 5.0
Glucagon				
4	85.5 ± 6.8	32.9 ± 5.7	121.3 ± 7.8	253.4 ± 47.9
7	96.6 ± 6.3	26.7 ± 5.0		
10	105.0 ± 5.9	20.0 ± 4.1		
15	113.8 ± 5.2	18.1 ± 4.2		
30	105.0 ± 5.7	11.7 ± 2.6		

*Data for normal children from Josefsburg et al.[72] Figure 19-4 shows graphic data as published, but specific mean values ± SEM were provided only for those time periods shown in Table 19-2. The insulin responses to glucose of normal children rise rapidly at 30 min and peak at 120 min with 58.1 ± 6.6 μU/ml; our data for CF children show lower insulin levels at all times in spite of higher blood glucose levels, but reach a peak of 33.6 ± 6.7 μU/ml at 90 min. In response to intravenous glucagon, normal children show a burst of insulin release to 253.4 ± 47.9 μU/ml in 2–4 min; CF children show blunted insulin responses, rising only to 32.9 μU/ml as a maximum. These data suggest that patients with cystic fibrosis show glucose intolerance with delayed insulin secretion in response to hyperglycemia and, in addition, show very poor insulin reserve to the maximal beta-cell stimulus of intravenous glucagon following oral glucose.

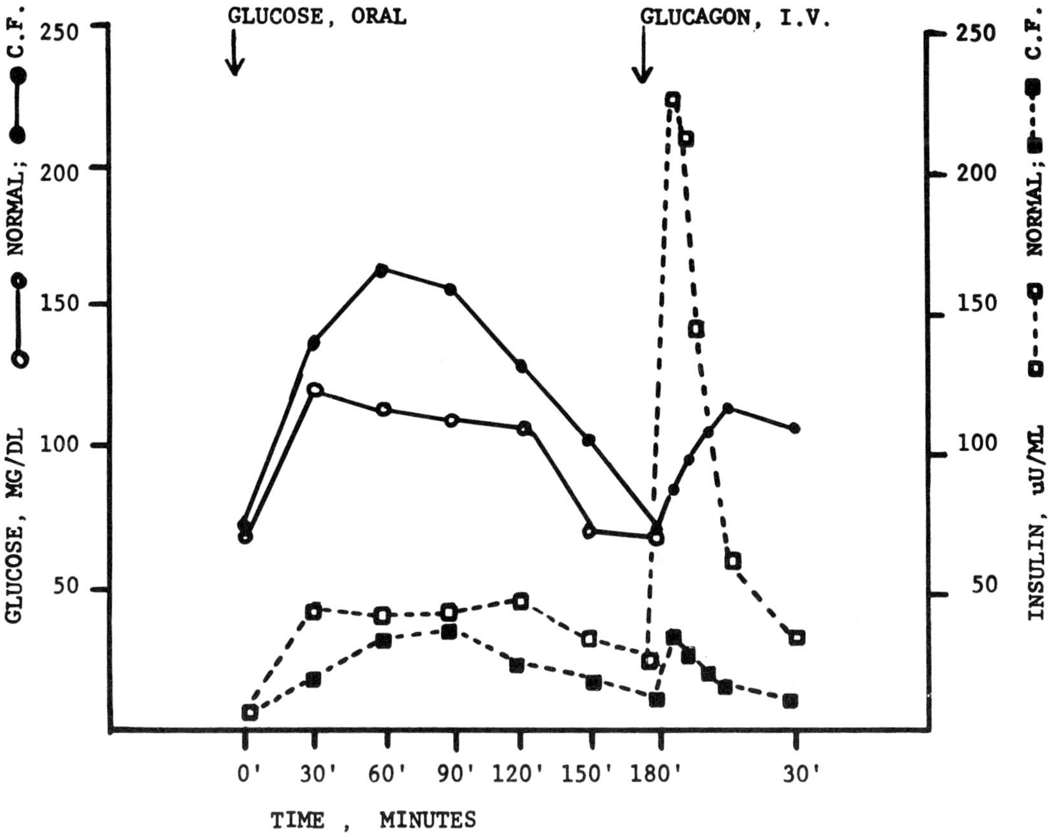

Figure 19-4 Intravenous glucagon given immediately after a 3-hr glucose tolerance test is a maximal stimulus to insulin release. The figure shows mean values for glucose and insulin responses to oral glucose (1.75 g/kg) in 16 patients with cystic fibrosis followed by intravenous glucagon (0.03 mg/kg) and continued sampling at 4, 7, 10, 15, and 30 min in 13 of the 16 patients. Responses for blood glucose in 16 CF patients (●——●) compared with normal children (○——○); simultaneous insulin responses (CF □----□) compared to normal responses (■----■). Normal values taken from published data.[72] Note that in spite of higher glucose levels in CF patients during the 3-hr glucose tolerance test, insulin levels at all times are lower than in normal children with lower glucose values. The insulin responses to glucagon in children with CF are minimal, indicating poor insulin reserve. Mean values only are plotted; actual values are listed in Table 19-2.

compared to the normal data of Josefsberg et al.[72] As shown in Table 19-2, normal children show a peak glucose response to oral glucose tolerance testing of 124.9 ± 5.1 mg/dl with peak levels at 30 min; cystic fibrosis patients show glucose intolerance to 162.6 ± 11.7 mg/dl as a peak level but a slow return to normal levels by 180 min; when intravenous glucagon is then given, normal children show an additional rise in glucose to 121.3 ± 3.8 mg/dl at 2–4 min and then a progressive return to normal by 30 min; cystic fibrosis patients show a slower glucose rise to 113.8 ± 5.2 mg/dl at 15 min and do not return to normal at 30 min. The insulin responses to intravenous glucagon in normal children show a hypersecretory rise to 253.4 ± 47.9 μU/ml whereas the cystic fibrosis patients show only a minimal response to 32.9 ± 5.7 μU/ml between 2 and 4 min after the injection. Thus, both the initial response to glucose and the reserve hypersecretory response to glucagon are deficient in these children when studied as a group. In considering the data individually, 10 of the 16 patients showed abnormal glucose tolerance in response to oral glucose loading as indicated in Table 19-2.

Sulfonylurea compounds (tolbutamide, chlorpropamide), given either orally or intravenously, will stimulate the production of insulin from the beta cell; the response varies from almost nil in type I diabetes to almost normal in type II diabetes and has been shown to correct glucose intolerance in some persons with MOD and MODY type II forms.[73] Sulfonylurea therapy has also been used temporarily to improve type I (JOD) diabetes in a few patients.[74] Several authors have utilized intravenous tolbutamide challenges in patients with cystic fibrosis and have reported variable insulin responses.[24,65,68] Those patients with the poorest glucose tolerance and lowest insulin response to glucose generally showed the poorer insulin responses to tolbutamide. Although not conclusive, it appeared that overall the insulin response to tolbutamide was better than to glucose. Nevertheless, these tests confirmed the impression that the glucose intolerance seen in cystic fibrosis patients was a result of insulin deficiency rather than peripheral resistance to normal levels of circulating insulin.

Wilmshurst[68] studied peripheral tissue responsiveness to insulin in his patients by analysis of the rate of fall of free fatty acids (FFA) and concluded that adipose tissue demonstrated an increased sensitivity to insulin in patients since the fall in FFA was accelerated over normal by comparable peripheral insulin levels. Increased peripheral sensitivity to insulin had been suggested in the study by Handwerger[24] and appears to have been confirmed by direct study of insulin receptors which have been found to be increased in number and affinity in children with cystic fibrosis.[75]

In contrast, infusion of insulin into patients with cystic fibrosis did not cause a drop in blood glucose comparable to normal responses.[71] When constant doses (0.01 unit/kg) of insulin were given, mean blood glucose values were at all times higher in patients with cystic fibrosis than in normals, although the differences were not statistically significant. Computing a ratio for insulin to glucose values did show highly significant differences, with normal ratios higher than those in patients with cystic fibrosis. These ratios were similar to those published by Wilmshurst,[68] where insulin-to-glucose ratios were calculated for glucose tolerance tests and tolbutamide tests. Such ratios, however, can be interpreted in two ways: (1) as indicating that for the same amount of insulin, blood glucose levels are lower in normals than in cystic fibrosis patients, or (2) for the same blood glucose value, insulin secretion is higher in normal than in cystic fibrosis patients. The authors selected the conclusion that insulin secretion was defective and later published studies indicating an increase in insulin receptors in peripheral monocytes of patients with cystic fibrosis.[75]

Clinical experience, however, with cystic fibrosis patients who require insulin therapy, as detailed later, suggests that some form of peripheral resistance to exogenous insulin is present. These apparently conflicting data imply that there may be some defect in insulin action within the peripheral target tissues beyond the receptor. Postreceptor defects have been described in several endocrine disorders such as pseudohypoparathyroidism[76] and diabetes insipidus.[77] A postreceptor defect could account for inadequate peripheral insulin action even in the presence of increased numbers of receptors. The question of whether patients with cystic fibrosis show increased sensitivity to insulin or whether they have a peripheral resistance to insulin action deserves further study.

Glucagon

It is now apparent that not only the beta cell but also the alpha cell of the islet of Langerhans is defective in secretory capability in children with cystic fibrosis.[69,71] Infusions of amino acids, in particular arginine, are potent stimulators of the alpha cell to produce glucagon as well as acting to stimulate the beta cell to produce insulin. These responses to arginine infusion in normal persons occur with very little change in blood sugar levels. In the first study reported,[69] 5 of 10 children with cystic fibrosis showed markedly decreased glucagon and insulin responses to arginine. These authors suggested that the decreased glucagon secretion could mask defective insulin secretion in terms of clinical glucose intolerance since glucagon and insulin are antagonists in carbohydrate metabolism; if beta-cell damage were to prevail, diabetes would then become clinically apparent. In addition, the glucagon deficiency could explain the relative absence of ketosis in these patients when diabetes supervened, since the usual forms of diabetes and ketosis are accompanied by elevations in plasma glucagon, and glucagon secretion is considered essential for the development of ketosis.[78]

When insulin and glucagon responses to both oral glucose and intravenous arginine were compared to normal children, patients with cystic fibrosis appeared to fall into two groups.[71] Those with normal oral glucose tolerance tests were classified as group I and showed subnormal insulin secretion to hyperglycemia, normal glucagon suppression to hyperglycemia, and a normal glucagon response to arginine. Those patients with glucose intolerance (group II) also showed subnormal insulin secretion and normal glucagon suppression to hyperglycemia, but responded poorly to arginine stimulation of glucagon secretion. These authors concluded that the blunting of the glucagon response in group II may be related to the progression of a generalized pancreatic abnormality not yet present in group I. The fact that abnormal hyperglycemia occurred in group II without concomitant elevations in glucagon clearly distinguished these patients from the usual forms of type II diabetes (MOD and MODY).

In summary, the studies involving combined alpha-cell and beta-cell secretion in patients with cystic fibrosis indicate that there may be progressive failure in both secretory systems with progressive disease of the exocrine pancreas. Failure of beta-cell function appears more consistent than failure of alpha-cell function, but the pattern of progressive failure is quite distinct from the usual forms of diabetes.

Management of Diabetes Mellitus in Patients with Cystic Fibrosis

As discussed earlier, testing with intravenous tolbutamide seems to indicate that almost all patients with cystic fibrosis have some residual capacity to secrete insulin. It would seem logical that oral therapy with tolbutamide and chemical derivatives would provide a method of prevention of hyperglycemia. This form of therapy has not been thoroughly discussed in the literature, and only one case report appears in detail.[79] Our limited experience would suggest that tolbutamide therapy is not a successful form of management in most patients. We have given therapeutic doses of tolbutamide to the 4 patients with the most serious glucose intolerance, and it was of value in only one in spite of responses to intravenous tolbutamide testing in all 4.

The responsive patient is presented in Table 19-3. This patient had a grossly abnormal glucose tolerance test in 1969. Treatment with oral tolbutamide, 0.25 g 3 times

Table 19-3
Oral Glucose Tolerance Before and After Sulfonylurea Therapy*

Date	Time (min) *0*	*30*	*60*	*120*	*180*	Comment
10/9/69	96	186	263	268	119	No therapy
10/16/69	76	127	160	125	52	Tolbutamide, 2 days
4/15/70	79	133	133	84	56	Tolbutamide, 6 months
10/22/70	71	116	153	113	48	No therapy, 6 months
12/17/74	74	164	191	210	140	No therapy, 4 years

*Patient P.K., CMH #043326, studied for glucose intolerance before and after oral therapy with tolbutamide for 6 months. Values are milligrams per deciliter. Treatment improved glucose tolerance with apparent prolonged effects after stopping the medication, but with return to glucose intolerance when evaluated 4 years later.

daily normalized the glucose tolerance test in 2 days. Treatment with tolbutamide continued for 6 months, and a repeat glucose tolerance test was again normal. Therapy was then discontinued voluntarily. Six months later, the oral glucose tolerance test was still normal. The family was advised to perform morning urinalyses for glucose, and these were negative for the ensuing 4 years. However, a repeat glucose tolerance test indicated that moderate intolerance had once again occurred. This is the only patient in our clinic who has been successfully treated with oral tolbutamide therapy. One lesson from this study indicates that morning testing for glycosuria is not a satisfactory method for detection of glucose intolerance and that patients should be instructed to test for glycosuria 2 hr after a meal. It also suggests that more patients should be receiving tolbutamide therapy when this type of glucose intolerance is discovered.

The management of patients with type I and type II diabetes in the past has been difficult because of poor techniques for evaluating control of hyperglycemia. A significant advance in evaluation of control occurred with the discovery that hemoglobin A will irreversibly combine with glucose when blood glucose levels are elevated above normal.[80] This process of glycosylation of normal hemoglobin will occur to a small degree in normal individuals without diabetes mellitus. The form of glycosylated hemoglobin usually measured is hemoglobin $A1_C$. This glycosylated hemoglobin has been found to be increased in undetected intermittent hyperglycemia prodromal to the development of clinical diabetes mellitus[81] and has been found mildly elevated in children with cystic fibrosis who have had normal fasting and postprandial glucose levels.[81,82] No studies of long-term management of children with cystic fibrosis and diabetes utilizing glycosylated hemoglobin as a measure of control have appeared in the literature.

Insulin therapy Earlier clinical studies[61,68] suggested that cystic fibrosis patients who developed the insulin-dependent form of diabetes required only low doses of insulin for adequate management. The only paper which mentioned doses and body weight[61] actually indicates large doses of insulin were required (0.6–3.3 units/kg/day). In most clinics where diabetic children (JOD) are managed, average insulin doses are 0.7 units/kg/day, and doses over 1.0 units/kg/day are usually found to be excessive and responsible for causing "brittle" management as well as the Somogyi phenomenon (posthypoglycemic hyperglycemia).[83] The study by Wilmshurst et al[68] did not actually involve insulin-dependent patients but is quoted as showing increased peripheral insulin sensitivity based upon indirect evidence from rates of fall of FFA, being more rapid in cystic fibrosis than in normals. The dilemma concerning whether or not peripheral resistance to insulin is present has been discussed earlier.

The incidence of insulin-dependent diabetes mellitus in the cystic fibrosis patient population appears to be in the range of 1%. The 1962 study of Rosan et al[61] indicated that there had been 10 patients out of 1300 who required insulin therapy in the dosage range of 0.6–3.3 units/kg. The study by Milner[65] mentions one insulin-dependent patient in a patient population of 105 children with cystic fibrosis. In our clinic of 422 patients with cystic fibrosis in the past 15 years, 4 patients have developed insulin requirements. Dosage has averaged 1.45 units/kg/day, suggesting some peripheral insensitivity to insulin. All studies have commented that patients with glucose intolerance and insulin-dependent diabetes mellitus have a very low incidence of ketosis. In one patient studied by us, ketosis was induced when fat content in the diet was increased and disappeared when fat content in the diet was reduced. Some workers have explained the lack of development of ketosis on the inability of the pancreas of these patients to secrete glucagon in amounts adequate to be associated with ketosis. It is also possible that the restriction of fat intake may reduce the tendency toward ketosis in this group of patients.

With the onset of insulin-dependent diabetes mellitus, one might suspect that the clinical course could rapidly deteriorate. In fact, this is not the case, as first pointed out by Rosan.[61] Three of the four patients on insulin therapy in our clinic survived more than 5 years after the diagnosis of insulin-dependent diabetes mellitus; however, only one survived 10 years.

Relationship between Diabetes Mellitus and Pancreatitis

Acute pancreatitis seldom leads to chronic pancreatitis, although it may relapse in the presence of gallstone disorders. Acute pancreatitis may be transiently associated with glucose intolerance but generally does not lead to permanent hyperglycemia. In contrast, chronic pancreatitis, especially that form called "chronic relapsing pancreatitis" is frequently associated with glucose intolerance and may progress to an insulin-dependent form of diabetes mellitus.[84] The pathology of chronic relapsing pancreatitis includes fibrosis, dilation of ducts, atrophy of ductal epithelium, eosinophilic protein plugs which frequently calcify, and perilobular and interlobular sclerosis with perineural inflammatory infiltration and nerve lesions in advanced stages. The most common cause in North America and Europe is chronic alcoholism. Chronic relapsing pancreatitis is likewise associated with low insulin levels. Low glucagon responses, however, are not seen until gross pancreatic destruction occurs.[85] Ketoacidosis is an infrequent complication but may be life-threatening when it occurs. These pathological findings and biochemical endocrine pancreatic responses are markedly similar to those seen in children with cystic fibrosis. Figure 19-5 demonstrates the presence of pancreatic

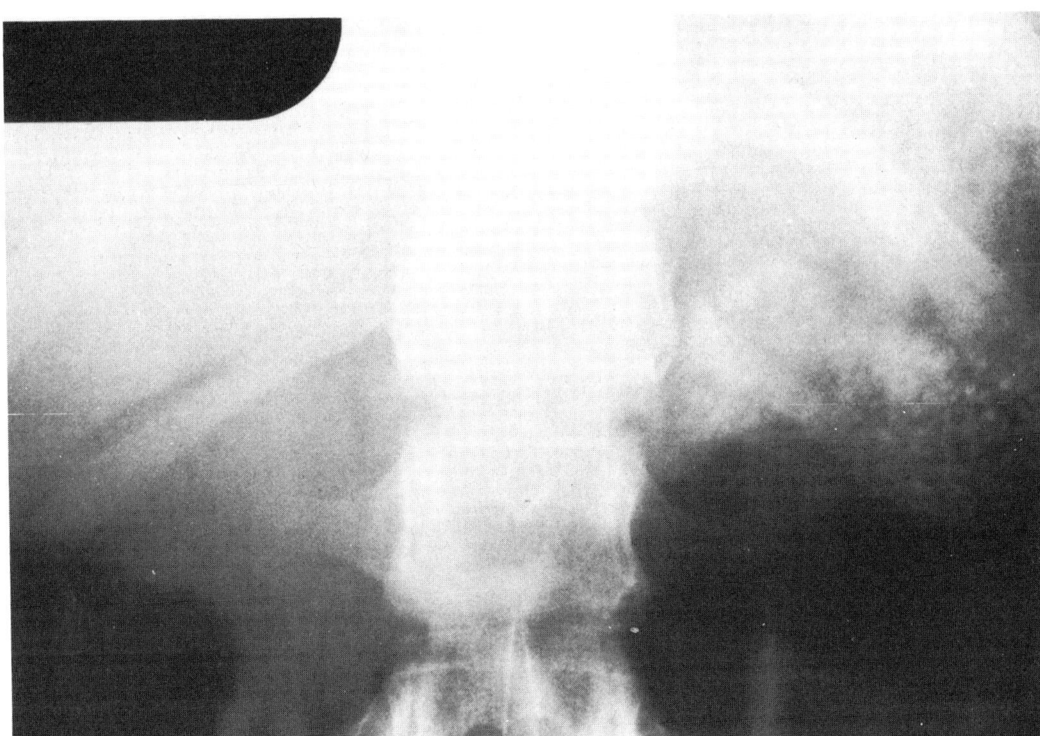

Figure 19-5 Radiograph of abdomen of 13-year-old boy (CMH #126182) with cystic fibrosis diagnosed since age 6 years and recent 2-month history of weight loss, polyuria and polydipsia. Blood glucose 642 mg/dl. Initial insulin requirements were 1.3 units/kg/day. Note fine flecks of calcification diffusely throughout the body and tail of pancreas; head of pancreas overlies spine and is difficult to define. Radiograph supplied through courtesy of Dr. Sandra Fernbach.

calcifications in a patient who developed insulin-dependent diabetes mellitus 7 years after the diagnosis of cystic fibrosis was established.

Another form of pancreatic diabetes associated with calcification in the pancreas has been described as a specific form of pancreatic diabetes in southern India.[86] It has been characterized as occurring in the younger age groups, especially children; it occurs in the lowest socioeconomic strata; the victims are malnourished, underweight, and grossly emaciated; there is no family history of diabetes mellitus; the patients are resistant to the development of ketosis; the pancreas is found to be fibrotic at autopsy; the etiology appears to be dietary in origin. The victims invariably have consumed large quantities of tapioca which is a cheap cereal substitute. This root appears to contain cyanide, which has been incriminated in the resultant damage to the endocrine pancreas.

The linkage between cyanide ingestion (tapioca), protein–calorie malnutrition, and diabetes appears to be well establised in that part of the world. The similarities between the form of diabetes associated with chronic relapsing pancreatitis and the diabetes associated with malnutrition and tapioca ingestion in southern India would suggest that toxic dietary substances might contribute to the type of diabetes that is found to develop in patients with cystic fibrosis. One might speculate that possible toxicity of various forms of therapy or deficiency states of trace minerals may be contributory toward beta-cell dysfunction. Further research in these areas might be productive.

Summation

The type of glucose intolerance and insulin dependence which develops in patients with cystic fibrosis is undoubtedly different from the usual forms of type I and type II diabetes melitus which are prevalent today and are genetically determined. The exact classification of diabetes associated with cystic fibrosis remains undetermined and may be placed either in the category of diabetes associated with genetic disorders or in the category of diabetes associated secondarily with pancreatic failure. The genetic forms of diabetes (type I, type II), however, are not associated with alpha-cell failure. The diabetes of cystic fibrosis appears to develop in those patients with the most serious forms of cystic fibrosis and pancreatic fibrosis and is accompanied by a failure of both alpha-cell and beta-cell function. We would prefer to include it in the category of "secondary diabetes" which includes chronic relapsing pancreatitis and the pancreatic diabetes of southern India.

Management of Glucose Intolerance

Apparently most clinics managing cystic fibrosis patients do not treat the various forms of glucose intolerance unless a definitive need for insulin control is present. We would suggest that a search for glucose intolerance be conducted on each patient by first obtaining routine glycosylated hemoglobin values, and when elevated, then instructing the families to test for glycosuria 2 hr after meals. If abnormal glucose tolerance is found, then treatment with oral hypoglycemic agents or insulin may be considered. The exact percentage of response to oral agents is presently unknown. Those patients who require insulin may need doses in excess of the usual child with type I diabetes mellitus, and the matter of peripheral insulin resistance has not been clarified. Few patients with insulin-dependent diabetes and cystic fibrosis have been reported, and none in detail.

Almost none of the patients live long enough to develop the vascular complications seen in the genetic forms of diabetes mellitus. The absence of ketoacidosis and vascular complications appears to have influenced the management of glucose intolerance in patients with cystic fibrosis, alleviating concern. Patients with type I (JOD) diabetes mellitus may suffer from increased susceptibility to bacterial infection and fungal infestation if hyperglycemia is poorly controlled. It would seem logical to conclude that high glucose content in the entrapped secretions of the lung in children with cystic fibrosis would predispose to these infectious complications and therefore it seems logical to suggest a more vigorous approach to discovery and control of postprandial hyperglycemia and diabetes mellitus in children with cystic fibrosis.

REFERENCES

1. Jost A: Fetal hormones and fetal growth, in Zondek T, Zondek LH (eds): *Fetal Endocrinology, Contributions to Gynecology and Obstetrics, Vol. 5.* London, S. Karger,1979, pp 1–20.
2. Boyer PH: Low birth weight in fibrocystic disease of the pancreas. *Pediatrics* 1955;76: 778–784.
3. Lloyd-Still JD, Hurwitz I, Wolff PH, et al: Intellectual development after severe malnutrition in infancy. *Pediatrics* 1974;54: 306–311.
4. Hill DE: Insulin and fetal growth, in New MI, Fiser RH (eds): *Diabetes and Other Endocrine Disorders During Pregnancy and in the Newborn.* New York, AR Liss, 1976, pp 127–139.
5. Pagliara AS, Karl IE, Kipnis DB: Transient neonatal diabetes; delayed maturation of the pancreatic beta cells. *J Pediatr* 1973;82:97–101.
6. Hirsch J, Farquhar JW, Ahrens EH Jr, et al: Studies of adipose tissue in man. *Am J Clin Nutr* 1960;8:499–511.
7. Sproul A, Huang N: Growth patterns in children with cystic fibrosis. *J Pediatr* 1964;65: 664–675.
8. Salmon WD Jr, Daughaday WH: A hormonally controlled serum factor which stimulates sulfate incorporation by cartilage in vitro. *J Lab Clin Med* 1957;49:825–836.
9. Van Wyk JJ, Underwood LE, Hintz RL, et al: The somatomedins: A family of insulin-like hormones under growth hormone control. *Rec Prog Horm Res* 1974;30:259–294.
10. Kemp SF, Rosenfeld RG, Liu F, et al: Acute somatomedin response to growth hormone: Radioreceptor assay versus radioimmunoassay. *J Clin Endocrinol Metab* 1981;52: 616–621.
11. Phillips LS, Vassilopoulou-Sellin R: Medical progress. Somatomedins. *N Engl J Med* 1980;302:371–380, 438–466.
12. Berlowitz M, Szabo M, Frohman LA, et al: Somatomedin-C mediates growth hormone negative feedback by effects on both the hypothalamus and the pituitary. *Science* 1981; 212:1279–1281.
13. Pimstone BL, Wittman W, Hansen JDL, et al: Growth hormone and kwashiorkor. Role of protein in growth hormone homeostasis. *Lancet* 1966;2:779–780.
14. Hintz RL, Suskind R, Amatayakul K, et al: Plasma somatomedin and growth hormone values in children with protein–calorie malnutrition. *J Pediatr* 1978;92:153–156.
15. Laron Z, Pertzelan A, Karp M, et al: Administration of growth hormone to patients with familial dwarfism with high plasma immunoreactive growth hormone: Measurement of sulfation factor, metabolic and linear growth responses. *J Clin Endocrinol Metab* 1971;33:332–342.
16. Wu A, Grant DB, Hambley J, et al: Reduced serum somatomedin activity in patients with chronic liver disease. *Clin Sci Mol Med* 1974;47:359–366.
17. Gluckman PD, Brinsmead MW: Somatomedin in cord blood: Relationship to gestational age and birth size. *J Clin Endocrinol Metab* 1976;43:1378–1381.
18. Ellis CE, Hill DE: Growth, intelligence and school performance in children with cystic fibrosis who have had an episode of malnutrition during infancy. *J Pediatr* 1975;87: 565–568.
19. Barclay RPC, Shannon RS: Trial of artificial diet in treatment of cystic fibrosis of pancreas. *Arch Dis Child* 1975;50:490–493.
20. Dooley RR, Moss AJ, Wright PM, et al: Norethandrolone in cystic fibrosis of the pancreas. *J Pediatr* 1969;74:95–102.
21. Dennis JL, Panos TC: Growth and bone-age retardation in cystic fibrosis. Response to an anabolic steroid. *JAMA* 1965;194:855–858.
22. Green OC, Fefferman R, Nair S: Plasma growth hormone levels in children with cystic fibrosis and short stature. Unresponsiveness to hypoglycemia. *J Clin Endocrinol Metab* 1967;27:1059–1061.
23. Biswas S, Norman AP, Baffoe G, et al: Prolactin, growth hormone and alpha-fetoprotein in children with cystic fibrosis. *Clin Chim Acta* 1976;69:541–542.
24. Handwerger S, Roth J, Gordon P, et al: Glucose intolerance in cystic fibrosis. *N Engl J Med* 1969;281:451–461.
25. Milunski A, Bray GA, Londono J, et al: Insulin, glucose, growth hormone and free fatty acids. Determinations in patients with cystic fibrosis. *Am J Dis Child* 1971; 121:15–19.
26. Lee JA, Dickinson LS, Kilgore BS, et al: Somatomedin activity in cystic fibrosis and reserpinized rats: Possible explanation for

growth retardation. *Ann Clin Lab Sci* 1980; 10:227–233.

27. Landon C, Rosenfeld RG, Hintz R., et al: Plasma somatomedin in cystic fibrosis adolescents is normal. *Pediatr Res* 1981;15: 634(A).
28. di Sant'Agnese PA, Davis PB: Cystic fibrosis in adults. 75 cases and a review of 232 cases in the literature. *Am J Med* 1979;66:121–129.
29. Knobil E: Patterns of hormonal signals and hormone action. *N Engl J Med* 1981;305: 1582–1583.
30. Green OC: Anabolic agents and childhood growth. Discussion of growth phases and significance of appropriate therapy. *Ohio State Med J* 1962;58:677–680.
31. Green OC: Sizing up the small child. *Postgrad Med* 1971;50:103–109.
32. Mitchell-Heggs P, Mearns M, Batten JC: Cystic fibrosis in adolescents and adults. *Q J Med* 1976;45:479–504.
33. Holsclaw DS, Perlmutter AD, Jockin H, et al: Genital abnormalities in male patients with cystic fibrosis. *J Urol* 1971;106:568–574.
34. Rosen SW, Weintraub BD: Monotropic increase of serum FSH correlated with low sperm count in young men with idiopathic oligospermia and aspermia. *J Clin Endocrinol Metab* 1971;32:410–416.
35. Denning CR, Sommers SC, Quigley HJ Jr: Infertility in male patients with cystic fibrosis. *Pediatrics* 1968;41:7–17.
36. Kaplan E, Shwachman H, Perlmutter AD, et al: Reproductive failure in males with cystic fibrosis. *N Engl J Med* 1968;279:65–69.
37. Taussig LM, Lobeck CC, di Sant'Agnese PA, et al: Fertility in males with cystic fibrosis. *N Engl J Med* 1972;287:586–589.
38. Frisch RE, McArthur JW: Menstrual cycles: Fatness as a determinant of minimum weight for height necessary for their maintenance or onset. *Science* 1974;185:949–951.
39. Moshang T, Holsclaw DS: Menarchal determinants in cystic fibrosis. *Am J Dis Child* 1980;134:1379–1412.
40. Oppenheimer E, Esterly JR: Observations in cystic fibrosis of the pancreas. VI. The uterine cervix. *J Pediatr* 1970;77:991–995.
41. Grand RJ, Talamo RC, di Sant'Agnese PA, et al: Pregnancy in cystic fibrosis of the pancreas. *JAMA* 1966;195:993–1000.
42. Cohen LF, di Sant'Agnese PA, Friedlander J: Cystic fibrosis and pregnancy. A national survey. *Lancet* 1980;2:842–844.
43. Flensborg EW, Johnsen SG: Significant changes in two 17-ketosteroid factors in cystic fibrosis. *Acta Paediatr Scand* 1972;61–62: 382.
44. Gray CE, Hamilton W: Excretion of dehydroepiandosterone in cystic fibrosis. *Acta Paediatr Scand* 1971;60:617.
45. Montalvo JM, McCaa CS, Cole WQ: Aldosterone metabolism in children with cystic fibrosis and their parents. *J Clin Endocrinol Metab* 1968;28:582–585.
46. Rapaport R, Levine LS, Petrovic M, et al: The renin–aldosterone system in cystic fibrosis. *J Pediatr* 1981;98:768–771.
47. Flensborg EW: Investigation of the effects of testosterone, dehydroepiandosterone, and dianabol on the electrolytes in the sweat in children with cystic fibrosis. *Acta Paediatr Scand* 1972;61:380–381.
48. Schaffner F, Popper H: Causation and consequences of cholestasis: An overview, in Goresky CA, Fisher MM (eds): *Jaundice.* New York, Plenum Press, 1974, pp 329–349.
49. Johnson FL, Lerner KG, Siegel M, et al: Association of androgenic–anabolic steroid therapy with development of hepatocellular carcinoma. *Lancet* 1972;2:1273–1276.
50. Abraham EH, Gerdes JS, Castillo RG, et al: Vitamin D deficiency rickets with abnormal liver function tests and myopathy as the presenting manifestations of cystic fibrosis. *Pediatr Res* 1981;15:625(A).
51. Simopoulos AP, Taussig LM, Murad F, et al: Parathyroid function in patients with cystic fibrosis (CF). *Pediatr Res* 1972;6:355(A).
52. Ruben BL, Crigler JF Jr, Berenberg W, et al: Hypothyroidism: A complication of iodide therapy in children with chronic respiratory involvement of cystic fibrosis. *Am J Dis Child* 1960;100:721–722.
53. Dolan TF, Gibson LE: Complications of iodide therapy in patients with cystic fibrosis. *J Pediatr* 1971;79:684–687.
54. Azizi F, Bentley D, Vagerakis A, et al: Abnormal thyroid function and response to iodides in patients with cystic fibrosis. *Trans Assoc Am Physicians* 1974;87:111.
55. Segall-Blank M, Vagerakis AG, Shwachman H, et al: Thyroid gland function and pituitary TSH reserve in patients with cystic fibrosis. *J Pediatr* 1981;98:218–222.
56. Moseley AJ, Fitzhugh FW, Hughes J, et al: Adrenal activity in thyroid dysfunction. *Am J Med* 1950;9:259–260.
57. Means MA, Dobson RL: Cytological changes in the sweat gland in hypothyroidism. *JAMA* 1963;186:113–115.
58. Gullo L, Labo G: Thyrotropic-releasing hormone inhibits pancreatic enzyme secretion in humans. *Gastroenterology* 1981;80: 735–739.
59. Andersen DH: Cystic fibrosis of the pancreas and its relation to celiac disease. *Am J Dis Child* 1938;56:344–399.
60. Wang C-I, Kwok S, Kogut MA: Insulin response to hyperglycemia, epinephrine and

glucagon infusion in cystic fibrosis (CF). *Clin Res* 1973;21:316.
61. Rosan RC, Shwachman H, Kulczycki LL: Diabetes mellitus and cystic fibrosis of the pancreas. *Am J Dis Child* 1962;104:625–634.
62. Lowe CU, May CD, Reed SC: Fibrosis of the pancreas in infants and children. *Am J Dis Child* 1949;78:349–374.
63. Shwachman H, Leubner H, Catzel P: Mucoviscidosis. *Adv Pediatrics* 1955;7:249–323.
64. Larsson Y: The islets of Langerhans in pancreatic fibrosis. *Pediatrics* 1958;21:893–902.
65. Milner AD: Blood glucose and serum insulin levels in children with cystic fibrosis. *Arch Dis Child* 1969;44:351–355.
66. Clodi HP, Pfeiffer EF: Mechanism of glucose intolerance in cystic fibrosis. *N Engl J Med* 1970;282:455–456.
67. Kjellman NIM, Larsson Y: Insulin release in cystic fibrosis. *Arch Dis Child* 1975;50:205–209.
68. Wilmshurst EG, Soeldner JS, Holsclaw DS, et al: Endogenous and exogenous insulin responses in patients with cystic fibrosis. *Pediatrics* 1975;55:75–82.
69. Stahl M, Girard J, Rutishauser M, et al: Endocrine function of the pancreas in cystic fibrosis: evidence for an impaired glucagon and insulin response following arginine infusion *J Pediatr* 1974;84:821–824.
70. Selden RF, Bennett MJ, Paulsen EP: Evidence for altered beta cell sensitivity to stimuli as a basis for poor insulin release in cystic fibrosis. *Cystic Fibrosis Club Abstr* 1976;17:17.
71. Lippe BM, Sperling MA, Dooley RR: Pancreatic alpha and beta cell function in cystic fibrosis. *J Pediatr* 1977;90:751–755.
72. Josefsburg Z, Flateau E, Doron M, et al: The influence of oral glucose loading on the insulin response to IV glucagon in children and adolescents. *Metabolism* 1976;25:277–280.
73. Fajans SS, Conn JW: Tolbutamide-induced improvement in carbohydrate tolerance of young people with mild diabetes mellitus. *Diabetes* 1960;9:83–88.
74. Mutch WJ, Stowers JM: Reversible mild diabetes in children after treatment with chlorpropamide. *Lancet* 1980;1:1158–1161.
75. Lippe BM, Kaplan SA, Neufeld ND, et al: Insulin receptors in cystic fibrosis: increased receptor number and altered affinity. *Pediatrics* 1980;65:1018–1022.
76. Drezner M, Neelon FA, Lebovitz HE: Pseudohypoparathyroidism type II: A possible defect in the reception of the cyclic AMP signal. *N Engl J Med* 1973;289:1060–1063.
77. Zimmerman D, Green OC: Nephrogenic diabetes insipidus type II. Defect distal to the adenylate cyclase step. *Pediatr Res* 1975;9:381(A).
78. Muller WA, Faloona GR, Unger RE: Hyperglucagonemia in diabetic ketoacidosis: Its prevalence and significance. *Am J Med* 1973; 54:52–57.
79. Peden VH, Powell KR, Rejent AJ: Glucose intolerance in a three-year-old child with cystic fibrosis. *Clin Pediatr* 1974;13:10–15.
80. Koenig RJ, Peterson CM, Jones RL, et al: Correlation of glucose regulation and hemoglobin $A1_C$ in diabetes mellitus. *N Engl J Med* 1976;295:417–420.
81. Spicer KM, Allen RC, Hallett D, et al: Synthesis of hemoglobin $A1_C$ and related minor hemoglobins by erythrocytes. In vitro study of regulation. *J Clin Invest* 1979;64:40–48.
82. Paulsen EP, Koury M: Hemoglobin $A1_C$ levels in insulin-dependent and -independent diabetes mellitus. *Diabetes* 1976;25(Suppl): 890–896.
83. Rosenbloom AL, Giordano' BP: Chronic overtreatment with insulin in children and adolescents. *Am J Dis Child* 1977;131:881–885.
84. Trapnell JE: Patterns of pancreatitis in Great Britain—with special reference to diabetes, in Podolsky S, Viswanathan M (eds): *Secondary Diabetes. The Spectrum of the Diabetic Syndromes.* New York, Raven Press, 1980, pp 77–88.
85. Vinik AI, Jackson WPU: Endocrine secretions in chronic pancreatitis, in Podolsky S, Viswanathan M (eds): *Secondary Diabetes: The Spectrum of the Diabetes Syndromes.* New York, Raven Press, 1980, pp 165–189.
86. Viswanathan M: Pancreatic diabetes in India: An overview, in Podolsky S, Viswanathan M (eds): *Secondary Diabetes: The Spectrum of the Diabetic Syndromes.* New York, Raven Press, 1980, pp 105–116.

20

Cystic Fibrosis in Adults

Pamela B. Davis

The need for a special chapter on adults with cystic fibrosis (CF) is in itself a kind of therapeutic triumph. When CF was first described in 1938, less than half its victims survived their first year. As recently as 1968, only 50% of the children born with CF in this country were expected to survive their 11th year, but by 1979 over half were expected to survive their 20th. Warwick and Pogue[1] estimate that if no improvements are made in case finding or survival, the equilibrium population of adults with CF in the United States will be 7000; however, if all patients with CF could be identified and mortality reduced by 50%, this population would number 54,000. This sizable population of patients with chronic and ultimately fatal illness cannot fail to have significant impact on the adult health-care delivery system. The unrecognized adults with CF provide us with diagnostic challenges, and the special, somewhat different character of CF in adults challenges us to extend our therapeutic strategies. This chapter will discuss making the diagnosis of CF in the adult, the character of CF in adult patients, the special complications of CF in adults, and the challenges of providing excellent care for the adult with CF (Figure 20-1).

DIAGNOSIS OF CYSTIC FIBROSIS IN ADULTS

The diagnosis of cystic fibrosis in adults, as in children, rests on demonstration of elevated sweat sodium and chloride in conjunction with chronic pulmonary disease,

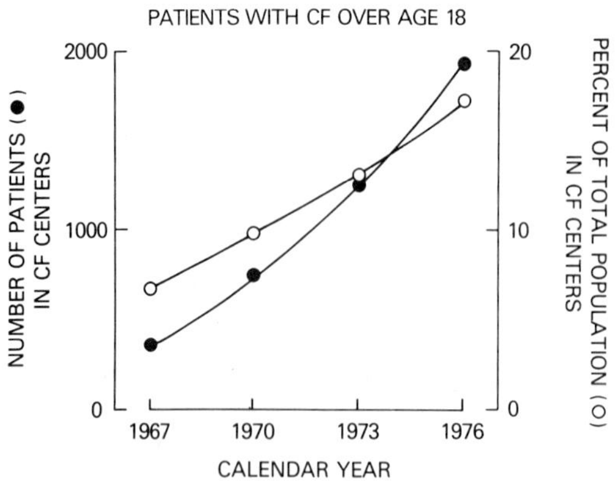

Figure 20-1 Patients with cystic fibrosis over the age of 18 years who are registered in Cystic Fibrosis Foundation-recognized centers. Graph shows actual number of patients (•) and proportion of adults in total CF population (○). Data are taken from Cystic Fibrosis Foundation patient registry.

pancreatic insufficiency, or both. The abnormal sweat chloride must occur in the appropriate clinical context for the diagnosis to be established, and conversely, even typical pulmonary and pancreatic disease must be associated with abnormal sweat electrolytes for a confirmed diagnosis of CF.

Although over 95% of new diagnoses of CF are made in children,[2] among those who reach age 18, over one fifth were diagnosed after the age of 15. Since patients diagnosed in adolescence or adulthood tend to be taller and heavier than those diagnosed earlier in life,[3] and most adults with CF ultimately achieve height and weight in the normal range,[3-5] normal stature should not deter evaluation for CF if other suggestive features are present. In adults, the etiologic spectrum of chronic obstructive pulmonary disease and pancreatic insufficiency is quite extensive, but because of the therapeutic, prognostic, and genetic implications of a diagnosis of CF, as well as its increasing prevalence, it is essential to maintain a high index of suspicion when adults present with symptoms compatible with CF.

The patterns of presentation of CF in adults are as protean as the disease itself. Respiratory complaints most often bring the patient to the physician's attention. Recurrent nasal polyposis and sinusitis or, more frequently, recurrent lower respiratory infections, chronic cough, or stubborn and atypical "asthma" are initial complaints. Symptoms directly referable to pancreatic insufficiency rarely begin in adulthood, but intestinal obstruction due to fecal impaction or intussusception (often initially misdiagnosed as periappendiceal abscess) may be the presenting complaint. Patients with some retained pancreatic function may present with pancreatitis. Occasionally, hepatic disease overshadows the involvement of other organs, and the patient presents with cirrhosis. A few individuals have no somatic symptoms and are identified in the course of evaluating siblings of a known patient with CF or, for some men, in the course of evaluation for infertility.[6]

Sweat Gland Involvement

The first part of the classical diagnostic triad for CF is the sweat electrolyte abnormality; demonstration of elevated sweat chloride has become the sine qua non for the diagnosis of CF. When properly performed, the sweat test has excellent discriminant power. False negatives are exceedingly rare and generally limited to acutely ill, edematous patients whose sweat chlorides revert to typical elevated values upon clinical recovery.[7] We have estimated, from available data in the literature, that fewer than one in 1000 CF patients has sweat chloride less than 50 mEq/liter and only 1–2% have chlorides between 50 and 60 mEq/liter.[8] Patients with normal exocrine pancreatic function tend to have lower sweat chlorides than those with full-blown pancreatic insufficiency, and many of the "borderline" values (50–60 mEq/liter) occur among these patients.[8] Over 98% of patients with CF have sweat chlorides greater than 60 mEq/liter. Very few healthy children (less than one in 1000) have sweat chlorides greater than 60 mEq/liter. The rare false-positive results occur in conditions readily distinguished clinically from CF, such as untreated adrenal insufficiency or nephrogenic diabetes insipidus.[99] Thus the sweat test is a remarkably good discriminant for CF in children.

However, normal adults have higher sweat chloride levels than normal children, and these values may overlap the CF range.[9] Elevated sweat chlorides have been reported to be particularly prevalent among adults with chronic bronchitis,[10] pancreatic insufficiency,[11] and obligate heterozygotes for cystic fibrosis,[10] precisely the groups for which the discriminant value of the sweat test is most important. Other series, however, indicate that the standard sweat test does retain its discriminant power in adults. Sekelj et al[12] analyzed unstimulated sweat from the hand for chloride content with an Orion electrode in 649 normal adults, 491 patients with chronic obstructive pulmonary disease, 355 patients with nonobstructive pulmonary disease, and other subjects with medical problems. Values greater than 40 mEq/liter were rechecked by the standard pilocarpine iontophoresis technique. All subjects had sweat sodium and chloride less than 65 mEq/liter, and 99% were below 50 mEq/liter. Jones[13] found that fewer than 5% of the 473 non-CF patients of all ages, including obligate heterozygotes for Cf, and patients with asthma and other pulmonary diseases, had sweat sodium >60 mEq/liter. Sweating was induced by pilocarpine iontophoresis and sodium measured by flame photometry. Two recent reports show that the standard pilocarpine iontophoresis sweat test with measurement of sodium and chloride separated a total of 130 diseased and healthy adults from 145 adults with CF almost without overlap[3,14] (Figure 20-2). Most cystic fibrosis centers encounter little practical difficulty in separating CF from non-CF adult populations with the standard pilocarpine iontophoresis sweat test method of Gibson and Cooke[15] (see Chapter 4).

The sweat electrolyte abnormality has clinical implications in addition to diagnostic significance: patients with CF suffer serious salt loss during periods of heavy sweating. Although infants are most susceptible to this complication because of their high surface area-to-volume ratio, young men who exercise vigorously in hot weather without adequate salt and water intake also appear to be at risk. Episodes of heat prostration were reported in 5% of American adult CF patients[3] (Table 20-1). Since cardiovascular collapse and death may follow soon after the first symptoms of salt depletion (listlessness and vomiting), rapid intravenous infusion of physiologic saline is essential. It is preferable to avoid the problem altogether by administering extra salt during periods of heavy sweating.

Pancreatic Disease

Pancreatic insufficiency is the second part of the classical diagnostic triad for cystic fibrosis. Its presence is usually established by noninvasive tests such as determination of elevated fecal fat excretion[16] or absence or marked reduction of the pancreatic isozyme of amylase in the serum.[17] However, if pancreatic status is in doubt and definitive determination is required, analysis of the trypsin, chymotrypsin, amylase, lipase, and bicarbonate content of the pancreatic secretion

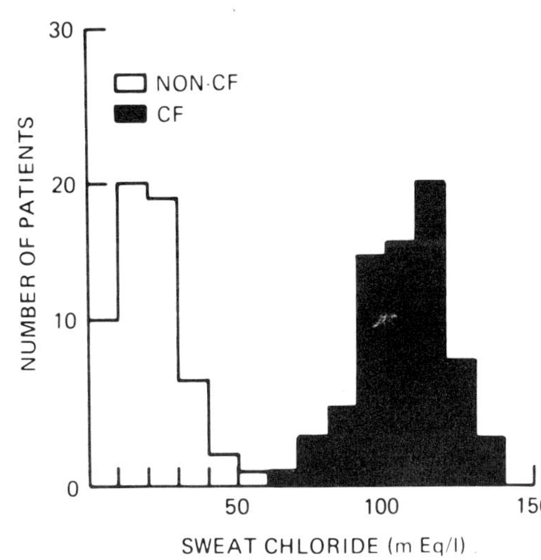

Figure 20-2 Distribution of values for sweat chloride in 75 adult patients with CF and 60 persons age 18–62 years old who do not have CF. Some of the non-CF group are healthy and some have other diseases such as diabetes mellitus, systemic lupus erythematosus, or chronic bronchitis.

Table 20-1
Complications of Cystic Fibrosis in Adolescents and Adults*

Complication	Number Affected†	Percent
Pulmonary disease	198/203	98
Hemoptysis		
Minor	147/286	52
Massive	18/234	8
Pneumothorax	47/280	17
Nasal polyps	114/280	41
Pancreatic insufficiency	156/165	95
Glycosuria	28/311	9
Intestinal obstruction	48/280	17
Cirrhosis	13/311	4
Heat prostration	7/145	5
Arthropathy	13/158	8

*Six series giving information about adolescent and adult patients were reviewed and the findings tabulated. The series were: di Sant'Agnese and Davis,[3] 75 patients over 18 yr; Shwachman et al,[14] 70 patients over 25 yr; Mitchell-Heggs et al,[4] 45 patients over 14 yr; Gracey and Anderson,[95] 31 patients over 12 yr; Howie and Stack,[96] 13 patients over 13 yr; Holsclaw,[73] 77 patients over 17 yr. Total, 311 patients.
†Denominator is total number patients for whom data are available; numerator is number affected.

before and after secretin stimulation remains the procedure of choice.[18,19] Although in a few patients with CF, the pancreas is histologically normal,[20] degeneration is progressive,[21] and most patients have anatomic pancreatic involvement by adulthood. Entirely normal pancreatic function is rare;[22] patients with normal pancreatic enzyme secretion are usually deficient in basal and secretin-stimulated bicarbonate secretion.[19,22] About 95% of adults have pancreatic insufficiency[3] (Table 20-1), compared to 80–90% for patients of all ages.[23] The deterioration of pancreatic function may be marked by recurrent episodes of pancreatitis.[24] In fact, some adults present in this manner, and unexplained recurrent pancreatitis should be an indication for sweat testing. In adulthood, although steatorrhea and azotorrhea continue unabated, symptoms directly referable to pancreatic insufficiency subside and unrestricted diet is usually well-tolerated.[3,16] Rectal prolapse is rare. However, since pancreatic insufficiency and malabsorption may contribute to the development of cholelithiasis,[25] intestinal obstructve complications,[26] nutritional deficiency,[27] and possibly to the progression of pulmonary disease as well,[100] pancreatic enzyme supplements should be continued in adults even though they may not be needed for symptomatic relief.

Respiratory Disease

The third member of the diagnostic triad for CF is chronic pulmonary disease, which is the major cause of morbidity and nearly the sole cause of mortality in adults. As in the child, this disease is chronic, suppurative, progressive, and eventually leads to bronchitis, bronchiectasis, respiratory insufficiency, cor pulmonale, and death. Only 2% of adults with CF lacked evidence of pulmonary disease by history or on chest roentgenogram or pulmonary function tests[3] (Table 20-1). Experience indicates that even these individuals will eventually develop pulmonary disease.

The pattern of disease in CF, with recurrent respiratory infections, may suggest disorders of the pulmonary defense mechanisms, and the differential diagnosis includes immunoglobulin deficiencies, immotile cilia syndrome, neutrophil or complement abnormalities, or even α_1-antitrypsin deficiency. Episodic exacerbations may suggest asthma, and the suppurative nature of the disease may suggest bronchiectasis of other etiologies. However, the roentgenographic, physiologic, and microbiologic features of the pulmonary disease in CF, taken together, constitute a distinctive pattern.

Chest Roentgenograms Typically, the chest x-ray in CF is abnormal before chronic respiratory symptoms appear. Table 20-2 summarizes the roentgenographic findings. Increased interstitial markings are seen on the roentgenograms of more than 98% of adults with CF. Cystic-bronchiectatic changes with ring shadows and honeycombing occur in 68%. Hyperinflation is common (about 67%) in adults and, unlike that in children, is invariably accompanied by parenchymal abnormalities. Other common findings include mucus plugging and lobar atelectasis. The right lung is involved more severely and more often than the left, and the upper lobes more so than the lower (Figure 20-3).

The chest roentgenogram in cystic fibrosis, with its upper lobe predominance and increased interstitial markings, may resemble that of tuberculosis, sarcoidosis, or eosinophilic granuloma. The cystic–bronchiectatic changes and mucus plugging may suggest bronchopulmonary aspergillosis or bronchiectasis of other etiologies. Hyperinflation and increased interstitial markings may suggest asthma, asthmatic bronchitis, or α_1-antitrypsin deficiency. These differential diagnoses can usually be eliminated by correlating the x-ray with history, pulmonary function tests, sputum flora, and of course, sweat chloride.

Pulmonary function tests As many as 10–15% of adults with cystic fibrosis may have normal routine spirometry,[3,28] although small-airways disease may be detected on more sensitive tests. Pulmonary function may remain normal for long periods of time, but deterioration is inevitable, and once begun, proceeds in an exponential fashion.[5,29,30] Although a few patients early in the course, may display a predominantly restrictive ventilatory defect, most patients develop an obstructive ventilatory impairment.[3,28,30] The forced expiratory volume in one second is strongly correlated with prognosis.[31] The diffusing capacity (corrected for age, alveolar volume, and hemoglobin) is normal or elevated until late in the course of the disease.[3] The P_AO_2 may remain in the normal range for long periods at the expense of hyperventilation; the a-AO_2 gradient is frequently widened. Hypercapnia is a late consequence of the CF pulmonary disease and is a poor prognostic sign.[3,31]

Table 20-2
Findings on Chest Roentgenogram in Adults with CF*

Abnormality	Number†	Percent
Increased interstitial markings	244/250	98
Cystic-bronchiectatic changes	169/250	68
Hyperinflation	165/250	66
Mucus plugging	24/75	32
Lobar atelectasis	50/250	20
None	4/200	2

*Four series giving x-ray information about adults with CF were reviewed and findings tabulated. The series were: di Sant'Agnese and Davis,[3] 75 patients over age 18 yr; Shwachman et al,[14] 70 patients over 25 yr; Schwartz and Holsclaw,[97] 55 patients over 17 yr; Friedman and Harwood,[98] 50 patients over 17 yr. Total 250 patients. †Denominator is total number of patients for whom data are available; numerator is number affected.

Sputum bacteriology Patients with CF have a chronic bacterial bronchitis which is never eradicated, even with intensive antibiotic therapy, and which contributes to progressive deterioration of pulmonary function. The most frequent offending organisms are *Staphylococcus aureus, Hemophilus influenzae,* and *Pseudomonas aeruginosa.*[3,32] The association of CF and *Pseudomonas aeruginosa* is particularly striking: over half the strains recovered from CF patients are mucoid, in contrast to less than 2% of strains recovered from non-CF patients.[33,34] Moreover, a single serotype, Homma 8, predominates.[34] Recovery of this organism from the respiratory tree suggests the diagnosis of cystic fibrosis.[35] The prevalence of *Pseudomonas aeruginosa* in sputum cultures from CF patients increases with age. Fink et al[28] report that the incidence of *Pseudomonas* recovery increased from age 18 to age 25 and reached 100% by age 28. similarly, Mitchell-Heggs et al[4] reported that during their 4½ year study, 10 of 45 adolescent and adult patients acquired *Pseudomonas aeruginosa* in their sputum, and none lost it. Discriminant analysis also indicates that the presence of *Pseudomonas aeruginosa* in the sputum is a poor prognostic sign.[36] The same study found that *Staphylococcus aureus* in addition to *Pseudomonas aeruginosa* in the sputum culture is a much less unfavorable prognostic indicator, but recovery of *Hemophilus influenzae* is an unfavorable prognostic sign.

Other gram-negative rods, such as *Escherichia coli, Pseudomonas cepacia, Pseudomonas maltophilia, Proteus,* or mucoid

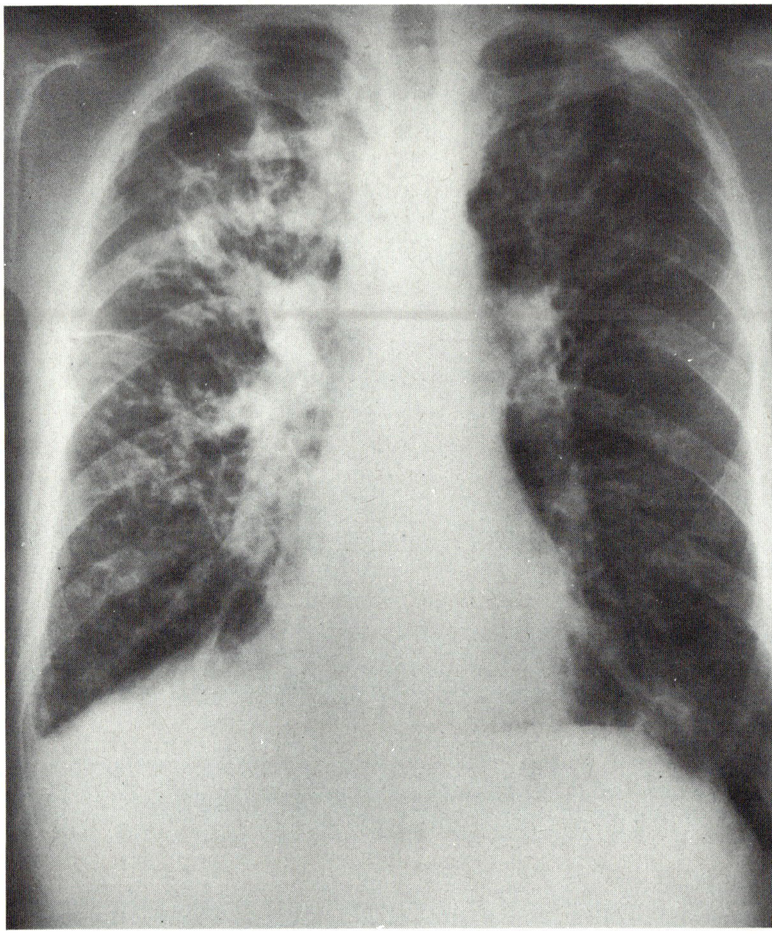

Figure 20-3 Chest roentgenograms of a 27-year-old man with cystic fibrosis illustrating increased markings, cystic-bronchiectatic changes, and hyperinflation: **A** Posteroanterior view.

Klebsiella species may be recovered from the sputum of adults with CF.[3,4,28,37] However, *Pseudomonas aeruginosa, Staphylococcus aureus,* and *Hemophilus influenzae* remain the principal pathogens for adults with CF, and with advancing age, *Pseudomonas* gradually supplants the others.

Pulmonary disease in CF and chronic bronchitis/emphysema As more patients with cystic fibrosis reach adulthood, comparison of their pulmonary disease with that of the chronic bronchitis/emphysema or chronic obstructive pulmonary disease patient is inevitable[38] (Table 20-3). The diseases share several features. Hypertrophy and hyperplasia of the mucus-secreting apparatus is prominent, and this leads to chronic productive cough. The pulmonary physiology is obstructive in both diseases, and prognosis is strongly related to the forced expiratory volume in one second.[31] Small-airways disease may be detected early in the course in both disorders, and air trapping and diminished flows are seen later. Hypoxemia and, eventually, respiratory insufficiency, cor pulmonale, and death result.

However, there are important differences between these two obstructive pulmonary diseases. CF is the direct consequence of an unknown genetic error, which causes abnormal mucus production and persistent respiratory infection. Despite therapy, progressive deterioration and respiratory death follow. Emphysema and chronic bronchitis, on the other hand, are produced largely by the host's response to chronic exposure to ir-

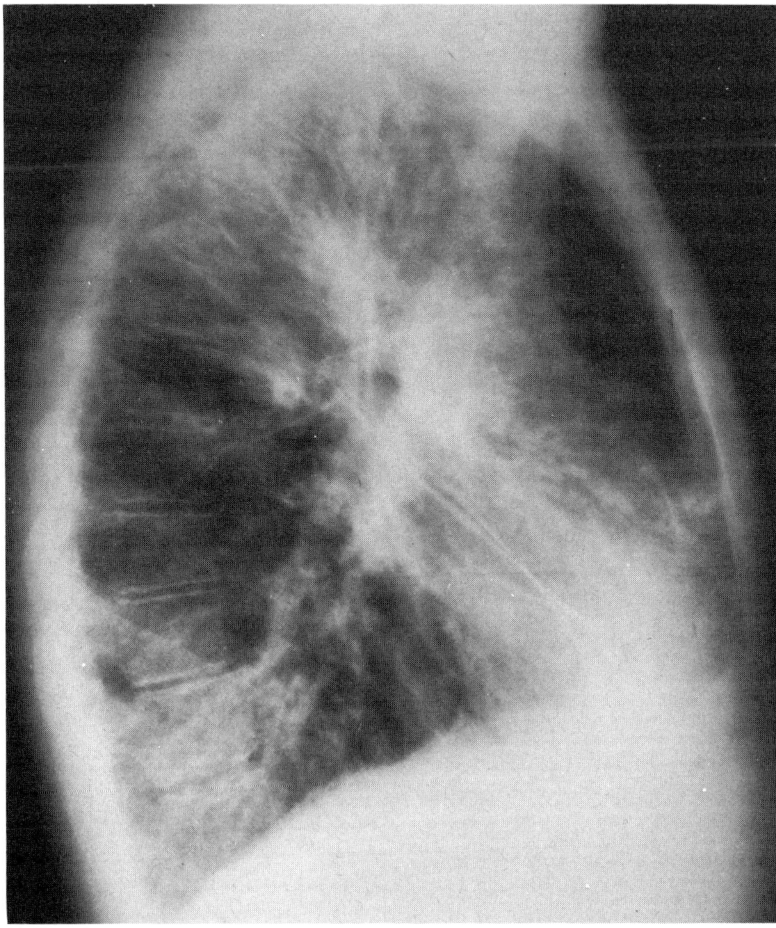

Figure 20-3B Lateral view.

ritants (usually tobacco smoke), although genetic predispositions to obstructive pulmonary disease almost certainly play some role in most patients and a substantial role in others (eg, α_1-antitrypsin deficiency). Sometimes, the emphysema/chronic bronchitis patient can retard or even arrest the progress of his disease by quitting smoking. Also, since serious pulmonary disease occurs later in life in chronic obstructive pulmonary disease, deaths unrelated to respiratory disease are frequent. Pathologically, in CF, initial lesions of bronchiolitis and bronchitis give way to bronchiectasis with little true emphysema but considerable anatomic alteration in pulmonary vasculature. In contrast, bronchiectasis is rare in chronic bronchitis/emphysema, but anatomic emphysema is common and extensive. The pulmonary vasculature is less prominently involved than is the case in cystic fibrosis. In CF, chronic bacterial bronchitis, never eradicated despite intensive therapy, undoubtedly contributes to the progression of the pulmonary lesion. Two organisms, *Staphylococcus aureus* and mucoid *Pseudomonas aeruginosa,* predominate. In contrast, in the emphysema/chronic bronchitis patient, *Streptococcus pneumoniae* and *Hemophilus influenzae* are most frequently recovered, and their role in the progression of the disease is uncertain.[39]

Because of these differences in etiology and pathophysiology, the preferred therapies are different. In CF, the chief objectives are to combat infection and remove

Table 20-3
Comparison of CF and Chronic Bronchitis

	Cystic Fibrosis	Chronic Bronchitis
Etiology	Genetic	Environmental; genetic predisposition
Pathology	Bronchiolitis, bronchitis, bronchiectasis	Bronchiolitis, bronchitis, emphysema
Physiology	Obstructive	Obstructive
Sputum flora	*S. aureus, Ps. aeruginosa*	*S. pneumoniae, H. influenzae*
Therapeutic emphasis	Removal of secretions, antibiotics	Bronchodilators, removal of secretions
Complications	Hemoptysis, pneumothorax, atelectasis	Polycythemia, pulmonary embolism
Extrapulmonary manifestations	Many: multisystem exocrinopathy	Few

secretions; antibiotics and postural drainage are therefore the principal therapeutic modalities. In emphysema/chronic bronchitis, the goal is to relieve reversible bronchial obstruction; bronchodilators are the primary treatment. Of course, these therapies are not mutually exclusive; some CF patients benefit from bronchodilators, and some emphysema patients benefit from antibiotics and postural drainage. However, the emphasis in the two disorders is clearly different. In addition, the course of CF is usually one of progressive decline of pulmonary function; by the time frank respiratory failure supervenes there is little reversible disease. Therefore, assisted ventilation is not often indicated for these patients.[40] In chronic bronchitis/emphysema, a course of exacerbation and remission is common, and some patients survive for years after assisted ventilation for respiratory failure.[41]

The complications of the two disorders differ as well. Minor hemoptysis occurs in both diseases, but massive hemoptysis and pneumothorax are much more frequent in CF. Hypoxemia in emphysema/chronic bronchitis is often complicated by polycythemia; this is rare in cystic fibrosis, probably because the chronic suppurative chest disease suppresses erythropoiesis. Lobar or segmental atelectasis is frequent in CF but unusual in emphysema/chronic bronchitis. On the other hand, pulmonary embolism, probably increased in incidence in chronic obstructive pulmonary disease patients, is unusual in cystic fibrosis. Hypertrophic pulmonary osteoarthropathy is probably more frequent in CF than in chronic obstructive pulmonary disease. Retention of CO_2 probably occurs at an earlier stage of disease in chronic bronchitis/emphysema than in CF.[31] Extrapulmonary manifestations of the disease process are, of course, more prominent in CF, a genetic multisystem disease, than in emphysema/chronic bronchitis, which is a primary pulmonary disorder.

Thus while CF and chronic bronchitis/emphysema share some important features, they are very different in others. Adults with CF constitute a special subset of patients with obstructive pulmonary disorders, and warrant special considerations in management.

In summary, the diagnosis of CF is established by elevated sweat chloride levels in a patient with either pancreatic insufficiency, chronic pulmonary disease of appropriate character, or, preferably, both (Table 20-4). Once the presence and nature of pulmonary and pancreatic involvement is established, confirmatory evidence for the diagnosis of CF may be obtained by demonstration of such ancillary findings as azoospermia in males, abnormal sinus roentgenograms, abnormal liver function studies, abnormal oral cholecystogram, or family history of CF.

It is important to diagnose CF correctly because of its genetic and prognostic implications. Siblings of a CF patient have a one in four chance of having the disease; children, one in 40. Knowledge of the correct diagnosis may permit anticipation, prevention, or early treatment of some complications such as heat prostration or intestinal obstructive phenomena. A specific diagnosis of CF is critical for intelligent patient management.

COMPLICATIONS OF CYSTIC FIBROSIS IN ADULTS

Just as making the diagnosis of CF presents special problems in the adult, as discussed above, the character of the disease changes somewhat with advancing age. Some complications appear for the first time in older patients, whereas others become less troublesome in adolescents and adults.

Respiratory Complications

Cor pulmonale In general, cardiac status is related to severity of pulmonary involvement: the more severe the hypoxemia, the worse the pulmonary hypertension and right-sided heart strain.[42] However, echocardiographic changes of increased right ventricular wall thickness and right ventricular dilation are seen even in patients with mild pulmonary disease.[43,44] For comparable degrees of pulmonary disease, adults, especially those with mild lung disease, have more severe echocardiographic abnormalities than the children.[44] This may reflect the cumulative effects of episodes of mild hypoxemia and nocturnal oxygen desaturation which occur even in minimally affected patients. It may be that as clinical experience with adults with CF accumulates, pulmonary hypertension and cor pulmonale may cause substantial difficulties in management (see Chapter 14).

Hemoptysis Even minor hemoptysis is unusual during the first decade of life, but blood streaking of the sputum occurs in over half of adults with CF and requires no specific treatment except that for the underlying pulmonary disease. Massive hemoptysis is also strongly related to age. In one series of 38 patients with massive hemoptysis, only two had their initial episode during the first

Table 20-4
Evaluation for Diagnosis of CF in Adults

Test	Expected Result in CF (% of adults with this result)
Sweat chloride and sodium	>60 mEq/liter (>98%)
Pulmonary evaluation	
Chest x-ray	Abnormal (98%) (see Table 20-2)
Pulmonary function tests	Obstructive ventilatory defect (>80%)
Sputum culture	*Staphylococcus aureus* (51%),* *Pseudomonas aeruginosa* (66%),* *Hemophilus influenzae* (34%)*
Pancreatic evaluation	
Duodenal drainage	Absent or reduced trypsin, chymotrypsin, amylase, lipase (95%)
Secretin test	Reduced HCO_3^- response (99%)
Stool fat	Elevated (95%)
Pancreatic isozyme of amylase in serum	Reduced or absent (95%)
Ancillary investigations	
Sinus x-rays	Abnormal (>95%)
Semen analysis	Azoospermia (>95% of men)

*Figures given are percent recovery of organism from 180 patients reported in four series: di Sant'Agnese and Davis,[3] Fink et al,[28] Mitchell-Heggs et al,[4] and Shwachman et al.[14]

decade of life; 71% were 15 years of age or older.[45] Nearly half the patients had recurrent episodes. Rarely, patients die during such episodes, by either exsanguination or drowning. An earlier report indicated that massive hemoptysis was an extremely poor prognostic indicator,[46] but later studies suggest that the prognosis of affected patients is comparable to that of nonaffected patients with the same degree of pulmonary disease.[3,45]

Because this complication is potentially lethal and frequently recurrent, definitive management, either by resection[3,47] or by Gelfoam embolization of the bleeding vessel,[48] is sometimes undertaken with good reported success. However, conservative management has also been effective.[45] A comparative study of methods of management has not been conducted.

Pneumothorax Pneumothorax also appears to be strongly associated with age. Among a total of 260 patients reported in four series, only one suffered an initial pneumothorax before the age of 10.[3,49-51] In combined series of adults, the incidence is 17%. Pneumothorax is recurrent in over half the cases, and in the two series that provided mortality data, 19% of the patients died during an episode of pneumothorax.[49,50] Because of the gravity of this complication, the persistence of underlying predisposing pulmonary pathology (usually subpleural blebs), and the frequency of recurrence, definitive management is frequently undertaken. Instillation of pleural sclerosing agents has resulted in good success in some centers[52] but most have turned to surgical procedures including pleurectomy, pleural abrasion, and oversewing of ruptured blebs[51,53] (see Chapter 21).

Arthropathy Clubbing is almost universal in patients with cystic fibrosis. Episodes of hypertrophic pulmonary osteoarthropathy, characterized by warmth and tenderness over the distal long bones, with or without effusions of the adjacent joints, and by periosteal elevation on roentgenograms, have been reported in patients with CF ranging in age from 9 to 25, with 7 of 10 patients over the age of 15.[3,54-56] Thus, it is likely that this complication increases in prevalence with advancing age. Pulmonary osteoarthropathy can be disabling for adults. Symptoms often vary in parallel with the pulmonary disease, and treatment of the pulmonary disease may be beneficial, as may salicylates.

Rhinosinusitis Roentgenographic abnormalities of the sinuses have been found in 92–100% of patients with CF of all ages.[3,57,58] The most common abnormality is pansinusitis, but in some cases more limited disease is found. Sinus flora were not correlated with sputum flora.[58] Acute sinusitis is rare. Symptoms are variable and are usually controlled by medical measures. The results of surgical intervention have often been disappointing, with a high recurrence rate.[58]

Nasal polyposis occurs in about 10% of children with CF,[57] compared to 41% of adults in combined series (Table 20-1). Recurrent nasal polyps may be the presenting complaint in previously undiagnosed patients with CF. Polyps tend to be multiple, may block the nasal passages, and tend to recur, sometimes rapidly, after resection,[58] presenting management problems for the adult patient with CF.

Intestinal Obstruction

The prevalence of intestinal obstructive complications in adults with CF is 17% in combined series.[3] The exact pathogenesis of the obstructive complications has not been determined, but the combination of maldigestion due to pancreatic insufficiency and abnormal intestinal gland secretions probably makes the fecal stream semisolid where it should be liquid.[26] Inspissated feces that adhere to the bowel wall may serve as a lead point for intussusception or as an accumulation point for more feces, leading to high fecal impaction, usually at the ileocecal junction (meconium ileus equivalent). The symptoms of these two conditions are similar—crampy abdominal pain and constipation, with or without nausea and vomiting. Even with intussusception, hematochezia is rare, and pain may be mild.

On physical examination, there is usually a tender, tubular mass in the right lower quadrant, although the mass occasionally occurs elsewhere in the abdomen. The intussusception is usually ileocolic, but colo-colic and ileo-ileal intussusceptions are also observed. Abdominal roentgenograms may reveal either a pattern typical of intestinal obstruction with dilated loops of bowel and air-fluid levels, or a nonspecific bowel gas pattern with a peculiar bubbly appearance of feces. The definitive diagnostic and therapeutic test is the Hypaque or Gastrografin enema. In addition to outlining the fecal impaction or the intussusception, these hypertonic enemas draw water into the gut and dislodge inspissated feces, and they help to reduce intussusceptions by hydrostatic pressure. If necessary these enemas may be repeated, with careful attention to fluid and electrolyte balance, until the obstruction is relieved. Although *N*-acetylcysteine by mouth and by enema or pancreatic enzyme supplements by mouth and by enema are occasionally successful, Hypaque or Gastrografin enemas are the treatment of choice.[3]

Surgery should be avoided if possible, for disastrous results may occur in the acute phase,[59] and it may predispose to future difficulties. Manipulation of the inflamed gut can lead to formation of adhesions, providing mechanical barriers that can cause future intestinal obstructions. Surgical reduction of intussusception with plication of ileum to cecum has failed to prevent recurrence.[3] Moreover, if resection is required, this may aggravate the malabsorption and nutritional deficit suffered by CF patients with pancreatic insufficiency. Therefore, conservative therapy is definitely preferable. Surgical intervention may, however, be necessary if the patient appears toxic, develops fever and leukocytosis, or fails to respond to conservative therapy.

Since intestinal obstruction tends to recur,[3] maintenance preventive therapy is indicated after the first episode or when fecal masses are repeatedly identified on physical examination. Large doses of dioctylsodiumsulfosuccinate, maintenance of adequate pancreatic enzyme replacement, or oral *N*-acetylcysteine may be helpful. Even with such prophylaxis, episodes recur in more than half of the patients.

Some adults with previously undiagnosed CF present with intestinal obstruction. These patients, because of their abdominal pain and tender right lower quadrant mass, may be misdiagnosed as having appendicitis or periappendiceal abscess. At surgery the correct diagnosis is suggested by viscid feces in the ileum and, if resection is undertaken, by the histologic appearance of the mucus glands of the appendix.[60] High fecal impaction is unusual in adults who do not have CF and who are not bedridden or immobilized. Similarly, intussusception is rare in adults, although diverticula may serve as lead points. Thus intussusception or high fecal impaction in young adults in the absence of other predisposing factors should arouse suspicion of CF.

Conversely, the frequency of right lower quadrant masses and abdominal pain in adults with CF may unduly divert suspicion from the appendix. Occasionally, periappendiceal abscess, subacute because of antibiotic therapy for lung disease, escapes detection for long periods in patients with CF.

Liver Disease

A distinctive type of focal biliary cirrhosis characterized by eosinophilic concretions in portal bile ductules, bile duct proliferation, inflammatory infiltrates, and sometimes scattered fibrosis is seen in CF necropsy specimens in over one fourth of patients.[61] Only a few patients (2–5%), however, go on to develop multilobular cirrhosis and exhibit the signs and symptoms of portal hypertension, such as ascites, varices, and hypersplenism, or the signs and symptoms of hepatic failure such as hypoalbuminemia, hypoprothrombinemia, and encephalopathy. Hepatic failure, accompanied by gastrointestinal hemorrhage, accounts for nearly all the nonpulmonary deaths due to cystic fibrosis beyond infancy. Portal-systemic shunting may be beneficial, and encephalopathy following shunting has not been a major problem.[62,63] The prevalence of focal and generalized cirrhosis probably increases with age[64] (see Chapter 18).

Gallbladder Disease

Microgallbladder is frequent in CF patients of all ages (16–18%),[64] but abnormalities on oral cholecystogram are most frequent in adults. Calculi occur in about 12% of patients.[65,66]

Cholelithiasis has been attributed to the formation of lithogenic bile by interruption of the enterophepatic circulation of bile acids in pancreatic insufficiency.[25] Pancreatic enzyme supplements reverse the bile acid malabsorption[25] and should be continued in adults even if they are no longer required for control of symptoms. Cholelithiasis may be complicated by cholecystitis, and surgical intervention has been undertaken with good success.

Glucose Intolerance

In CF increasing pancreatic fibrosis probably causes mechanical disruption and "strangulation" of the islets, producing endocrine pancreatic dysfunction.[67] Insulinopenia, glucagonopenia, altered peripheral sensitivity to insulin, and insulin receptor abnormalities contribute to a form of glucose intolerance which rarely produces ketoacidosis and is seldom complicated by diabetic vasculopathy, despite long-standing hyperglycemia.[67–71] Diabetic control is easily achieved with small doses of insulin. The prevalance of hyperglycemia is probably higher in adults with CF than in children; some 9% of adults have frank glycosuria (Table 20-1). Moreover, the results of sensitive tests suggests a higher prevalence of diabetic vasculopathy than previously suspected.[72] Since in the usual diabetes mellitus, development of vasculopathy depends on duration of hyperglycemia (among other factors), it may be expected that with increasing survival of cystic fibrosis patients, more diabetic nephropathy, retinopathy, and vasculopathy will indeed be observed (see Chapter 19).

Reproductive Complications

Women In women with CF menarche is delayed by about two years,[73] but eventually, normal menstrual cycles are established and normal secondary sexual characteristics and libido develop. Menstrual irregularities, anovulatory cycles, and secondary amenorrhea are relatively common during exacerbations of the pulmonary disease and probably contribute to the relative infertility of women in CF. Although anatomically the female reproductive tract is normal, the cervical mucus of women with CF has reduced water content and may not undergo the normal midcycle viscosity change that favors sperm penetration. This thick desiccated cervical mucus forms a mechanical barrier to sperm and may also contribute to reduced fertility.[74,75]

Vaginitis appears to be frequent among women with cystic fibrosis. Antibiotics administered for pulmonary infection and glucose intolerance predispose to *Candida* infection, although nonspecific vaginitis also appears to be frequent. Cervicitis, cervical erosions, and mucous gland hyperplasia in the cervix are common pathologic findings.[76] For these reasons, gynecologic consultation is important in the management of women with CF.

Despite their apparently reduced fertility, women with CF can become pregnant. A survey of North American Cystic Fibrosis Centers identified 129 pregnancies.[77] Therapeutic abortion was performed in 25 pregnancies. No maternal deaths during pregnancy were recorded. Of the women who carried to term, 12% died within 6 months of delivery, a figure not significantly different from the age-adjusted expected mortality rate for CF women. Over one fourth of deliveries were premature, and fetal wastage occurred in 11%: these complications were significantly associated with maternal mortality within 2 years of term. Pregnancy was complicated by congestive heart failure in 13% of cases and by poor weight gain (< 10 lb) in 41%. Both complications probably reflect the maternal pulmonary disease. An abnormal right heart may decompensate from the dramatic blood volume increase during the second trimester, and relative underweight in CF is strongly associated with pulmonary status.[78] These results, taken together, suggest that pregnancy is hazardous for the woman with CF with poor pulmonary status and for her fetus. Also, serious pulmonary disease during pregnancy may necessitate use of drugs potentially harmful to the fetus, although no instances of drug-related fetal injury were recorded in the survey. (See Chapter 23 for a discussion of goiter in the fetus following maternal iodide ingestion.) In addition, all children of women with CF will be obligate heterozygotes, and one in 40–50 will have the disease.

On the other hand, the data of Cohen et al [77] show that 85 of 97 (88%) women with CF completed pregnancies and had viable and apparently healthy infants. Major congenital malformations, exept for one case of CF, were not observed. Therefore, successful outcome of pregnancy is usual in CF, particularly if the mother has only mild pulmonary involvement. Because of these considerations, counseling for the patient and her partner must be individualized, and the prospects for and the potential hazards of pregnancy should be made clear.

Voluntary infertility is frequent among women with CF who are concerned with the potential hazards of pregnancy, the genetic implications for the infant, and the possibility that the child might lose a parent prematurely. Contraception may pose problems for these patients. Barrier methods (condoms or diaphragm) are often the most suitable but require assiduous compliance. The intrauterine device may not be suitable for some nulliparous women. Oral contraceptives may cause pulmonary exacerbation, aggravate or even cause polypoid cervicitis,[79] and are associated with hepatic and thrombogenic dysfunction. However, they may be used, in as low a dosage as possible, when gynecologic and pulmonary follow-up is assured. Sterilization may be undertaken in carefully selected and counseled women.

Men Like women with CF, men may have delayed growth and sexual maturation, but the pituitary–gonadal axis is intact,[80] and normal libido and secondary sexual characteristics develop eventually. The capacity for sexual performance is normal. However, unlike women, most male patients have an anatomic abnormality of the reproductive tract: atretic vasa deferentia with absent or abnormal bodies and tails of the epididymes and seminal vesicles.[81–83] Although active spermatogenesis is present in the testes, no sperm appears in the ejaculate because of mechanical obstruction of the vas. The prostate gland appears normal. It is estimated that over 95% of men with CF have azoospermia; however, a few do have a normal sperm count and have fathered children,[84] and intact male reproductive tracts have been identified at necropsy.[85]

Because a few men with CF are fertile, semen analysis must be performed before counseling is undertaken. Ordinarily, semen analysis is done when sexual maturation is reached but before intercourse has begun, although this plan can be modified to meet individual needs. The infertile man with CF typically has small ejaculate volume, usually less than 2 ml and frequently less than 1 ml, and no sperm are found.[86] Because of the small volume of ejaculate, sometimes no further studies can be obtained, but, if possible, obstructive azoospermia should be confirmed by documenting reduced fructose content. Other abnormal findings include low pH, elevated citric acid content, and elevated acid phosphatase.[81,86] Most fertile males with CF have normal semen analysis,[84] but one is reported to have normal sperm count with reduced volume, pH, and fructose content.[87]

Counseling of the fertile man with CF should include information about the genetics of his disease. The infertile man with CF should be encouraged to inform his partner. If the couple wishes to raise children, adoption or artificial insemination of the wife are alternatives. Reconstruction of the vas has not been reported in men with CF.

Psychosocial Complications

Chronic illness and the limitations it imposes on the patient's potential can clearly pose psychosocial problems for patients with CF.[88-90] Conversely, attitude and philosophy affect the medical progression of CF so strongly that they are included in prognostic scores.[91] The psychosocial complications of CF change with age because the normal progression of psychological maturation brings new concerns with each developmental stage.

Many of the psychosocial consequences and concomitants of CF are those of most chronic illnesses with onset in childhood: the child grows up looking and feeling different.[92,93] In adolescence, physical deviation from the norm is often poorly tolerated by the individual and the peer group. The patient with CF may be distinguished from his classmates by short stature, underweight, barrel chest, or delayed sexual development, or by the pills he takes and the physical therapy he performs. Development of peer group relations may therefore be difficult.

Sexual adjustment may be complicated by the delay in sexual maturation, embarrassment about other physical stigmata of disease, multiple gynecologic difficulties in women, and infertility in both sexes. Nevertheless, most patients over 25 do marry and more than 80% of the marriages reported in two series were intact.[3,14] Thus despite potential and real difficulties, many patients with CF achieve successful heterosexual relationships.

Occupation strongly contributes to identity, especially among men but increasingly among women. Patients with CF must often make educational and vocational concessions to their present or potential physical limitations. Some environments and irritants such as dust, fumes, or smoke may aggravate lung disease, and the patient's physical capacity to work may decline in the future. Thus a sedentary occupation is preferable to one requiring physical labor. Although these considerations limit the selection of occupations, adults with CF have achieved remarkable educational and vocational success[3,14] and score well on scales of strength of commitment to vocational choice and work values.[94] Even those individuals who obtain and hold satisfying jobs may face staggering medical expenses which jeopardize their financial security. In some cases patients must waive health insurance benefits to secure a job, yet the income from the job renders them ineligible for public assistance. Financial difficulties are a major stress for the productive adult with CF.

Because the child with CF depends heavily upon his parents for the day-to-day management of a complex treatment regimen, establishment of independence may be difficult. Struggles over independence have the potential to be acted out in destructive ways, including noncompliance with medical advice and risk-taking behavior such as smoking and discontinuing the treatment program. Adjustment in the separation–individuation phase appears to be strongly related to the willingness of family to discuss cystic fibrosis in the preadolescent and adolescent years.[92]

Success in adult life depends heavily on the psychological health of parents. If they encourage development of self-esteem from more cognitive–intellectual or affective attainments, the patient has good opportunity to maintain self-esteem in spite of disease or disability. If they encourage independent functioning while remaining concerned, the patient can develop a reasonable life style, while assuming responsibility for his own treatment program.

Although the identity challenges of adolescence may be prolonged in CF patients, their confrontation with mortality occurs earlier. In the process of dying and death, patients gradually disassemble the bonds to spouse, parents, and peers. In addition to being concerned with themselves, the patients worry about the financial and emotional well-being of their survivors. Increasing attention, both scientific and lay, to the issues and process of dying has made much information available to physicians and families about how best to help the patient. Provision of emotional and medical support during the process of dying is a major obligation of the physician who cares for patients with cystic fibrosis.

ROLE OF THE INTERNIST

As we have seen in the preceding pages, CF in adults differs somewhat from CF in children. Although the complaints related to pancreatic insufficiency diminish in adulthood, new complications arise, such as massive hemoptysis, pneumothorax, or hypertrophic osteoarthropathy. Other complications, such as nasal polyposis, diabetes, intestinal obstruction, and cholelithiasis, become more prevalent or more distressing. Two problems unique to adults occur—reproductive difficulties and special psychosocial problems. Women develop gynecologic and even obstetric complaints; men need semen analyses; both sexes need reproductive counseling. In the psychosocial area, issues of sexuality become important. But even more pressing may be financial burdens—paying medical bills when one is no longer eligible for crippled children's or for parent's health insurance. Finally, issues of selection of occupation and finding a job loom large for the adult with CF. These adults do constitute a special subgroup of CF patients. They make a transition to adult life which is fraught with special medical, developmental, and financial difficulties.

In normal children in the United States development as an autonomous individual is accompanied by a transition to medical care by adult medical specialists—gynecologists, internists, or sometimes family practitioners. Medical care is no longer "brokered" by parents; the patient assumes responsibility for himself. His concerns and complaints are those of an adult, not a child. His doctor expects him to become an active participant in his own health care.

In Great Britain and Australia, sometime during adolescence, by mutual agreement between patient and physician, the CF patient begins to visit an internist, who gradually assumes full responsibility for his care. Although the initial transition to adult care was difficult in some clinics, once orderly mechanisms were established and an interested physician identified, this transfer presented little problem. The principles of care of CF which evolved in pediatric clinics, such as availability of a dedicated physician or provision of appropriate ancillary and consultative services, guide the workings of these adult clinics as well.

However, in the United States, most of the care rendered to adults with CF is delivered by pediatricians in a pediatric setting. In 1981, a survey of U.S. CF centers found that fewer than half have internists participating in outpatient care of CF adults, and one quarter have no internal medicine involvement in inpatient care. One third of centers hospitalize adults in pediatric hospitals, and another one fourth house these patients on pediatric wards of general hospitals. This use of pediatric facilities is contrary to hospital policy in over half the cases. In the past, only a few patients with CF attained adulthood, and these scattered survivors could easily be cared for in pediatric centers. Now, however, 20% of the total U.S. CF population is over age 18, and this proportion is steadily increasing. This large number of adult patients with chronic, progressive, and ultimately fatal illness cannot fail to stress pediatric facilities. It may not be feasible to expect facilities designed for children to cater to the special needs of adults with CF.

However, because in the United States adults with CF have been followed in pediatric facilities, very few internists have had substantial experience with these patients. Since most medical learning takes place during supervised rendering of care, internists without experience with CF patients may be ill-prepared to care for them. This unfamiliarity with CF is unfortunate, for in many ways the internist (and particularly the pulmonologist) is an appropriate primary physician for these patients. His expectation that the patient will be an autonomous participant in his own care may encourage resolution of the difficult separation-individuation conflict in the patient. The internist is familiar with the non-CF medical problems an adult may encounter. He deals regularly with reproductive issues and complaints. The pulmonologist is familiar with pulmonary physiology and pathophysiology and may draw upon this background in his approach to the CF patient. His extensive technological armamentarium should be available for appropriate and compassionate application to the care of CF patients. Because he is trained to deal with older patients, he is familiar with the wearing effects of chronic illness and with death. He deals regularly with multisystem disease and degeneration. Such a physician would be a valuable member of the health-care team for adults with CF. Every effort should be made to recruit and train such physicians and to ensure exposure of internal medicine as well as pediatric house officers to inpatient and outpaient care of CF patients.

SUMMARY

The increasing number of adults with CF is evidence of the progress of the last 40 years in managing this disease. Not only has the duration of life been extended, but its quality has improved as well. Most patients can remain active and productive until shortly before their deaths.[3,14] However, their lives are still short, and they are complicated by complex and demanding treatment regimens which are palliative at best. The challenge for the next 40 years is clear: identification of the basic defect so that specific therapies can be designed. Failing that, or if identifying the basic defect does not lead to better treatment (as has been the case for many genetic disorders), we must critically examine our therapeutic program. We must discard the ineffective measures and develop scientifically validated, streamlined treatment regimes designed to maximize benefits while minimizing inconvenience. Better health will allow the adult with CF to lead a fuller and richer life.

REFERENCES

1. Warwick WJ, Pogue RE: Cystic fibrosis, an expanding challenge for internal medicine. *JAMA* 1977;238:2159–2162.
2. Cystic Fibrosis Foundation: Survival Studies of Patients with Cystic Fibrosis. 1978 Report. Rockville, Maryland.
3. di Sant'Agnese PA, Davis PB: Cystic fibrosis in adults: 75 cases and a review of 232 cases in the literature. *Am J Med* 1979;66:121–132.
4. Mitchell-Heggs P, Mearns M, Batten JC: Cystic fibrosis in adolescents and adults. *Q J Med* 1976;45:479–504.
5. Corey ML, Longitudinal studies in cystic fibrosis, in Sturgess J (ed): *Perspectives in Cystic Fibrosis.* Mississauga, Ontario, Imperial Press Ltd., 1980, pp 246–255.
6. Stern RC, Boat TF, Doershuk CF, et al: Cystic fibrosis diagnosed after age 13. *Ann Intern Med* 1977;87:188–191.
7. MacLean WE, Trippe RW: Cystic fibrosis with edema and falsely negative sweat test. *J Pediatr* 1973;83:86–88.
8. Davis PB, Hubbard VS, di Sant'Agnese PA: Low sweat electrolytes in a patient with cystic fibrosis. *Am J Med* 1980;69:643–649.
9. Anderson CM, Freeman M: Sweat test results in normal persons of different ages compared with families with fibrocystic disease of the pancreas. *Arch Dis Child* 1960;34:581–587.
10. di Sant'Agnese PA, Powell GF: The eccrine sweat defect in cystic fibrosis of the pancreas (mucoviscidosis). *Ann NY Acad Sci* 1962;93: 555–599.
11. Bank S, Marks IN, Novis B: Sweat electrolytes in chronic pancreatitis. *Am J Dig Dis* 1978;23:178–181.
12. Sekelj P, Belmonte M, Rasmussen K, et al: Survey of electrolytes of unstimulated sweat from the hand in normal and diseased adults. *Am Rev Respir Dis* 1973;108:603–609.
13. Jones JD, Steige H, Logan GB: Variations of sweat sodium values in children and adults with cystic fibrosis and other disorders. *Mayo Clin Proc* 1970;45:768–773.
14. Shwachman H, Kowalski M, Khaw KT: Cystic fibrosis: A new outlook. *Medicine* 1977;56:129–149.
15. Gibson LE, Cooke RE: A test for concentration of electrolytes in sweat in cystic fibrosis of the pancreas utilizing pilocarpine by iontophoresis. *Pediatrics* 1959;23:545–549.
16. Lapey A, Kattwinkel J, di Sant'Agnese PA, et al: Steatorrhea and azotorrhea and their relation to growth and nutrition in adolescents and young adults with cystic fibrosis. *J Pediatr* 1974;84:328–334.
17. Taussig LM, Wolf RO, Wood RE, et al: Use of serum amylase isoenzymes in evaluation of pancreatic function. *Pediatrics* 1974;54:229–234.
18. Hadorn B, Zoppi G, Shmerling DH, et al: Quantitative assessment of exocrine pancreatic function in infants and children. *J Pediatr* 1968;73:39–50.
19. Hadorn B, Johansen PG, Anderson CM: Pancreozymin secretin test of exocrine pancreatic function in cystic fibrosis and the

significance of the result for the pathogenesis of the disease. *Can Med Assoc J* 1968;98: 377–385.

20. Oppenheimer EH: Absence of pancreatic lesions in cystic fibrosis. *Birth Defects, Orig Art Ser* 1972;8:108–113.
21. Kopito LE, Shwachman H, Vawter GF, et al: The pancreas in cystic fibrosis chemical composition and comparative morphology. *Pediatr Res* 1976;10:742–749.
22. Gaskin K, Forstner G: Volume and HCO_3-secretion in CF patients, in Sturgess, J (ed): *Perspectives in Cystic Fibrosis.* Mississauga, Ontario, Imperial Press Ltd., 1980, p 15a.
23. Wood RE, Boat TF, Doershuk CT: Cystic fibrosis. *Am Rev Respir Dis* 1976;113:833–876.
24. Shwachman H, Lebenthal E, Khaw KT: Recurrent acute pancreatitis in patients with cystic fibrosis with normal pancreatic enzymes. *Pediatrics* 1975;55:86–92.
25. Roy CC, Weber AM, Morin CL, et al: Abnormal biliary lipid composition in cystic fibrosis. Effect of pancreatic enzymes. *N Engl J Med* 1977;297:1301–1305.
26. Mullins F, Talamo R, di Sant'Agnese PA: Late intestinal complications of cystic fibrosis. *JAMA* 1965;192:741–746.
27. Forstner G, Gall G, Corey M, et al: Digestion and absorption of nutrients in cystic fibrosis, in Sturgess, J (ed): *Perspectives in Cystic Fibrosis.* Mississauga, Ontario, Imperial Press Ltd., 1980, pp 137–148.
28. Fink RJ, Doershuk CF, Boat TF, et al: Pulmonary function and morbidity in 40 adult patients with cystic fibrosis. *Chest* 1978;74: 643–647.
29. Menendez R, Mather F, Waring WW: Long-term patterns of obstructive lung disease in cystic fibrosis. *Chest* 1980;77:321–323.
30. Corey M, Levison H, Crozier D: Five- to seven-year course of pulmonary function in cystic fibrosis. *Am Rev Respir Dis* 1976;114: 1085–1092.
31. Wagener JS, Taussig LM, Burrows B, et al: Comparison of lung function and survival patterns between cystic fibrosis and emphysema or chronic bronchitis patients, in Sturgess, J (ed): *Perspectives in Cystic Fibrosis.* Mississauga, Ontario, Imperial Press Ltd., 1980, pp 236–245.
32. Mearns MB, Hunt GH, Rushworth R: Bacterial flora of respiratory tract in patients with cystic fibrosis 1950–1971. *Arch Dis Child* 1972;47:908–913.
33. Doggett RG: Incidence of mucoid Pseudomonas aeruginosa from clinical sources. *Appl Microbiol* 1969;18:936–937.
34. Zierdt CH, Williams RL: Serotyping of *Pseudomonas aeruginosa* isolates from patients with cystic fibrosis of the pancreas. *J Clin Microbiol* 1975;1:521–526.
35. Reynolds HY, di Sant'Agnese PA, Zierdt CH: Mucoid *Pseudomonas aeruginosa,* a sign of cystic fibrosis in young adults with chronic pulmonary disease? *JAMA* 1976;236: 2190–2192.
36. Knoke JD, Stern RC, Doershuk CF, et al: Cystic fibrosis: The prognosis for five-year survival. *Pediatr Res* 1978;12:676–679.
37. Blessing J, Walker J, Maybary B, et al: *Pseudomonas cepacia* and *maltophilia* in the cystic fibrosis patient. *Am Rev Respir Dis* 1979; 119:262.
38. Boat TF, Petty TL: Chronic bronchitis and cystic fibrosis: Two chronic obstructive lung diseases of adults. *Am Rev Respir Dis* 1977; 116:1–2.
39. Tager I, Speizer FE: Role of infection in chronic bronchitis. *N Engl J Med* 1975;292: 563–570.
40. Davis PB, di Sant'Agnese PA: Assisted ventilation for patients with cystic fibrosis. *JAMA* 1978;239:1851–1854.
41. Rogers RM, Weiler C, Ruppenthal B: Impact of the respiratory intensive care unit on survival of patients with acute respiratory failure. *Chest* 1972;62:94–97.
42. Siassi B, Moss AJ, Dooley RR: Clinical recognition of cor pulmonale in cystic fibrosis. *J Pediatr* 1971;78:794–805.
43. Allen HD, Taussig LM, Gaines JA, et al: Echocardiographic profiles of the long term cardiac changes in cystic fibrosis. *Chest* 1979; 75:428–433.
44. Lester LA, Egge AC, Hubbard VS, et al: Echocardiography in cystic fibrosis: A proposed scoring system. *J Pediatr* 1980;97:742–748.
45. Stern RC, Wood RE, Boat TF, et al: Treatment and prognosis of massive hemoptysis in cystic fibrosis. *Am Rev Respir Dis* 1978;117: 825–828.
46. Holsclaw DS, Grand RJ, Shwachman H: Massive hemoptysis in cystic fibrosis. *J Pediatr* 1970;76:829–834.
47. Levitsky S, Lapey A, di Sant'Agnese PA: Pulmonary resection for life-threatening hemoptysis in cystic fibrosis. *JAMA* 1970; 213:125–127.
48. Fellows KE, Khaw KT, Schuster S, et al: Bronchial artery embolization in cystic fibrosis: technique and long-term results. *J Pediatr* 1979;95:959–963.
49. Luck SR, Raffensperger JG, Sullivan HJ, et al: Management of pneumothorax in children with chronic pulmonary disease. *J Thorac Cardiovasc Surg* 1977;74:834–839.
50. Boat TF, di Sant'Agnese PA, Warwick WJ, et al: Pneumothorax in cystic fibrosis. *JAMA* 1969;209:1498–1504.

51. Knight RK, Batten JC: Pneumothorax in cystic fibrosis, in Sturgess, J (ed): *Perspectives in Cystic Fibrosis.* Mississauga, Ontario, Imperial Press Ltd., 1980, pp 376–381.
52. Kattwinkel J, Taussig LM, McIntosh CL, et al: Intrapleural instillation of quinacrine for recurrent pneumothorax. *JAMA* 1973;226: 557–559.
53. Stowe SM, Boat TF, Mendelsohn H, et al: Open throracotomy for pneumothorax in cystic fibrosis. *Am Rev Respir Dis* 1975;111: 611–617.
54. Athreya BH, Borns P, Rosenlund ML: Cystic fibrosis and hypertrophic osteoarthropathy in children. *Am J Dis Child* 1975;129:634–637.
55. Matthay MA, Matthay RA, Mills DM, et al: Hypertrophic osteoarthropathy in adults with cystic fibrosis. *Thorax* 1976;31:572–575.
56. Grossman H, Denning CF, Baker DH: Hypertrophic osteoarthropathy in cystic fibrosis. *Am J Dis Child* 1964;107:39–44.
57. Shwachman H, Kulczycki L, Mueller H, et al: Nasal polyposis in patients with cystic fibrosis. *Pediatrics* 1962;30:389–401.
58. Jaffe BF, Strome M, Khaw KT, et al: Nasal polypectomy and sinus surgery for cystic fibrosis—a 10 year review. *Otolaryngol Clin North Am* 1977;10:81–90.
59. Hodson ME, Mearns MB, Batten JC: Meconium ileus equivalent in adults with cystic fibrosis of pancreas: A report of six cases. *Br Med J* 1976;2:791–792.
60. Shwachman H, Holsclaw DS: Examination of the appendix at laparotomy as a diagnostic clue in cystic fibrosis. *N Engl J Med* 1972;286: 1300–1301.
61. di Sant'Agnese PA, Blanc WA: A distinctive type of biliary cirrhosis of the liver associated with cystic fibrosis of the pancreas. *Pediatrics* 1956;18:387–409.
62. Stern RC, Stevens DP, Boat TF, et al: Symptomatic hepatic disease in cystic fibrosis: Incidence, course, and outcome of portal systemic shunting. *Gastroenterology.* 1976; 70:645–649.
63. Schuster SR, Shwachman H, Toyama WM, et al: The management of portal hypertension in cystic fibrosis. *J Pediatr Surg* 1977;12: 201–206.
64. Roy CC: Gastrointestinal and hepatobiliary complications: Changing pattern with age, in Sturgess, J (ed): *Perspectives in Cystic Fibrosis.* Mississauga, Ontario, Imperial Press Ltd., 1980, pp 190–197.
65. L'heureux PR, Isenberg JN, Sharp HL, et al: Gallbladder disease in cystic fibrosis. *Am J Roentgenol* 1977;128:953–956.
66. Hubbard VS, Head GL, Shawker TH, et al: Radiological and ultrasound evaluation of the gallbladder in patients with cystic fibrosis. *Pediatr Res* 1978;12:324.
67. Handwerger S, Roth J, Gorden P, et al: Glucose intolerance in cystic fibrosis. *N Engl J Med* 1969;281:451–461.
68. Lippe BM, Kaplan SA, Neufeld ND, et al: Insulin receptors in cystic fibrosis: Increased receptor number and altered affinity. *Pediatrics* 1980;65:1018–1022.
69. Wilmshurst EG, Soeldner JS, Holsclaw DS, et al: Endogenous and exogenous insulin responses in patients with cystic fibrosis. *Pediatrics* 1975;55:75–82.
70. Lippe B, Sperling MA, Dooley RR: Pancreatic alpha and beta cell functions in cystic fibrosis. *J Pediatr* 1977;90:751–755.
71. Stahl M, Girard J, Rutishauser M, et al: Endocrine function of the pancreas in cystic fibrosis: Evidence for an impaired glucagon and insulin response following arginine infusion. *J Pediatr* 1974;84:821–824.
72. Rodman HM, Matthews LW, Nussbaum E, et al: Chronic complications of diabetes in CF patients, in Sturgess, J (ed): *Perspectives in Cystic Fibrosis.* Mississauga, Ontario, Imperial Press Ltd., 1980, p 31a.
73. Holsclaw DS: Cystic fibrosis: Overview and pulmonary aspects in young adults. *Clin Chest Med* 1980;1:407–423.
74. Kopito LE, Kosasky HS, Shwachman H: Water and electrolytes in cervical mucus from patients with cystic fibrosis. *Fertil Steril* 1973;24:512–516.
75. Oppenheimer EH, Case AL, Esterly JR, et al: Cervical mucus in cystic fibrosis: A possible cause of infertility. *Am J Obstet Gynecol* 1970;108:673–674.
76. Oppenheimer EH, Esterly JR: Observations on cystic fibrosis of the pancreas. VI. The uterine cervix. *J Pediatr* 1970;77:991–995.
77. Cohen LF, di Sant'Agnese PA, Friedlander J: Cystic fibrosis and pregnancy; a national survey. *Lancet* 1980;2:842–844.
78. Kraemer R, Rudenberg A, Hadorn B, et al: Relative underweight in cystic fibrosis and its prognostic value. *Acta Paediatr Scand* 1978; 67:33–37.
79. Dooley RB, Braunstein H, Osher AB: Polypoid cervicitis in cystic fibrosis patients receiving oral contraceptives. *Am J Obstet Gynecol* 1974;118:971–974.
80. Rosen SW, Weintraub BD: Monotropic increase of serum FSH correlated with low sperm count in young men with idiopathic oligospermia and aspermia. *J Clin Endocrinol Metab* 1971;32:410–416.
81. Kaplan E, Shwachman H, Perlmutter AD, et al: Reproductive failure in males with cystic fibrosis. *N Engl J Med* 1968;279:65–69.
82. Holsclaw DS, Perlmutter AD, Jockin H, et al: Genital abnormalities in male patients

with cystic fibrosis. *J Urol* 1971;106:568–574.
83. Oppenheimer EH, Esterly JR: Observations on cystic fibrosis of the pancreas. V. Developmental changes in the male genital system. *J Pediatr* 1969;75:806–811.
84. Taussig LM, Lobeck CC, di Sant'Agnese PA, et al: Fertility in males with cystic fibrosis. *N Engl J Med* 1972;287:586–589.
85. Landing BH, Wells TR, Wang CL: Abnormality of epididymis and vas deferens in cystic fibrosis. *Arch Pathol* 1969;88:569–580.
86. Rule AH, Kopito L, Shwachman H: Chemical analysis of ejaculates from patients with cystic fibrosis. *Fertil Steril* 1970;21:515–520.
87. Feigelson J, Pecau Y, Shwachman H: A propos d'une paternité chez un malade atteint de mucoviscidose: Études des fonctions génitales et de la filiation. *Arch Fr Pediatr* 1969;26:937–944.
88. Lewiston NJ: Saturday's children: Adolescents and adults with cystic fibrosis in today's society, in Sturgess, J (ed): *Perspectives in Cystic Fibrosis.* Mississauga, Ontario, Imperial Press Ltd., 1980, pp 266–274.
89. Gayton WF, Friedman SB: Psychosocial aspects of cystic fibrosis: A review of the literature. *Am J Dis Child* 1973;126:856–859.
90. Rosenlund ML, Lustig HS: Young adults with cystic fibrosis: The problems of a new generation. *Ann Intern Med* 1973;78:959–962.
91. Taussig LM, Kattwinkel J, Friedewald WT, et al: A new prognostic score and clinical evaluation system for cystic fibrosis. *J Pediatr* 1973;82:380–385.
92. Boyle IR, di Sant'Agnese PA, Sach S, et al: Emotional adjustment of adolescents and young adults with cystic fibrosis. *J Pediatr* 1976;88:318–326.
93. Strauss GD, Pedersen S, Dudovitz D: Psychosocial support for adults with cystic fibrosis. *Am J Dis Child* 1979;133:301–305.
94. Goldberg R, Isralsky M, Shwachman H: Vocational development and adjustment of adolescents with cystic fibrosis. *Arch Med Rehab* 1979;60:369–374.
95. Gracey M, Anderson CM: Cystic fibrosis of the pancreas in adolescence and adulthood. *Aust Ann Med* 1969;18:91–101.
96. Howie AD, Stack BHR: Cystic fibrosis in adolescents and young adults. *Scot Med J* 1979;24:193–198.
97. Schwartz EE, Holsclaw DS: Pulmonary involvement in adults with cystic fibrosis. *Am J Roentgenol Radium Ther Nucl Med* 1974;122:708–718.
98. Friedman PG, Harwood I: Adult cystic fibrosis: Radiologic findings and pathologic correlation, in Sturgess, J (ed): *Perspectives in Cystic Fibrosis.* Mississauga, Ontario, Imperial Press Ltd., 1980 p 15a.
99. Report of the committee for a study for evaluation of testing for cystic fibrosis. *J Pediatr* 1976;88:711–734.
100. Gaskin E, Gurwitz D, Corey M, et al: Improved pulmonary function in Cystic Fibrosis patients without pancreatic insufficiency, in Sturgess J (ed): *Perspectives in Cystic Fibrosis.* Mississauga, Ontario, Imperial Press Ltd., 1980, pp 226–230.

21

Surgical Problems in Cystic Fibrosis

John G. Raffensperger

Children with cystic fibrosis of the pancreas are prone to several complications which may require surgical intervention; meconium ileus and meconium peritonitis are the most common. Older children develop a similar syndrome due to inspissated stool in the cecum and terminal ileum. The relentless progress of the disease occasionally leads to pneumothorax, hemoptysis, bronchiectasis, and bleeding from esophageal varices during later years which may require surgical intervention. Finally, children with cystic fibrosis have a higher than normal incidence of appendicitis and inguinal hernias. Although these children have poor pulmonary function and suboptimal nutrition, with proper attention to pulmonary toilet, fluid and electrolyte management, and postoperative pain control, they will tolerate a major operation surprisingly well.

MECONIUM ILEUS

Meconium ileus is a mechanical obstruction of the distal ileum by thick, inspissated meconium which affects approximately 8% of patients born with cystic fibrosis.[1-3] This thickened meconium is primarily the result of abnormal mucus production in the intestine rather than a deficiency in pancreatic secretions.[4] The terminal ileum is contracted for 10–15 cm proximal to the ileocecal valve (Figure 21-1). In this portion of the bowel, meconium forms hard, grey concretions. The more proximal ileum is dilated to three to four times its normal size and contains

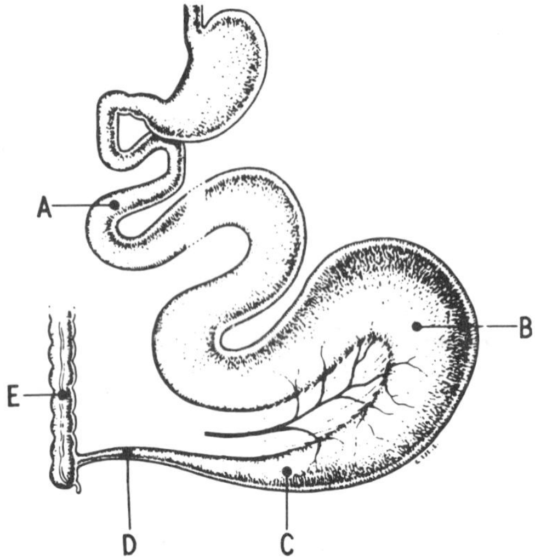

Diagram showing appearance of intestine at different levels. *A,* progressive hypertrophy and dilatation down the small intestine; *B,* maximally enlarged loop, elongated mesentery ± volvulus; *C,* tapering segment of bowel with putty-like contents; *D,* distal ileum contracted, containing meconium concretions; *E,* unexpanded large bowel.

Figure 21-1 Details on diagram. Reproduced from Holsclaw et al: *Am J Dis Child* 1965;109:104 (reference 2), with permission. Copyright 1965, American Medical Association.

thick, tenacious dark green meconium (Figure 21-2).

The heavy dilated loops of intestine may form a volvulus, and distention may result in ischemic necrosis and perforation with extravasation of meconium into the peritoneal cavity. Approximately a third of our own cases of meconium ileus have been complicated by intestinal gangrene or perforation. In addition, a rare infant with cystic fibrosis may have an intestinal atresia. Distal to the atresia, the bowel is filled with particularly hard concretions of meconium. Currently in our neonatal unit, every baby with an intestinal obstruction has a sweat test for cystic fibrosis before he is sent home from the hospital.

Diagnosis

Any infant with a low intestinal obstruction may have meconium ileus. Typically, these infants are born with abdominal distention. Within a few hours after birth, as air is swallowed, the distention increases and the baby commences to vomit bile-stained material. There will either be no stool passage or at most there will be a small plug of meconium which will be obtained on rectal examination. There are frequently firm, dilated loops of bowel palpable through the abdominal wall. Abdominal roentgenograms will demonstrate dilated loops of small bowel, especially in the upper abdomen. Unlike other forms of intestinal obstruction, upright x-rays fail to demonstrate air-fluid levels, because the meconium is too thick to layer out.[5] Air bubbles which are forced into the thick meconium in the terminal ileum result in a ground-glass or granular appearance in the right lower quadrant of the abdomen on plain roentgenograms. This sign is also occasionally seen in an infant with Hirschsprung's disease; therefore, it is not specific for meconium ileus. A barium enema which demonstrates a small unused colon with dilated proximal loops of small bowel is suggestive only of an obstruction in the terminal ileum. However, if contrast material can be forced into the terminal ileum to demonstrate meconium concretions, the diagnosis can be made with considerable certainty. Tests for intestinal enzymes and sweat chloride determinations are rarely of help on the first day or so of life, when a decision concerning an operation must be made.

Treatment

As soon as the diagnosis of neonatal intestinal obstruction is suspected, the baby is placed in a warm, humidified isolette, given intravenous fluids, antibiotics, and an oral-gastric tube is passed. These measures should be commenced before the baby is sent for roentgen studies. When the clinical examination and initial x-rays support the diagnosis of an uncomplicated meconium ileus, the ideal treatment consists of Gastrografin enemas administered under x-ray control. Gastrografin is an aqueous contrast solution containing 76% sodium methylglucamine diatrizoate and a wetting agent,

Tween 80. This is a very hyperosmotic solution, and it draws fluid from the circulation of the bowel lumen.

Noblitt described a technique in which 50–100 ml of undiluted Gastrografin is administered through a straight, soft 8 French rectal tube.[7] The buttocks must be firmly taped together to prevent leakage of the solution and increments of 20–30 ml are given with a syringe until the contrast material fills the colon and distal ileum. Progress is followed with fluoroscopy, and the procedure is terminated when the dilated ileum is outlined. In some cases, liquefied meconium is returned immediately. More often, it is necessary to repeat the procedure at intervals of 12–24 hr. In addition to the Gastrografin enema given in the x-ray department, the floor nurses administer further enemas consisting of 1% N-acetylcysteine or Mucomyst. Ten milliliters of 1% N-acetylcysteine is also injected into the gastric tube every 4 hr. The tube is then clamped for 15–20 min and left open on gravity drainage.

During this entire period, the infant's urinary output and vital signs are closely monitored. It is usually necessary to give 20 ml/kg of plasma or serum albumin over and above maintenance fluids to replace secretions lost into the intestinal lumen. In most cases, the abdominal distention is relieved within two or three days. When the abdomen is soft, flat, and stool is being passed, oral feedings are offered. If there is no passage of stool and continued abdominal distention after 48 hr, or if there is any abdominal tenderness, free fluid, or pneumoperitoneum, an operation is indicated.

A variety of operations have been recommended for meconium ileus. These include resection of the dilated bowel with a double-barreled Mikulicz ileostomy and simple enterotomy with irrigation of the bowel followed by anastomosis; The Bishop-Koop operation involves resection of the dilated ileum, irrigation of the bowel at the operating table, and then establishment of intestinal continuity with Roux-en-Y anastomosis.[8–10] The distal ileum is exteriorized so that irrigations of the distal ileum can be carried out in the postoperative period. This technique has given excellent

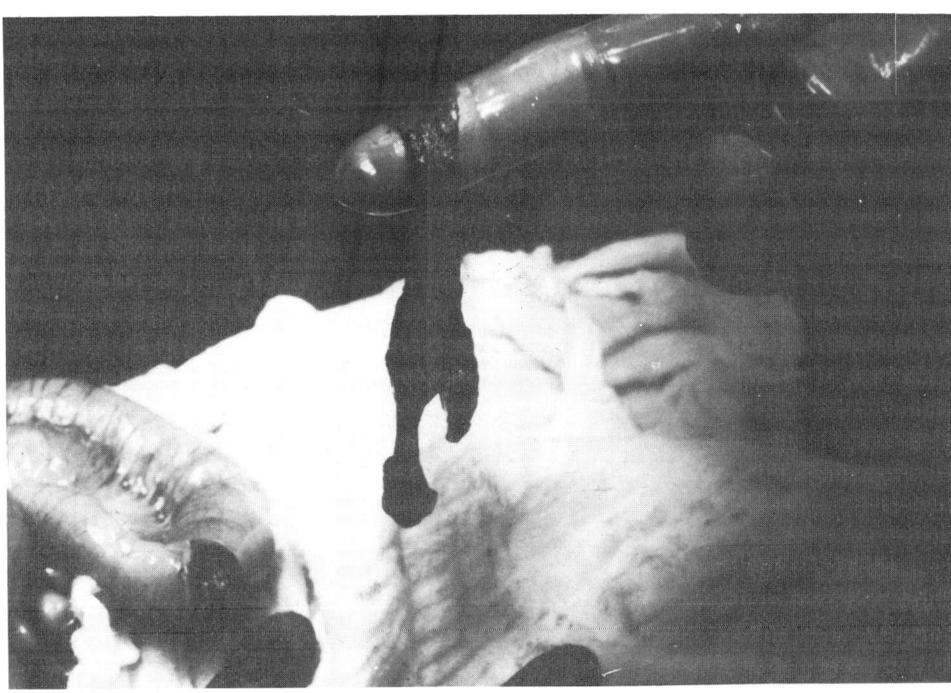

Figure 21-2 Typical thick meconium found in meconium ileus.

results. In our series of 15 patients, 1 has recovered with enemas, and 14 required an operation; 93% of these infants have survived (Table 21-1). Recently, Harberg and his colleagues have described a simpler operation in which a T-tube is sutured into the terminal dilated ileum without resection or exteriorization.[11] Pancreatic enzymes are then instilled through the tube in the postoperative period. The tenacious meconium is liquefied and expelled. Ten of his 11 patients survived.

Regardless of the initial treatment for meconium ileus, it is necessary to commence postural drainage and pulmonary physiotherapy in the immediate postoperative period. We use humidity and parenteral antibiotics during the first 5–7 days following an operation. Further antibiotics are given only for specific pulmonary infections. Initial feedings consist only of glucose and water. Thereafter, the mother's breast milk is given if it is available, otherwise we commence feeding with a protein hydrolysate formula, such as Pregestimil or Nutramigen. At this time, all infants born with an uncomplicated meconium ileus should survive. The long-term prognosis of these children is similar to that for others who have cystic fibrosis without meconium ileus.

MECONIUM PERITONITIS

An intrauterine intestinal perforation from a volvulus, ischemic necrosis, or an atresia results in leakage of meconium in to the peritoneal cavity. An early perforation causes an inflammatory reaction, adhesions, and calcifications which result in an adherent, twisted mass of bowel. Usually at the time of birth the liquid meconium has been absorbed, but leaves the inflammatory reaction and an intestinal obstruction. Abdominal roentgenograms demonstrate dilated loops of intestine and calcifications (Figure 21-3). At operation, the original perforation is usually sealed by adhesions. When the perforation occurs later in intrauterine life, the infant is born with a hugely distended, fluid-filled peritoneal cavity. The abdomen is dull to percussion, the flanks bulge, and the scrotum is often distended with fluid (Figure 21-4).

Table 21-1
Incidence of Meconium Abnormalities at Children's Memorial Hospital, 1970–1980*

	Total	CF	CF (%)
Meconium plug	25	6	25
Meconium ileus	15	12	80
Meconium peritonitis	8	4	50

*Note the variable percentages accounted for by cystic fibrosis. Data from Olsen et al.[34]

Roentgenograms demonstrate an opaque abdomen with little air in the intestine. Typically, loops of bowel are floating in the mid-abdomen and the diaphragms are elevated. An abdominal paracentesis which returns opalescent green fluid is diagnostic for meconium peritonitis. All possible fluid is aspirated with a syringe and needle to relieve respiratory distress secondary to the elevated diaphragms. The infant is then given intravenous fluids, antibiotics, and prepared for an operation. Usually, the perforation is found in the ileum or colon. Depending on the baby's general condition, the perforation may be exteriorized or the involved intestine may be resected and a Bishop-Koop type of anastomosis performed. Meconium peritonitis is usually, but not always, associated with cystic fibrosis of the pancreas. There should be a high index of suspicion. If the initial sweat chloride tests are not diagnostic, several more determinations should be carried out. During the past 10 years we have operated upon 8 babies with meconium peritonitis and all have survived. Four (50%) of these infants had cystic fibrosis (Table 21-1).

MECONIUM PLUG SYNDROME

The meconium plug syndrome is often confused with meconium ileus. These infants have mild abdominal distention and fail to pass a stool at the time of birth. A barium enema outlines a cast of meconium in the distal colon.[12] Frequently the plug is expelled following the barium or a saline enema. After the plug is expelled, the infant passes normal meconium and has no further difficulties. Unfortunately, some children who were originally diagnosed as having meconium plug syndrome turned out to have CF or Hirschsprung's disease.[13] For this reason, we feel that a sweat chloride test should always be done to rule out cystic fibrosis in a child with meconium plug syndrome, and in addition they must either be followed very carefully for further signs of Hirschsprung's disease, or a rectal suction biopsy should be performed before they leave the hospital. Hypothyroidism should also be considered. Of our 25 patients seen with meconium plug syndrome, 6 (25%) had cystic fibrosis (Table 21-1).

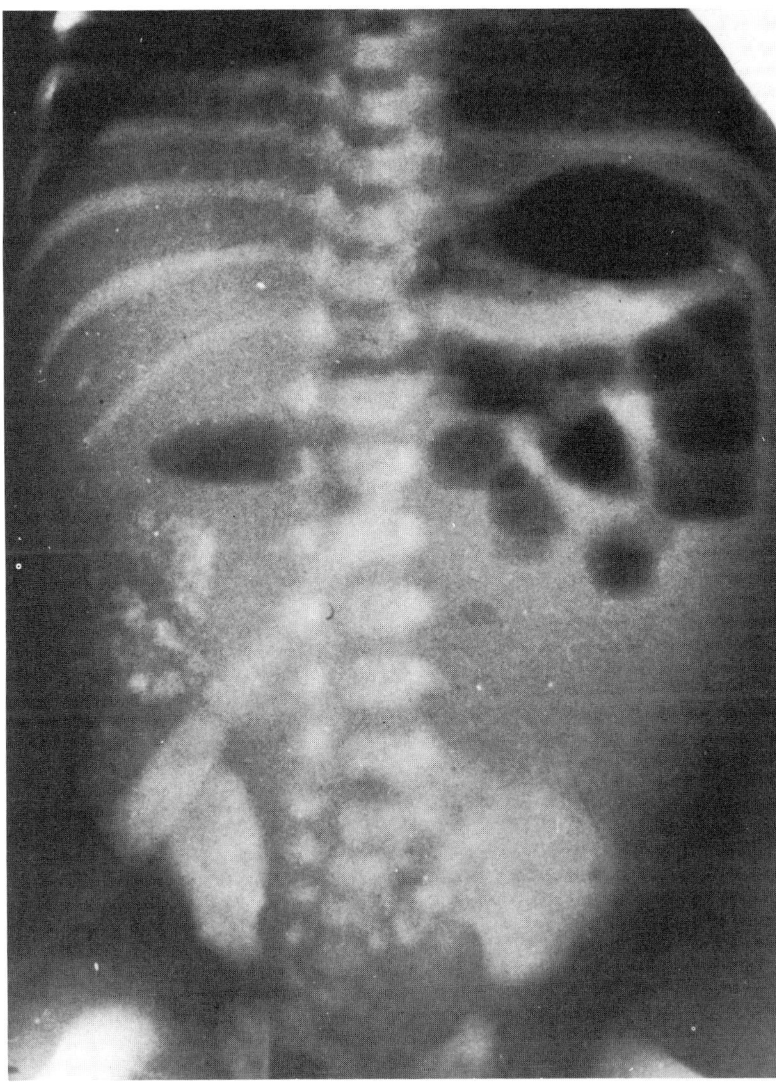

Figure 21-3 Meconium peritonitis calcifications in the right upper quadrant, with dilated small bowel.

ABDOMINAL PAIN AND INTESTINAL OBSTRUCTION IN THE OLDER CHILD

The three most important diagnoses which must be considered in cystic fibrosis patients who develop acute or recurrent bouts of abdominal pain are meconium ileus equivalent syndrome, appendicitis, and intussusception. Any one of these conditions may precede the diagnosis of cystic fibrosis. Indeed, the finding of thick inspissated stool in the ileum or colon or the characteristic microscopic findings of cystic fibrosis in the appendix may be the tipoff to the correct diagnosis of cystic fibrosis. Since the thick, inspissated fecal matter is the most important etiology in the latter two diagnoses, we shall consider all three in this section.

Meconium Ileus Equivalent

In the 1950s and early 1960s, older children with cystic fibrosis and mechanical bowel obstruction due to thick, inspissated fecal matter were first reported.[14–17] At operation or autopsy, the ileum and colon were found to be distended with thick, putty-like material which was adherent to the wall of the bowel. This syndrome may develop in children of any age, and it has been reported in adults.[18] There is often a history of inadequate oral intake or even cessation of pancreatic enzyme ingestion. The patient then develops recurrent bouts of colicky abdominal pain, constipation, and finally an intestinal obstruction with abdominal distention. Characteristically, there is an indentable, firm, nontender mass in the right lower quadrant. Plain roentgenograms will demonstrate bubbly material distending the cecum and dilated loops of small bowel. The barium enema typically reveals an intraluminal accumulation of feces and perhaps hyperplastic mucosal folds.

Initial therapy consists of intravenous fluids, nasogastric tube suction, and intensive pulmonary toilet. When fluids and electrolyte deficits have been corrected, a Gastrografin or Hypaque enema is given as described for meconium ileus in the neonate. Therapy with Gastrografin, however, should not be undertaken until intussusception or appendicitis have been completely ruled out. In addition to the contrast enemas, pancreatic enzymes or N-acetylcysteine is given through the gastric tube. Ten of 12 patients reported by the Mayo Clinic were successfully treated with medical therapy.[19] It is necessary, however, to examine these patients at frequent intervals for abdominal tenderness, fever, or an elevated white count, or for failure to improve on medical treatment. Glick and associates found Hypaque was as effective as Gastrografin in the treatment of meconium ileus equivalent.[20] After successful treatment of an obstruction episode, the dosage of pancreatic extract should be reassessed and increased if necessary.

Intussusception

A 1% incidence of intussusception was found in children with cystic fibrosis.[21] The average age of 9 years is well over that for the usual child with intussusception. Adherent, solid masses of stool form the lead point. This may be either in the ileum or colon. These children also develop crampy abdominal pain, vomiting, and abdominal distention. Unlike the usual case of intussusception, only 25% of the patients of Holsclaw et al had rectal bleeding. The contrast enema is most important in differentiating meconium ileus equivalent from intussusception. An attempt should be made to reduce the intussusception by hydrostatic pressure during the barium enema. The barium container is held no more than 3 ft above the patient, and no manipulation of the abdomen is made in order to avoid perforation of the bowel. If reduction cannot be achieved with a barium enema, an operation is indicated. Clearly, if manual reduction can be accomplished, this is all that is necessary. If there is gangrene of the bowel or perforation, an intestinal resection and anastomosis are indicated.

Appendicitis

The right lower quadrant pain seen in children with thick, inspissated feces im-

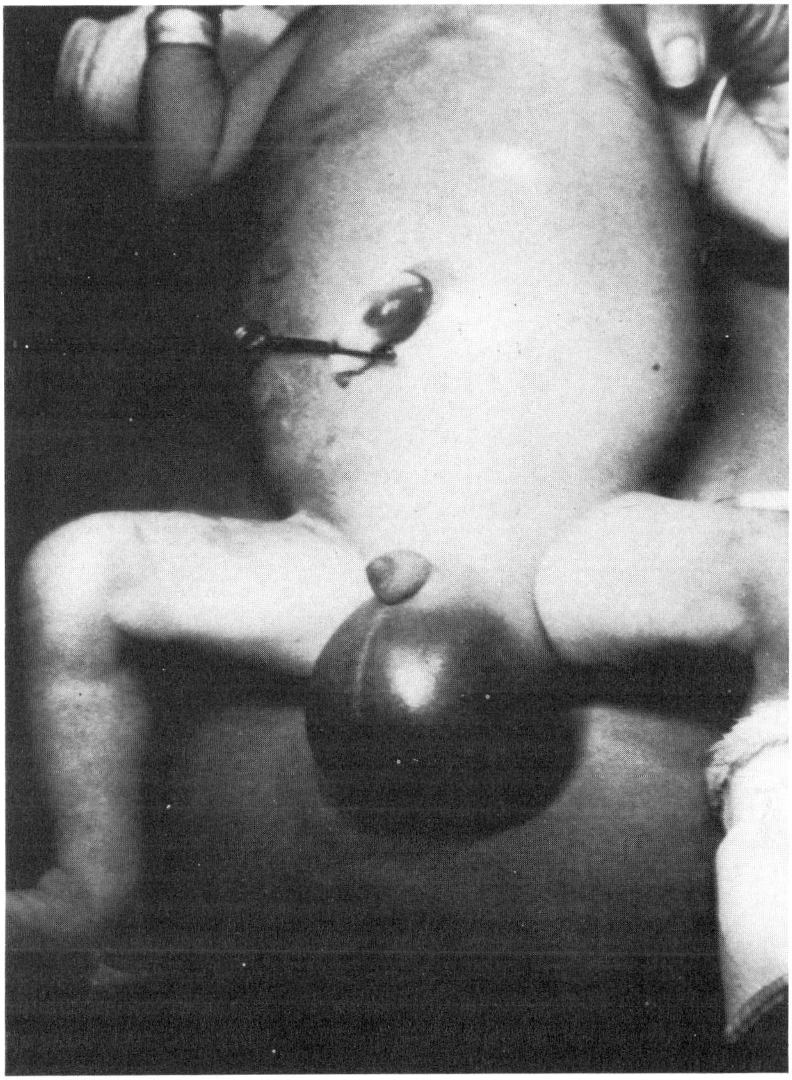

Figure 21-4 Huge distended abdomen causing a respiratory arrest; 400 ml of meconium had exuded from a perforation of the transverse colon.

pacted in the distal ileum or cecum can mimic appendicitis. The correct diagnosis of meconium ileus equivalent may not be made preoperatively, especially if cystic fibrosis has not been previously suspected. If the appendix is removed, the gross findings of the lumen of the appendix distended with firm stool should lead the surgeon to suspect the correct diagnosis.[20] Furthermore, if microscopic examination of the appendix demonstrates an increase in the goblet cells which are swollen with retained secretions, together with mucus streaming into the crypts and dilatation of the crypts, the diagnosis of cystic fibrosis is further supported.[22,23]

On the other hand, since chronic abdominal pain is so common in a child with known cystic fibrosis, the diagnosis of appendicitis may be overlooked. Also, chronic antibiotic treatment for pulmonary infections may mask the symptoms of appendicitis.

Holsclaw described three patients who developed appendiceal perforation or abcess formation while they were being evaluated and treated for abdominal pain in the hospital.[24] The correct diagnosis was made after observation in all of these patients, but his paper points up the difficulties in differentiating appendicitis from meconium ileus equivalent syndrome. Localized tenderness together with a positive Rovsing's sign is the most valuable physical finding which will differentiate appendicitis from other noninflammatory problems. In doubtful cases, a barium enema should be administered. If this demonstrates obstruction of the appendiceal lumen or indentation of the cecum by an abscess, appendicitis is the likely diagnosis and an exploratory laparotomy should be performed.

On the other hand, if the contrast enema demonstrates a large amount of solid fecal material in the colon, some time should be spent with Gastrografin enemas to effect an evacuation of this material. If the symptoms and signs are promptly relieved, this is all that is necessary. However, if there is persistent tenderness and pain together with fever and elevation of the white count, an operation is indicated. In most cases, appendectomy and drainage are all that are necessary. If, however, the surgeon finds appendicitis together with distention of the cecum and ileum with hard feces, it may be desirable to insert a catheter through the stump of the appendix, which is then brought out as an appendecostomy. Postoperative irrigations with N-acetylcysteine can then be carried out without difficulty.

RECTAL PROLAPSE

Rectal prolapse occurred in 22.6% and was the initial complaint in 12 of 386 patients.[25] The prolapse is usually only mucosa and is readily replaced by manual manipulation. It usually occurs between one and two years of age and stops spontaneously with treatment of the cystic fibrosis and as nutrition improves. The author has never found it necessary to operate on a child with rectal prolapse and cystic fibrosis.

SURGICAL MANAGEMENT OF PULMONARY COMPLICATIONS

Pneumothorax

Pneumothorax is one of the most common pulmonary complications of cystic fibrosis. At the University of Minnesota, 6.4% of 444 patients experienced 52 episodes of pneumothorax between 1963 and 1977.[26] In our own patients, the risk of pneumothorax increased to 12.5% when patients over 10 years of age were studied.[27] More than half the initial pneumothoraces occurred in children between the ages of 11 and 15 years. The relentless progress of disease results not only in areas of atelectasis, fibrosis, and microabscesses, but in apical subpleural bullae. These bullae, which may become quite large, rupture into the pleural cavity.

A pneumothorax further reduces pulmonary function by direct pulmonary compression and in addition causes pain, shallow breathing, and reluctance to cough. Since the patient is confined to bed, any form of treatment interferes with postural drainage and chest physiotherapy, resulting in increased retention of purulent sputum. These factors hasten the patient's downhill course. Furthermore, prolonged hospitalization seriously interferes with schooling and the child's quality of life. These factors must be taken into consideration when deciding upon a course of treatment. The diagnosis of a pneumothorax is easily made if a chest roentgenogram is taken on a patient who has developed acute pleuritic-type chest pain and increasing dyspnea.

Treatment The initial treatment of a pneumothorax is the insertion of a chest tube by closed thoracotomy. The chest wall is carefully prepared with an antiseptic such as Povidone iodine and draped with sterile towels. The midaxillary line in the 5th or 6th intercostal space is chosen for the tube insertion site. The skin at the intercostal space is liberally infiltrated with a local anesthetic. The chest tube, such as a size 16–20 French plastic tube, is inserted through a small skin incision and tunneled through the subcutaneous tissue for 2-3 cm, then passed through an intercostal space. Care must be taken to hug the superior surface of a rib in order to avoid the intercostal bundles. The subcutaneous tunnel is important to prevent an air leak around the tube and to prevent leakage of air into the chest cavity when the tube is removed. The tube is then connected to a water seal with −1 to −20 cm of water suction. It may be very difficult to expand a stiff fibrotic lung and, if there is a residual pleural space, either the insertion of more chest tubes or an operation should be considered. More suction may be required if there is a persistent air leak. If the lung reexpands within 24−48 hr and if the air leak stops, no further therapy is necessary. Unfortunately, persistent air leaks and recurrent pneumothoraces are common.

In our series, 25 episodes of pneumothoraces were initially treated only with chest tube drainage. Three of these patients died, and two eventually required thoracotomy. Twenty of the pneumothoraces resolved, but 50% of them recurred. Consequently, when there is a prompt lung reexpansion but no further air leak, a sclerosing solution should be instilled in the pleural cavity in order to promote adhesions which hopefully will prevent a recurrent pneumothorax. Various agents such as 50% dextrose, quinacrine, and nitrogen mustard have all been used for this purpose. We prefer to instill 1-1½ g of tetracycline into the pleural cavity. Any of these agents cause severe pain, but this can be ameliorated by injecting 1% lidocaine into the pleural cavity through the chest tube. The tube is clamped and, half hour later, the tetracycline and 100 ml of saline are injected. The tube is again clamped, and then after several hours again reconnected to the water seal.

Unfortunately, the recurrence rate following sclerotherapy is almost as high as that following tube drainage alone. When there is a persistent air leak after 4-5 days, particularly if there is incomplete expansion of the lung, an operation is indicated to suture the leaking apical blebs and to perform a pleurodesis. Although there is great reluctance to subject a patient with poor lung function to an operation, this has proved to be a very successful procedure which prevents recurrent episodes of pneumothoraces and shortens the patient's hospital course. It does not diminish pulmonary function in the long term.

Preoperatively, specific antibiotics are given based on a sputum culture, and every effort is made to clear the patient of pulmonary secretions. During anesthesia, a complete pulmonary lavage is carried out with saline irrigations and suctioning through the endotracheal tube. This in itself is most helpful. The operation is carried out through a "mini" anterior thoracotomy. The apical blebs are sutured, thus stopping the air leak. The entire pleural surface of the lung and the parietal pleura are then vigorously rubbed with dry gauze to create a pleuritis and adhesions. Finally the intercostal nerves are infiltrated with a long-acting local anesthetic agent. This allows the child to cough and to become ambulatory almost immediately after the operation. As soon as the lung has expanded, the chest tubes are removed, and the patient is discharged from the hospital. In our own series of patients, we have not seen a recurrent pneumothorax following this procedure.

Pulmonary Resection

The resection of localized areas of atelectasis or bronchiectasis may reduce the volume of sputum and slow the progression of fibrosis and pulmonary sepsis. When one lobe or segment has failed to reexpand despite maximum medical therapy over a period of 6 months, and if the rest of the lung fields are reasonably clear, resection may offer definite benefit. A patient with localized atelectasis which has resisted vigorous outpatient therapy with postural drainage, pulmonary physiotherapy, antibiotics, and aerosol inhalations should be admitted to the hospital for bronchoscopy and a bronchogram. It is beneficial to combine these two procedures since the bronchoscopic aspiration and lavage allows the removal of thick purulent secretions.

This procedure in itself is of benefit to the patient, but it also allows better filling of the bronchiectatic spaces by the contrast material. Often only 5–6 ml of a contrast material such as aqueous Dionsil is required to map the tracheobronchial tree in suspicious areas. The contrast material is introduced under fluoroscopy by a catheter through the endotracheal tube. Small amounts of contrast are injected into the orifice of the atelectatic lobe and into any other suspicious area of the lung. When roentgenograms are completed, the tracheobronchial tree is again aspirated and lavaged by way of the endotracheal tube. When performed in this fashion, the procedure is safe and often the aspiration lavage provides temporary improvement. Computerized tomography is presently being evaluated to replace bronchiography.

Schuster[28] performed pulmonary resection in 21 patients. Eighty percent experienced a decrease in symptoms and nine patients were completely free of symptoms for a prolonged period. Mearns and her associates carried out 23 resections in children aged 11 months to 15 years.[29] They concluded that the resection should be done at an early age, particularly if the localized atelectasis occurs before 2 years. The surgical specimens in their cases demonstrated complete collapse, obliteration of the airway by fibrous tissues, and endobronchial abscesses. One of their patients who had a fulminant lung abscess died in the immediate postoperative period.

Twenty-one of the 22 survivors were improved and 6 were completely free of symptoms for prolonged periods of time. There were seven late deaths from 3 to 8 years postoperatively. In order for pulmonary resection to be carried out safely, a prolonged period of postural drainage and pulmonary physiotherapy is required to clear the tracheobronchial tree of purulent secretions. In the most severe cases a preoperative tracheostomy may be required to remove the secretions by suction. Unfortunately, tracheostomies carry their own complications and prevent the patient from coughing. We prefer intensive medical treatment, perhaps combined with tracheobronchial lavage through an endotracheal tube or bronchoscopy.

Hemoptysis

Hemoptysis is a sudden, terrifying event which brings the specter of death to patients with chronic suppurative pulmonary disease. With the advance of cystic fibrosis, the bronchial arteries become enlarged, tortuous, and thin-walled in response to the chronic inflammation and peribronchiolar granulation tissue. Bronchial arteriography has demonstrated this enlargement and tortuosity, as well as direct shunts between the bronchial and pulmonary circulation.[30,31] Erosion of these bronchial vessels leads to hemoptysis.

Schuster and Fellows have observed excellent correlation between bronchoscopy and selective arteriography in localizing the source of hemorrhage.[32] Bronchoscopy is most useful when the initial massive hemorrhage has slowed to a "trickle," because endoscopy is not only dangerous but unrewarding when the tracheobronchial tree is filled with blood. Selective bronchial arteriography will demonstrate the large, tortuous vessels and, if the study is performed during a major hemorrhage, extravasation of contrast will specifically localize the bleeding site.

The initial treatment of hemoptysis includes bed rest, sedation, and transfusions to maintain blood volume. In the rare instance when bleeding is localized to the bronchiectatic lobe, and if the remaining lung is relatively clear, pulmonary resection provides suitable treatment for the hemoptysis and the localized purulent focus. Unfortunately, most of these patients have advanced, diffuse disease. In these cases, bronchial artery embolization may be performed concomitantly with arteriography. Schuster and Fellows[32] reported success with Gelfoam embolization through a bronchial artery catheter. Embolization was carried out in eight of their patients. Bleeding was controlled in all. Unfortunately, two patients died within one month with respiratory failure. Two patients required multiple embolization before cessation of the massive hemoptysis occurred. There is a risk of transverse myelitis with this form of therapy because the emboli may occlude the vertebral arteries.

Portal Hypertension

Focal biliary cirrhosis with plugging of bile ductules by inspissated secretions occurs very early in the course of cystic fibrosis of the pancreas. These liver changes may progress to severe biliary cirrhosis, cholangitis, and biliary stasis in the older patients. This progressive, extensive liver pathology is the basis for portal hypertension which leads to the esophageal varices and hypersplenism occasionally seen in teenagers and young adults. Schuster and his associates have now reviewed 48 patients with cystic fibrosis and portal hypertension.[33] This represents a 2% incidence among 2500 patients who were followed over 25 years. Portal hypertension develops insidiously but should be suspected in any patient with a firm liver and an enlarging spleen. Although hypersplenism as measured by a decreased platelet, white, or red blood cell count is a common laboratory finding, in our experience the hypersplenism secondary to portal hypertension has rarely presented serious problems. Massive upper gastrointestinal hemorrhage is often the first clinical symptom. The sudden onset of hematemesis often follows a febrile illness associated with the ingestion of aspirin.

The differential diagnosis consists of peptic ulcer and gastritis. The presence of a palpably enlarged spleen strongly suggests portal hypertension and esophageal varices. Fortunately, the bleeding from any of these lesions will stop with bed rest, antacids, and lavage of the stomach with an iced solution of 1% sodium bicarbonate. Transfusions, preferably with fresh whole blood, are given to replace losses as measured by the vital signs and urinary output. When the bleeding has stopped, an esophagogram and an upper gastrointestinal roentgen study will demonstrate the varices. Although endoscopy will confirm the diagnosis, in our hands roentgenographic studies are less traumatic and will demonstrate the varices as accurately as endoscopy. On the other hand, if varices are not demonstrated and if the roentgen studies do not indicate the site of bleeding, flexible endoscopy is indicated to study the esophagus, stomach, and duodenum in order to determine the source of hemorrhage.

Several operations will reliably control portal hypertension in older children. A portocaval shunt will completely divert blood away from the liver, and is most effective in lowering portal pressure. A splenorenal shunt will also decompress the portal system. If neither of the above operations is feasible, a mesocaval shunt between the end of the divided inferior vena cava and the side of the superior mesenteric vein is also satisfactory. Although all of these operations will lower portal pressure and prevent future episodes of bleeding, one must weigh the potential benefits of a major difficult operation against the possible deleterious effects on pulmonary function. In addition, diversion of blood away from the liver may decrease liver function and certainly increases the risk of hepatic encephalopathy.

Schuster and his associates feel that a shunt operation should be performed on patients with portal hypertension with a "good pulmonary status." They would operate on a patient who had had one episode of variceal hemorrhage or on a patient with hypersplenism who had not yet bled. With this aggressive approach they have operated on 25 patients; 16 have survived for 1 month to 15 years, 9 patients died early following the operation, and 11 others survived from 9 months to 11 years. Deaths in their series were due to progressive pulmonary failure, postoperative bleeding, and hepatic decompensation.

Currently in our own practice, we have treated these patients conservatively with antacids, a bland diet, and strict avoidance of aspirin. We have reserved operations for those children with recurrent or life-endangering hemorrhage. Our choice is a side-to-side splenorenal shunt with preservation of the spleen. (See Chapter 18 for further discussion of this topic.)

REFERENCES

1. Donnison AB, Shwachman H, Gross RE: A review of 164 children with meconium ileus seen at the Children's Hospital Medical Center, Boston. *Pediatrics* 1966;37:833–850.
2. Holsclaw DS, Epstein HB, Nixon HH: Meconium ileus 20 year review of 109 cases. *Am J Dis Child* 1965;109:101–113.
3. 1976 Report on Survival Studies of Patients with Cystic Fibrosis. Atlanta, Georgia, Cystic Fibrosis Foundation, 1978, p 3.
4. Thomaidis TS, Arey JB: Intestinal lesions in cystic fibrosis of the pancreas. *J Pediatr* 1963;63:444–453.
5. White H: Meconium ileus new roentgen sign. *Radiology* 1956;66:567–571.
6. Neuhauser EB: Roentgen changes associated with pancreatic insufficiency in early life. *Radiology* 1946;46:319–328.
7. Noblitt HR: Treatment of uncomplicated meconium ileus by Gastrografin enema—a preliminary report. *J Pediatr Surg* 1969;4: 190–197.
8. Gross RE: *The Surgery of Infancy and Childhood.* Philadelphia, WB Saunders, 1953.
9. Swenson O: *Pediatric Surgery.* New York, Appleton, Century, Crofts, 1958.
10. Bishop HC, Koop CE: Management of meconium ileus. *Ann Surg* 1957;145:410–414.
11. Harberg FJ, Senekjian EK, Pokorny WJ: Treatment of uncomplicated meconium ileus via T tube ileostomy. *J Pediatr Surg* 1981;16:61–63.
12. McKity VG, Hoogman JE, Paciulli J: Meconium blockage syndrome. *Radiology* 1967;88:740–744.
13. Ellis DG, Clatworthy HW: The meconium plug syndrome revisited. *J Pediatr Surg* 1966;1:54–61.
14. Levy EA: Case of fibrocystic disease of the pancreas with intestinal obstruction. *Arch Dis Child* 1951;26:335–339.
15. Birse EL: Intestinal obstruction as a late complication of fibrocystic disease of the pancreas. *Br Med J* 1956;2:286–287.
16. Jensen KG: Meconium ileus equivalent in a 15-year-old patient with mucoviscidosis. *Acta Paediatr* 1962;51:344–348.
17. Cordonnier JK, Izant RJ: Meconium ileus equivalent. *Surgery* 1963;54:667–672.
18. Spiro RK, Landman ME: Meconium ileus equivalent. *Am J Gastroenterol* 1978;69: 302–306.
19. Matseshe JW, Go VL, DiMagno E: Meconium ileus equivalent complicating cystic fibrosis in young adults—report of 12 cases. *Gastroenterology* 1977;72:732–736.
20. Glick SN, Kressel HY, Laufer I, et al: Meconium ileus equivalent—treatment with Hypaque enema. *Diagn Imaging* 1980;49: 149–152.
21. Holsclaw DS, Rocmans L, Shwachman H: Intussusception in patients with cystic fibrosis. *Pediatrics* 1971;48:51–58.
22. Shwachman H, Holsclaw DS: Examination of the appendix at laparotomy as a diagnostic clue in cystic fibrosis. *N Engl J Med* 1972; 286:1300–1301.
23. Holsclaw DS, Rocmans L, Shwachman H: Abdominal complaints and appendiceal changes leading to the diagnosis of cystic fibrosis. *J Pediatr Surg* 1974;9:867–873.
24. Holsclaw DS, Habboushe C: Occult appendiceal abscess complicating cystic fibrosis. *J Pediatr Surg* 1976;11:217–221.
25. Kulczycki L, Shwachman H: Studies in cystic fibrosis of the pancreas, occurrence of rectal prolapse. *N Engl J Med* 1958;259:409–412.
26. Rich RH, Warwick WJ, Leonard AS: Open thoracotomy and pleural abrasion in the treatment of spontaneous pneumothorax in cystic fibrosis. *J Pediatr Surg* 1978;13(3): 237–241.
27. Luck SR, Raffensperger JG, Sullivan HJ, et al: Management of pneumothorax in children with chronic pulmonary disease. *J Thorac Cardiovasc Surg* 1977;74(6):834–839.
28. Schuster S, Shwachman H, Harris BC, et al: Pulmonary surgery for cystic fibrosis. *J Thorac Cardiovasc Surg* 1964;48(8):750–760.
29. Mearns M, Hodson CJ, Jackson A, et al: Pulmonary resection in cystic fibrosis—results in 23 cases, 1957–1970. *Arch Dis Child* 1972;47:499–508.
30. Fellows KE, Stigol L, Schuster S, et al: Selective bronchial arteriography in patients with cystic fibrosis and massive hemoptysis. *Radiology* 1975;114:551–556.
31. Liebow AA, Hales MR, Lindskog GE: Enlargement of the bronchial arteries and their anastomoses with the pulmonary arteries in bronchiectasis. *Am J Pathol* 1949;25:211–231.
32. Schuster SR, Fellows KE: Management of major hemoptysis in patients with cystic fibrosis. *J Pediatr Surg* 1977;12:889–896.
33. Schuster SR, Shwachman H, Toyama W, et al: The management of portal hypertension in cystic fibrosis. *J Pediatr Surg* 1977;12(2): 201–206.
34. Olsen M, Luck S, Lloyd-Still JD, et al: The spectrum of meconium disease in infancy. *J Pediatr Surg* 1982;17(5):479–482.

22

Neurological Complications in Cystic Fibrosis

Lawrence G. Tomasi

Approaching cystic fibrosis as a neurologist requires little, if any, consideration of its basic genetic defect but rather an appreciation of the neurological syndromes associated with chronic malnutrition, intractable respiratory infections and, ultimately, pulmonary insufficiency. These syndromes represent involvement of the central nervous system secondary to extracranial processes that are encountered frequently in a variety of common medical diseases. Thus, their signs and symptoms are well described in the literature, even if their incidence and prevalence in cystic fibrosis remain somewhat uncertain. There is a suggestion from recent reports on adolescents and young adults with cystic fibrosis, however, that modern management techniques have increased the frequency of these central nervous complications in addition to increasing life expectancy.

PULMONARY INSUFFICIENCY

Because chronic obstructive pulmonary disease is the major cause of morbidity and mortality in cystic fibrosis patients that survive infancy,[1,2] an understanding of the metabolic encephalopathy associated with pulmonary insufficency is useful in the management of these patients. The mechanisms by which this altered cerebral function occurs has not been fully explained, and the encephalopathy, in most instances, is a summation of the cerebral signs in hypoxemia,[3] congestive heart failure,[5] systemic infection,[6] and neuromuscular fatigue. Of these variables, the degree of CO_2 retention correlates most closely with the neurological symptoms.[7] In addition, at a given P_aCO_2 those patients whose pulmonary insufficiency is chronic have significantly less cerebral dysfunction, suggesting an increase in the brain's capacity to buffer the excess bicarbonate. In these cases, the severity of neurological symptoms is better correlated with the degree of acidosis within the cerebral spinal fluid, reflecting brain P_aCO_2, than with the arterial P_aCO_2.[8]

The mental changes usually begin insidiously with symptoms of insomnia, nervousness, low frustration tolerance, and dull diffuse headaches which may progress to confusion, disorientation, lethargy, and stupor. More rapid progression of these symptoms is commonly associated with acute systemic or pulmonary infections but also frequently may be precipitated by sedatives and/or tranquilizers inappropriately prescribed for treatment of the initial symptoms. Seizures are rare. The pupils are small and briskly reactive unless hypoxia is significant, in which case they are dilated and fixed. Infrequently, distended ophthalmic veins and papilledema are noted on funduscopic examination, reflecting the increased intracranial pressure associated with chronic hypercarbia and hypoxia. Other prominent neurological signs commonly noted include multifocal myoclonus and asterixis. Muscle tone is normal to mildly increased with depressed deep tendon reflexes. Bilateral positive Babinski signs are frequent.[9]

The diagnosis of hypercapnic–hypoxic encephalopathy is not difficult when a patient's chronic obstructive pulmonary disease is near its terminal stages. A greater diagnostic problem occurs, however, if a patient with previously compensated but marginal pulmonary function becomes encephalopathic as a result of a large bronchial mucous plug, hemoptysis, pneumothorax, systemic infection, or excessive sedation. The headaches, confusion, and somnolence may attract more attention than the signs of respiratory decompensation.[10] If such a patient also demonstrates the previously described neurological signs suggestive of increased intracranial pressure, it is easy to see how a physician could incorrectly arrive at the diagnosis of a brain abscess or some other intracranial catastrophe, subjecting the patient to unnecessary diagnostic studies.

In the management of pulmonary insufficiency, two associated conditions closely related to CO_2 narcosis often exacerbate the neurological dysfunction. One is hypoxemia, and the other is metabolic alkalosis secondary to aggressive management. As noted previously, the severity of the encephalopathy is more closely related to the degree and acuteness of the hypercapnia than to the hypoxia. The severity of cerebral dysfunction associated with increasing hypoxia is described in Figure 22-1. Cerebral blood flow (CBF) progressively increases with arterial P_aO_2s of less than 50 mm Hg and coma secondary to hypoxia rarely occurs until the arterial P_aO_2 approaches 30 mm Hg. Hypoxia of this magnitude must be corrected because of the threat of immediate irreversible damage to the central nervous system.[11] Overzealous treatment, however, frequently removes the hypoxemia-stimulated respirations, resulting in further CO_2 retention and exacerbation of the neurological symptoms. On the other hand, the encephalopathy also may become more severe by the rapid correction of the CO_2 narcosis by artificial ventilation with the development of a metabolic alkalosis. Although usually asymptomatic, it has been associated with the development of multifocal myoclonic seizures and death,[12] perhaps related to the decreased cerebral blood flow secondary to intense cerebral vasoconstriction associated with the hypocapnia.

The development of an encephalopathy also has been related to a massive loss of salt and water in the sweat of patients with cystic fibrosis.[1,2] Classically, the development of a dilutional hyponatremia was both more common and dangerous in infants. With improved medical care, this complication also has become frequent in adult cystic fibrosis

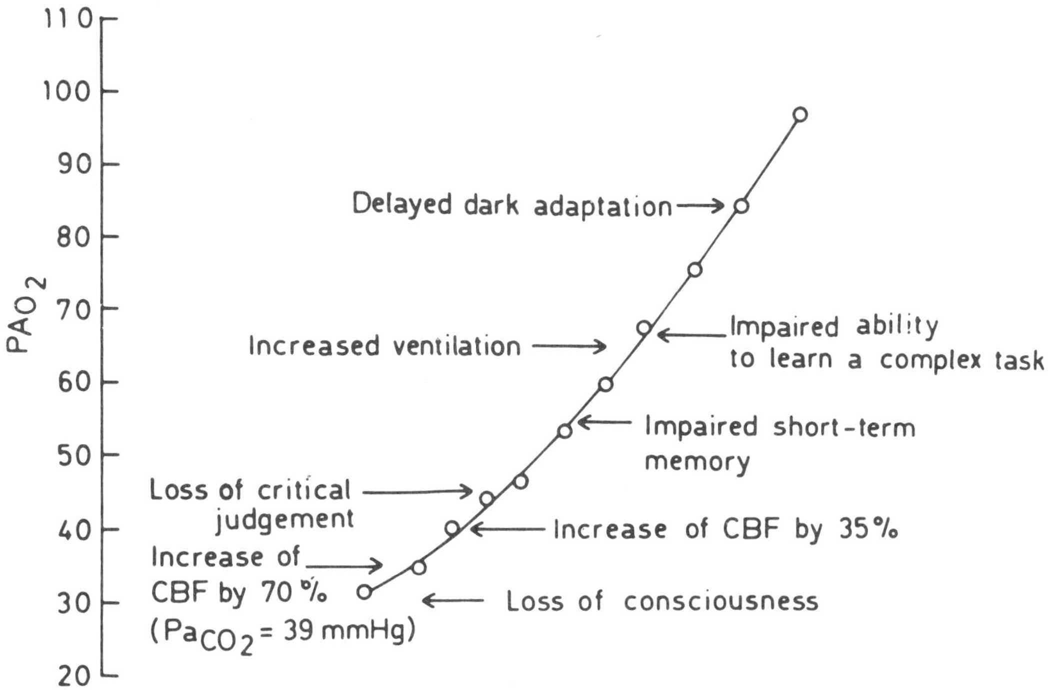

Figure 22-1 Behavioral responses to hypoxia. Reproduced with permission of Siesjö OK, Johannsson H, Fjungren B, et al: Brain dysfunction in metabolic disorders, in Plum F (ed): *Research Publication Association of Nervous and Mental Disorders* (reference 11), New York, Raven Press, 1974.

patients with a recently reported incidence of 6%.[2] The syndrome of inappropriate antidiuretic hormone secretion also has been described.[13] The neurological symptoms of dilutional hyponatremia result from the excess accumulation of water within the cells of the central nervous system, hence the term water intoxication, and are caused by altered excitability of the neuronal membranes.[14] Neurological symptoms are related both to the absolute serum sodium concentration and the rapidity with which the dilutional hyponatremia developed.[15] In a group of 65 patients with hyponatremia,[16] the mean serum sodium concentration at which symptoms of confusion, stupor, coma, and seizures occurred were 120 mEq/liter, 114 mEq/liter, 112 mEq/liter, and 110 mEq/liter, respectively (Figure 22-2). Although these results demonstrated a highly significant overall correlation between the serum sodium and neurological dysfunction, the substantial overlap that existed was related to the etiology of the hyponatremia and the rapidity of its development. One would anticipate that modern management techniques improving the physical endurance of cystic fibrosis patients also could result in an increased incidence and prevalence of water intoxication if appropriate salt supplementation is not provided (see Chapter 4).

RESPIRATORY INFECTIONS

An intractable lifelong bacterial bronchitis and sinusitis is a hallmark of cystic fibrosis. Recent reviews of adults with cystic fibrosis indicate that the destructiveness of the bacterial infection continued to progress with increasing age as evidenced by pulmonary complications such as minor hemoptysis (60%), massive hemoptysis (7%), and pneumothorax (16%), all of which are rare in childhood.[2] Severe sinusitis and nasal polyps also were increasingly prevalent.[1,2]

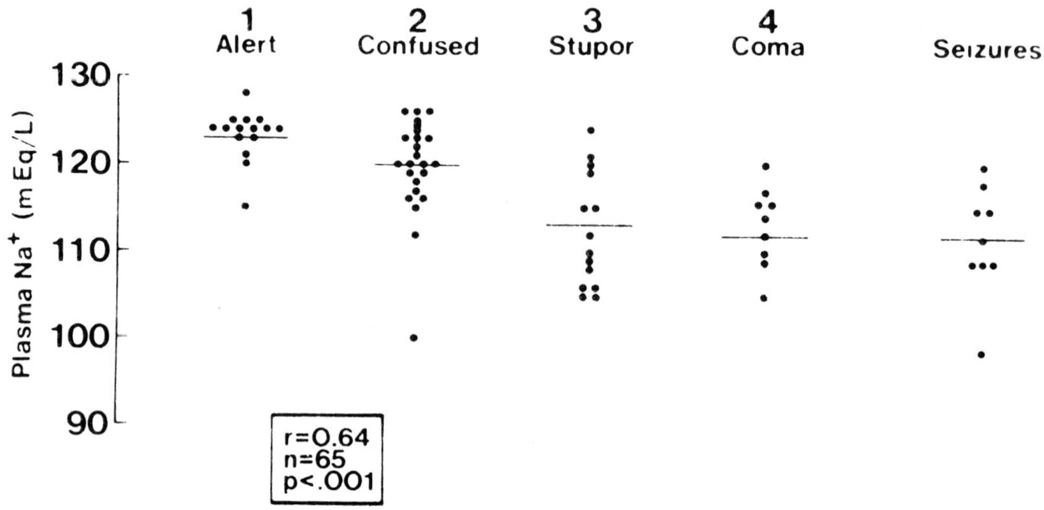

Figure 22-2 The relationship between plasma sodium concentration and depression of sensorium in 65 patients with plasma sodiums of 128 mEq/liter or less. All patients who developed seizures had plasma sodiums of less than 122 mEq/liter. Reproduced with permission of Arieff AI, Flach F, Massry SG: Neurological manifestation and morbidity of hyponatremia: correlation with brain water and electrolytes. *Medicine* 1976;55:121–129.

Considering the increased life expectancy of cystic fibrosis patients and the destructive nature of their chronic respiratory infection, the reports[17,18] describing four young adults who developed a brain abscess could have been anticipated, despite the fact that they are unknown in childhood. Each presented with the classical symptoms and signs of increased intracranial pressure associated with an expanding intracranial mass lesion. They were treated by conventional therapy, and the three patients that survived have minimal neurological sequelae. In one patient, the organism isolated from the abscess also was isolated extracranially and the source was determined to be the oral cavity.[17] Since the pathogenesis, diagnosis, and treatment of brain abscesses in cystic fibrosis are similar if not identical to that described in other diseases with chronic bacterial respiratory infections, the general concepts required for diagnosis and treatment will be reviewed. In older cystic fibrosis patients, a high index of suspicion, early diagnosis, and modern nonsurgical management can convert the presence of a brain abscess from a terminal complication of their chronic obstructive pulmonary disease to one with little if any neurological sequelae.

Except in cases associated with trauma, the occurrence of a brain abscess should always be considered secondary to a focus of suppuration elsewhere in the body.[19] An appreciation of the means by which the organisms reach the brain is an essential requirement in the understanding of the etiology of brain abscesses and other intracranial infectious processes, such as epidural and subdural empyema, from which they must be distinguished. In the preantibiotic era, mastoiditis and sinusitis accounted for more than 50% of the cases[20] and even now are recognized as a frequent source of the infection.[21] The infection commonly reaches the nervous system by direct extension which may be documented by an associated osteomyelitis and/or empyema. In other cases, the mode of extension is via the diploic veins which provide a direct route from the infected sinuses to the leptomeninges. The most frequent route in the development of an intracranial abscess, however, is via a bacteremia whose source is either the mouth, nasal sinuses, or lungs.[19,22]

It has been demonstrated that the injection of bacteria into normal brain tissue will rarely create an abscess and that cerebral circulatory dysfunction, especially embolic infarction, is a prerequisite for its development.[23] Ischemia of nervous system tissue is considered necessary for the breakdown of the blood–brain barrier, providing the offending organisms direct access to nervous tissue. The lack of collateral circulation and relatively poor inflammatory response within the nervous system are ideal for proliferation of anaerobic organisms. Multiple organisms are frequently recovered with anaerobic streptococcus isolated in up to 50% of the cases.[24] In another series,[25] anaerobic organisms were isolated alone or in combination with aerobic organisms in 63% and 26% of the cases, respectively. In only 11% were aerobic organisms the principal infectious agent.

Considering the pathogenesis of cerebral abscesses, one can only speculate as to the reasons for their low incidence in cystic fibrosis. In the four patients reported,[17,18] the presence of multiple abscesses in three patients and the remoteness from the paranasal sinuses in the fourth suggests the mechanism of bacteremia and embolic infarction. Factors common to cystic fibrosis patients that may depress the occurrence of a bacteremia include high titers of locally produced IGA,[26] hypergammaglobulinemia,[27] and high specific antibody titers to the infecting organisms.[28] Perhaps, even more important than these physiological mechanisms is the routine management of cystic fibrosis patients with prophylactic broad-spectrum antibiotics. With respect to the vascular system, it is not certain that pulmonary right-to-left shunts occur in cystic fibrosis and significant atherosclerosis within the cerebral circulation would be unlikely in these patients based on their age and nutrition. The relative abscence of dental caries,[29] a common source of bacteremia, also may be a mitigating factor.

The symptoms and signs of a brain abscess are characteristically those of an expanding intracranial mass lesion. The inital symptoms are most often a dull nondescript headache. In about half the patients, the headache is more severe on one side, which helps to localize the abscess. Seizures are less frequent. The headache increases in severity and later is accompanied by other symptoms of increased intracranial pressure such as nausea, morning vomiting, and lethargy. Papilledema and focal neurological signs occur relatively late in the course of the illness. Often the focal neurological signs tend to be obscured by the patient's drowsiness and general ill health. Visual-field deficits and frontal lobe release signs such as the grasp and suck reflexes are important to note, although a hemiparesis is frequently described in ambulatory patients.

A common misconception is that cerebral abscesses, like abscesses elsewhere in the body, will provoke fever, leukocytosis, and increased sedimentation rate. In fact, only if the abscess is adjacent to or involves the leptomeninges are systemic manifestations of the infectious illness noted, the most frequent being nuchal rigidity. As a general rule, abscesses are within the brain at the grey–white matter junction with symptoms and signs of an expanding intracranial mass lession such as a tumor providing few clues of its infectious etiology.

Neither routine skull x-rays nor a lumbar puncture are helpful in excluding an abscess, but the latter commonly is associated with herniation and death in their presence. Signs of increased intracranial pressure such as split sutures, silver-beaten markings, and erosion of the sella are uncommon in such rapidly expanding lesions. Osteomyelitis, even if present, is rarely demonstrated on routine skull films. In those patients in whom a lumbar puncture inadvertently was performed, a moderate increase in CSF pressure, pleocytosis (20–300 cells), a mild elevation in protein, and a normal glucose are the rule. The EEG may be considered a useful screening procedure, demonstrating disturbances in electrical activity in the majority of patients (68%). These disturbances, however, are frequently nonspecific and the unilateral high-voltage slow-wave activity of less than 2 cycles per second described as specific for brain abscess (Figure 22-3) was detected in only 38% of the patients.[30]

Both the brain scan and the CT scan (Figure 22-4) have been major advances in the diagnosis of cerebral abscesses. Although the brain scan may be slightly more sensitive in establishing the diagnosis, both demonstrate an accuracy that approaches 100%. More importantly, the CT scan has revolutionized management of cerebral abscesses, significantly decreasing their morbidity and mortality, and is perhaps the most significant advance in their management since antibiotics.[31] Utilizing the CT scan to determine the number of abscesses as well as for the stereotactic placement of a needle through a small burr hole for drainage and cultures has resulted in the nonsurgical management of these patients in the majority of cases.[32–34] Frequent follow-up CT scans while the patient is being treated with antibiotics and Decadron can demonstrate quantitatively the response to therapy. Such therapy spares injury to the surrounding edematous but normal brain tissue (Figure 22-4) and results in minimal neurological sequelae in those patients diagnosed early.

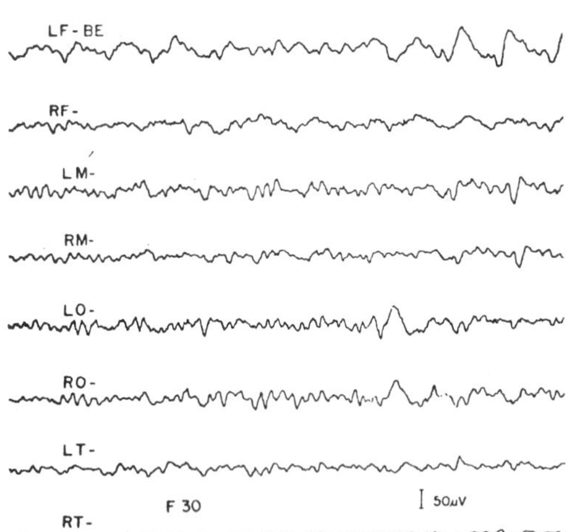

Figure 22-3 Electroencephalographic localization of an abscess in the frontal aspect of the left cerebral hemisphere. Note rhythmic delta activity of 1–2 cycles per second occurring in the left frontal leads (LF-BE) in comparison to the recording from the right frontal leads (RF). More nonspecific delta waves are present in other areas of the recording with disorganization of the background activity. Reproduced with permission of Kooi KA, Tucker RT, Marshall RE: *Fundamentals of Electroencephalography.* New York, Harper & Row, 1978.

In the majority of cases, this neurological complication is readily distinguished from the encephalopathy of pulmonary insufficiency. In difficult cases, however, the CT scan or brain scan is an important neurodiagnostic test to exclude the presence of an abscess. In the single cystic fibrosis patient who died during treatment, there was associated intracranial bleeding. Such a complication might be more frequently encountered in cystic fibrosis, considering the vasodilatation and hypervolemia associated with carbon dioxide retention as well as clotting abnormalities associated with hepatic dysfunction and vitamin K deficiency. The importance of cultures in these patients cannot be overemphasized, considering that the organism almost certainly will be partially resistant to the antibiotics utilized for therapeutic management.

MALNUTRITION

A major advance in the management of cystic fibrosis was the prevention of protein–calorie malnutrition utilizing pancreatic supplements. More recent nutritional concerns are related to the potential consequences of selective dietary deficiencies such as trace metals and fat-soluble vitamins. The diagnosis of cystic fibrosis must be considered, however, before these management techniques are utilized, and a recent clinical pathological conference[35] grimly outlines the failure to thrive, dehydration, and hypoglycemia that may occur in the undiagnosed infant. Although not mutually exclusive, the neurological manifestations of malnutrition in the infant and older child with cystic fibrosis are sufficiently distinct that they will be discussed separately.

Infancy

Central nervous system growth and maturation during the first year of life may

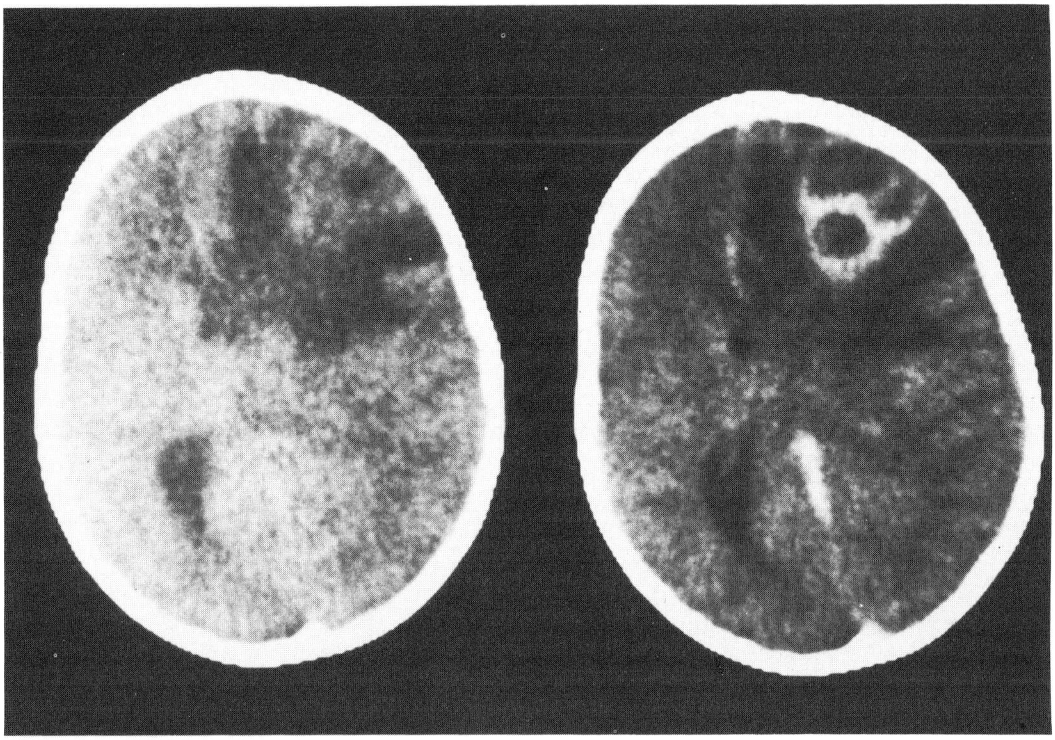

Figure 22-4 Computerized tomogram (CT) scans in a patient with a right frontal lobe abscess. Scan prior to contrast infusion (left) demonstrates a large irregular hypodense zone within the right frontal area with ventricular distortion. Scan following contrast infusion (right) demonstrates a large abscess with ring enhancement and daughter abscesses anteriorally. The capsule of the abscesses demonstrated by the contrast enhancement are emphasized by the hypodense neucrotic core within the ring as well as the hypodense lesion of cerebral edema surrounding the abscess (donut sign).

be estimated by means of the occipital frontal circumference (OFC) of the skull, but the true rapidity of brain growth may only be appreciated by the fact that brain weight is related to the OFC by the following exponential function[36]:

$$\text{Brain weight (g)} = \frac{x^3}{100} - \frac{3000}{2x}$$

where x = OFC (cm).

Thus, brain weight is doubled at 6 months of age and almost triples by 1 year reaching 80% of its adult weight, whereas the extracranial mass of a 1-year-old infant is less than 15% of adult proportions.[37] Morphologically, this growth spurt of the central nervous system consists of glial multiplication, myelination, dendritic growth, and establishment of synaptic connections.[38] During infancy, only the granular neurons of the cerebellum increase in number early in the neonatal period; the neurons of the cerebral cortex achieve adult numbers by the middle of gestation.

The belief that "malnutrition spares the brain" is based on observations in adults dying of malnutrition and is not directly applicable to infants. In experimental animal models, protein–calorie undernutrition results in a modest decrease in brain weight in association with the marked decrease in somatic growth. Numerous studies in humans from preindustrialized countries with malnutrition have demonstrated similar reductions in brain weight.[39–41] Cell number as estimated by DNA[42] also is reduced, although for the most part it is the glial and not the neuronal population.

Biochemically, there is a reduction in brain lipids,[43–45] with a concomitant reduction in the enzymes necessary for their synthesis. The lipids were predominantly constituents of myelin membranes, and their ratios indicated an absolute reduction in myelin rather than an altered composition.[43,45] Alterations in amino acid patterns in the neurotransmitters also have been described. There is no definable neuropathology in the traditional sense, but clearly, during development, undernutrition has the potential to adversely influence cell division, migration, and elaboration of synaptic connections. For the most part, however, it would appear that these developmental changes are of a quantitative nature, with no striking distortion in either the morphology of the cells or the complexity of their connections, and have been viewed more in terms of a retardation in the normal developmental process. On the other hand, utilizing these same morphological and neurochemical techniques, it is virtually impossible to differentiate the nervous tissue of a genius from that of an idiot.

Clinically, malnourished infants are apathetic, irritable, and weak, with marasmic children suffering a greater reduction in head circumference than those with kwashiorkor.[46,47] On examination, these infants may demonstrate an increased transillumination of the head, considered to be the result of an excess accumulation of subarachnoid fluid over the cerebral hemispheres.[49] Proximal muscle wasting with weakness is associated with muscular hypotonia and hyporeflexia in 40–50% of the older infants.[50,51]

Neurophysiologically, abnormalities have been demonstrated in the electroencephalogram,[52] evoked potentials,[53] and nerve conduction studies.[54] Following treatment, the majority of these abnormalities revert to normal; head circumference is an exception. Similar to the morphological data, these findings are abnormal primarily in that they reflect a delay in the normal maturation of the nervous system rather than a neuropathological pattern. Normalization of these parameters upon follow-up indicates that this developmental delay is not irreversible, but such parameters have little relationship to the adequacy of higher cortical functions in adulthood.

In conclusion, major objective parameters of growth and maturation of the nervous system are delayed by undernutrition in infancy, with brain size perhaps representing the only persistent deficit in the adult. Inasmuch as intellectual function may bear some relationship to brain size, numerous studies have reported on the patterns of motor and cognitive development in these children. The vast majority of these studies, utilizing children from preindustrialized countries, agree that in early childhood a deficit in standardized developmental tests may be demonstrated, but intellectual deficits persisting into later life are much less frequently reported. The few studies that have been performed on children with chronic malnutrition since birth secondary to intestinal malabsorption rather than protein–calorie deprivation are of greater relevance. They report delays in early childhood but were unable to demonstrate deficits persisting into later childhood.[55,56] At 6½–7 years of age, children with cystic fibrosis or prior ileal resection in the neonatal period performed similar to controls in the Goodenough-Harris drawing test.[55]

Perhaps, the most pertinent study for our purposes was the report of the 41 patients[56] who were malnourished in the first year of life secondary to cystic fibrosis (34 cases), protracted diarrhea (4 cases), and ileal atresia (3 cases). The mean weight for these patients during the first 6 months of life correspond to the 70th percentile malnutrition on the Wellcome classification,[57] whereas if the lowest individual weight for each infant during this same period is utilized, 58% of the infants had evidence of third-degree malnutrition.[58] At the time of their evaluation, 2–21 years later, the mean head circumference of the group was in the 12th percentile, whereas their heights and weights were all between the 3rd and 25th percentile.

The standardized tests of intelligence utilized were dependent on the patients' age and included the Merrill-Palmer scale (18–72 months of age); the Wechsler intelligence scale for children (WISC) (5–15 years of age), and the Wechsler adult intelligence scale (WAIS) (14 years to adulthood). Sensory motoric abilities were estimated by the Lincoln-Oseretsky test of motor ability (5–15 years of age), and social adaption was estimated utilizing the Vineland scale of social maturity. The control group consisted of 41 siblings who were not matched for age or position in the family. An estimate of parental IQ and social-economic classification also was reported.

Significant differences between the malnourished infants and sibling controls upon follow-up were statistically significant only between 2 and 5 years of age on the Merrill-Palmer intelligence test (Figure 22-5) and

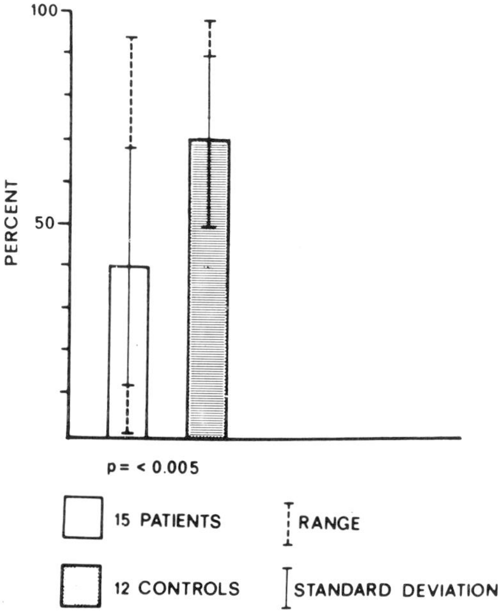

Figure 22-5 Performance on the Merrill-Palmer intelligence test of children between 2 and 5 years of age that were undernourished in infancy because of chronic malabsorption. Comparison to sibling controls. Reproduced with permission of Lloyd-Still JD, Hurwitz I, Wolff PH, et al: Intellectual development after severe malnutrition in infancy. *Pediatrics* 1974;54:306–311 (reference 56). Copyright 1974, American Academy of Pediatrics.

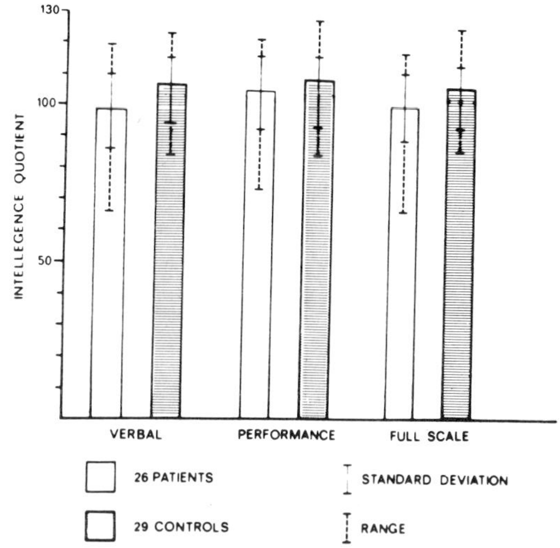

Figure 22-6 Performance on the WISC and WAIS intelligence tests of children greater than 5 years of age that were undernourished in infancy because of intestinal malabsorption. Comparison with sibling controls. Reproduced with the permission of Lloyd-Still JD, Hurwitz I, Wolff PH, et al: Intellectual development after severe malnutrition in infancy. *Pediatrics* 1974;54: 306–311 (reference 56). Copyright 1974, American Academy of Pediatrics.

not, in later childhood, on either the WISC or WAIS (Figure 22-6). There were no significant differences between the groups in the Lincoln-Oseretsky test of motor development or the Vineland scale of social maturity. Although numerous postulates have been advanced to explain these findings, perhaps the simplest is that infant intelligence tests, which evaluate primarily sensory and motor functions, are more heavily dependent on the physical health of the child than the standardized intelligence tests utilized at later ages, which depend on language development and the ability to abstract and reason.

In conclusion, the effects of protein-calorie undernutrition during infancy on central nervous system maturation has been demonstrated morphologically, neurochemically, clinically, neurophysiologically, and developmentally. By these parameters, this deficit is best viewed as a delay in the normal nervous maturation rather than any neuropathological alteration. Reversal of these maturational deficits has been demonstrated clinically, neurophysiologically, and developmentally, with a possible deficit in the brain mass as a significant nagging exception. Despite appropriate continuing concern that deficits in higher cortical function may be a result of protein–calorie undernutrition during infancy, such a deficit has been difficult to substantiate, especially in those countries for which the intelligence tests are standardized.

The psychological trauma associated with protein–calorie undernutrition in infancy and continuing in childhood which has not been discussed may be a more significant factor in dulling the intellectual behavior of these children in adulthood, but such parameters are difficult to examine with standardized intelligence tests. Further research may clarify these problems, but at the present time the level of protein–calorie undernutrition common in cystic fibrosis patients should not be considered as an etiology for delayed central nervous system maturation.

That early restitution for protein–calorie malnutrition can result in "catch-up brain growth" during early infancy has been inferred by reports of increased intracranial pressure in deprived normal infants[59,60] and patients with cystic fibrosis following appropriate therapy.[61,62] In the majority of reports, the only sign suggestive of increased intracranial pressure was a bulging anterior fontanelle occurring within the first week of treatment. Rarely has an elevated cerebral spinal fluid pressure been recorded upon lumbar puncture,[62] and convincing evidence of a significant increase in the OFC during this period has not been reported. The bulging anterior fontanelle disappears during the second week of therapy with the infant's neurological evaluation remaining unchanged throughout the entire time of the episode. Although one could speculate that the etiology of this presumed increased intracranial pressure is improved cerebral blood flow and a transient increase in intracranial blood volume rather than accelerated brain growth, the latter explanation is more satisfying and emphasizes the importance of early diagnosis in cystic fibrosis.

In contrast to the syndrome of presumed "catch-up brain growth" associated with improved nutrition, two other syndromes should be considered in the cystic fibrosis infant with a bulging anterior fontanelle. One is that associated with tetracycline therapy and the other is vitamin A deficiency. This unusual complication of tetracycline therapy is usually noted within the first few days after initiation of the drug and has been reported to occur after a single dose.[63,64] Unless recognized, the infant may develop signs of increased intracranial pressure, including lethargy, vomiting, and opisthotonic posturing. Meningitis is often suspected in such children until the lumbar puncture is performed. The mechanism by which tetracycline creates this increased intracranial pressure has not been established, but rapid resolution of the symptoms and signs is associated with withdrawal of the medication. Although now infrequently utilized in infancy because of the permanent staining of the secondary teeth, such symptoms of increased intracranial pressure have also been reported in older children[65] and in adults.[66]

The influence of vitamin A on the developing nervous system is impressive, with more than 70 types of malformations cataloged primarily associated with hypervitaminosis A exposure during gestation.[67] Controversy concerning the pathogenesis of hypervitaminosis A centers on whether the neuroepithelium or supporting mesoderm are primarily affected through alterations in mitochondrial metabolism.[68] Surprisingly, both an excess[69] and a deficiency[70,71] of vitamin A have been associated with increased intracranial pressure, although the postulated mechanisms differ.

In hypervitaminosis A, symptoms are more common in infancy, although an adolescent being treated for acne vulgaris also has been reported.[72] The postulated mechanism is cerebral edema secondary to an increased capillary permeability of the brain.[73] On the other hand, the increased intracranial pressure secondary to vitamin A deficiency is related to a decreased absorption of cerebral spinal fluid (CSF), with radiological studies consistent with a communicating hydrocephalus.[70,71] Experimental studies in vitamin A-deficient animals have demonstrated that CSF production is normal but absorption is decreased.[74] This decrease in CSF absorption is thought to be related to thickening of the dura secondary to an accumulation of mucopolysaccharides.[75]

Clinically, although vitamin A intoxication could potentially occur in cystic fibrosis with overzealous therapy, vitamin A deficiency is the major concern in infancy, with neurological signs of increased intracranial pressure[70,71] and rarely an associated facial nerve paralysis.[71,76] Neurological symptoms in childhood include blindness with xerophthalmia.[77] Associated systemic signs of vitamin A deficiency are a generalized epithelial metaplasia, anemia, growth retardation, and gynecomastia. Such a constellation of signs with the demonstration of a low serum vitamin A or carotene level virtually assures the diagnosis. Symptoms and signs rapidly resolve with vitamin A therapy. In fact, the prophylactic administration of vitamin A to patients with cystic fibrosis has so reduced the incidence of this neurological complication that in the most recent report, a bulging fontanelle was the presenting sign of cystic fibrosis in an undiagnosed infant.[70]

Considering that restitution of adequate nutrition, tetracycline therapy, and vitamin A deficiency as etiologies for a bulging fontanelle have been so well described in cystic fibrosis, it is surprising that we continue to see these patients and other infants with malabsorption syndromes subjected to neuroradiological investigations to rule out an intracranial catastrophe.

Childhood and Adult

At 2 years of age, the physical mass of the central nervous system approaches adult levels and there is virtually no concern as to the effect of chronic continued protein–calorie undernutrition on brain maturation. Studies in adult human volunteers, however, have demonstrated significant alterations in their attitude and motivation with similar dietary restrictions. In one study, 36 normal young adult males were placed on a semistarvation diet for 6 months during which time they lost an average of 25% of prior body weight.[78] These men reduced physical activities to a minimum, complained that thinking was "too much bother," and described themselves as mentally dull and unable to concentrate. Their subjective concerns, however, were not documented on standardized intelligence tests which were not significantly altered from control values. It is not known whether the attitudes of patients with chronic malabsorption are altered similarly, but such studies may be helpful in understanding the frequently altered family dynamics in cystic fibrosis.[56]

On the other hand, selected deficiencies in vitamins and/or trace metals do result in central nervous system dysfunction, some of which are irreversible. The initial signs of neurological dysfunction in individuals on a hunger strike are related to a deficiency in the water-soluble B vitamins.[79] Symptoms of strabismus, nystagmus, ataxia of gait, and mental changes such as apathy and global confusion are primarily attributed to thiamine deficiency. This syndrome, termed Wernicke's encephalopathy, if untreated, can progress to an irreversible amnesic state with confabulations termed Korsakoff's psychosis.[80] The etiology of this neurological syndrome is thought to be the result of a decrease in decarboxylation reactions, primarily inhibition of pyruvate decarboxylase which requires a thiamine derivative as an essential cofactor.[81]

Chemical confirmation of a thiamine deficiency is made by demonstrating low levels of red blood cell transketolase,[82] but a dramatic recovery during the acute stage following parenteral administration of less than 5 mg of thiamine also is an important factor in establishing the specific etiology of the encephalopathy.[80] A diffuse polyneuropathy coexists with the Wernicke–Korsakoff syndrome in greater than 80% of these patients. The etiology of the polyneuropathy is considered to be multiple B-vitamin deficiencies, primary pyridoxine and pantothenic acid, rather than a specific thiamine deficiency. The complete caloric deprivation in individuals on a hunger strike, with its associated protein catabolism, results in death secondary to a cardiomyopathy prior to any symptoms of fat-soluble vitamin deficiencies.

The fat- and water-soluble vitamin status of cystic fibrosis patients most recently has been investigated in both England[83] and the United States.[84] The majority of patients in both studies received vitamin supplementation, pancreatic enzymes, and the high-protein, high-energy, low-fat diet utilized in the modern management of these patients. Neither study reported a significant difference in the blood levels of water-soluble vitamins between cystic fibrosis patients and controls. Both studies,[83,84] however, confirmed previous findings of deficiencies in fat-soluble vitamins despite the reocommended vitamin suplementation.[85,86] Low plasma levels of vitamins A and E, both of which are associated with specific neurological syndromes, were extremely prevalent.

Vitamin A Dietary sources of vitamin A include animal fats and liver as well as the β-carotene of colored vegetables that is converted to vitamin A within the body. Absorption of this vitamin via the thoracic duct requires the presence of bile salts in the intestinal tract. The liver stores greater than 90% of the vitamin A reserves from which it is transported throughout the body by a retinol-binding protein.[87,88] Except in infancy, night blindness is the major neurological symptom of vitamin A deficiency.[77] Rhodopsin (visual purple), a compound important for dark adaption and rod function within the retina, requires a continuing supply of vitamin A.

In both recent studies, the plasma vitamin A concentration in cystic fibrosis was significantly less than normal controls. In 18 cystic fibrosis patients, ages 6–18 years (mean age 11 years), the mean plasma level of vitamin A was 30.7 μg/dl in comparison to a mean control value of 36.9 μg/dl.[84] In three of these patients, the plasma vitamin A was greater than three standard deviations below mean control levels. Evidence of a deficiency in zinc also was reported in this series of patients, perhaps secondary to impaired absorption, as has been demonstrated in patients receiving pancreatic supplements.[89] The importance of an associated zinc deficiency in these patients is related to the recent observation that zinc is necessary in maintaining normal plasma concentrations of vitamin A.[90]

The recent series from England,[83] which included 36 younger cystic fibrosis patients, also described significantly depressed plasma vitamin A levels despite supplementation with up to 4000 IU/day. In this series, 43% of the patients had values greater than two standard deviations below the mean for the controls. Levels of retinol-binding protein (RBP) also were examined and found to be significantly lower in cystic fibrosis patients (34 ± 1.8 μg/ml) than in controls (60.7 ± 4.3 μg/ml). In 67% of these patients, the RBP was greater than two standard deviations below control levels. Plasma vitamin A levels were significantly correlated with the RBP levels but not to the severity of steatorrhea in these patients.

The interrelationship of malabsorption, zinc deficiency, retinol-binding protein, and low plasma vitamin A levels in cystic fibrosis is complex. The plasma vitamin A level in cystic fibrosis remains low despite its fourfold greater concentration within the liver.[87] It has been postulated that a zinc deficiency results in low plasma vitamin A levels by decreasing the transport of this vitamin from the liver to the tissues via retinol-binding protein.[88] On the other hand, daily oral supplementation for a two-week period with 4000 IU of water-miscible vitamin A to 14 cystic fibrosis patients resulted in an increase in their mean vitamin A levels from 1.68 to 3.09 μm/liter.[83]

Vitamin E As with vitamin A, vitamin E is ubiquitous within the diet and requires bile acids for absorption. Although deficiency syndromes in experimental animal models have been known for over 60 years, the direction of research as well as the unsubstantiated claims in preventing diseases of man had convinced most physicians that its importance lay within animal nutrition, not in human disease states. A number of studies both in experimental animals and humans within the last decade, however, has significantly altered this impression. It now appears that vitamin E is intimately involved with cellular and subcellular membranes, where it functions as the first line of defense against peroxidation of vital phospholipids.[91–93] In this role, observations that the dietary requirements for vitamin E are dependent on numerous other factors are understandable considering that the exposure of the animal to peroxidants and antioxidants varies with diet and other environmental circumstances.

The relationship of vitamin E to selenium also has been clarified. Selenium is an essential trace element necessary for the enzymatic activity of glutathione peroxidase, whose primary role in cellular metabolism also is to neutralize these same peroxides.[94–96] Thus, the observation that an animal's requirement for a fat-soluble vitamin may be at least partially replaced by a trace metal is explainable since they are essential for separate cellular systems that have an identical function, ie, the neutralization of peroxides.

In general, the signs of vitamin E deficiency appear directly related to a tissue's reparative and regenerative potential. The first sign of vitamin E deficiency in man and animals is a chemical abnormality in erythrocyte metabolism that may be quantified by increased erythrocyte susceptibility to hydrogen peroxide.[97–99] The shortened erythrocyte life span is easily compensated by an increase in the bone marrow production of reticulocytes. Of greater clinical significance is the neurological dysfunction secondary to the myopathy and the irreversible loss of neurons and their processes. The progressive neuromuscular syndrome of vitamin E deficiency has been demonstrated in more than 25 diverse animal species distributed over the phylogenetic tree from shark to monkey to man.[98]

The myopathy of vitamin E deficiency has been studied for over 40 years, with many recent investigators utilizing the rabbit experimental model. As with most nutritional deficiencies, the rapidly maturing young animal is most suitable. In the late stages of the deficiency syndrome, the animal has a severe painless paralysis with extensive muscular degeneration and atrophy. Microscopically, the muscle is characterized by hyaline or Zenker's degeneration of the actin–myosin complex, sarcolemmal tube formation, dystrophic calcifications, and macrophagic invasion with phagocytosis of the degenerated sarcoplasm.[100]

In earlier stages or a less acute degree of vitamin E deficiency, evidence of regeneration as well as repair of muscle fibers is described. An equilibrium appears to develop with degeneration and regeneration coexisting chronically in atrophic muscles despite continued vitamin E deficiency.[100,101] Other studies have demonstrated the rehabilitating effect of vitamin E therapy when initiated during the early stages of the myopathy.[102,103]

During the earlier stages, morphological abnormalities include streaming of the Z-disc, degenerative mitochondria, fragmented sarcoplasmic reticulum, and development and aggregation of membranes termed myelin figures. Initially, there is sporadic involvement of the muscle fibers. Following treatment with vitamin E, the morphological picture returns to near normal, with only isolated residual abnormalities. Biochemically, evidence of regeneration occurring during the myopathic process includes increased number of ribosomes, increased protein synthesis, and elevations in the serum creatinine phosphokinase (CPK).[104] With the increased protein synthesis, there also is evidence of a dedifferentiation of the muscle fibers based on a partal return to a fetal CPK enzyme pattern.[105]

During these early stages, mitochondrial dysfunction is noted, with an increased oxygen uptake and a decreased phosphorylative capacity within the muscle.[102] This is consistent with the observation that the mitochondria contain a significant proportion of the vitamin E within the cell,[92,106] as well as about 25% of the cell's lipid, a considerable portion of which is unsaturated and susceptible to peroxidation. It is uncertain at what tissue level of vitamin E the destructive parameters of the myopathy overwhelm the regenerative capacity of muscle in the young animals.

The rehabilitative effects of vitamin E have been demonstrated in the immature animal. In older animals, however, the rapidity of these pathological changes is decreased, with less evidence for regeneration and the morphological appearance of a more nonspecific generalized atrophy. This may be related to the decreased regenerative capacity of mature muscle and the fact that, as in the nervous system, there is little, if any, ability to replace lost muscle fibers through mitosis. Hypertrophy of remaining muscle fibers is the only means to compensate for muscle fiber destruction in the mature animal. Evidence of central nervous system manifestations in vitamin E deficiency influencing the myopathy has been suggested by the histochemical changes in the fast and slow muscles in rabbits.[107]

A much longer time on a vitamin E-deficient diet is required to develop the characteristic central nervous system pathology.[108,109] Differences in species, vulnerability to the myopathy is an important factor, since a rapidly progressive myopathy may result in the animal's death in the absence of central nervous system lesions. The most common experimental animal utilized to study the neuropathology of vitamin E deficiency is the rat.[110–112]

Rats were maintained on a vitamin E-deficient diet for periods ranging from 5 to 12 months. Studies that utilized a shorter time period of deficiency exacerbated the absence of vitamin E in the diet by the addition of polyunsaturated fatty acids such as those in "stripped" corn oil,[111] emphasizing the recurring observations that the severity of the neuromuscular syndrome is related both to the extent and duration of vitamin E deficiency as well as other environmental variables.

The neuropathological lesions described are identical to those recently reported in the rhesus monkey[113] and will be outlined in greater detail. Ten sexually immature rhesus monkeys weighing approximately 3 kg each were fed a vitamin E-deficient diet for periods from 30 to 33 months. Three of the monkeys served as controls receiving 300 mg of α-tocopherol acetate per week by mouth. Serum vitamin E concentrations in the three supplemented control animals varied between 1200 and 1600 μg/dl throughout the study. During the first 24 months, the vitamin E-deficient monkeys gained weight, appeared healthy, and were difficult to distinguish from control animals. In the third year, however, at least one of the following signs of vitamin E deficiency appeared in each animal: up to a 30% weight loss, generalized muscle weakness, and anemia.

Following 30 months on the vitamin E-deficient diet, two monkeys were repleted for 3 months with α-tocopherol acetate, 300 mg weekly by mouth. In both animals, the weight loss, anemia, and generalized muscle weakness resolved over 3 months with a return of the serum vitamin E to control levels at the time of sacrifice. Histological changes in the muscle were reminiscent of a chronic myopathy with variation in fiber size, vacuolations, and occasional necrosis (Figure 22-7). Neuropathologically, the extent and severity of the lesions within the central nervous system were not correlated with the duration of markedly reduced vitamin E levels, the severity of the anemia, the extent of the weight loss, or the degree of muscle weakness. In addition, the neuropathological lesions in the two vitamin E-repleted monkeys paralleled those in the unrepleted monkeys, despite a reversal of the peripheral manifestations of vitamin E deficiency.

The characteristic loss of axons and myelin sheaths in the posterior columns of the spinal cord, most prominent within the cervical regions, is shown in Figure 22-8. Swollen dystrophic axons (spheroids) were present in their greatest number within the posterior horns of the spinal cord (Figure 22-9). Moderate axonal loss within the posterior (sensory) roots was described, the

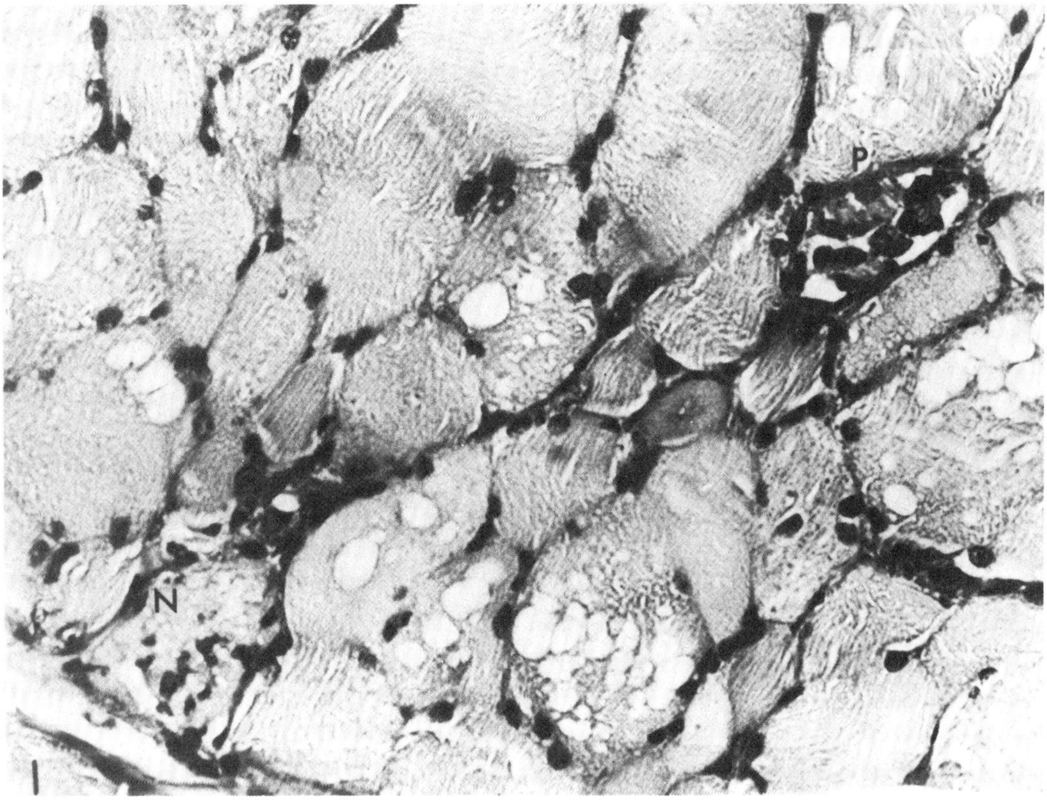

Figure 22-7 Myopathy of the quadriceps muscle in monkey following 33 months on a vitamin E-deficient diet. There is a variation in fiber size, vacuolated fibers, necrotic fibers (N), and evidence of phagocytosis (P). Hematoxylin and eosin stain, × 250. Reproduced with permission of Nelson JS, Fitch CD, Fischer VW, et al: Progressive neuropathologic lesions in vitamin E-deficient rhesus monkeys. *J Neuropathol Exp Neurol* 1981;40:166–186 (reference 113).

extent of which was proportional to, but not as severe as, the axonal loss in the adjacent posterior columns. The anterior (motor) roots were intact. Intracranially, similar but less severe neuropathological lesions were described in the trigeminal roots. Loss of neurons within the spinal cord was much less extensive than axonal loss, with degeneration of nerve cell bodies both in the dorsal ganglia and anterior horns of the spinal cord. Accumulation of lipopigment was evident within the neurons, the severity of which in any single animal was not proportional to the axonal loss. Examination of the peripheral nervous system yielded abnormalities primarily in the distal peripheral nerves with a decrease in the larger sensory fibers (6–12 μm) and evidence of segmental demyelination.

In man, the two most common chronic diseases associated with low plasma vitamin E levels and the characteristic neuropathology of vitamin E deficiency as outlined in the monkey experimental model[113] are cystic fibrosis[114,115] and biliary atresia.[116] As might be expected, the frequency and severity of these neuropathological lesions is much greater in biliary atresia than cystic fibrosis, being present in 100% of infants surviving to one year of age.[116,117]

Recently, the incidence of these lesions was examined retrospectively in two large series of cystic fibrosis patients at autopsy.[117,118] Both series utilized the number of dystrophic axons (spheroids) as a means of quantifying the neuropathological severity and grouped patients according to age by decade. In addition, an attempt was made to determine

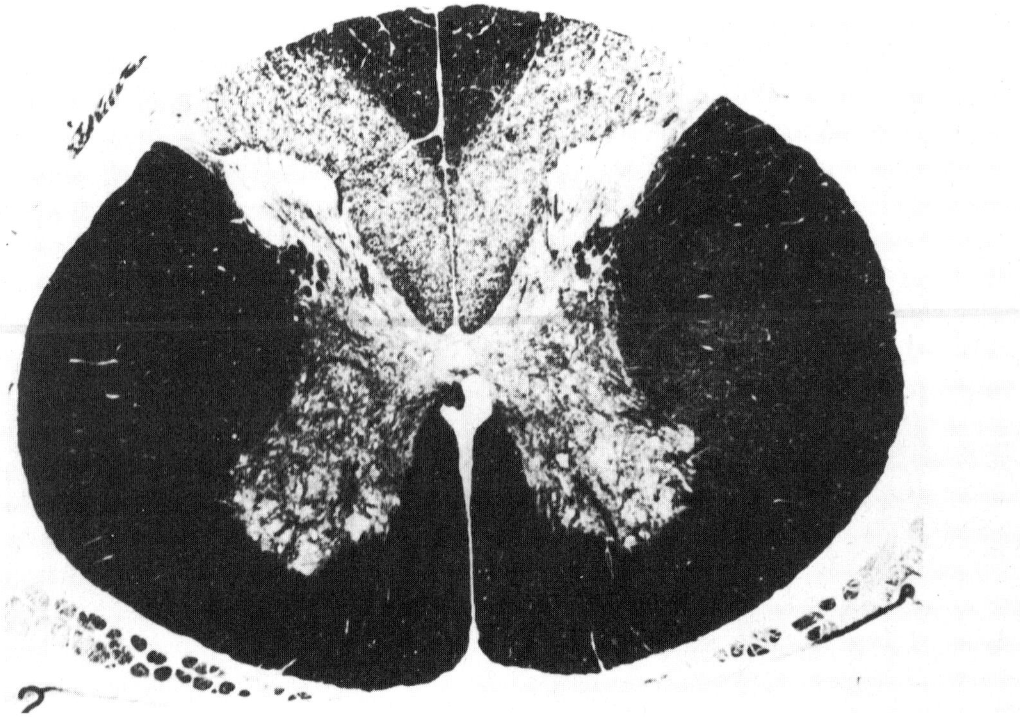

Figure 22-8 Cervical spinal cord of a monkey following 33 months on a vitamin E-deficient diet. Marked degeneration of the posterior columns as evidenced by lack of uptake of the myelin stain (white areas) in the fasciculus cuneatus (lateral area) with lesser involvement of the fasciculus gracilis (medial). Normal uptake of the myelin stain within the corticospinal tracts (lateral). Loyez stain, × 10. Reproduced with permission of Nelson JS, Fitch CD, Fischer VW, et al: Progressive neuropathologic lesions in vitamin E-deficient rhesus monkeys. *J Neuropathol Exp Neurol* 1981;40:166–186 (reference 113).

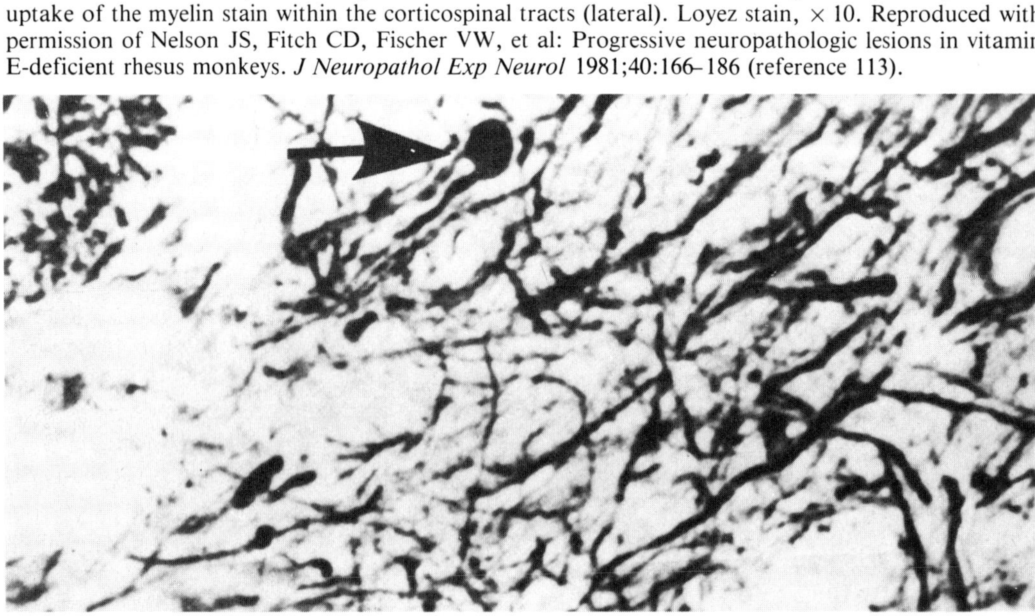

Figure 22-9 The posterior horn of the cervical spinal cord in a monkey on a vitamin E-deficient diet for 33 months. There is moderate axonal loss and the development of dystrophic axons (spheroids, arrows). Studies have utilized the number of spheroids in gauging the severity of the myelopathy. Sevier-Munger stain, × 250. Reproduced with permission of Nelson JS, Fitch CD, Fischer VW, et al: Progressive neuropathologic lesions in vitamin E-deficient rhesus monkeys. *J Neuropathol Exp Neurol* 1981;40:166–186 (reference 113).

whether vitamin E supplementation affected either the incidence or severity of these lesions by grouping the patients as to the year of their death on the assumption that vitamin E supplementation was more prominent in those patients that recently died. As could be anticipated from the animal studies, both the incidence and severity of axonal dystrophy increased with age in the 47 cystic fibrosis patients from 30% in the first decade to greater than 80% in the third decade[117] (Figure 22-10).

The data from the second series of 38 patients are remarkably similar, with an incidence of zero, 80%, 90%, and 100% in the first, second, third, and fourth decades, respectively.[118] The variability in the incidence during the first decade between the two series may be related to the time period from which the cases were obtained. In the series in which the incidence in the first decade was 30%, the time period examined was from 1952 to 1980 (Figure 22-10), whereas the time period examined in the second series was from 1967 through 1979. This difference in the time period from which the cases were obtained also may explain the discrepancy between the two series as to the efficacy of vitamin E supplementation in preventing these neuropathological lesions.

In the series which described patients from 1952 through 1980 (Figure 22-11), data were presented indicating that there has been a decrease in the incidence of these neuropathological lesions presumably related to vitamin E supplementation. In the series in which the cases were obtained between 1967 and 1979,[118] no decrease was noted in the incidence or severity of these lesions. Unfortunately, neither neurological examinations nor plasma vitamin E levels were available to correlate with these retrospective neuropathological findings on autopsied cystic fibrosis patients.

The clinical syndrome of vitamin E deficiency in man has been best described in children with long-standing cholestatic liver disease. The author first described a 7-year-old boy with severe malabsorption since

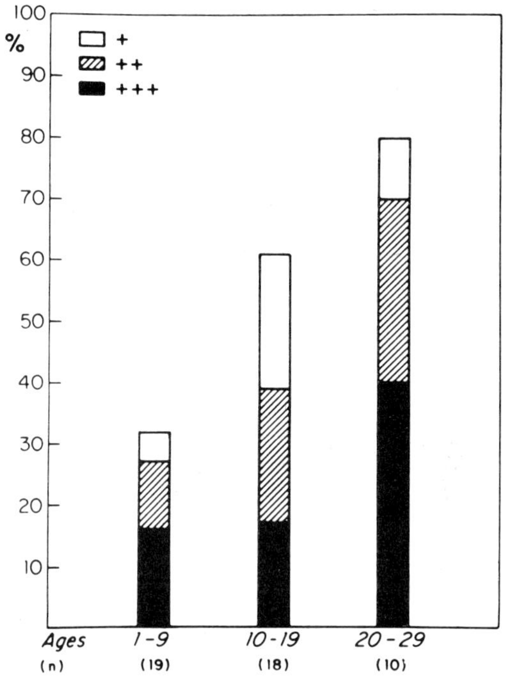

Figure 22-10 Incidence and severity of dystrophic axons (spheroids) in the gracile nucleus of the cervical spinal cord in patients by age. Severity was estimated by the number of spheroids as follows: minimal 1–5 (+); moderate 6–10 (+ +); and severe 11–20 (+ + +). Reproduced with permission of Sung JH, Park SH, Mastri AR, et al: Axonal dystrophy in the gracile nucleus in congenital biliary atresia and cystic fibrosis (mucoviscidosis): Beneficial effect of vitamin E therapy. *J Neuropathol Exp Neurol* 1980;39: 584–597 (reference 117).

birth and the clinical syndrome now associated with vitamin E deficiency in man.[119] Symptoms were a progressive external ophthalmoplegia and proximal muscle weakness (Figure 22-12). Upon examination, a progressive exotropia of the left eye and bilateral ptosis were present. The weakness was of a proximal distribution with greater involvement of the lower extremities than the upper extremities. A bilateral foot drop was present. Muscle bulk was generally decreased, as was muscle tone. Deep tendon reflexes were absent in the lower extremities and hypoactive in the upper extremities. The plantars were extensor bilaterally. Sensory abnormalities included a decreased response

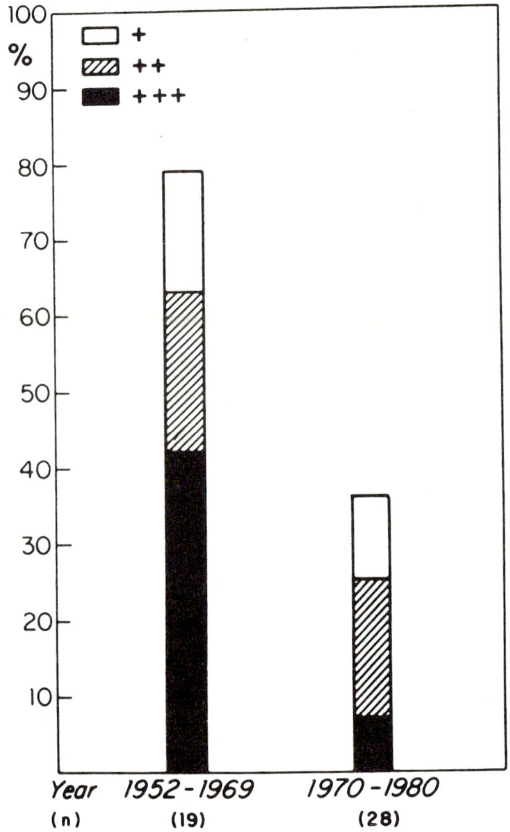

Figure 22-11 The incidence and severity of dystrophic axons (spheroids) in the gracile nucleus of the cervical spinal cord in cystic fibrosis patients grouped as to the time of the autopsy. Severity was estimated by the number of spheroids as follows: minimal 1-5 (+); moderate 6-10 (+ +); and severe 11-20 (+ + +). Reproduced with permission of Sung JH, Park SH, Mastri AR, et al: Axonal dystrophy in the gracile nucleus in congenital biliary atresia and cystic fibrosis (mucoviscidosis): Beneficial effect of vitamin E therapy. *J Neuropathol Exp Neurol* 1980;39: 584–597 (reference 117).

in the lower extremities to light touch, vibration, and position, with a normal response to pain and temperature. The hematocrit was 25%. Electromyography and nerve conduction velocities were normal, with the exception of slowed distal sensory latencies. Muscle biopsy demonstrated an absence of an inflammatory response, but muscle fibers were atrophic and occasional pyknotic nuclei were noted. Electron microscopy was normal, with the exception of occasional areas of

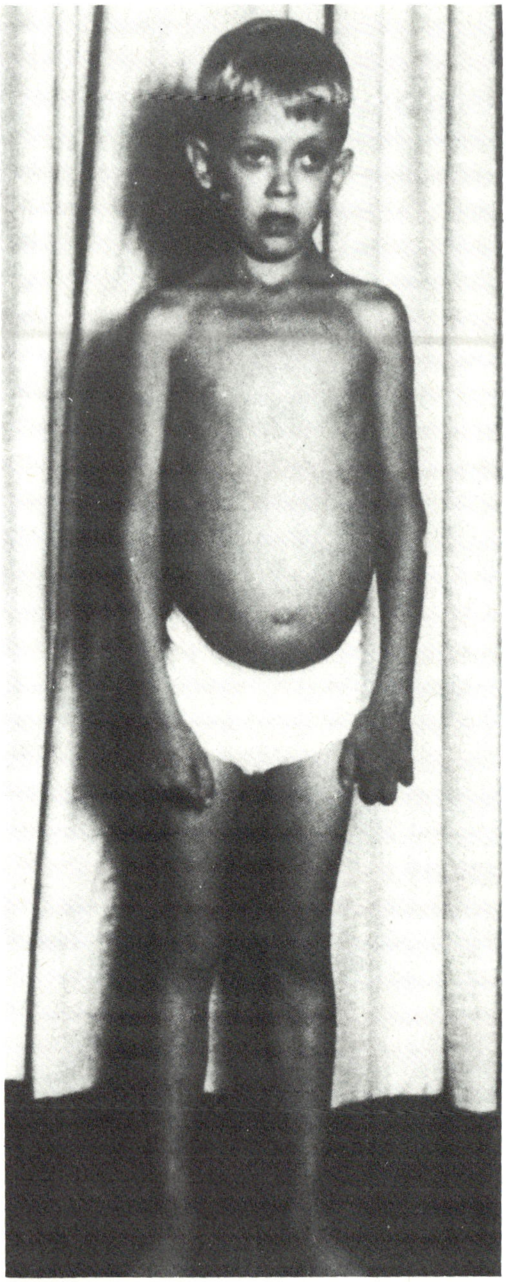

Figure 22-12 Child with severe vitamin E deficiency secondary to chronic cholestasis syndrome. Note decreased muscle mass, lumbar lordosis, clubbing of the digits, myopathic facies, and external ophthalmaplegia. Plasma vitamin E level was 8 μg/dl. Reproduced with permission of Tomasi LG: Reversibility of human myopathy caused by vitamin E deficiency. *Neurology* 1979;29:1182–1186 (reference 119).

Z-band smearing. Serum CPK and aldolase were two and a half and three times the upper limits of normal, and the plasma α-tocopherol was 8 μg/dl.

The patient was treated with water-solubilized vitamin E as the only therapeutic variable and remained on this therapy until his death 3 years later. Follow-up chemical studies during the first 16 months of therapy are outlined in Table 22-1. There was a gradual return of the muscle enzymes to normal levels which was associated with the elevation in the plasma α-tocopherol. The massive dose of vitamin E required to elevate his plasma tocopherol was thought to be related to his daily dose of cholestyramine (1.8 g/kg) inhibiting bile acid and vitamin E absorption. The remarkably low level of vitamin E in this patient was related to the chronic usage of cholestyramine since 18 months of age.

After four months of therapy, an objective improvement could be demonstrated in his myopathy. He gained weight and had no further deterioration in his neurological status for the 3 years prior to his death from gram-negative sepsis and liver failure. The hyporeflexia, bilateral Babinski's, and abnormalities of his sensory examination persisted, with the neuropathological examination demonstrating the characteristic lesions of vitamin E deficiency.

As suggested by the monkey experimental model,[113] the peripheral manifestations of vitamin E deficiency including hyporeflexia, bilateral Babinski signs, and abnormalities on sensory examination were irreversible. More recently, 6 children were reported with similar long-standing cholestatic liver disease and neurological abnormalities.[120] Neuropathological examination in 3 patients demonstrated the lesions characteristic of vitamin E deficiency, including the peripheral nerve abnormalities as described in the monkey experimental model with the papers sharing common authors.

Symptoms and signs consistent with the neuromuscular syndrome of vitamin E deficiency rarely have been reported in cystic fibrosis. In a series of 70 adults, a peripheral neuropathy was reported as a complication in one patient, although further details are lacking.[1] A study of the muscular performance in 20 cystic fibrosis patients concluded that there was no significant correlation to the serum vitamin E level.[121]

Recently, the author evaluated 40 patients in a cystic fibrosis clinic with the single selection criteria of being able to cooperate for a detailed neurological examination.[122] The mean age of this patient population was 8.4 years. Abnormalities on the neurological evaluation were noted in 10 patients (25%) whose mean age was 13 years. Evidence of a peripheral neuropathy as manifested by a decreased vibratory sense was demonstrated

Table 22-1
Response of Serum CPK and Aldolase to α-Tocopherol Therapy in a Child with Severe Vitamin E Deficiency*

	Months						
	0	*2*	*4*	*6*	*9*	*12*	*16*
Dose vitamin E (mg/24 hr)		200	400	400	400	800	800
Dose vitamin E (mg/kg/24 hr)†		9(26)	18(51)	17(49)	16(46)	32(92)	32(92)
CPK (33–184)‡	613	305	144	201	136	120	71
Aldolase (2–12)‡	34	18	15	18	14	13	2
Plasma α-tocopherol (550–1500 μg/dl)‡	8	22	68	115	138	278	350

*Reproduced with permission of Tomasi LG: Reversibility of human myopathy caused by vitamin E deficiency. *Neurology* 1979;29:1182–1186.
†Average adult daily intake (0.2–0.5 mg). Numbers in parentheses indicate the multiple of average daily intake.
‡Range of normal values.

in 7 patients, 3 of whom had symptoms of paresthesias. In one patient, ataxia, not of cerebellar orgin, was noted. The 3 remaining patients all had varying degress of an external ophthalmoplegia, and one of these also had a mild seventh cranial nerve palsy. Detailed nerve conduction velocities on these 10 patients demonstrated low normal motor nerve conduction velocities (5 patients), absence of sural nerve sensory potential (2 patients), and prolonged latencies of the sural nerve (3 patients). Electromyographic studies were normal, except one patient demonstrated myopathic responses of the ocular muscles. Serum CPK values were normal in all patients. The mean plasma vitamin E was significantly decreased in all 40 patients, the severity of which did not correlate with the neurological abnormalities.

The chemical abnormalities of vitamin E deficiency were investigated in 50 cystic fibrosis patients whose mean plasma vitamin E level was 125 μg/dl, range 23–410 μg/dl (control mean 730 μg/dl, range 550–960 μg/dl).[97,123] In these patients, the susceptibility of red blood cells to hemolysis showed a sigmoidal relationship to the plasma vitamin E level. Determination of ^{51}Cr-labeled red blood cell survival documented an improved survival curve following supplementation with vitamin E. A myopathy evidenced by creatinuria was present in 13 of 25 patients studied, with the total group demonstrating an average creatine excretion of 200 mg/24 hr (normal mean 20 mg/24 hr). Elevated plasma aldolase and CPK were demonstrated in two patients. Creatinuria is a common feature of muscle disease and has been demonstrated to be an early sign of vitamin E deficiency myopathy in the monkey experimental model responding to vitamin E therapy.[124]

There is universal agreement that significantly low levels of plasma vitamin E exist in cystic fibrosis which partially responds to supplemental vitamin E therapy. Recent studies[125,126] have demonstrated normal blood levels of selenium and glutathione peroxidase activities. Neuropathological studies demonstrate conclusively that lesions characteristic of vitamin E deficiency are present in cystic fibrosis patients, and their incidence increases with the chronological age of the patient.[117,118] A few clinical studies have demonstrated chemical abnormalities[97,123] and neurological abnormalities[122] consistent with vitamin E deficiency. What remains uncertain is the incidence and severity of this neurological syndrome within the cystic fibrosis population. Its development is insidious, with clinical signs easily overlooked in a population of patients whose underlying disease results in a chronic progressive debilitating clinical course.

There have been few, if any, symptoms of vitamin E intoxication reported to date,[127] and additional vitamin E supplementation as well as a more complete neurological evaluation may help clarify this problem in the future. It is entirely possible that the peripheral neuropathy previously attributed to vitamin B-complex deficiencies and chloramphenicol were symptoms and signs of vitamin E deficiency. Vitamin E, in addition to vitamin A, is required for normal retinal function.[128,129] It could be postulated that low vitamin E levels are synergistic with chloramphenicol to produce the optic neuropathy, limiting the usefulness of this broad-spectrum antibiotic.

Among the antibiotics that have been utilized chronically in cystic fibrosis, the optic neuropathy associated with chloramphenicol is perhaps the most significant neurological complication of therapy.[130–132] Although described in diseases other than cystic fibrosis, it is included in this section because vitamin deficiencies have been implicated to be synergistic with chloramphenicol in its pathogenesis.[133,134] The vast majority of patients who developed this complication were adolescents or young adults with rather advanced pulmonary disease who had received chloramphenicol for months to years at doses ranging from 30 to 60 mg/kg/day.

Characteristically, symptoms of this toxic reaction developed acutely with loss of visual acuity, disturbances in color vision, complaints of orbital pain, and transient further reduction in visual acuity with reading

(Uhthoff's symptom). On examination, signs included sluggishly reactive pupils, an enlarged blind spot, central scotoma, and significant difficulty with the Ishihara color plates. On funduscopic examination, the picture is that of a papillitis, as reflected by hyperemic indistinct optic disk margin and edema of the fundus. Occasionally, the disk is normal, but with the other symptoms and signs, the diagnosis of a retrobulbar neuritis is easily made. Neurophysiologically, abnormalities have been demonstrated in the electroretinogram and visual evoked responses, reflecting retinal dysfunction and optic nerve damage respectively.[131] Morphological studies confirm abnormalities of the ganglion cells of the retina in addition to the optic nerve.[135,136]

Management of this complication has been somewhat variable. In all patients in whom the chloramphenicol was discontinued, visual function rather promptly improved, although in some cases follow-up evaluations demonstrated less than normal visual acuity and the development of optic atrophy.[131,132] In other patients, the drug was continued and therapy was directed at providing therapeutic doses of the B vitamins as well as vitamin E. In those patients, visual acuity also improved. In still others, the chloramphenicol was discontinued until visual acuity improved, after which it was reinstituted without a further exacerbation of their optic neuropathy.

The majority of patients who developed this complication were on the recommended additional vitamin therapy, although the adequacy of the blood levels was rarely documented. In the few patients in which chloramphenicol blood levels were obtained, excessively high serum concentrations were not encountered.[132] A number of patients also had associated symptoms of painful parasthesias in their fingers and toes which also remitted with discontinuation of the chloramphenicol. Considering the rapidity of development of the visual symptoms, it is not at all certain that they can be anticipated. There is a suggestion that the painful parasthesias may precede the visual complaints,[132] and the role of the electroretinogram (ERG) and visual evoked responses in predicting those patients who may develop the optic neuropathy has not been determined. In those cases in which these neurophysiological studies have been performed, however, they appeared to normalize prior to the return of visual acuity.

Chloramphenicol clearly is the major perpetrator of the optic neuropathy, since such complications have not been observed in cystic fibrosis in the absence of this drug. On the other hand, the role of hypoxia, hypercapnia, and the vitamin deficiencies, especially vitamin A and vitamin E, have not been thoroughly examined. This complication has only occurred in older patients with advanced pulmonary disease, and degeneration of the neurons within the retinal layer has been demonstrated in experimental animals subjected to chronic vitamin E deficiency.[128,129] It has been recommended that patients receiving chloramphenicol receive frequent examinations of their visual acuity and be taught to utilize a hand-held card for self-examination. The utility of this recommendation has not been documented.

REFERENCES

1. Shwachman H, Kowalski M, Khaw K-T: Cystic fibrosis: A new outlook: 70 patients above 25 years of age. *Medicine* 1977; 56:129–149.
2. di Sant'Agnese PA, Davis PB: Cystic fibrosis in adults: 75 cases and a review of 232 cases in the literature. *Am J Med* 1979;66:121–132.
3. Siesjö BK, Plum F: Pathophysiology of anoxic brain damage, in Gaull GE (ed): *Biology of Brain Dysfunction.* New York, Plenum Publishing, 1972.
4. Siesjö BK: *Brain Energy Mechanisms.* New York, John Wiley & Sons, 1978.
5. Eisenberg S, Madison L, Sensenbach W: Cerebral hemodynamic and metabolic studies in patients with congestive heart failure II. Observations in confused subjects. *Circulation* 1960;21:704–709.
6. Simmons RL: The role of the central nervous system in septic shock II. Hemodynamic, respiratory and metabolic effects of intracisternal or intraventricular endotoxin. *Ann Surg* 1968;167:158–167.
7. Siekes HO, Hickam JB: Carbon dioxide intoxication. *Medicine* 1956;35:389–423.

8. Posner JB, Swanson AG, Plum F: Acid-base balance in cerebrospinal fluid. *Arch Neurol* 1965;12:479–496.
9. Plum F, Posner JB: *Diagnosis of Stupor and Coma*. Philadelphia, FA Davis, 1966.
10. Austen FK, Carmichael MW, Adams RD: Neurologic manifestations of chronic pulmonary insufficiency. *N Engl J Med* 1957;257: 579–590.
11. Siesjö BK, Johannsson H, Fjungren B, et al: Brain dysfunction in metabolic disorders, in Plum F (ed): *Research Publication of the Association of Nervous Mental Disorders*. New York, Raven Press, 1974.
12. Rotherman EB Jr, Safar P, Robin EB: CNS disorder during mechanical ventilation in chronic pulmonary disease. *JAMA* 1964; 189:993–996.
13. Cohen LF, di Sant'Agnese PA, Taylor A, et al: The syndrome of inappropriate anti-diuretic hormone secretion as a cause of hyponatremia in cystic fibrosis. *J Pediatr* 1977;90:574.
14. Katzman R, Pappius HM: *Brain Electrolytes and Fluid Metabolism*. Baltimore, Williams and Wilkins, 1973.
15. Rymer MM, Tishman RA: Protective adaptation of brain to water intoxication. *Arch Neurol* 1973;28:49–54.
16. Arieff AI, Flach F, Massry SG: Neurological manifestation and morbidity of hyponatremia: Correlation with brain water and electrolytes. *Medicine* 1976;55:121–129.
17. Fischer EG, Shwachman H, Wepsic JG: Brain abscess and cystic fibrosis. *J Pediatr* 1979;95:385–388.
18. Duffner PK, Cohen ME: Cystic fibrosis with brain abscess. *Arch Neurol 1979;36: 27*–28.
19. Victor M, Banker BQ: Brain abscess. *Med Clin North Am* 1963;47:1355–1370.
20. Evans W: Pathology and etiology of brain abscess. *Lancet* 1931;1:1231–1234.
21. Jefferson AA, Keogh AJ: Intracranial abscesses: A review of treated patients over 20 years. *Q J Med* 1977;46:389–400.
22. Garfield J: Management of supratentorial intracranial abscess: A review of 200 cases. *Br Med J* 1969;2:7–11.
23. Molinari GF, Smith L, Goldstein MD, et al: Brain abscess from septic cerebral embolism. *Neurology* 1973;23:1205–1212.
24. Brewer NS, MacCarty CS, Wellman WE: Brain abscess: A review of recent experience. *Ann Intern Med* 1975;82:571–576.
25. Brook I: Bacteriology of intracranial abscess in children. *J Neurosurg* 1981;54:484–488.
26. Martinez-Tello FJ, Braun DG, Blanc WA: Immunoglobin production in bronchial mucosa and bronchial lymph nodes, particularly in cystic fibrosis of the pancreas. *J Immunol* 1968;10:989–1003.
27. Schwartz RH: Serum immunoglobin levels in cystic fibrosis. *Am J Dis Child* 1966;11: 408–411.
28. Neter E: *Pseudomonas aeruginosa* infection and humoral antibody response of patients with cystic fibrosis. *J Infect Dis* 1974;130 (Suppl):132–133.
29. Jagels AE, Sweeney EA: Oral health of patients with cystic fibrosis and their sibling. *J Dent Res* 1976;55:991–994.
30. Michel B, Gastaut JL, Bianchi L: Electroencephalographic cranial computerized tomographic correlations in brain abscess. *Electroencephalogr Clin Neurophysiol* 1979; 46:256–273.
31. Rosenblum ML, Hoff JT, Norman D, et al: Decreased mortality from brain abscesses since advent of computerized tomography. *J Neurosurg* 1978;49:658–668.
32. Kamin M, Biddle D: Conservative management of focal intracerebral infection. *Neurology* 1981;31:103–106.
33. Weisberg LA: Nonsurgical management of focal intracranial infection. *Neurology* 1981;31:575–580.
34. Berg B, Franklin G, Cuneo R, et al: Nonsurgical cure of brain abscess: Early diagnosis and follow-up with computerized tomography. *Ann Neurol* 1978;3:474–478.
35. Balistreri WF, Buchino JJ: Dehydration, seizures, and hypoglycemia in a 4-month-old child. *J Pediatr* 1980;97:689–694.
36. Dobbing J, Sands J: Head circumference, biparietal diameter and brain growth in fetal and post-natal life. *Early Hum Dev* 1978;2: 81–92.
37. Brandt I: Postnatal growth of preterm and full term infants, in Johnston FE, Roche AF, Suzanne C (eds): *Human Physical Growth and Maturation: Methodologies and Factors*. New York, Plenum Press, 1980.
38. Dobbing J: Nutrition and brain development, in Thalhamer O, Baumgarten K, Pollak A (eds): *Perinatal Medicine, 6th European Congress*. Stuttgart, Thieme, 1979.
39. Winick M, Rosso P: The effect of severe early malnutrition on cellular growth of human brain. *Pediatr Res* 1969;3:181–189.
40. Canosa CA, Salomon JB, Klein RE: The intervention approach: The Guatemala study, in Moore WM, Silverberg MM, Read MS (eds): *Nutrition, Growth and Development of North American Indian Children*. DHEW Publication No. 26, Washington, DC, Government Printing Office, 1972.
41. Lechtig A, Delgado H, Martorell R, et al: Effect of maternal nutrition on infants' growth and mortality in a developing country, in

Rooth G, Bratteby LE (eds): *Perinatal Medicine, 5th European Congress.* Stockholm, Almquist & Wiksell International, 1976.

42. Winick M, Rosso P, Waterlow J: Cellular growth of cerebrum, cerebellum and brain stem in normal and marasmic children. *Exp Neurol* 1970;26:393–400.
43. Rosso P, Hormazábal J, Winick M: Changes in brain weight, cholesterol, phospholipid, and DNA content in marasmic children. *Am J Clin Nutr* 1970;23:1275– 1279.
44. Fishman MA, Prensky AL, Dodge PR: Low content of cerebral lipids in infants suffering from malnutrition. *Nature* 1969;221:552–553.
45. Fox JH, Fishman MA, Prensky AL, et al: The effect of malnutrition on human central nervous system myelin. *Neurology* 1972;22: 1213–1216.
46. Graham G, Morales E: Studies in infantile malnutrition I. Nature of the problem in Peru. *J Nutr* 1963;79:479–486.
47. Pretorius PJ, Novis H: Nutritional marasmus in Bantu infants in the Pretoria area II Clinical and pathological aspects. *S Afr Med J* 1965;39:501–509.
48. Engsner G, Belete S, Sjögren I, et al: Brain growth in children with marasmus. A study using head circumference measurement, transillumination and ultrasonic echo ventriculography. *Uppsala J Med Sci* 1974;79: 116–122.
49. Mönckeberg F: The effect of malnutrition on physical growth and brain development, in Prescott JW, Read MS, Coursin DB (eds): *Brain Function and Malnutrition: Neuropsychological Methods of Assessment.* New York, John Wiley & Sons, 1975.
50. Sachdev KK, Taori GM, Pereira SM: Neuromuscular status in protein–calorie malnutrition. *Neurology* 1971;21:801–805.
51. Platt BS, Heard CRC, Stewart RJC: Experimental protein–calorie deficiency, in Munro HN, Allison JB (eds): *Mammalian Protein Metabolism, Vol. 2.* New York, Academic Press, 1964.
52. Engel R: Abnormal brain wave patterns in kwashiorkor. *Electroencephalogr Clin Neurophysiol* 1956;8:489–502.
53. Beck EC, Dustman RE: Developmental electrophysiology of brain function as reflected by changes in evoked response, in Prescott JW, Read MS (eds): *Brain Function and Malnutrition: Neurophysiological Methods of Assessment.* New York, John Wiley & Sons, 1975.
54. Taori GM, Pereira SM: Electroencephalograms and nerve conduction in survivors of kwashiorkor. *Br J Nutr* 1974;31:59–62.
55. Valman HB: Intelligence after malnutrition caused by neonatal resection of ileum. *Lancet* 1974;1:425–427.
56. Lloyd-Still JD, Hurwitz I, Wolff PH, et al: Intellectual development after severe malnutrition in infancy. *Pediatrics* 1974;54: 306–311.
57. Classification of infantile malnutrition (editorial). *Lancet* 1970;2:302–303.
58. Gomez F, Galvan R, Frenk S, et al: Mortality in second and third degree malnutrition. *J Trop Pediatr* 1956;2:77–84.
59. DeLevie M, Nogrady MD: Rapid brain growth upon restoration of adequate nutrition causing false radiologic evidence of increased intracranial pressure. *J Pediatr* 1970;76:523–528.
60. Sondheimer FK, Grossman H, Winchester P: Suture diastasis following rapid weight gain. *Arch Neurol* 1970;23:314–318.
61. Bray PF, Herbst JJ: Pseudotumor cerebri as a sign of "catch-up" growth in cystic fibrosis. *Am J Dis Child* 1973;126:78–79.
62. Roach ES, Sinal SH: Increased intracranial pressure following treatment of cystic fibrosis. *Pediatrics* 1980;66:622–623.
63. O'Doherty NJ: Acute benign intracranial hypertension in an infant receiving tetracycline. *Dev Med Child Neurol* 1965;7: 677–680.
64. Fields JP: Bulging fontanel: A complication of tetracycline therapy in infants. *J Pediatr* 1961;58:74–76.
65. Maroon JC, Mealy JJ: Benign intracranial hypertension. Sequel to tetracycline therapy in a child. *JAMA* 1971;216:1479–1480.
66. Kock-Weser J, Gilmore EB: Benign intracranial hypertension in an adult after tetracycline therapy. *JAMA* 1967;200: 345–347.
67. Schenefelt RE: Animal model: Treatment of various species with a large dose of vitamin A at known stages of pregnancy. *Am J Pathol* 1972;66:589–592.
68. Morris GM: The ultrastructural effects of excess maternal vitamin A on the primitive streak stage rat embryo. *J Embryol Exp Morphol* 1973;30:219–242.
69. Feldman MH, Schlezinger NS: Benign intracranial hypertension associated with hypervitaminosis A. *Arch Neurol* 1970; 22:1–7.
70. Abernathy RS: Bulging fontanelle as presenting sign in cystic fibrosis. *Am J Dis Child* 1976;130:1360–1362.
71. Keating JP, Feigin RD: Increased intracranial pressure associated with probable vitamin A deficiency in cystic fibrosis. *Pediatrics* 1970;46:41–46.
72. Lascari AD, Bell WE: Pseudotumor cerebri due to hypervitaminosis A. Toxic consequence of self-medication of acne in a girl.

Clin Pediatr 1970;9:627–628.
73. Maddux GW, Foltz FM, Nelson SR: Effect of vitamin A intoxication on intracranial pressure and brain water in rats. *J Nutr* 1974;104:478–482.
74. Calhoun MC, Hurt HD, Eaton HD, et al: Rates of formation and absorption on cerebrospinal fluid in bovine hypovitaminosis A. *J Dairy Sci* 1967;50:1486–1494.
75. Cousins RJ, Eaton HD, Rousseau JE Jr, et al: Biochemical constituents of the dura mater in vitamin A deficiency. *J Nutr* 1969;97:409–448.
76. Bass MH, Fisch GR: Increased intracranial pressure with bulging fontanelle: A symptom of vitamin A deficiency in infants. *Neurology* 1961;11:1091–1094.
77. Petersen RA, Petersen VS, Robb RM: Vitamin A deficiency with xeropthalmia and night blindness in cystic fibrosis. *Am J Dis Child* 1968;116:662–665.
78. Keys A, Brozek J, Henshel A, et al: *The Biology of Human Starvation, Vol. 2.* Minneapolis, University of Minnesota Press, 1950.
79. Young VR, Scrimshaw NS: The physiology of starvation. *Sci Am* 1971;225:14–21.
80. Victor M, Adams RD, Collins GH: The Wernicke-Korsakoff syndrome: A clinical and pathological study of 245 patients, 82 with post-mortem examinations, in Plum F, McDowell FH (eds): *Contemporary Neurology Series, No. 7.* Philadelphia, FA Davis, 1971.
81. Dreyfus PM, Hauser G: The effect of thiamine deficiency in the pyruvate decarboxylase system of the central nervous system. *Biochim Biophys Acta* 1965; 104:78.
82. Brin M: Erythrocyte transketolase in early thiamine deficiency. *Ann NY Acad Sci* 1962;98:528–529.
83. Congden PJ, Bruce G, Rothburn MM, et al: Vitamin status in treated patients with cystic fibrosis. *Arch Neurol* 1981;56: 708–714.
84. Solomons NW, Wagonfeld JB, Rieger C, et al: Some biochemical indices of nutrition in treated cystic fibrosis patients. *Am J Clin Nutr* 1981;34:462–474.
85. Shwachman H, Khaw K-T: Cystic fibrosis, in Shirkey HC (ed): *Pediatric Therapy.* St. Louis, CV Mosby, 1968.
86. Mearns M: Cystic fibrosis. *Br J Hosp Med* 1974;12:497–506.
87. Underwood BA, Denning CR: Blood and liver concentrations of vitamins A and E in children with cystic fibrosis of the pancreas. *Pediatr Res* 1972;6:26–31.
88. Jacob RA, Sandstead HH, Solomons NW, et al: Zinc status and vitamin A transport in cystic fibrosis. *Am J Clin Nutr* 1978;31: 638–644.
89. Aggett PJ, Thorn JM, Delves HT, et al: Trace element malabsorption in exocrine pancreatic insufficiency. *Monogr Paediatr* 1979;10:8–12.
90. Smith JC Jr, McDaniel EG, Far FF, et al: Zinc: A trace element essential in vitamin A metabolism. *Science* 1973;181:954–955.
91. Kornbrust DJ, Mavis RD: Relative susceptibility of microsomes from lung, heart, liver, kidney, brain and testis to lipid peroxidation: Correlation with vitamin E content. *Lipids* 1980;15(5):315–322.
92. Murphy DJ, Mavis RD: A comparison of the in vitro binding of α-tocopherol to microsomes of lung, liver, heart and brain of the rat. *Biochim Biophys Acta* 1981;663: 390–400.
93. Reddy JK, Lalwani ND, Dabholkar AS, et al: Increased peroxisomal activity in the liver of vitamin E deficient rats. *Biochem Int* 1981;3(1):41–49.
94. Hafeman DG, Sunde RA, Hoekstra WG: Effect of dietary selenium on erythrocyte and liver glutathione peroxidase in the rat. *J Nutr* 1974;104:580–587.
95. Rotruck JT, Pope AL, Ganther HE, et al: Selenium: Biochemical role as a component of glutathione peroxidase. *Science* 1973; 179:588–590.
96. Chow CK, Reddy K, Tappel AL: Effect of dietary vitamin E on the activities of the glutathione perioxidase system in rat tissues. *J Nutr* 1973;103:618–624.
97. Farrell PM, Bieri JG, Fratantoni JF, et al: The occurrence and effects of human vitamin E deficiency. A study in patients with cystic fibrosis. *J Clin Invest* 1977;60:233–241.
98. Mason KE, Horwitt MK: Effects of deficiency in animals, in Sebrell WH, Harris RS (eds): *The Vitamins.* New York, Academic Press, 1972.
99. Horwitt MK, Century B, Seman AA: Erythrocyte survival time and reticulocyte levels after tocopherol depletion in man. *Am J Clin Nutr* 1963;12:99–107.
100. VanVleet JF, Hall BV, Simon J: Vitamin E deficiency. A sequential light and electron microscopic study of skeletal muscle degeneration in weanling rabbits. *Am J Pathol* 1978;52:1067–1079.
101. VanVleet JF, Hall BV, Simon J: Vitamin E deficiency: A sequential study by means of light and electron microscopy of the alterations occurring in regeneration of skeletal muscle of affected weanling rabbits. *Am J Pathol* 1967;51:815–830.
102. Heffron JJA, Chan AC, Gronert GA, et al: Decreased phosphorylative capacity and

respiratory rate of rabbit skeletal muscle mitochondria in vitamin E dystrophy. *Int J Biochem* 1978;9:539–543.

103. Dahlin KJ, Chan AC, Benson ES, et al: Rehabilitating effect of vitamin E therapy on the ultrastructural changes in skeletal muscles of vitamin E deficient rabbits. *Am J Clin Nutr* 1978;31:94–99.

104. Olson RE: Creatine kinase and myofibrillar proteins in hereditary muscular dystrophy and vitamin E deficiency. *Am J Clin Nutr* 1974;27:1117–1129.

105. Armstrong JB, Lowden JA, Sherwin AL: Brain isoenzyme of creatine kinase III. Active and inactive forms in dystrophic muscle of vitamin E deficient rabbit. *J Biol Chem* 1977;252:3117–3120.

106. Wins O, Bunnell RH, Gloor U. Absorption and distribution of vitamin E in the tissue. *Vitam Horm* 1962;20:441–442.

107. Parry DJ, Motpetit VJA: Histochemical changes in fast and slow muscles of nutritionally dystrophic rabbits. *J Neuropathol Exp Neurol* 1978;38(3):231–243.

108. Einarson L: Criticizing review of the concepts of the neuromuscular lesions in experimental vitamin E deficiency, preferably in adult rats. *Acta Psychol Neurol Scand (Suppl)* 1952;78:8–76.

109. Einarson L: Deposits of fluorescent acid-fast products in the nervous system and skeletal muscles of adult rats with chronic vitamin E deficiency. *J Neurol Neurosurg Psychiatr* 1953;16:98–109.

110. Lampert P, Blumberg JM, Pentschew A: An electron microscopic study of dystrophic axons in the gracile and cuneate nuclei of vitamin E deficient rats. *J Neuropathol Exp Neurol* 1964;23:60–77.

111. Machlin LJ, Filipski R, Nelson J, et al: Effects of a prolonged vitamin E deficiency in the rat. *J Nutr* 1977;107;1200–1208.

112. Towfighi J: Effects of chronic vitamin E deficiency on the nervous system of the rat. *Acta Neuropathol* 1981;54:261–267.

113. Nelson JS, Fitch CD, Fischer VW, et al: Progressive neuropathologic lesions in vitamin E deficient rhesus monkeys. *J Neuropathol Exp Neurol* 1981;40:166–186.

114. Sung JH: Neuroaxonal dystrophy in mucoviscidosis. *J Neuropathol Exp Neurol* 1964; 23:567–583.

115. Geller A, Gilles F, Shwachman H: Degeneration of fasciculus gracilis in cystic fibrosis. *Neurology* 1977;27:185–187.

116. Sung JH, Stadlan E: Neuroaxonal dystrophy in congenital biliary atresia. *J Neuropathol Exp Neurol* 1966;25:341–361.

117. Sung JH, Park SH, Mastri AR, et al: Axonal dystrophy in the gracile nucleus in congenital biliary atresia and cystic fibrosis (mucoviscidosis): Beneficial effect of vitamin E therapy. *J Neuropathol Exp Neurol* 1980;39:584–597.

118. Cavalier SJ, Gambetti P: Dystrophic axons and spinal cord demyelination in cystic fibrosis. *Neurology* 1981;31:714–718.

119. Tomasi LG: Reversibility of human myopathy caused by vitamin E deficiency. *Neurology* 1979;29:1182–1186.

120. Rosenblum JL, Keating JP, Prensky AL, et al: A progressive neurologic syndrome in children with chronic liver disease. *N Engl J Med* 1981;304:503–508.

121. Darby CW, Davidson AGF, Desai ID: Muscular performance in cystic fibrosis patients and its relation to vitamin E. *Arch Dis Child* 1973;48:72–75.

122. Chabria S, Tomasi LG, Lloyd-Still JD: Neurological manifestations of cystic fibrosis: Lack of relationship to vitamin E deficiency. *Ann Neurol* 1978;4:194.

123. Farrell PM, Fratantoni JC, Bieri JG, et al: Effects of vitamin E deficiency in man. *Acta Paediatr Scand* 1975;64:150–151.

124. Dinning JS, Day PL: Vitamin E deficiency in the monkey. I. Muscular dystrophy hematologic changes and the excretion of urinary nitrogenous constituents. *J Exp Med* 1957; 105:395–402.

125. Castillo R, Landon C, Eckhardt K, et al: Selenium and vitamin E status in cystic fibrosis. *J Pediatr* 1981;99:583–585.

126. Lloyd-Still JD, Ganther HE: Selenium and glutathione peroxidase levels in cystic fibrosis. *Pediatrics* 1980;65:1010–1012.

127. Roberts HW: Perspective on vitamin E as therapy. *JAMA* 1981;246(2):129–131.

128. The effect of deficiency of vitamins E and A on the retina. *Nutr Rev* 1980;38:386–389.

129. Amemiya T: Photoreceptor outer segment and retinal pigment epithelium in vitamin E deficient rats. *Graefes arch Ophthalmol* 1981;216:103–109.

130. Harley RD, Huang NN, Macri CH, et al: Optic neuritis and optic atrophy following chloramphenicol in cystic fibrosis patients. *Trans Am Acad Ophthalmol Otolaryngol* 1970;74:1011–1031.

131. Godel V, Nemet P, Lazar M: Chloramphenicol optic neuropathy. *Arch Ophthalmol* 1980;98:1417–1421.

132. Huang NN, Harley RD, Promadhattanedi V, et al: Visual disturbances in cystic fibrosis following chloramphenicol administration. *J Pediatr* 1966;68:32–44.

133. Keith GG: Optic atrophy induced by chloramphenicol. *Br J Opthalmol* 1964;48:567–569.

134. Joy JT, Sealettar R, Sodie DB: Optic and

peripheral neuritis: Probable effect of prolonged chloramphenicol therapy. *JAMA* 1960;173:1731–1734.

135. Leitman PS, di Sant'Agnese PA, Wong VG: Optic neuritis in cystic fibrosis of the pancreas: Role of chloramphenicol therapy. *JAMA* 1964;189:924–927.

136. Wong VG, Collins E: Optic atrophy in cystic fibrosis of the pancreas. *Am J Ophthalmol* 1965;59:763–768.

23

Cystic Fibrosis—Iatrogenic Complications* and Related Issues

Harry Shwachman

When a new drug or physical mode of therapy is introduced for a relatively new disease such as cystic fibrosis, there is a period of evaluation, the duration depending on how often the disorder occurs and how many patients and physicians are willing to participate. Cystic fibrosis occurs in approximately 1 in 1600 white births. First clearly described as a fatal disease in 1938, it remains one of the unsolved congenital metabolic disorders. Under these circumstances it is natural to expect a variety of therapies, many of them empirical and safe, others perhaps ineffective or harmful. An estimated 12% of hospital admissions to intensive care units are due to iatrogenic disease.[1,2]

Before discussing the iatrogenic complications or those which we, as physicians, are responsible for producing, it might be well to list the complications which reflect the natural course of the disease. Those involving the pancreas and gastrointestinal tract include meconium ileus, volvulus, rupture of the gut, meconium peritonitis, neonatal jaundice, loss of bile, rectal prolapse, malabsorption, glucose intolerance, diabetes mellitus, vitamin deficiencies, cirrhosis of the

*See reference D'Arcy, Griffen: *Iatrogenic Diseases*. New York, Oxford University Press, 1979.

liver, portal hypertension, hypersplenism, intussusception, fecal impaction, failure to grow, bone demineralization, and pneumotosis intestinalis. In the male the anatomical defects in the derivatives of the wolffian ducts cause sterility in the great majority of patients.

Of grave significance are the events which occur in natural sequence in the respiratory system of the untreated patient. These complications, also considered features of the disease, include chronic cough, bronchitis, atelectasis, respiratory tract infection superimposed on chronic obstructive pulmonary disease, pneumonia, bronchiectasis, empyema, lung abscesses, pneumothorax, hemoptysis, and cor pulmonale. Upper respiratory tract involvement includes sinusitis and nasal polyposis. Finally the sweat gland defect may, under certain circumstances, result in dehydration, heat stroke, and death.

Of great significance are those failures made by physicians who do not recognize this disease in early life or make incorrect diagnoses, notably celiac disease, asthma, or tuberculosis. What occurs more frequently is the making of the diagnosis of CF in a child who does not have the disease. A false diagnosis of CF may result in restricting family size and subject the patient to costly and unnecessary treatment. Errors made in laboratory diagnosis are numerous, and the physician must be critical of all laboratory tests. An elevated value of electrolytes in sweat does not by itself make the diagnosis. Cystic fibrosis remains a clinical diagnosis confirmed by laboratory tests. Harm to the patient's family can also result from no or inadequate education; this pertains to genetic counseling, the dangers of heat exposure, air travel, or staying at very high altitudes; and neglecting to provide influenza vaccine under appropriate circumstances.

ANTIBIOTICS

The most common iatrogenic complications include reactions to a host of antibiotics used to treat the pulmonary infections, whether it be bronchitis or extensive bronchiectasis[3] (Table 23-1). Almost all antibiotics may produce side effects, even when given in the proper dose. Allergic or hypersensitivity reactions may involve many systems and may occur in those who do not have CF as well as in those who do. The effects may be febrile, dermatological, gastrointestinal, hematologic, neurological, or nephrotoxic. The incidence of allergy in the CF population is about 16–20%, the same as in the healthy child population.

The appearance of *Pseudomonas* in sputum and bronchial secretions from patients with CF is commonly ascribed to the prior administration of antibiotics. This view is not fully shared by some investigators. The conversion of the rough to smooth strain of *Pseudomonas* is characteristic in patients with CF and is rarely encountered in other disorders. Secondary and superimposed fungal infections are also ascribed to prolonged antibiotic therapy.

We strongly recommend that before prescribing a drug, the brochure which accompanies it be examined carefully to avoid an overdose and to become familiar with the possible ill effects. In all cases, justification for the use of the drug must be balanced by the positive beneficial effect expected. One should not administer a drug merely because it will do no harm. One must have evidence that it will do good.

Sulfisoxazole is frequently prescribed along with one of the antistaphylococcal agents in our therapy. This is one of the safest drugs, and the complications of hematuria, drug rash, or nausea are rare, the incidence being an estimated 1 per 1000.

The tetracyclines deserve special mention.[4,5] Some children with CF in whom *Staphylococcus aureus* was present in sputum and throat cultures were given oral chlortetracycline (Aureomycin) or oxytetracycline (Terramycin) in small doses over a long period. When the permanent teeth erupted a number of years later, they were noticeably stained. What is more, under ultraviolet light the stained teeth fluoresced. (Staining of bone also was observed in our postmortem studies.)

Table 23-1
Iatrogenic Complications

Incorrect diagnosis	Drugs
False positive	Anabolic agents—androgenic effects, cholestasis, hepatotoxicity
False negative	Iodides—goiter, hypothyroidism, skin rashes
Antibiotics, general	Steroids—metabolic, diabetes, cataract
Hypersensitivity	Improper feeding
Gastrointestinal disturbances	Soy formula—anemia, hypoproteinemia, malnutrition
Dermatological disturbances	Whole milk—intestinal obstruction
Fever	Selenium supplements—toxicity
Superinfection	Fad diets—malnutrition
Neurotoxicity	Medium-chain triglyceride oil—diarrhea
Ototoxicity	Failure of prevention
Renal toxicity	Heat prostration—salt loss
Venous thrombosis	Influenza—missed vaccination
Antibiotics, specific	High-altitude hypoxemia
Tetracycline	Surgical considerations
Dental staining	Sympathetic denervation of the pancreas
Deposition in bone	Pulmonary lavage
Retardation of bone development	Tracheostomy
Photosensitivity	Rectal prolapse (surgical reduction)
Bulging fontanel	Enemas in newborn intestinal obstruction
Gastrointestinal disturbances	Intravenous alimentation
Chloramphenicol	Sepsis
The gray syndrome	Deficiencies, especially metabolic
Loss of vision	Cholestasis and liver dysfunction
Peripheral neuritis	Pancreatic replacement
Bone-marrown depression, agranulocytosis	Allergy to pork—diarrhea
Aminoglycosides	Overdose of pancreatin—fecal impaction
Ototoxicity	Asthmatic attacks caused by inhaled powder
Renal toxicity	Bacterial contamination *(Salmonella)*
Neurotoxicity	Hyperuricemia and kidney stones
Long-acting "sulfa"	Aerosols/Mist
Encephalitis	IPPB (intermittent positive-pressure breathing) —dissemination of infection, pneumothorax
Synthetic penicillin	Mucomyst—bronchospasm, bleeding
Allergic reactions	3% salt mist— irritation and bleeding
Gastrointestinal disturbances	Mist—pulmonary edema, increased risk of infection, psychological
Electrolyte disturbance	
Sulfisoxazole	
Bone-marrow depression	
Nephrotoxicity	
Gastrointestinal disturbances	

The discolored teeth posed social and behavioral problems. Affected children tried not to open their mouths. They hardly ever spoke up in school or smiled, and they were taunted by classmates who accused them of not brushing their teeth. At first we resorted to capping those of the stained teeth that could be seen when the children smiled. Finally, the psychological trauma was abated when a bleaching method was found to decrease the stain.

Because the tetracyclines are incorporated during the time of tooth calcification in the first 6 years of life,[7-9] we can prevent this staining by avoiding the use of tetracyclines in patients under 6 years of age. Tetracyclines should also be avoided in women during the second half of pregnancy because the drugs effect fetal bone growth and because they are incorporated in bone and tooth buds.

Another undesirable effect of the tetracyclines in photosensitivity. When patients on tetracyclines are exposed to the sun, regardless of age, they may develop a tan or burn of the exposed parts. To avoid this type of reaction, we avoid prescribing the tetracyclines during the summer. The undesirable gastrointestinal effect of the tetracyclines appear to be uncommon in our population.

Chloramphenicol is a useful antibiotic in the treatment of the pulmonary infection in cystic fibrosis. A report on its use for more than 3 years of daily therapy was issued by our clinic in 1963.[10] No toxic effect was noted in the 50 patients studied or in the 23 records culled from the postmortem file. Since that time we have encountered one patient who developed fatal aplastic anemia. A more common complication, blindness, occurred in more than 25 patients following varying months of daily therapy.[11,12] Optic neuritis was reported by many other observers, who also noted rapid recovery when chloramphenicol was discontinued. Huang and colleagues[13] have seen 20 patients with CF develop optic neuritis with no blood dyscrasia. Central scotoma was noted. There were no hematological changes. The retina may appear normal in most of these patients. We have been impressed with the noticeable decrease of this complication since we began prescribing large amounts of vitamin B complex whenever we give chloramphenicol.

Another rare complication of chloramphenicol therapy is peripheral neuritis. This can be a painful and distressing complaint. The weight of the sheet in bed may be painful to the lower extremities, and there may be a burning sensation in the soles of the feet. The nerve conduction time in the affected limb may be delayed. Recovery is relatively slow and may take two or three months (see Chapter 22).

All aminoglycosides are widely used, including streptomycin, amikacin, gentamicin, tobramycin, and a host of newer drugs. These drugs are generally administered intravenously or intramuscularly in doses varying from 4 to 8 mg/kg/day, as specified in the accompanying brochures. Much larger dosages have been used with safety. One must be aware of ototoxic and nephrotoxic effects. Tobramycin is less nephrotoxic than gentamicin. We have not observed these effects in our patients. Usually a semisynthetic penicillin compound is administered at the same time, such as carbenicillin or ticarcillin because of the synergistic effect on *Pseudomonas*. Sensitivity reactions following the use of these drugs have been noted. Many intravenous agents are apt to cause a burning sensation, pain, and erythema at the site of the injection and, rarely, thrombosis of the vein. The semisynthetic penicillins may cause transient elevations of some liver function tests and an increase in the sodium load, since many of the preparations are sodium salts.

OTHER DRUGS

A variety of anabolic agents have been employed to increase growth and general well-being with varying degrees of suceess.[14,15] We have employed Nilevar, Winstrol, and Dianabol daily for as long as two or three months and found these drugs useful, although we are not altogether enthusiastic. The main side effect is masculinization. We have had to stop the drug in small boys because of penile erections. In females the drug can cause hoarseness, hirsutism, acne, and enlargement of the clitoris. Cholestasis and hepatotoxicity are potential complications.

Attempts to "thin" bronchial secretions with iodides have met with mixed success. At the Yale Clinic, hypothyroidism resulted when the iodides were used extensively.[16] We have also noted this complication.[17] Since iodine passes readily through the placenta, we do not prescribe iodides to our pregnant women. We have encountered one premature infant who had a huge goiter at delivery, born to a mother with CF. This mother had taken iodides during the first 3 months of her pregnancy before she advised us that she was pregnant. In a recent report, Cohen et al[18] records finding no evidence of toxic complications when the aminoglycosides were given to homozygous pregnant women. Our limited experience is in agreement.

IMPROPER FEEDING

Vitamin and fatty acid deficiencies are uncommon in our patients since we prescribe twice the recommended dose of multivitamins on empirical grounds based on the poor absorption of the fat-soluble vitamins and the permissive use of small amounts of fats in patients with pancreatic insufficiency. However, the failure to give fat-soluble vitamins may result in deficiencies in vitamins A, D, E, and K. We have encountered two infants with rickets owing to vitamin D deficiency, a number of patients with vitamin K deficiency, and three recent patients with vitamin A deficiency, manifested by night blindness and low levels of serum vitamin A. We have seen no clinical features of vitamin E deficiency, even when the blood level of tocopherol is low, except for hemolytic anemia of prematurity. Serum vitamin E may correlate partly with the degree of steatorrhea as well as with creatinuria, ceroid deposition, muscle weakness, and increased serum creatine phosphokinase. Excess administration of vitamin A can result in skeletal lesions with bone pain, fever, increased intracranial pressure, and rash.

In patients born into CF families the diagnosis can be established with certainty by performing the sweat test. A positive sweat test in the neonatal period indicates cystic fibrosis. Other helpful tests include examining the meconium, pancreatic fluid, or stool trypsin. There is a strong misconception that babies under 6 weeks cannot be properly sweat tested. This is fallacious. We have succeeded in performing the sweat test in close to 95% of babies under 6 weeks, although we must admit poor success in sweat testing premature babies. Pancreatic fluid analysis, formerly a routine diagnostic procedure, is no longer considered necessary because the sweat test is more reliable and easier to perform. At present the meconium test for albumin may be considered a good screening test since it can pick up many, but not all, infants with CF. The stool trypsin test is a useful procedure in infants and children under 4 years of age. This test refers to the functional condition of the pancreas, recognizing the fact that as many as 15% to 20% of all patients with CF may have adequate pancreatic exocrine function.

Since we cannot offer a cure for CF, parents may listen to anyone who offers them hope or a successful mode of therapy; in rare instances patients and parents may retreat into some religious world. Recently a veterinary pathologist asserted that CF was not an inherited disease but was due to a deficiency of selenium. No experimental evidence was offered; the theory was based on the pathological changes in one monkey that was observed only after death. This person suggested a gluten-free diet with added selenium. Many parents pinned their hopes on this person's theory. Even more damaging was the advice to mothers with CF children that if selenium was taken during the next pregnancy, CF could be prevented in the next child. There is no evidence that selenium plays any more significant role than does copper, zinc, or magnesium in the treatment of cystic fibrosis.[19,20]

Improper feeding in the undiagnosed infant with CF may bring on anemia, hypoproteinemic edema, and other metabolic derangements. Formula changes in the treatment of diarrhea in infancy, common in pediatric practice, are frequent in CF. A soy preparation may be poorly tolerated and has led to anemia, malnutrition, and hypoproteinemia in some infants with CF.

The use of whole-milk formulas for the baby recovering from meconium ileus surgery or for the newborn with CF may cause hard casein curds that could be the source of intestinal obstruction.[21] A formula of low-curd tension will avoid this uncommon complication.

FAILURE OF PREVENTION

Physicians who are familiar with the disease will provide certain warnings to patients and parents; failure to heed them could put the CF patient's life in jeopardy. In this category is the warning to prevent sunstroke or undue exposure to heat, which results in loss of electrolytes and fluid through sweat and leads to shock. It is noteworthy that Dorothy Andersen was aware of this fatal outcome in babies with CF prior to the demonstration of the sweat defect, having observed that a hot spell in New York City proved fatal to babies with CF.[22]

Residing even for short periods at elevations above 5000 feet may increase respiratory distress. One severely ill patient with CF was sent from Boston to a pulmonary center in Denver for further care. Upon arrival in Denver he was sent home with the warning that the elevation of Denver would be hazardous. We recall advising one patient, early in her pregnancy, to move from an elevation of 6000 feet to sea level. This advice was given on the basis of arterial blood gas determinations under conditions equivalent to these two elevations. The patient heeded the advice, and her pregnancy ended satisfactorily with a healthy full-term infant.

Physicians will recommend immunization against influenza in the fall when an increased incidence is predicted. They will not recommend vaccination against the *Pneumococcus* because the *Pneumococcus* rarely invades the respiratory tract in CF, and furthermore the patients are generally on antibiotics that are effective in eradicating the *Pneumococcus*. One might make an exception when dealing with the splenectomized patient.

SURGICAL CONSIDERATIONS

One must be aware of medical or surgical reports that provide dangerous or risky recommendations. The report by Ochsner and his colleagues falls in this category. In 1950 Ayers et al[23] described a new method of treatment consisting of sympathetic denervation of the pancreas by splanchnicectomy block with procaine hydrochloride and complete splanchnicectomy on the right side. They reported five treated patients with CF who showed spectacular immediate results. They also proposed a theory of neuroeffector mechanisms which we were unable to comprehend. One patient died following surgery and the remaining four patients were discharged on the seventh and eighth days following surgery. One patient developed a postoperative pneumothorax.

Shortly after this report, many parents from around the country asked that their CF children be treated in this way, and a number of ill patients were subjected to surgery and died.

The following year Ayers et al[24] reported on 24 patients, 20 of them under 4 years of age and many of them bad risks for surgery. This time they stated that the operation did not improve pancreatic function as was noted in the first patient. They did find some improvement in the respiratory component of the disease. Only one patient had a mild clinical manifestation of the disease, and 23 had advanced bronchiectasis. Three patients were considered to have improved. There were nine deaths within one year following splanchnicectomy. The postoperative course was difficult to evaluate because the patients were treated with chlortetracycline which had been shown to be therapeutically effective.[5] It is noted that no further reports concerning this operation have appeared in the 30 years since these were published.

A procedure which we have performed in the past in patients with moderate pulmonary disease—pulmonary lavage with *N*-acetylcysteine—we no longer advocate. The aim of this therapy is straightforward: to clear the plugged bronchi. Success with this type of therapy was initially advocated by Reas. The number of enthusiasts for this procedure has diminished over the years. According to our experience with 35 patients over a 15-year-period,[25] this procedure offers little benefit. A variety of modifications have been introduced, such as in the nature of the anesthetic agent, in the nature and volume of solutions, in the selection and type of patient, in the number of segments treated, and in the positions used. This procedure is difficult to evaluate and reproduce.

Another surgical procedure which we do not find necessary is the reduction of the prolapse of the rectum. We have been able to reduce recurrent prolapse in all cases stemming from CF by reducing the total fat in the diet and giving an adequate pancreatic preparation with each meal. On rare occasions we have had to resort to temporary mechanical strapping of the buttocks.

Another surgical procedure worth considering is tracheostomy to permit bronchial drainage. We have recommended and performed tracheostomies prior to major surgery involving the chest or abdomen. This procedure is excellent for temporarily clearing the bronchi of mucopurulent material. However, there are undesirable reactions. One that is common, but not serious, is subcutaneous emphysema, which generally involves the neck and face and rarely more of the body. A more serious risk is that of accidentally producing a pneumothorax. A tracheostomy to provide better drainage in a CF patient with extensive bronchiectasis is something most of us prefer not to recommend lightly. In the past we have had successful tracheostomies in a 16-year-old patient for over 5 months and in another patient 28 years of age for over 5 years when she died at age 33. This latter patient became an advocate of this procedure. We feel it has its place, but most of us shy away from making a strong recommendation. Hyperalimentation is a relatively new procedure which we hesitate to recommend in patients with CF because the benefit may appear dramatic but is usually short lived.

PANCREATIC REPLACEMENT

Pancreatic preparations have been marketed for many years, and the products available in this country have improved markedly over the past 30 years. The pig pancreas is the major source of pancreatin. One rare complication noted in England was salmonellosis[26,27] from contaminated pancreatin. We have not encountered a contaminated product in this country.

Our use of pancreatin is limited to patients with pancreatic insufficiency. This includes about 80% of our patients with CF, all our patients with the Shwachman syndrome, and the rare surgical extirpation in cases of nesidioblastosis. We found Viokase powder and tablets, introduced in about 1950, to be an effective preparation. In a small number of families, the healthy adult caretakers developed acute asthmatic symptoms when exposed to the powdered preparation. A less-effective beef pancreatin was substituted in such cases. We have not encountered this type of asthmatic reaction in a child with CF. A rare patient may be allergic to pork and may react by having diarrhea. We have found pancreatic preparations made from vegetable sources are less effective than those from the pig or cow.

About four years ago Johnson & Johnson put a new preparation, Pancrease, on the market; this product comes in the form of microspheres packed in a capsule. Each microsphere is coated so that when it reaches the stomach, it is not inactivated by gastric juice. One to three capsules can be taken per meal—depending on the nature and size of the meal—rather than 10 or more Viokase tablets. The newest product made available by Organon, Cotazym-S, is of a similar nature. A rare untoward effect of Pancrease has been the development of fecal impaction following its sudden introduction with each meal. We have not seen this reaction if the change to Pancrease is made gradually over a period of about one month. A rare patient will refuse this product because of increased flatulence, or an unpleasant odor from the urine.

A complication initially ascribed to pancreatin preparations was hyperuricosuria, with the risk of stone formation. This created a stir because all pancreatic preparations had a high purine content.[28] The alarm did not unsettle us since we were unable to consider this a serious complication. In a study carried out in our clinic,[29] we did not find inordinately high blood uric acid or kidney stones. The Toronto clinic, where huge amounts of pancreatin were used, did not have an epidemic of renal problems owing to elevated uric acid. What this original study accomplished was to alert us to the need to use pancreatin in the smallest effective dose (see Chapter 17).

Intestinal impaction, wrongly called "meconium ileus equivalent," has been noted more frequently in the older patient. This may result from dietary indiscretion, from a change in the nature of the pancreatic preparation, an increase in dose per meal, or from no detectable alteration in eating habits.

AEROSOLS AND MISTS

Intermittent positive-pressure breathing (IPPB) is sometimes employed for the delivery of solutions by aerosol, including wetting agents, *N*-acetylcysteine, bronchodilators, antibiotics, and saline or various mixtures both in the home and in the hospital. There is controversy as to whether this mode of therapy is effective. Furthermore the indiscriminate use of IPPB at home may result in pneumothorax, especially if the pressure is greatly increased.

The use of a mist tent at night has been advocated in the past on the following assumptions: it will help thin out secretions and make chest bronchial drainage more effective, it will decrease water loss from the lung, and it may make the patient more comfortable. The scientific evidence for benefit is very meager. When we gradually eliminated this form of therapy, most patients and parents were happy, especially since they were not able to notice any significant changes when the child slept in or out of the tent. This subject is not closed, especially since a small number of excellent people still advocate this form of therapy. However, mist tent therapy was one of the factors involved in aggravating the psychological problems of these children[30] (see Chapter 12.)

REFERENCES

1. Trunet P, LaGall JR, Lhoste F, et al: The role of iatrogenic disease in admissions to intensive care. *JAMA* 1980;244:2617–2620.
2. Boston Collaborative Drug Surveillance Program: Hospital admissions due to adverse drug reactions. *Arch Intern Med* 1974;134: 219–223.
3. Borda IT, Slone D, Sick H: Assessment of adverse reactions within a drug surveillance program. *JAMA* 1968;205:645–647.
4. Shwachman H, Schuster A: The tetracyclines: Applied pharmacology. *Pediatr Clin North Am* 1956;3:295–303.
5. Shwachman H, Crocker AC, Foley CE, et al: Aureomycin therapy in pulmonary involvement of pancreatic fibrosis (mucoviscidosis). *N Engl J Med* 1949;241:185–192.
6. Zegaralli SV, Denning CR, Kutchen AH, et al: Discoloration of teeth in patients with cystic fibrosis of the pancreas. *Clin Pediatr* 1963;2:329–331.
7. Wallman IS, Hilton HB: Teeth pigmented by tetracycline. *Lancet* 1962;1:827–829.
8. Grossman ER, Walchek A, Freedman H, et al: Tetracyclines and permanent teeth: The relation between dose and tooth color. *Pediatrics* 1971;47:567–570.
9. Jagels AE, Sweeney EA: Oral health of patients with cystic fibrosis and their siblings. *J Dent Res* 1976;55:991–996.
10. Lloyd AVC, Grimes G, Khaw KT, et al: Chloramphenicol for long-term therapy of cystic fibrosis. *JAMA* 1963;184:1001–1006.
11. Cooke JG Jr, Brown RE, Geppert LJ: Optic neuritis with prolonged use of chloramphenicol. *J Pediatr* 1966;68:27–31.
12. Denning CR, Bruce GM, Spalter HF: Optic neuritis in chloramphenicol-treated patients with cystic fibrosis. *Pediatrics* 1968;41:7–17.
13. Huang NN, Harley RD, Promadhattavedi V, et al: Visual disturbances in cystic fibrosis following chloramphenicol administration. *J Pediatr* 1966;68:32–44.
14. Good TA, Bessman SP: Anabolic steroids in cystic fibrosis of the pancreas. *Am J Dis Child* 1966;111:272–277.
15. Dooley RR, Moss AJ, Wright PM, et al: Norethandrolone in cystic fibrosis of the pancreas. *J Pediatr* 1969;74:95–102.
16. Dolan TF, Gibson LE: Complications of iodide therapy in patients with cystic fibrosis. *J Pediatr* 1971;79:684–687.
17. Ruben BL, Crigler JF Jr, Berenberg W, et al: Hypothyroidism, a complication of iodide therapy in children with chronic respiratory involvement of cystic fibrosis. *Am J Dis Child* 1960;100:721–722.
18. Cohen LF, di Sant'Agnese PA, Friedlander J: Cystic fibrosis and pregnancy. *Lancet* 1980;2:842–844.
19. Lloyd-Still JD, Ganther HE: Selenium and glutathione peroxidase levels in cystic fibrosis. *Pediatrics* 1980;65:1010–1012.
20. Hubbard JS, Barbero G, Chase HP:

Selenium and cystic fibrosis. *J Pediatr* 1980; 96:421–422.

21. Donnison AB, Shwachman H, Gross RE: A review of 164 children with meconium ileus seen at the Children's Hospital Medical Center, Boston. *Pediatrics* 1966;37:833–850.
22. Kessler WR, Andersen DH: Heat prostration in fibrocystic disease of the pancreas and other conditions. *Pediatrics* 1951;8:648–656.
23. Ayers WB, Stevens D, Ochsner A: Fibrocystic disease of the pancreas. Treatment by sympathetic denervation of the pancreas and presentation of a theory of neuroeffector mechanisms. Preliminary report of five cases. *JAMA* 1950;142:7–12.
24. Ayers WB, Stevens D, Ochsner A, et al: Splanchnicectomy for pancreatic fibrosis. *Pediatrics* 1951;8:657–663.
25. Khaw KT, Roura AA, Shwachman H: A controlled study of pulmonary lavage in patients with cystic fibrosis. *Cystic Fibrosis Club Abstr* 1965;6:17.
26. Glencross EJG: Pancreatin as a source of hospital-acquired salmonellosis. *Br Med J* 1972;2:376–378.
27. Forrester RM, Keen JH: Pancreatin as a source of *Salmonella*. *Br Med J* 1972;3:472.
28. Nousia-Arvanitakis S, Stapleton PB, Linshaw MA, et al: Therapeutic approach to pancreatic extract induced hyperuricosuria in cystic fibrosis *J Pediatr* 1977;90:302–305.
29. Adeniyi-Jones S, Khaw KT, Gordon D, et al: Uric acid metabolism in children with cystic fibrosis. *Cystic Fibrosis Club Abstr* 1977; 18:22.
30. McCollum AT, Gibson LE: Family adaptation to the child with cystic fibrosis. *J Pediatr* 1970;77:571–598.

SECTION THREE

PSYCHOLOGIC, SOCIAL AND ECONOMIC FACTORS

24

Psychological Functioning of Cystic Fibrosis Patients

John V. Lavigne

For many cystic fibrosis (CF) patients, the disease requires a demanding regimen of daily treatments and close monitoring of the child's physical state. CF children experience physical symptoms, deviant growth patterns, and physical limitations that are not shared by their healthy counterparts. Since there are daily and sometimes almost continuous reminders of the disease, CF is not a condition that the patient can readily ignore. As the life span of CF patients increases, the psychological impact of the disease and the quality of life of the CF patients will demand increasing attention from the professionals who provide their care.

The interested professional—whether a clinician or researcher—who turns to the literature on the psychosocial aspects of CF may be struck by the methodological problems in many of the studies, and also by the contradictory reports about the psychological functioning of the CF patients. This review is being written with two purposes in mind: first, to summarize the results of studies which have been published on the psychological funtioning of CF children and adolescents; and second, to review the methodology employed in these studies. Studies which have only included CF patients will be examined first, along with general reviews and impressionistic reports on CF patients. Following this, studies employing comparison groups will be presented. Studies of single cases will not be reviewed. The reports that are discussed were located through searches of *Index Medicus* and *Psychological Abstracts,* along with examining the bibliographies of articles discovered through such searches. With regard to single-group studies, the reviews are not exhaustive, but the major papers have been presented. An effort has been made to present all the papers that use more sophisticated methodology involving the use of control or comparison groups.

SINGLE-GROUP STUDIES

In the single-group studies, the authors were primarily concerned with the description of a single sample of CF patients and not with comparisons of those patients with other samples of ill or healthy children. In these studies, any subdivisions of the CF group into smaller samples were made according to age of the patient or the severity of the illness.

CF patients of various ages have been studied in this manner. Studies by Drotar,[1] McCollum and Gibson,[2] Falkman,[3] Tropauer et al,[4] Lawler et al,[5] and Spock and Stedman[6] have included both children and adolescents in their sample. A single-group study by Boyle et al[7] examined adolescents and young adults ages 13–30 years, and the studies by Cytryn et al[8] and Kulczycki et al[9] included only children below the ages of 9 years and 10 years, respectively. Table 24-1 includes a summary of sample sizes in each study.

While data collection procedures varied, each study included an interview with the child, parent, or both. In addition, three of the studies[5,7,8] included standard projective tests (Thematic Apperception Test, Rorschach, or both) with the patient. Abbreviated projective tests, using human figure drawings or the house–tree–person technique, were included in the data collection procedures of other studies.[3,6–8] A parent questionnaire was included in the study by McCollum and Gibson,[2] but information on its reliability and validity were not presented. Intelligence tests were included in several studies.[3,5,6,8,9]

The major findings of the individual studies are summarized in Table 24-1. Although the results are not uniform across all of these studies, a composite picture emerges of the types of adjustment problems that CF patients can display in childhood and adolescence. Overt behavior problems have been noted among CF children when they first enter school,[2] including problems of inattentiveness, daydreaming, restlessness, and disruptive classroom behavior. Such behavior was reported in 44% of the sample studied by McCollum and Gibson,[2] one of the few single-group studies in which any results were quantified. Anxiety, depression, intrapsychic conflicts, and psychosomatic complaints have been noted across a wide spectrum of ages in various studies.[1,5–7] Likewise, global, nonspecific emotional indicators on abbreviated projective tests at a variety of ages have been reported.[3] Among school-age children, problems with academic work, noncompliance, and discipline have been described.[1,5] Among children under 12, the tendency to ask questions about the disease and to show concern about death increased with age. Also increasing with age was the tendency for the patients to show shame and embarrassment about having CF and some of its distasteful symptoms, such as frequent coughing.[2,4] Maladaptive use of the defenses of denial, fantasy, regression, and repression have also been reported.[5] The IQs of CF patients seemed to be normal, with several studies suggesting levels of performance in the average range[3,6,8,9] or slightly higher.

Psychological problems were especially prominent among adolescents with CF. Questions and concerns about death seemed to occur more frequently during this developmental period than before. Likewise, the adolescent with CF was even more sensitive to feelings of being different and alienated from peers than the younger children. Questions about and fear of death increased in frequency,[2,4] and dissatisfaction with one's physical appearance accelerated during this time. There were indications that concerns about sexuality, growth, and development became more common—aided, of course, by the fact that many CF patients showed delays in these areas. Conflicts about independence and dependence, common even among healthy adolescents, were thought to be intensified in the CF adolescents, chiefly because the demands of the disease heighten dependency at a time when the person is striving to become independent. There was also an increased tendency among the adolescents to balk at medical care.[1,2]

This rather pessimistic profile of the functioning of CF children is similar to that reported in other literature reviews and impressionistic reports of CF patients.[10–14] This profile may be an artifact of the methods employed in these studies. Few of the studies report the frequency with which the various psychological problems exist among the CF patients. For example, Tropauer et al[4] reported that "preoccupation with death and ultimate disability was seen more frequently with adolescents" (p 426), but the frequency, intensity, and debilitating effects of such thoughts were not described. Thus, the potential problems of the CF patients are highlighted but not placed in the proper context. Also contributing to this pessimistic profile are those studies which only describe the psychological functioning of CF patients who have been referred for psychotherapy because they were not coping well with their disease.[1] From studies which lack representative samples, frequency data, or control groups, the reader can readily develop the notion that psychological problems characterize these children when, in fact, they may characterize only a minority of CF patients.

Cytryn et al[8] reported a single-group study which conveys a different view of the functioning of CF children than that of the composite picture described above, partly because these authors do report the frequency of psychological problems among the CF children. These authors report that a majority of the children (not adolescents) were functioning well and generally using defenses in an adaptive fashion. They report that 41% of their sample showed no disturbance; 17%, mild disturbance; 28%, moderate disturbance; and 14%, severe disturbance. These results differ markedly from other single-group studies which tend to emphasize the adjustment problems of the CF children. Of course, the Cytryn et al[8] study only included children, whereas many of the other studies examined adolescents as well, and the age differences as well as methodology may contribute to the differences in the findings.

Other methodological problems plague all of these studies. In all but one report, control or comparison groups were not included in the designs at all—an obvious and significant weakness. Without such controls, it is impossible to determine whether the characteristics of the children are unique to the CF population, or even whether the problems described occur more frequently among the CF patients than other ill or healthy children. In the one exception,[3] comparison groups from a different study were used for only two of the multiple measures reported. On a projective measure of emotional adjustment, the CF children were not significantly different from diabetic children, but they did show more signs of emotional problems than the children selected for being well-adjusted. Unfortunately, the comparison groups were not well described, and it is questionable whether these samples were adequately matched with the CF children on such relevant variables as sex, age, and socioeconomic status.

Another significant problem involves the description and validation of the assessment methods used in these studies. The studies tended to rely upon interview and projective techniques to assess the personalities of the CF patients. Uniformly, the authors failed to report on the reliability and validity of the interview procedures employed. In each of the studies, the results are a function of the skills and predilections of the individual interviewers. Unfortunately, without reliability

Table 24-1
Single-Group Studies

Author	Sample	Method	Results
Drotar, 1978[1]	N = 32 CF patients ages 5–19 years; all referred for psychological problems	Interviews with children and parents	Patients showed academic problems related to emotional stress, discipline problems (including noncompliance with medications), psychosomatic complaints, anxiety reactions (especially related to fear of death). Among adolescents, problems resolving independence–dependence conflicts.
McCollum and Gibson, 1970[2]	N = 65 CF patients from 56 families; children and adolescents included from a variety of SES backgrounds.	Maternal interviews and questionnaires, plus information gathered in a support group.	44% of children had behavior problems in first year of school (inattentive, restless, disruptive). Between ages 8 and 12 years, children concerned about differences from peers; increased frequency of questions about death and shame about the disease. Adolescents feel isolated from peers, struggle over independence–dependence issues, and show decreased compliance with medical regimen.
Falkman, 1977[3]	N = 52 CF patients, ages 4.6–15.1 years; N = 22 preschoolers, N = 30 school age; Diabetic and well-adjusted controls available on some measures	Maternal interview, medical evaluation and teacher report on the children; WISC or Leiter IQ on the children; also Bender-Gestalt and human figure drawings	Children ranged in awareness of the disease. Children asked first question about the disease between 3 and 15 years. 75% of parents felt they let the child have his/her own way often. 30% of school-age children were enuretic. Only 2 of 22 teachers who completed the questionnaire thought the child was overprotected; 8 teachers thought the child was embarrassed by symptoms (coughing). On Bender, CF patients showed perceptual–motor problems but did not differ from controls on emotional indicators. On HFD, CF patients equaled diabetics on number of emotional indicators, and showed more emotional indicators than children who were chosen for being well-adjusted.

Author	Sample	Method	Results
Tropauer et al, 1970[4]	N = 20 CF patients ages 5–20 years	Interview with mother; interview and house-tree-person drawings with the children	15 children understood illness. There was a general absence of overt depression. ⅓ of the children had expressed concern with dying. Young children were most concerned with interruption of play, diet, physical limitations. More concern with death among adolescents. Behavioral difficulties included: discipline problems, independence–dependence conflicts in adolescents; adolescents overly sensitive about the disease, and ashamed about having CF. The child's emotional adjustment related to communication and emotional support in family.
Lawler et al, 1965[5]	N = 11 CF patients ages 4–19 years	Psychiatric interviews with patient and parent; preschoolers given Stanford-Binet and CAT; school-age children given WISC, a reading test, Rorschach	Marked anxiety and preoccupation with death noted; depression noted in all patients; oral conflicts common. IQs were average or above. Common defenses were denial, excessive use of fantasy, hostility turned inward leading to depression, hostility toward others, repression, repressed aggression.
Spock and Stedman, 1967[6]	N = 34 CF patients ages 3–16 years	Interviews, draw-a-person, Peabody picture vocabulary test, Bender-Gestalt	Mean IQ = 104. Children appeared highly verbal in response to anxiety. Anxiety reflected in drawings and interviews.
Boyle et al, 1976[7]	N = 27 CF patients ages 13–30 years	Interviews, WISC or WAIS, drawings, TAT, Rorschach	Patients generally functioning well on a daily basis, but with high levels of depression and anxiety. Patients showed dissatisfaction with physical appearance, poor interpersonal relations, family conflicts including overdependence, and heightened awareness of the future.

Table 24-1 (continued)

Author	Sample	Method	Results
Cytryn et al, 1973 [8]	N = 29 CF patients 8 months to 9 years of age	Analysis of fantasy material, drawings, Rorschach, Bayley scales, Stanford-Binet	Patients showed concern about bodily integrity, but a majority were functioning well. 41% showed no disturbance; 17%, mild disturbance; 28%, moderate disturbance; 14%, severe disturbance. Among those with severe problems, small stature and poor family backgrounds were overrepresented. Defenses observed usually were adaptive. Defenses used in a healthy manner included reaction formation, striving for academic success, fantasy. Less healthy defenses included regression, withdrawal, avoidance (especially in preschool group).
Kulczycki et al, 1969 [9]	N = 26 CF patients all under 10 years of age	Psychiatric interview with children and parents; psychological evaluation with children	Mean IQ = 105 (test not specified). The accuracy of the child's conception of the disorder varied widely.

data and adequate descriptions of methods, the reader cannot really be confident that another set of interviewers might not have reached different conclusions (for example, the results of the Cytryn et al[8] study differ so much from those of other studies using similar assessment techniques). Similarly, the reliability of the rating systems used in analyzing the projective tests is not described in these studies; once again, this is highly problematic since the reliability of these measures is not established, and the validity of these techniques is often questioned.[15]

The descriptions of the CF patients in these studies are very rich and detailed, but without confidence in the methods being employed, the results of these studies must be accepted with serious reservations. It seems best for the clinician to consider these results as examples of how CF children may sometimes present and the kinds of concerns they may sometimes have, but not as representations of the personality traits and problems that typify CF patients. The researcher may find this material to be helpful for generating hypotheses about CF children and adolescents which require further testing.

CONTROL- AND COMPARISON-GROUP STUDIES

There are only a few studies of CF children using either control groups of normal, healthy children or comparison groups of other children with chronic illnesses or handicaps. These studies have tended to use measures of intelligence or personality which could be quantified and for which reliability and validity measures are available. Each of these studies is discussed separately and summarized in Table 24-2.

Four of the studies have examined one or two specific areas of the child's functioning (narrow-band studies), while several others have examined a broader range of personality variables or indices of psychopathology (broad-band studies).

Narrow-Band Studies

Ellis and Hill[16] compared the intellectual abilities of 7- to 10-year-old CF patients who had been malnourished during the first years of life versus CF patients who had not been malnourished during that time. The intelligence test administered was the Wechsler Intelligence Scale for Children (WISC). There were no differences between the malnourished and control groups on the full-scale IQ, verbal scale IQ, or performance scale IQ. Similar to the results of most of the single-group comparison studies, the mean IQs of these CF patients were in the average range of ability (the mean full-scale IQ for the control group was 104.1, and for the malnourished group, 99.3). Among the various subscales, a significant difference was found only among the backward digit span subtest. There were also no differences between the malnourished and control groups on a measure of academic achievement, the Wide-Range Achievement Test.

In two other studies, Goldberg and his colleagues examined the vocational adjustment of children with CF. One study[17] included 25 CF children and 25 healthy children from a public school. The children ranged in age from 12 to 18 years. The measure was a structured vocational interview for which measures of reliability and validity were available. Among the children ages 12–16 years, the CF patients showed lower levels of realism and less specificity in their plans for vocations. However, the CF patients were higher in the amount of commitment they displayed and the amount of information they had acquired about the vocation. At age 17, the CF patients were higher than the controls in all categories of vocational adjustment except realism. By age 18, the CF patients were lower than the healthy controls on realism, educational planning, work values, and initiative, but higher on vocational awareness. The only consistent deficit the CF patients displayed was in the area of realism, "the ability to plan while bearing in mind one's limitations as well as environmental constraints." Actually, for many of the CF patients, avoiding the reality of the physical condition may have been a coping device which enabled them to continue to develop their career plans, and it may not

Table 24-2
Control/Comparison Group Studies

Author	Subjects	Method/Measures	Results
Ellis and Hill, 1975[16]	N = 22 CF patients malnourished in 1st year of life; N = 16 CF patients not malnourished (= controls)	Administered WISC between 7 and 10 years of age; wide-range achievement test	No significant IQ differences except on backward digit span subtest. Full-scale IQs: malnourished *Ss* = 99.3; control *Ss* = 104.1. No differences on wide-range achievement test.
Goldberg et al, 1979[17]	N = 25 CF patients, N = 25 healthy patients; all ages 12–18 years	All administered a structured vocational interview	Between ages 12 and 16, the CF group was lower than the healthy group on specificity of plans and realism. CF patients scored higher on strength of commitment and awareness of career information. At 17, CF patients higher on all areas except realism. At 18, CF patients higher on vocational plans and awareness, but lower on educational plans, work values, realism, and initiative.
Goldberg and Johnson, 1978[18]	N = 170 normal, healthy children; N = 25 CF patients; N = 33 burn patients; N = 30 congenital heart disease patients; N = 225 delinquents; N = 193 physically handicapped patients; all ages 11–19 years (grades 6–12)	Structured vocational interview	For CF patients only: CF patients ranked ahead of all other patient groups on vocational development. CF patients performed comparably to the healthy children when age and grade were controlled.
Kucia et al, 1979[19]	N = 15 well-adjusted CF patients; N = 15 poorly adjusted CF patients	Two structured family interaction tasks	Among well-adjusted group: families were more creative; fathers were more creative and supportive than among the poorly adjusted group. Among poorly adjusted group: mothers were more creative; children had more success on the tasks and better communication; families had more success on the tasks. No significant differences between groups on family measures of support and communication.

Author	Subjects	Method/Measures	Results
Gayton et al, 1977[20]	N = 33 CF patients; N = 31 siblings; ages 5–18	Missouri children's picture series (MCPS); Holtzman inkblot; Piers-Harris self-concept scale	For children ages 5–13, no difference between groups on MCPS or self-concept measures. Only one of 22 differences on Holtzman significant. Data for older children not formally analyzed.
Tavormina et al, 1976[22]	N = 30 CF patients; N = 20 asthma patients; N = 78 diabetics; N = 16 hearing-impaired patients; ages 5–19 years	Missouri children's picture series (MCPS); Nowicki-Strickland locus of control scale; Piers-Harris self-concept scale; Junior Eysenck personality inventory; psychological screening inventory	CF children more immature and dependent than the standardization sample of the MCPS. CF patients do not differ from standardization samples on the measures of self-concept, neuroticism, locus of control, or MCPS measures of aggression, inhibition, sleep disturbances, somatization.
Kellerman et al, 1980[24]	N = 23 CF patients; N = 30 oncology patients; N = 30 cardiology patients; N = 30 diabetic patients; N = 25 nephrology patients; N = 30 rheumatology patients; N = 349 healthy children; adolescents	State-trait anxiety inventory; Rosenberg self-esteem scale; Wallston et al health locus of control scale	For CF patients, CF patients did not differ from other groups on measures of anxiety or self-esteem. CF patients higher on internal locus of control measure than other illness groups and comparable to the healthy controls on this measure.
Zeltzer et al, 1980[25]	Same as Kellerman et al	Illness impact questionnaire	CF adolescents reported that they thought about their disease while feeling healthy more than adolescents with other chronic illnesses. CF patients expressed more feelings of treatment-related problems than healthy adolescents.

have been a maladaptive trait at all. The results of the second study[18] were consistent with the first, with only the CF patients among five groups of handicapped adolescents approaching the level of vocational adjustment of healthy children.

In the fourth narrow-band study, Kucia et al[19] compared family interaction patterns among the families of 15 CF children who were nominated by their physicians as being well-adjusted and 15 CF children who were considered to be poorly adjusted. The CF children in the study ranged from 6 to 17 years old. On two family interaction measures, the families of the well-adjusted children appeared to be more creative when considered as a unit. The fathers in particular were more creative and supportive. Paradoxically, the mothers of the children who were poorly adjusted were more creative than the mothers of the well-adjusted CF children. Both the poorly adjusted children and their families had more successes on the tasks. The poorly adjusted children were higher on measures of effective communication than the well-adjusted children. The families of well- and poorly adjusted children did not differ on family measures of communication or positive support. The pattern of results is quite interesting because the poorly adjusted children and their families often did better than the well-adjusted children. The basis for these paradoxical findings is not clear.

In these four studies, the methodology is quite clear and the controls were adequate. In two of the studies,[16,19] CF children were compared to other CF children who differed on some important characteristic. This approach has two major advantages: (1) no other illness group can provide as complete a match for CF patients as other CF patients; and (2) the approach of comparing subgroups of CF patients is most likely to help us understand the variables which contribute to different degrees of adjustment among this patient group.

Broad-Band Studies

Gayton et al[20] conducted a study using objective personality measures (eg, paper-and-pencil tests) to assess the degree of emotional upset experienced by CF children. The study included 33 CF children and 31 of their siblings, with the latter serving as the comparison group. The ages of the children ranged between 5 and 18 years. In the data analysis, the children were divided into groups—younger children between ages 5 and 13 years and older children. All children between 5 and 13 were administered the Piers-Harris self-concept scale, the Missouri children's picture series, and the Holtzman inkblot scale. There were 23 patients and 26 siblings in this age group. The older children were given the Tennessee self-concept scale, the Rotter locus of control, Holtzman inkblot, and Minnesota multiphasic inventory (MMPI).

Among the younger children (ages 5–13 years), no differences were reported between the CF children and their siblings on either the self-concept scale (Piers-Harris) or the Missouri children's picture series. Only one difference emerged on the Holtzman inkblot test out of 22 comparisons, and this would be expected by chance. When individual comparisons were made with the norms on these tests, few children differed by even one standard deviation from the norms on any of the measures.

The results for the older children were not formally analyzed, but "subjective inspection" suggested no differences between CF patients and either the siblings or the normative data. However, there were only 10 older CF patients and 5 siblings in this part of the study.

Two methodological problems emerge in this design. First, it is questionable whether siblings constitute an adequate control group because these siblings offer increased emotional problems of their own. For example, in one study,[21] the siblings of chronically ill children displayed more signs of social withdrawal and irritability than healthy controls at all ages; among the younger age group (3–6 years old), the siblings of chronically ill children displayed more symptoms of emotional problems overall than did the healthy controls. Second, there are certain criteria which must be met before the data collected from the study sample and from the standardization sample can be compared, and these criteria were not met. The same problem arises in the study by Tavormina et al[22] and will be discussed below.

In the study be Tavormina et al[22] children ages 5–19 years with CF (N = 30), asthma (N = 20), diabetes (N = 78), and hearing impairments (N = 16) were examined. These children were administered the Piers-Harris self-concept scale, the Eysenck personality scale for children, the Nowicki-Strickland locus of control scale, and the Missouri children's picture series (MCPS). The CF children did not differ from the normative sample on the Piers-Harris, Eysenck, or locus of control measures. On the MCPS the CF children were less mature, less conforming, and more dependent than the normative sample. Dependency was inferred from the tendency of the CF patients to score in the feminine direction on a measure of masculinity–femininity. On the psychological screening inventory, no differences between the normative sample and CF adolescents emerged.

The validity of the Gayton et al[20] and the Tavormina et al[22] studies depends upon the appropriateness of comparing data collected from a specific sample of CF patients with the standardization data from each of the various personality measures. This approach can only be valid if the samples of CF patients do not differ from the standardization sample on relevant characteristics such as age of the children, racial and sex composition, and socioeconomic status. Neither study demonstrated the comparability of the CF sample and the standardization sample on such variables. In the Gayton et al[20] paper, the demographic characteristics of the sample were not adequately described, and it is impossible to determine if the CF sample is comparable to the standardization sample.

In the Tavormina et al[22] study, the sample is well described but not necessarily comparable to the standardization samples of each of the personality measures used. For example, the manual for the Missouri children's picture series[23] does not indicate the social class of the children in the standardization sample or whether the children came from urban or rural schools. Obviously, without such information, it cannot be determined whether the CF patients were comparable to the standardization group. Also, 50% of the standardization sample were girls; in the Tavormina et al[22] study, 63% were girls. This sex difference is important in two regards. First, five of the nine MCPS scales were developed using only male subjects, and the validity of these scales for girls is questionable. Second, the authors concluded that CF patients were more dependent than healthy children because the CF patients tended to score in the feminine direction on the MCPS masculinity–femininity scale. Because a femininity scale was used as a measure of dependency, the overrepresentation of girls in the CF sample may have biased the results in the direction of increased dependency. Most of the methodological problems in both of these studies could have been circumvented by the inclusion of a matched control group.

A somewhat better controlled series of studies has been presented by Kellerman et al[24] and Zeltzer et al.[25] Their studies included 349 healthy adolescents and 168 adolescents with various illnesses. Oncology, cardiology, diabetic, nephrology, rheumatology, and CF patients were included. There were 23 CF patients. The groups were matched on sex, previous illnesses other than the primary diagnosis, and number of siblings. There were group differences in race, with CF patients having the highest proportion of white patients. The differences in socioeconomic status (SES) paralleled the race differences, with white patients enjoying higher SES levels. To control for race and SES effects, the data were reanalyzed without including the black patients. The authors report that the results were essentially the same in both instances. The studies included measures of anxiety, self-esteem, and a measure of health locus of control (ie, the individual's feelings of control over his or her own health). A high internal locus of control reflects the individual's belief that he or she has a high degree of control over his or her health. An external locus of control reflects a belief in extraneous factors controlling one's health.

For the anxiety and self esteem measures, there were no differences between the groups. On the measure of locus of control, the CF group did not differ from healthy children or diabetics in their belief about having control over their health, whereas other illness groups tended to have a more externalized sense of control over their health. The authors suggest that this may be due to the fact that the CF patient exercises "some degree of control over his illness and symptoms." CF patients also reported that they thought about their illness more often while feeling healthy than did patients with other diseases.

Summary of Control and Comparison Studies

With the exception of the Kucia et al [19] and Ellis and Hill [16] studies, the other studies using comparison groups have all attempted to determine whether CF patients differ from normal, healthy children on various personality or psychopathology measures. While most of the single-group comparison studies suggest that the CF children do differ from healthy children in significant ways, the comparison group studies suggest that the CF patients are essentially the same as healthy children. Collectively, the latter studies indicate no differences between CF patients and healthy children on measures of self-esteem and self-concept, locus of control, anxiety, aggression, inhibition, sleep disturbances, neuroticism, and most areas of adolescent vocational adjustment. They do suggest higher levels of immaturity, dependence, and worry (about their disease), and less realism about career planning.

Just as the methodological problems demand that the reader be circumspect in interpreting the results of the single-group studies, so do these limitations force the reader to be cautious in accepting the many findings of no differences in the controlled studies. Serious methodological shortcomings are present in the studies by Gayton et al [20] and Tavormina et al.[22] The data in the Kucia et al [19] study seem contradictory and nonintuitive, and there is no acceptable rationale to explain how poorly adjusted children score better than well-adjusted children in many areas. If one only considers the few other reasonably well-controlled studies we have located—those by Kellerman et al,[24] Ellis and Hill,[16] Zeltzer et al,[25] and Goldberg et al [17,18]—then the number of confirmed findings about the personality and adjustment of CF patients is extremely small: they do not differ from healthy children and adolescents on intelligence, anxiety, self-esteem, and most areas of vocational adjustment, but they do worry more about their disease than children with other types of illness. Their sense of control over their health is more internalized than among children with other illnesses, and they seem to be like healthy children in this regard. Obviously, the range of questions about the functioning of the CF children and adolescents which remain to be explored using solid research methods is considerable.

RESEARCH NEEDS

As this review shows, we have very little reliable information about the psychological functioning of CF children. At the same time, the single-group studies provide many interesting ideas about the thoughts, fears, conflicts, and concerns of the CF children and adolescents. These studies serve as sources of hypotheses about the personalities of CF children that deserve closer examination in studies using better methodology. The research needs are many. There is a strong need for reliable observations of CF children's behavior, social skills, worries, and adjustment problems. It is important to determine the frequencies of the problems which occur in these areas, and also which characteristics and behavior patterns distinguish the CF children from healthy children at different ages. For example, it would be useful to know how frequently independence–

dependence problems and noncompliance occur among CF children at various ages; whether CF children exhibit more behavior problems in school than healthy children; how many CF children express concern about death at various ages; and how strong are the school-age and adolescent CF patients' concerns about their physical appearance. There is also very little information about the personality and adjustment of young adults with CF.

Questions about the behaviors that characterize CF children should be just a starting point, however. Research must also address how the various characteristics of the patient and the family are interrelated within the CF population. For example, are CF children with short stature or delayed sexual development more depressed or anxious than other CF children? Is open communication about CF related to good adjustment? Do children who feel different from their peers cease taking their medication or balk at other forms of therapy? Is parental overprotection (or other parental behavior) related to vocational adjustment among the CF patients? What temperamental traits influence the adjustment of CF patients? Answering such questions often will require comparisons among subgroups of CF patients who differ on certain characteristics (eg, concern about physique) to determine whether the traits are related to other psychologically relevant traits.

Finally, while there are a few studies describing treatment procedures using psychotherapy and support groups with CF patients,[26,29] they are purely descriptive reports. Studies examining intervention strategies for psychosocial support would be very helpful, although clearly very difficult to do.

REFERENCES

1. Drotar D: Adaptational problems of children and adolescent with cystic fibrosis. *J Pediatr Psychol* 1978;3(1):45–50.
2. McCollum AT, Gibson LE: Family adaptation of the child with cystic fibrosis. *J Pediatr* 1970;77:571–578.
3. Falkman C: Cystic fibrosis—a psychological study of 52 children and their families. *Acta Paediatr Scand Suppl* 1977;269:1-93.
4. Tropauer A, Franz MN, Dilgard VW: Psychological aspects of the care of children with cystic fibrosis. *Am J Dis Child* 1970;119:424–432.
5. Lawler RH, Nakielny W, Wright NA: Psychological implications of cystic fibrosis. *Can Med Assoc J* 1966;94:1043–1046.
6. Spock AM, Stedman DJ: Psychologic characteristics of children with cystic fibrosis. *NC Med J* 1966;27:426.
7. Boyle IR, di Sant'Agnese PA, Sack S, et al: Emotional adjustment of adolescents and young adults with cystic fibrosis. *J Pediatr* 1976;88:318–362.
8. Cytryn L, Moore P, Robinson ME: Psychological adjustment of children with cystic fibrosis, in Anthony EJ, Koupernik C (eds): *The Child in His Family, Vol. 2. The Impact of Disease and Death.* New York, John Wiley & Sons, 1973, pp 37–47.
9. Kulczycki LL, Robinson ME, Berg CM: Somatic and psychological factors relative to management of patients with cystic fibrosis. *Clin Proc Child Hosp DC* 1969;25:320.
10. Rosenstein BJ: Cystic fibrosis of the pancreas: Impact on family functioning, in Debuskey M, Dombro RH (eds): *The Chronically Ill Child and His Family.* Springfield, Illinois, Charles C Thomas, 1970, pp 23–32.
11. Lewiston NJ: Saturday's children: Adolescents and adults with cystic fibrosis in today's society. In *Proceedings of the 8th International Conference on Cystic Fibrosis.* Toronto, Canadian Cystic Fibrosis Foundation, 1980, pp 266–274.
12. Bronheim SP: Pulmonary disorders: Asthma and cystic fibrosis, in Magrab PR (ed): *Psychological Management of Pediatric Problems, Vol I.* Baltimore, University Park Press, 1978, pp 309–344.
13. Gayton WF, Friedman SB: Psychosocial aspects of cystic fibrosis. *Am J Dis Child* 1973;126:856–859.
14. Patterson PR: Psychosocial aspects of cystic fibrosis, in Patterson P, Denning C, Kutscher A (eds): *Psychosocial Aspects of Cystic Fibrosis.* New York, Columbia University Press, 1973, pp 3–12.
15. Anastasi A: *Psychological Testing.* New York, Macmillan, 1968.
16. Ellis CE, Hill E: Growth, intelligence, and school performance in children with cystic fibrosis who have had an episode of malnutrition during infancy. *J Pediatr* 1975;87:565–568.
17. Goldberg RT, Isralsky M, Shwachman H: Vocational development and adjustment of

adolescents with cystic fibrosis. *Arch Phys Med Rehabil* 1979;60:369–374.

18. Goldberg RT, Johnson BD: A comparative study of five groups of handicapped children in vocational rehabilitation. *Scand J Rehabil Med* 1978;10:215–220.
19. Kucia C, Drotar D, Doershuk CF, et al: Home observation of family interaction and childhood adjustment to cystic fibrosis. *J Pediatr Psychol* 1979;4:189–196.
20. Gayton WF, Freedman SB, Tavormina JF, et al: Children with cystic fibrosis: I. Psychological test findings of patients, siblings, and parents. *Pediatrics* 1977;59:888–894.
21. Lavigne JV, Ryan M: Psychologic adjustment of siblings of children with chronic illness. *Pediatrics* 1979;63:616–627.
22. Tavormina JB, Kastner LS, Slater PM, et al: Chronically ill children: A psychologically and emotionally deviant population? *J Abnorm Child Psychol* 1976;4(2):99–110.
23. Sines JO, Pauker JD, Sines LK: *Missouri Children's Picture Series Manual.* Iowa City, Psychological Assessment and Services, Inc., 1974.
24. Kellerman J, Zeltzer L, Ellenberg L, et al: Psychological effects of illness in adolescence. I. Anxiety, self-esteem, and perception of control. *J Pediatr* 1980;97:126–131.
25. Zeltzer L, Kellerman J, Ellenberg L, et al: Psychologic effects of illness in adolescence. II. Impact of illness in adolescents—crucial issues and coping styles. *J Pediatr* 1980;97:132–138.
26. Winder A, Medalie M: Support for growth in cystic fibrosis teenagers, in Patterson P, Denning C, Kutscher A (eds): *Psychosocial Aspects of Cystic Fibrosis.* New York, Columbia University Press, 1973, pp 103–112.
27. Strauss GD, Pedersen S, Dudovitz D: Psychosocial support for adults with cystic fibrosis. *Am J Dis Child* 1979;133:301–305.

25

The Patient, the Family, and the Community

Dorothy M. Lloyd-Still

John D. Lloyd-Still

The diagnosis of cystic fibrosis presents numerous problems which test the coping abilities of the afflicted child, the parents, the siblings, and the extended family. Furthermore, the disease places demands upon the community and the human service system.

Lavigne (see Chapter 24) discussed the lack of controlled studies about the psychological implications of CF for the individual patient. The literature is similarly limited in discussing the implications for family and community systems. Indeed, work in this area seems to be largely based upon clinical impressions. In reviewing this literature, we have excluded most articles that present no data.

A patient with CF and the family face a continual series of crises starting at diagnosis, and continuing through the crises associated with normal developmental stages, to physical deterioration and finally death. Apart from these well-documented crises, an increasingly critical problem is presented by the burgeoning population of adults with cystic fibrosis. Adults now comprise over 20% of the total population registered with the CF data registry.[1] As patients with CF reach adulthood with varying stages of physical impairment, we find a group of individuals who have outlived our present level of expertise. Most CF centers do not have provisions for meeting the special needs of adult patients, and many pediatric-oriented practitioners have difficulty relating to these needs (see Chapter 20).

Certain clinics describe a high percentage of families with problems in functioning,[2-4] while other clinic populations appear to have more effective coping mechanisms.[5,6] Effective coping may be related to superior patient management or may be a function of other intervening variables. Variables relating to the nature of the clinic may include the size of the clinic population, percentage of multiproblem families, the philosophy of the center director, community resources, and the availability of support systems such as involvement with chapter activities. Patient characteristic variables may include age, number of siblings (especially if others have CF), socioeconomic status, religion, ethnic background, availability of care-givers, and family stability.

DIAGNOSIS

In a classic study of family adaptation to CF, McCollum and Gibson[7] present data obtained from 56 families with 65 living children with cystic fibrosis. Their methodology included a multiple-choice questionnaire by which all quantified data were obtained, social work interviews, and monthly group meetings with a physician and a social worker. They described a "prediagnostic" stage which spans the time between arousal of concern about the child's health and the establishment of a correct diagnosis; the mean duration of this phase was 17.5 months. Parents characteristically sought medical advice on repeated occasions because continuation of the symptoms led to mistrust and hostility toward physicians.

The nature of the developing parent-child relationship was of concern, as the infants demonstrated feeding disturbances (84%), fussiness, and difficulty in being comforted. As a result, mothers experienced self-doubt and self-reproach, often coupled with despair and hostility toward the infant. This hostility, often reinforced by other unpleasant symptoms (eg, foul-smelling stools, cough), can intensify parental guilt during the following stage.

The "confrontational stage," as described by McCollum et al,[7] is reached with the confirmation of the diagnosis of cystic fibrosis. The threat of a potentially fatal illness produces an acute, anticipatory mourning reaction, as the central issue facing the parents is the possible loss of their child. Other issues often presented are concern about further reproduction, possible disease in other family members, the adequacy of the patient's physical environment, the adequacy of financial resources, and the therapeutic techniques to be mastered. All of these tangential issues, critical in themselves, can become the focus of parental concerns instead of the potentially fatal illness itself.

Defenses initially demonstrated include denial, isolation, avoidance, and repression. Affective responses are manifested in the form of sleep and appetite disturbances, intense grief, guilt, and anger. Anxiety at this stage is related to feelings of helplessness, intensity of affective responses, and awareness of the parents' own mortality.

McCollum and Gibson's[7] findings are supported by Burton's[4] survey of 53 CF families in Northern Ireland. Data were obtained by the use of structured interview schedules administered during an average of four home visits for an average total interview time of 20 hours per family. Burton[4] describes the normal parental need to care for and to protect one's children. As the diagnosis of CF threatens the fulfillment of this need, the internal integrity of the parents is challenged. Initial shock gives way to defense mechanisms, including denial. Burton[4] found that with an average postdiagnosis time of 4½ years, 26% of mothers and 39% of fathers doubted the implications of their child's disease and questioned the competence of the physicians. When defenses fail, despair, lack of self-esteem, and self-criticism are manifested. Burton[4] found that the longer the prediagnostic phase and the older the child, the more likely are the parents to experience severe shock at diagnosis. Following diagnosis, classic symptoms of grief were noted, with depression reported by 44% of mothers and 33% of fathers, accompanied by nervousness and sleep and appetite disorders.

The pattern of professional contact during the diagnostic period is described by Blumenthal,[8] who conducted a mental health survey which compared the parents of CF children with the parents of mentally retarded children. The families of 69 CF children were studied with the use of a structured interview schedule. Blumenthal's[8] data do not support the myth of parents "shopping" for a diagnosis. During diagnosis, the CF families had an average of 4.74 professional contacts per person. Examples of the average contact per case by type of physician were: pediatrician 2.6, general practitioner 1.02, internist 0.21, and surgeon 0.15. In discussing the importance of the physician-family relationship in the management of the diagnostic phase, Blumenthal[8] describes the physician characteristics that parents perceived as important and helpful: level of supportiveness and interest, ability of physician in enabling parents to ventilate feelings, and ability in bringing parents to the point of understanding the implications of the disease. Parents at this stage were more concerned about receiving treatment for their child than they were about receiving information.

Coolidge[9] outlined some suggestions for physicians when telling parents about a diagnosis of CF: choose a comfortable, private room; choose words that are easily comprehended; when the tears come and anger and intense feelings come—stay. Dare to "feel and care with the family," to answer questions, to eventually introduce the family to appropriate team members.

Our own experience with the diagnosis of CF is generally consistent with the reported observations. Ten to 15% of patients with CF present with meconium ileus in the newborn period. According to the CF data registry, the majority (75%) of patients with CF are now diagnosed under 3 years of age. In our center, over 600 sweat tests are performed annually and 15–20 new patients with cystic fibrosis are diagnosed. When there is a positive family history, parents are usually familiar with the diagnosis. Other families may never have heard of the disease and, under these circumstances, reaction to diagnosis is likely to be more prolonged. Shock upon hearing the diagnosis may be followed by disbelief and anger at themselves for the genetic implications and at the physicians for delay in making the diagnosis. During the diagnostic phase, the parents behavior may be characterized by anxiety and depression until they have been able to resume some equilibrium in their lives. Parents vary in their reactions to bad news, and the physician and associates must allow time for parents to begin to learn about the disease and the therapeutic program. Moreover, the status of the patient may vary from a severely ill postsurgical neonate whose survival may be in doubt to a normal, healthy-appearing toddler whose only symptom is a rectal prolapse.

Certain principles apply to the interview, which in our clinic is usually held with physician, social worker, and parents together. First, it should take place in comfort and privacy so that the parents may be able to show their emotions without feeling constrained. Second, the interview must be unhurried, and time should be available to pursue discussion in depth if the parents so desire. Third, arrangements must be made for ongoing education, depending on the family's readiness. Many families are unable to comprehend detailed explanations about CF at the initial interview. During this interview, the parents may be given appropriate selections from the excellent pamphlets published by the CF Foundation, including "The Genetics of Cystic Fibrosis," "Your Child and Cystic Fibrosis," "A Teacher's Guide to Cystic Fibrosis," and "Living With Cystic Fibrosis, A Guide for the Young Adult." Some parents request information regarding research. It may be appropriate to inform them about the CF Foundation and the address of their local chapter.

At the next interview the parents can be introduced to other team members such as the nurse and nutritionist. Respiratory therapists will begin educating the parents in therapy, and arrangements are made for registering with the state crippled children's program. Most families are anxious to meet with other parents and see other children with cystic fibrosis. Parents can be introduced to the CF clinic during the initial inpatient admission and will then feel more familiar with the physical facilities and the personnel of the clinic.

There are considerable advantages to an initial hospital admission for all newly diagnosed patients with CF, with the possible exception of siblings of already diagnosed patients. We have found that when this practice is followed, the families have had more support in coping with the diagnostic phase, perhaps related to the greater time available to educate them in the therapeutic program. Moreover, it is considerably more difficult to conduct prolonged, undisturbed interviews in the setting of a busy CF clinic than during hospitalization. In our experience, families whose children were never hospitalized at initial diagnosis find it more difficult to accept the proffered professional support and react more frequently by isolating themselves or by seeking other consultations.

An important aspect of the diagnostic phase is the gathering of baseline data about family functioning, and the laying of critical groundwork for professional support and intervention. In a prospective study of 40 families of leukemia patients using data from social work interviews, Kaplan et al[10] found that early coping responses are predictive of stress outcomes. Statistically significant differences in the number of child, marital, and grief problems were found between adaptive and maladaptive families. Criteria for adaptive responses are: ability to comprehend the nature of the disease, ability of the parents to communicate the seriousness of the illness to all members of the immediate family, and the ability of the parents to respond to the diagnosis with appropriate feelings of grief and sadness without inhibiting expression of these feelings in themselves or others. Failure to meet each of these criteria is classified as maladaptive. Kaplan et al[10] believe that the optimal point for intervention with maladaptive families occurs during the early, acute stage of crisis, immediately following confirmation of the diagnosis. This is a time when families are making those decisions which are associated with maladaptive coping and poor stress outcomes.

THE SCHOOL-AGE CHILD

As the child enters school, the problem of integrating into and adapting to an environment designed for "normal" children is faced. McCollum and Gibson[7] reported that 44% of the children in their study had adjustment problems in the first year of school. These problems included inattentiveness, daydreaming, restlessness, and disturbing classroom behavior. Although no control figures for adjustment problems were given, these figures would be well above the national average and much higher than other studies on the social functioning of chronically ill children.[11]

The developmental task for children between the ages of 4 and 7 years is the lessening of parental attachments and the development of a capacity for independent functioning outside of the home, a task complicated by the physical manifestations of cystic fibrosis. Of the study parents, 47% acknowledged that they had permitted their child less independence than a healthy child. Only one study child had a significant school avoidance problem. In another study [12] comparing patients with CF aged between 5 and 13 years with siblings, the results did not support previous estimates of an increased incidence of emotional disturbance in children with cystic fibrosis.

Between the ages of 8 and 12 years, children develop a heightened awareness of and sensitivity to differences from their peers. Children with cystic fibrosis at this age begin to demonstrate shame about the perceptible manifestations of the disease and an emerging awareness of their prognosis. Embarrassment is felt relative to flatulence and stool odor, the need to take medications, dietary limitations, spasms of coughing, the presence of a mist tent, and reduced physical stamina. McCollum and Gibson[7] found that 72% of the school-age children in their study raised questions to their parents about the disease, the treatment, or the prognosis. Yet one third of the study parents had avoided giving any information to the child about the illness, and parents of 28% of the study children reported that their children had not asked questions.

Burton[4] reported that of the 30 study children attending school, 26% had initial adjustment problems, and only 20% were reported by their parents to have subsequently experienced problems in going to school. She speculated that this relatively positive response to school may have been explained by two factors. School attendance may reassure the children about their normality, and the children may respond positively to being in a freer environment than they experienced at home. Overall IQ testing of the study children showed normal intellectual development with the Weschler intelligence test having a mean of 104 and a range of 72–137; 50% of the girls and 37% of the boys scored significantly better on the vocabulary subtest than on any other IQ scale item. However, when attainment tests (Schonell reading test, Schonell spelling test, Vernon arithmetic–mathematics test) were performed, all but one of the CF children were retarded in one subject. Fifty-five percent of the study boys and 66% of the study girls were tested as below normal in two or more basic subjects.

Burton[4] speculated that in spite of good behavioral adjustment in school, children with cystic fibrosis have anxiety about their social acceptability and essential security and therefore are not able to pay attention to classroom work. Also, 25% of the 97 parents interviewed acknowledged having lower expectations for school achievement because of the illness. There were indications as well that some teachers reduced their standards for the study children. When compared with a control group, children with CF were found by their classroom teachers to be more unsettled, particularly in the realm of passivity. Other studies of IQ by the Weschler scale in CF do not confirm these findings, and the results were in the normal range for verbal and performance standards.[2,5,13,14]

In Sweden, where a registry of all patients with cystic fibrosis is maintained, surveys of all the registry families were conducted in 1970 and 1978. Kollberg[15] reported that although most patients with CF were absent from school more than their classmates, the proportion may be decreasing. In 1970, 66% of children with CF were absent more frequently than their classmates, and in 1978, 55% of children with CF were absent more frequently. In the 1978 survey, 14% of parents reported that their children had problems with their school work, and 24% of patients had received extra tutoring. Of the patients with CF surveyed, 88% had continued their studies to the high school level. No details of attainment or performance were given.

Drotar[6] used a study design whereby four groups were compared. The groups were composed of (1) 91 cystic fibrosis patients, (2) 47 patients with other chronic diseases, (3) 71 physically healthy cystic fibrosis siblings, and (4) 61 physically healthy children. Questionnaires were administered to the parents of all the study children; the children were between the ages of 3 and 13 years. The study showed that children with CF achieved an age-adequate level of adjustment at home and school. The level of adjustment was largely unrelated to the severity of the cystic fibrosis. The authors concluded that the adjustment of children as rated by parents and teachers is not consistently different from that of comparison groups.

These widely differing results could be explained by the different therapeutic modalities practiced in these dissimilar environments. The reassuring results achieved in Cleveland,[6] Rochester, and Baltimore[12] may be related to a more sophisticated approach to the therapy of the disease. These high standards are probably not attained in most other CF centers, where the results from the Burton[4] study could more accurately reflect the status of these children.

In an effort to avert some of these problems that can arise on entry into school, most CF center personnel have used an educational approach. Before the start of school, the family is given a pamphlet published by the CF foundation ("A Teacher's Guide to Cystic Fibrosis") to give to the school staff. This pamphlet explains the disease, the need for and details of medication, and the problems related to coughing and malabsorption. If parents report school problems developing, the nurse or social worker usually contacts either the school nurse or teacher and in most cases the problem is resolved. Rarely is it necessary to pursue further detailed psychological evaluation. In those rare circumstances where resistance is encountered, the clinic staff must work with the parents to enable them to act as advocates on behalf of their child. When children are severely incapacitated, a home tutor may be more appropriate. In general, emphasis should be placed on supporting the parents and child to integrate into the school environment, with the least possible restrictions.

THE ADOLESCENT AND ADULT PATIENT

Most cystic fibrosis clinics now care for adolescent and adult patients. McCollum and Gibson[7] reported that adolescence for their study patients was marked by several characteristics. They reported that the retardation of growth and sexual development intensified the patient's deviance and isolation from peers. Age-appropriate strivings for independence were thwarted by realistic dependence upon adults for physical care. There was a marked variation in the capacity of parents to support their adolescents in seeking gratification through independent social, intellectual, and physical activities. The study found that compliance with the full therapeutic regimen was typically not sustained throughout adolescence. Parents acquiesced to the patient's protests against therapy, manifesting underlying feelings of hopelessness about the prognosis.

Tropauer et al[3] studied 20 children (ages 5–20 years) with cystic fibrosis and 23 mothers, using psychiatric interviews and psychological testing. The authors concluded that the relative invalidism and necessity for daily care prolonged the dependent relationship between the patient and parents. The vicissitudes of the illness interfered with the peer relationships that are important in helping the adolescent gain independence. Hopes and plans for school and career may thus be thwarted by the disease.

Boyle et al[14] studied 27 patients with CF aged 13–30 years. Data were obtained from psychiatric interviews and psychological testing. Although two thirds of the patients studied functioned adequately, they often demonstrated impaired emotional adjustment. The authors identified four main sources of stress, similar to the findings of McCollum and Gibson.[7]

Altered physical appearance was significant, as patients were acutely aware of looking different from others of their age groups. Interpersonal relations were strained; patients had a sense of isolation and few friends. Of the seven married patients included in this study, the authors characterized only one as stable. Conflicts in upbringing were demonstrated as few parents were able to discuss CF and its implications with the patient. The young adults studied were often overprotected and infantilized by their mothers, while the fathers were typically withdrawn and unavailable. As patients with CF grow older, they demonstrate an increased awareness of the future. The adolescents studied were anxious about their disease and unable to tolerate discussion about the future. The young adults studied either avoided thoughts about the future or looked back rather than ahead. Although all patients used the mechanisms of denial and avoidance, these defenses break down at times, particularly as decreasing physical capacity is noted.

The authors make some suggestions for professionals. Fathers should be supported in being more involved with their children, while mothers should be supported in allowing their children to be more independent and responsible. Both parents and patients should be enabled to communicate about cystic fibrosis. Patients should be encouraged to continue at school or work. Specific issues such as sterility, pregnancy, genetic counseling, and adoption need to be discussed and explained.

Warwick and Pogue[1] warned that cystic fibrosis will present a major challenge for internists in the next decade. These patients present a variety of issues traditionally unfamiliar to CF professionals—eg, employment, vocational rehabilitation, insurance coverage, psychosexual functioning, independent living, and marriage. The social worker can play a major role in enabling patients to utilize available resources. The young adult consumer services committee of the CF Foundation is addressing many of these issues and acts as an advocate for adolescent and adult patients. The CF Foundation has published a position paper recognizing the role of the internist in the care of these patients and encouraging the participation of internists in the establishment of adult CF clinics.

The task force on adult care of the CF Foundation conducted an adult-care consumer survey in 1981.[16] A sample of 450 adults with CF was randomly selected from a nationwide mailing list of 650 adults. Completed questionnaires were received from 55% of the sample. The age range of the respondents was from 16–43 years (mean 25 years). In response to questions about outpatient CF care, 98.1% reported receiving care within the same facility as children, and 89.8% reported receiving care at the same time as the children. Only 7.6% reported that they attend a special adult clinic, but 94.1% indicated that they would attend a CF adult-care center if it were available. Access to a social worker familiar with CF was reported by 67.3% of the respondents; the importance of this access was ranked very important by 17.3%, important by 33.5%, and unimportant by 35.9%. Psychological counseling was ranked very important by 23.8%, important by 27.6%, and unimportant by 37.1%. Genetic counseling was ranked very important by 28.1%, important by 34.3%, and unimportant by 27.6%. Vocational counseling was seen as very important by 28.6%, important by 29.1%, and unimportant by 32.9%. In response to a question about whether the CF clinic staff had explained the reproductive complications of CF, 69% of the respondents replied yes and 29.4% no.

Studies on sexual functioning in adult patients with CF are limited. Levine and Stern[17] used a structured interview and questionnaire to investigate the sexual functioning of 30 married patients with cystic fibrosis. The study patients included 19 females with an average duration of marriage of 3.25 years and 11 males with an average duration of marriage of 5 years. Nine of the 30 patients had serious sexual problems manifested as decreased desire. No control figures were quoted. The authors concluded that although severe cystic fibrosis makes serious sexual problems due to physical illness more likely, their study results indicate that physicians can assure adult patients with CF that they have a reasonable chance for normal sexual functioning.

Decisions about career choices are as critical for adults with CF as they are for the general population, and these decisions are made more complex by the necessity to reconcile the patient's goals with realistic career choices. Ideally, appropriate vocational counseling should be built into the entire secondary educational experience. Each state operates a vocational rehabilitation agency whose major purpose is to assist disabled clients towards pursuit of gainful occupations. A CF center caring for adolescent and adult patients should establish an effective liaison with the appropriate state agency.[18,19] Wide variations exist among states in terms of actual services provided, but should include evaluation, medical expenses, job training, and college tuition.

The young adult services committee of the Cystic Fibrosis Foundation conducted a nationwide survey on vocational and life adjustment problems of young adults with cystic fibrosis.[20] The study was conducted in two stages. The pilot study surveyed patients 13 years of age and older in CF centers in three geographic areas. In a second phase, patients 15 years and older were surveyed in five additional geographic areas. The methodology included written questionnaires completed by patients, parents, and physicians. A sample of 62 young adults were personally interviewed.

The study revealed that one of the most consistent and critical problems was the lack of financial assistance for medical care for people over 21 who were only partially disabled or not currently disabled. The majority of patients studied were still in school. One third were employed. School records showed that 80% were in age-appropriate regular classes, 6% were in special classes, and 5% had dropped out of high school. Subsequent to this study intensive lobbying efforts were conducted in many states by CF parents, center directors and staff, and consumers, with the result that at present over 20 states now have programs for patients over 21 years of age. Information about specific programs are available from the Cystic Fibrosis Foundation.

FAMILY IMPACT

Attempts to document the extent to which a child with CF impacts negatively on family functioning have produced a range of results. Meyerwitz and Kaplan[21] interviewed 111 families with CF children using a structured interview schedule. The interview included items relating to social history, current familial status and functioning, and reactions to the disease. A chi-square analysis was used to test the significance ($P < 0.05$) of the relationship between any two variables. The authors concluded that the results indicated "universal and severe" emotional reactions to the occurrence of CF. An inability to accept the child's condition was reported in 11% of the families, feelings of immobilization were reported in 10%, anxiety in 8%, and thinly veiled hostility in 17%.

That cystic fibrosis causes maladjustment in patterns of interaction and role definitions is indicated by the fact that 54% of the mothers had been employed prior to the diagnosis, and only 26% were so employed following diagnosis. Furthermore, one third of the fathers had been forced to accept a reduction in occupational status or were unable to accept a transfer, promotion, or other special opportunity. As family role patterns shift, the readjustment process dilutes the family's capacity to meet the emotional needs of its members.

A dilution is also seen in the family's relationship with the community. Negative attitudes were attributed to relatives by 37% of the families; negative attitudes were attributed to the broader community by 41%; negative attitudes were attributed to one or both by 54%. The social structure was viewed as positive and accepting by only 46% of the families. Not only is the level of support available from the community to help with the crises a factor, but the community may itself create stress by the nature of its responses.

The authors identified variables that were significant in explaining differential responses to the disease. Analysis of variables related to patient role and attitudes indicate that stress reactions are more likely to be manifested (1) when the child is active in seeking information about his/her prognosis, (2) when the child engages in activities outside of the home that are perceived to be potentially harmful, (3) when the child is younger, (4) when the diagnosis has been delayed, and (5) when there are two or more children with CF in the family.

Variables related to parental roles and attitudes that cause differential responses include the way in which difficulties are perceived, the nature of parental attempts at adjustment, and the affective responses to these adjustments. Variables relative to parental attributes and roles prior to diagnosis include the age of the parents and whether or not the mother was employed.

Analysis of variables relative to the family structure indicates that stress reactions are more likely when parents display anxiety about the effects of the disease attributes upon the well children. Denial, avoidance, and overemphasis on the negative ramifications of CF are more likely to be manifested when there is only one CF child in the family and when the family has previously lost a child to CF. The only extrafamilial variable identified as significant indicates that families with no religious affiliation are more likely to demonstrate psychophysiological manifestations of stress.

Turk[22] used a questionnaire with both forced-choice and open-ended questions in a study of 25 families with CF children. The results indicated that parents felt deprived of time and energy to engage in leisure-time activities, time to be alone with a spouse, time and energy to engage in adult activities, and time for self. Finances were a source of conflict between parents. Families experienced a breakdown in their ability to communicate between parents and children about important family issues.

Twenty children with CF and 23 mothers were studied by Tropauer et al.[3] Psychiatric interviews were conducted with all subjects, and a modified house–tree–person technique was used with the children. Only three mothers were found to be clinically depressed, although eight others had frequent periods of dejection and discouragement. Most mothers, however, retained the ability to continue functioning in a supportive role for the child, despite significant emotional conflicts and personal suffering. Open communication and mutual support were found to be significant factors in the extent to which the child's illness had a disruptive impact on the family unit.

In reviewing the registry of all CF families in Sweden, Kollberg[15] reported that 90% of the families were intact, demonstrating no tendency towards increased divorce. One fourth of the families had made a geographical move since the diagnosis, either to housing more appropriate for the management of CF or to be closer to services. "Many" of the mothers were unemployed, had cut down to part-time, or had changed jobs, almost all due to the need to treat the CF child.

Burton's study[4] included questions about the behavior and attitudes of well siblings. Fifty of the 58 CF children had well siblings living at home; there was a total of 112 with brothers and sisters. All but 23% of the study families reported "change" in the attitude of the well children toward the sick child. Positive, protective responses were reported from about half of the older siblings. Younger siblings, however, were more likely to demonstrate jealousy and other negative reactions. The well children were described as "left out" or "resentful" by 39% of the mothers and 26% of the fathers. Parents of 43% of the older children reported that their children felt responsible for the CF child's well being. Problem behavior on the part of the well sibling was described by 37% of the mothers and 28% of the fathers. The problems reported ranged from "rebelliousness" to nightmares. Communication patterns were significant in the Northern Ireland study, with 53% of the mothers stating that they had not discussed the illness with the well children. Only 43% of the mothers and 27% of the fathers reported that they had been asked about CF by their well children.

Blumenthal[23] used the parents of patients with CF as a control group in a study designed to measure the susceptibility to mental illness of parents of children with phenylketonuria (PKU) and of parents of children with nonphenylketonuric mental retardation. A standard interview schedule was administered to 121 parents of children with CF, 108 parents of children with PKU, and 102 parents of children with non-PKU mental retardation. The interviews were coded, and mental health was evaluated by a set of indices constructed by assigning numerical values to certain items in the code. Analysis of variance was used to evaluate the data.

The mental health indices included an alcohol index, a depression index, a nervous breakdown index, a professional persons index (consultations with physicians relative to mental health problems), and a hospitalizations (for mental problems) index. Functional indices included a total illnesses index, medications (for mental health) index, job stability index, divorce index, accident (automobile) index, and a mobility (social) index. No statistically significant differences were found between the three groups. Interestingly, on the divorce index, the mean score for CF parents is significantly lower than the score for the other two groups.

The impact of chronic disease on normal siblings was studied by Breslau et al.[24] The study included 370 Cleveland families of children with CF, cerebral palsy, myelodysplasia, or multiple handicaps; 49 of the families had a CF child. Data obtained from 1034 randomly selected children in Manhattan were used as controls. Of the families interviewed, 239 had normal children between 6 and 18 years old. The mothers completed a self-administered instrument that measured the behavior problems of a randomly selected sibling in the age group. Inventories were used to measure the sibling's adjustment, the level of disability of the identified patient, and the mother's perception of the effect of the disease on the sibling. Results showed that the diagnostic category of the patient had no statistically significant effect, and the level of disability of the patient had no relationship to the adjustment of the normal sibling.

In a critical review of the psychosocial literature on CF, Frydman[25] describes the methodological shortcomings of most research to date. Findings are anecdotal in nature, overemphasize negative consequences, and lack an appropriate theoretical framework. Future research, he suggests, needs to focus on coping strategies and identifying barriers to adjustment. The objective of research should shift from defining the despair and the grim consequences of CF to defining strategies for preventing poor adaptation. Research may well point to a need for systemic change in patterns of health-care delivery. To define the success of family functioning as dependent on its own structure is perverse, and neglects the role of the social structure in effecting that functioning.

In summary, there seems good evidence that the family responsibilities of having a CF child cause adjustments and restrictions in the occupations of both parents. Stress reactions are more likely with questions about prognosis, harmful outside activities, younger children, delayed diagnosis, and when more than one child in the family has cystic fibrosis. In certain noncommunicative families the effects of CF on the non-CF siblings can be detrimental. Most studies of the psychosocial effects on the siblings of these patients showed no differences from control groups. Future research needs to be directed towards techniques for enabling families to develop more effective coping mechanisms. The importance of care-givers working with the family to facilitate and to enhance communication among family members is highlighted in the research to date.

DEATH

The final and ultimate crisis for patients with CF and their families comes as death approaches. The psychosocial process of death and dying has been well documented.[26] The five stages include denial and isolation, anger, bargaining, depression, and acceptance. The stages of grief are similar for CF and other diseases. Bronheim[27] identifies uncertainty about life expectancy as an added source of stress with cystic fibrosis. Patients die at different ages and stages of the disease. Death is often a lingering process, with repeated "final" episodes from which the patient rebounds (the so-called Lazarus syndrome). The accompanying anger, confusion, and guilt can present challenges to the coping abilities of families.

Virtually all published literature about the psychosocial aspects of the dying process for patients with CF is anecdotal in nature (eg, Patterson et al[28]). Most of the scientific studies in this area have concerned children with cancer. Cystic fibrosis is distinguished from cancer by its genetic basis, which may lead to an additional burden of guilt for parents, and anger of the patient directed at the parents. Differential responses, coping mechanisms, and interventions are avenues for future research in distinguishing cystic fibrosis from other fatal diseases.

The issue of home care for the terminally ill patient with CF is another area where research is indicated. Fagan and Harwood[29] report that more than two thirds of the patients at the San Diego Cystic Fibrosis Center chose to die in their homes. The advantages of this approach are identified as continued involvement with family and friends; more normal interaction with siblings; access to special pets, belongings, favorite foods; diminished feelings of impotence on the part of the parents; and more honest and open grieving. The disadvantages are identified as increased staff time, difficulty in obtaining autopsies, medical complications, and the separation of the family from the active hospital support system.

Waechter[30] conducted a study with 64 children between the ages of 6 and 10; the subjects were divided into four groups matched for age, race, social class, and family background. In one group were 16 terminally ill children, including 6 with cystic fibrosis. The second group included chronically ill children with a good prognosis. Children in the third group were hospitalized with an acute illness. A fourth group of nonhospitalized children were selected at an elementary school. A general anxiety scale for children, projective testing, and parent interviews were administered.

Analysis of the results of the general anxiety scale showed that the total scores of the children with fatal illness were twice as high as the scores of the other hospitalized children. Although only 2 of the 16 fatally ill children had discussed their concerns about death with their parents, the proportion of stories related to death on projective testing was 63%. This suggests that an awareness of their prognosis is conveyed to children by their perception of nonverbal cues. A highly significant correlation was found between the total score on the projective tests and the degree to which the child had been given an opportunity to discuss fears and prognosis. This suggests that open communication does not heighten death anxiety, but rather decreases feelings of isolation, alienation, and a perception that the disease is too terrible to talk about. Similar findings have been reported by Spinetta and Maloney[31] in work with leukemic children.

In a handbook for parents[32] and a similar publication for health professionals,[33] the authors identified issues that must be addressed as all family members prepare emotionally for the death.

The level at which children are able to conceptualize about death varies with age and developmental level, according to the authors. For children under 3, anxiety about separation is pervasive; there is no comprehension of death per se. During the preschool years, between about 3 and 5 years of age, most children begin to develop an understanding of death as something that happens to others and not to themselves. An understanding of death evolves slowly. Children under the age of 10 begin to conceptualize about death, but have generally not developed a full understanding. By about age 11, most children have developed the ability to grasp the concepts of the universality and permanence of death.

Communication with the child is identified as a critical factor, with process (how something is said) meaning more to the child than content (what is said). The authors suggest points that can be discussed with children, as appropriate for the individual child's age and level of readiness.

1. Death, like birth, is a part of the natural order of things.
2. Death has a social significance.
3. Death is a separation on both sides.
4. The loss is never complete. The deceased lives on in some special way.
5. The child will not be alone at death and after death.
6. At the time of death, people

need to know that they have done all they could do with their lives.
7. The child needs to be reassured that it is all right to cry and feel sad.
8. The child needs to be reassured that silence is acceptable.
9. When death finally comes, it will not hurt.
10. When someone we love dies, it is important for us to be able to say good-bye.
11. Adults sometimes do not know very much about death either.

The importance of preparing ahead of time for necessary physical and legal matters is emphasized, including discussions regarding autopsy and burial, and, important to the child, decisions about disposing of treasured possessions.

In contrast to the consistency of approach to the families of a newly diagnosed child with CF, in practice there is considerable inconsistency in how the death of a patient with CF is managed. Important variables include the age of the patient, how long the patient has been critically ill, the strengths and weaknesses of the particular family, family support systems, religious philosophy and support, previous experience with CF, number of siblings and whether or not they have the disease, other disorders such as alcoholism which may be present in the family, and numerous other characteristics that may distinguish us as individuals. The team approach has many advantages in view of the importance of listening and communication that is required when the child is seriously ill. The feelings of mutual support from such an approach far outweigh any perceived lack of individual involvement. Indeed, the team approach is important in preventing the family from feeling isolated.

The publication "Guide to Diagnosis and Management of Cystic Fibrosis"[34] discusses almost every complication of the disease except death. There are a variety of alternative approaches that different individuals have found most advantageous, and until someone analyzes these different methods, it is not possible to make more than subjective recommendations. Most of the CF health care team have known the families of the dying patient for a number of years, and this helps considerably with mutual communication and trust.

The importance of the family being physically present during this period must be stressed, and if the patient dies at home this presence is ensured. Infants and children may need to be held, and this is easily accomplished despite the oxygen and other technical apparatus. Families need to be assured after the death of a child that they did everything possible for the child; this is one of the times when the guilt of having produced a child with CF is particularly acute for parents. Other responses to death are similar to those for parents of children with other diseases and have been well documented.[32,33] At some variable interval after the death of a child, the family should be given an opportunity to discuss any questions, concerns, anxieties, or other problems that may have arisen. Other families may not wish to avail themselves of this opportunity, and recommendations should be individualized and adapted to the different needs of different families.

SUMMARY

This chapter has identified crisis points for the patient with CF and the family. Each of these crises presents a natural point of intervention for the professional team to work with the family towards the shared objective of life enhancement. The challenge remains with CF care-givers to assess to what extent current human services systems (eg, vocational rehabilitation, financial assistance, schools, health care delivery, etc) have a functional or dysfunctional effect on the mental health of the CF family.

REFERENCES

1. Warwick WJ, Pogue RE: Cystic fibrosis—an expanding challenge for internal medicine. *JAMA* 1977;238:2159–2162.
2. Lawler RH, Nakielny W, Wright NA: Psychological implications of cystic fibrosis.

Can Med Assoc J 1966;94:1043–1046.

3. Tropauer A, Franz MN, Dilgard VW: Psychological aspects of the care of children with cystic fibrosis. *Am J Dis Child* 1970; 119:424–432.
4. Burton L: *The Family Life of Sick Children. A Study of Families Coping with Chronic Childhood Disease.* London, Routledge and Kegan Paul, 1975.
5. Kulczycki LL, Regal D, Tantisunthorn C: The impact of cystic fibrosis on the parents and patients, in Patterson PR, Denning CR, Kutscher AH (eds): *Psychosocial Aspects of Cystic Fibrosis.* New York, Columbia University Press, 1973.
6. Drotar D, Doershuk CF, Stern RC, et al: Psychosocial functioning of children with cystic fibrosis. *Pediatrics* 1981;67:343.
7. McCollum AT, Gibson LE: Family adaptation to the child with cystic fibrosis. *J Pediatr* 1970;77:571–578.
8. Blumenthal MD: Experiences of parents of retardates. *Arch Gen Psychiatr* 1969;21: 160–171.
9. Coolidge CB: The dying of Robin: A mother's reflections. *J Pediatr Psychol* 1977; 2:79–81.
10. Kaplan DM, Grobstein R, Smith A: Predicting the impact of severe illness in families. *Health Soc Work* 1976;1:71–82.
11. Pless IB, Roghmann KJ: Chronic illness and its consequences: Observations based on three epidemiologic surveys. *J Pediatr* 1971; 79:351–359.
12. Gayton WF, Friedman SB, Tavormina JF, et al: Children with cystic fibrosis: Psychological test findings of patients, siblings and parents. *Pediatrics* 1977;59: 888–894.
13. Lloyd-Still JD, Hurwitz I, Wolff PH, et al: Intellectual development after severe malnutrition in infancy. *Pediatrics* 1974;54:306–311.
14. Boyle IR, di Sant'Agnese PA, Sack S, et al: Emotional adjustment of adolescents and young adults with cystic fibrosis. *J Pediatr* 1976;88:318–326.
15. Kollberg H: Cystic fibrosis in Sweden: A ten-year sociomedical follow up, in *Proceedings of Eighth International Congress of Cystic Fibrosis.* Toronto, Canadian Cystic Fibrosis Foundation, 1980, pp 256–261.
16. *Adult Care Consumer Survey.* Cystic Fibrosis Foundation, 6000 Executive Boulevard, Suite 309, Rockville, Maryland 20852, 1981.
17. Levine SB, Stern RC: Sexual function in cystic fibrosis. *Cystic Fibrosis Club Abstr* 1981;22:130.
18. Goldberg RT, Johnson BD: A comparative study of five groups of handicapped children in vocational rehabilitation. *Scand J Rehabil Med* 1978;10:215–220.
19. Goldberg RT, Isralsky M, Shwachman H: Vocational development and adjustment of adolescents with cystic fibrosis. *Arch Phys Med Rehabil* 1979;60:369–374.
20. Educational and Vocational Counseling for Young Adults with Cystic Fibrosis. Pamphlet published by Cystic Fibrosis Foundation, 3379 Peachtree Road NE, Atlanta, Georgia 30326 (now in Rockville, Maryland).
21. Meyerwitz JH, Kaplan HB: Familial responses to stress: The case of cystic fibrosis. *Soc Sci Med* 1967;1:249–266.
22. Turk J: Impact of cystic fibrosis on family functioning. *Pediatrics* 1964;34:67–71.
23. Blumenthal MD: Mental illness in parents of phenylketonuric children. *J Psychiatr Res* 1967;5:59–74.
24. Breslau N, Weitzman M, Messenger K: Psychologic functioning of siblings of disabled children. *Pediatrics* 1981;67:344–353.
25. Frydman MI: Implications of cystic fibrosis for health services and the afflicted. *Soc Sci Med* 1979;13A:147–150.
26. Kubler-Ross E: *On Death and Dying.* New York, Macmillan, 1969.
27. Bronheim SP: Pulmonary disorders, asthma and cystic fibrosis, in Magrab PR (ed): *Psychological Management of Pediatric Problems, Vol. 1.* Baltimore, University Park Press, 1978, pp 309–344.
28. Patterson PR, Denning CR, Kutscher AH: *Psychosocial Aspects Of Cystic Fibrosis.* New York, Columbia University Press, 1973.
29. Fagan E, Harwood I: Home care for the dying patient, in *Proceedings of Eighth International Congress of Cystic Fibrosis.* Toronto, Canadian Cystic Fibrosis Foundation, 1980, pp 275–278.
30. Waechter EH: Children's awareness of fatal illness. *Am J Nurs* 1971;71:1168–1172.
31. Spinetta JJ, Maloney LJ: Death anxiety in the outpatient leukemic child. *Pediatrics* 1975;56:1034–1037.
32. Spinetta JJ, Deasey-Spinetta P: *Emotional Aspects of Life-Threatening Illness in Children. A Handbook for Parents.* Cystic Fibrosis Foundation, 6000 Executive Boulevard, Suite 309, Rockville, Maryland 20852, 1980.
33. Spinetta JJ, Deasey-Spinetta P: *Talking with Children with a Life Threatening Illness. A Handbook for Health Care Professionals.* Cystic Fibrosis Foundation, 6000 Executive Boulevard, Suite 309, Rockville, Maryland 20852, 1980.
34. *Guide to Diagnosis and Management of Cystic Fibrosis.* Cystic Fibrosis Foundation, 6000 Executive Boulevard, Suite 309, Rockville, Maryland 20852, 1979.

26

The Cystic Fibrosis Foundation

Robert J. Beall

Sherry L. Keramidas

The Cystic Fibrosis Foundation is a private, voluntary health agency whose mission is directed toward finding the means to effectively treat, control, and prevent cystic fibrosis. Through its direct support of programs and interaction and collaboration with other voluntary and professional groups, government agencies, and private institutions, the CF Foundation has become a focal point for CF research, care, training, and education.

Founded in 1955 as the National Cystic Fibrosis Research Foundation (NCFRF),* the foundation grew out of the hopes and efforts of a small group of dedicated parents, physicians, and volunteers. From its inception, the foundation focused on research and education. Following successful efforts to organize a group interested in CF, the NCFRF began a period of rapid growth. New divisions and departments took shape, and the foundation began to broaden its interests and program support base.

In 1960, a major decision was made to develop a nationwide network of CF centers, partially supported by the foundation, which would offer specialized expertise in the diagnosis and treatment of CF. Subsequently,

*The foundation shortened its name to the Cystic Fibrosis Foundation in 1972.

research and training programs were expanded to include grants, fellowships, scholarships, and traineeships. The CF Foundation also began a clinical fellowship program to help train the urgently needed cadre of physicians specializing in CF treatment.

A computerized registry of CF patient information was initiated to provide a disease-oriented data base for statistical, epidemiological, and clinical studies. Finally, consumer-oriented programs were established to identify and deal with the psychosocial, educational, and financial problems which arise in the lives of those affected by CF. During the interval from 1955 to 1980, the CF Foundation has allocated $49 million in support of its medical and scientific programs.

ORGANIZATION OF THE CF FOUNDATION

The organization of the CF Foundation brings together the volunteer community—both lay and medical—and professional staff to develop and implement the foundation's policies and programs. The key units in the foundation's organization are: the board of trustees, which is comprised of volunteers and is responsible for setting policy; the field, which includes chapters and areas, representing volunteers and professional staff who are involved in implementing many of the nonmedical activities; and the national office, whose professional staff is responsible for the design and implementation of many of the CF Foundation's programs. The overall organization of the foundation is schematically shown in Figure 26-1.

The CF Foundation's field is one of the principal means for outreach to the general public. Presently, this field encompasses 60 professionally staffed chapters throughout the country; an additional 10 chapters are run solely by volunteers. Chapter members include CF families, health care professionals, educators, community leaders, and other interested individuals from the general public. These local groups are the instruments by which volunteers contribute their efforts to the fight against CF through three primary chapter functions: carrying out public education programs in local communities; conducting year-round fund-raising events; and, developing and conducting nonmedical care service programs for CF parents and families. A listing of local chapters is available through the foundation's national office.

Although the CF chapters are autonomous groups, there is a strong link between chapters and the national office through direct working relationships and through the area directors who are part of the national staff. In addition, representatives from chapters sit on the foundation's board of trustees and are thereby involved in determining foundation policies.

The national office, with its professional staff, is the vehicle for implementing the programs and policies established by the foundation's board of trustees. The national office also serves as the liaison among CF patients and families, other volunteers, the general public, the scientific and health-care communities, and the various federal agencies and legislative groups concerned with health care. Programmatically, the foundation seeks to achieve its goal through a wide variety of activities conducted in the five major areas of the national office: medical and scientific, public policy, field services, resource development, and public relations and communications. The medical/scientific program is the focal point of the foundation, the vehicle through which the CF Foundation goal may be realized. However, the other programs provide the base for supporting medical/scientific activities by increasing public awareness of the problems and challenges of CF, raising funds for research, training, and care; and coordinating the foundation's outreach activities.

Medical/Scientific Program

Cystic fibrosis is a complex disease which has proven not to be amenable to singular approaches in research or care. Recognizing

CFF ORGANIZATION DIAGRAM

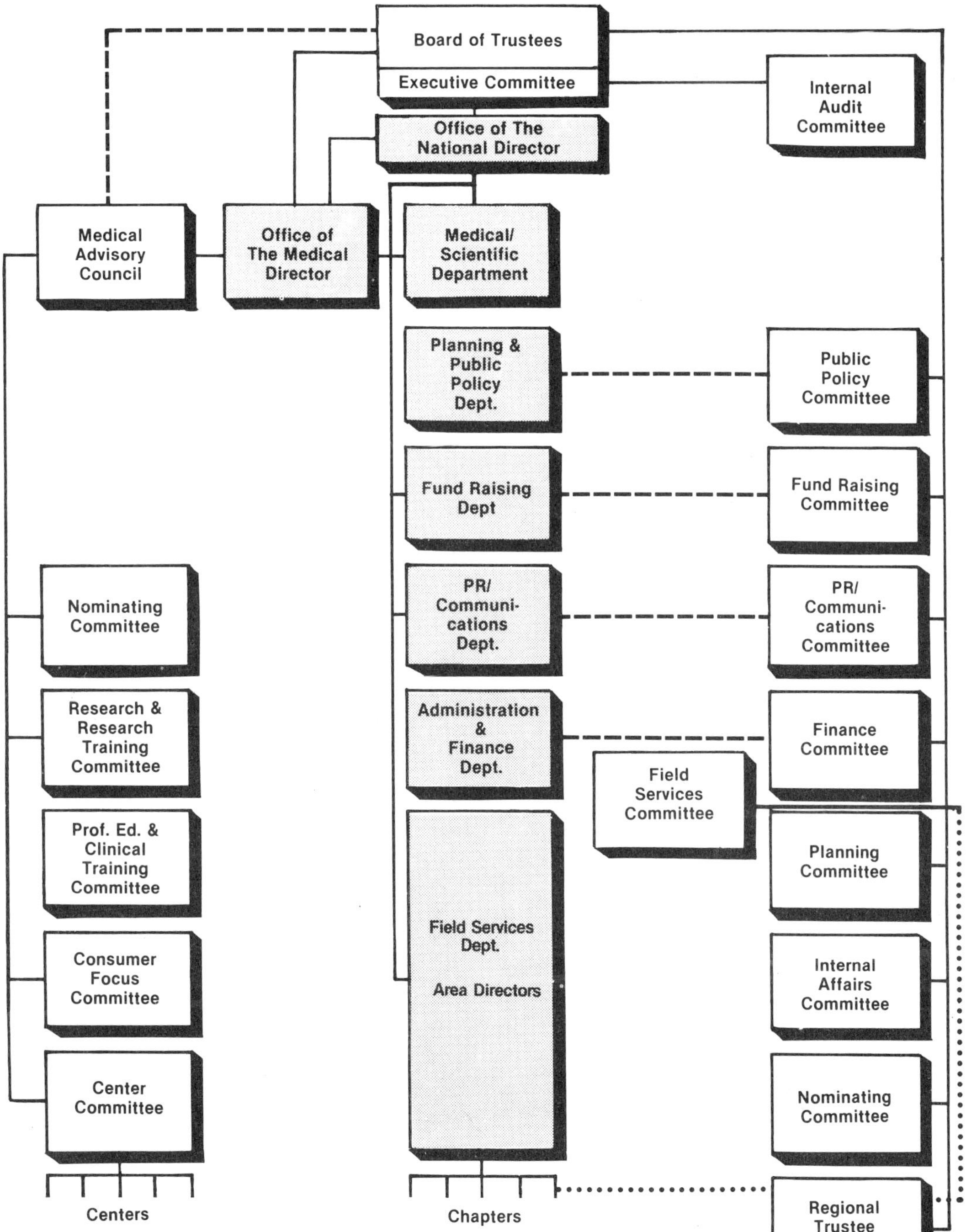

- shaded areas represent professional staff; unshaded areas represent volunteers;
- the lay volunteers are represented on the right-hand side of the chart; the medical volunteers on the left; and

——— functional   – – – – advisory   • • • • • • • • • liaison

Figure 26-1

this, the foundation has sought to establish a medical/scientific program which is multifaceted, responsive to the needs of the biomedical community, and flexible to enable changes in directions and/or support as needed. In designing and updating its medical and scientific activities, the foundation has maintained close ties with the National Institutes of Health (NIH), other research-sponsoring agencies, and medical institutions to ensure that the CF activities of the foundation are complementary to these other programs.

The medical/scientific program is organized into five major components: research and research training, centers (health care), professional education and clinical training, the patient registry, and consumer focus activities.

A major focus of the medical/scientific program is ongoing support of research and research training. Through its grant and fellowship awards, the foundation supports basic and clinical research in a diverse range of biomedical disciplines and specialties. In addition to direct, peer-reviewed funding of research, the foundation has devoted considerable effort to increasing awareness of the challenges and opportunities in CF research and stimulating new research. This is accomplished through a number of vehicles including: support of scientific conferences; interaction with professional societies, such as the American Thoracic Society, American Society for Microbiology, American Academy of Pediatrics, etc; and preparation of newsletters and other publications directed to the research community. Similar mechanisms also are applied for the professional education/clinical training and consumer focus components.

The foundation's health care delivery component, the CF center program, was established to furnish accurate case-finding and early diagnosis; comprehensive, specialized care; and long-term follow-up. The network of foundation-approved centers numbers over 125 nationwide. Most centers are located within medical schools or teaching hospitals and offer a range of inpatient and outpatient care and counseling services. Many centers also provide an environment for clinical training of health care professionals and conducting clinical research.

The foundation's patient registry is a longitudinal data base containing general demographic and background information on each patient seen in the CF center network. The registry currently is used to generate yearly demographic and actuarial statistics. Efforts to include basic treatment history of patients are being explored, as is the use of the registry as a tool for clinical research studies.

The consumer focus component is a rather unique element of the medical/scientific program, coordinating medical and related needs of consumers, education, and outreach activities. Further, the activities are closely related to consumer-oriented elements of the public policy program.

The planning and assessment of activities of the medical/scientific program reflect coordinated efforts between professional staff and volunteers representing the research and health care communities and consumers. The success of the program perhaps has been best demonstrated through the growth of medical/scientific activities, the ever-increasing number of biomedical professionals involved in CF research and care, and the evolution of innovative support mechanisms which complement federal and institutional programs. In planning its future, the foundation will strive to maintain the responsiveness and flexibility of this key program area.

Public Policy Department

The foundation, through its public policy program, participates in development of legislation at the federal and state levels which promotes and protects the interests and needs of the CF consumers and families, the research and health care communities, and the foundation. This is accomplished through a range of activities undertaken by the professional staff, including:

1. Developing and maintaining open communication between

the foundation and federal and state governments.

2. Providing advice and counsel to the legislative and executive branches of federal and state governments in the development of legislation and the subsequent rules and regulations as they relate to the CF constituency.
3. Encouraging and fostering government funding for CF and related research and professional training by actively participating in the authorization and appropriations for the National Institutes of Health (NIH) and facilitating the development of strong working relationships among the foundation, NIH, and other government agencies.
4. Assisting in improving the quality, accessibility, and availability of government-supported health care services to CF consumers and families by maintaining strong working relationships with the government agencies, such as the Office of Maternal and Child Health and other Department of Health and Human Services agencies; communicating the needs and concerns of the CF community; encouraging congressional and state support for programs and services.
5. Organizing the CF constituency into a volunteer legislative network which participates in the above activities.

Within the last five years, the CF Foundation's public policy program has come to the forefront among voluntary health agencies. Through the efforts of the staff, members of the foundation have been invited to testify before congressional committees considering health-care issues and budget appropriations for health care and biomedical research. The program has called national attention to CF problems and challenges through the establishment of a presidentially mandated National CF Week (in mid-September), as well as through the establishment of CF research as a trans-institute issue at the National Institutes of Health. Foundation legislative and policy efforts will continue at the national, state, and local levels. At the state and local fronts, public policy programs now are implemented through the parents and other volunteers and through a consumer representative program, a network of adult CF patients who are working to bring the needs and issues of the patient population to public attention.

Resource Development Department

The CF Foundation's programs are supported entirely through funds raised from the private sector. The foundation's resource development department is responsible for planning, implementing, and coordinating activities and projects to obtain the fiscal resources needed to maintain CF Foundation programs.

Resource development efforts are planned and implemented through the foundation's national office and through its network of chapters. Implemented in communities across the country, the foundation sponsors several fund-raising campaigns, including the "bowl-for-breath," bike-a-thons, and direct mail to the public.

Funds donated to the foundation through wills and bequests, pooled income funds, unitrusts, annuity trusts, gift annuities, and similar sources are coordinated by the national office which offers assistance to donors contributing through such programs. Finally, to support the continued growth of the medical/scientific programs, the foundation also has implemented a program for seeking support from private foundations, corporations, clubs, and organizations.

Public Relations/ Communications Department

Reaching the general public on the nature of CF, the needs of patients, and the efforts to meet such needs is coordinated by the foundation's public relations/communications department. In conjunction with the foundation's other departments, its medical advisors, and the board of trustees, this arm of the CF Foundation works with chapters, centers, and the mass media to educate and inform communities of developments and directions in CF-related research and care. It also is the responsibility of the public relations/communications department to determine the public's need for information and to develop materials to meet these needs. Finally, this department helps to maintain the foundation's clearinghouse of materials for the professional and lay communities.

INTERNATIONAL COORDINATION

In an effort to provide care to CF patients worldwide and to coordinate research on this disease, the CF Foundation in the United States actively participates in international professional and lay programs. International programs are supervised by the International Cystic Fibrosis (Mucoviscidosis) Association (ICFMA, Robert D. McCreery, president, 3567 East 49 Street, Cleveland, Ohio 44105).

For the professional communities, the ICFMA sponsors conferences and symposia on issues and directions of CF research and care. Every four years, this group sponsors a large-scale international conference which addresses multiple aspects of CF, encompassing clinical care, research, psychosocial aspects of the disease, access to care, and other public policy and consumer concerns. This conference includes professional and lay-oriented sessions. Smaller, more focused, meetings are held annually.

FUTURE DIRECTIONS OF THE CF FOUNDATION

In an era of rapid change, it is often difficult to conclusively plot a future course. In the coming years, the foundation will continue to pursue its overall mission and goal—to improve the length and quality of life of those affected by CF and to ultimately find the means to cure and prevent CF—through support of an innovative medical/scientific program.

This will include continuation of research, training, and health-care delivery support. In the coming years, the foundation also will seek to bolster its support of CF research through establishment of a network of specialized research centers. Finally, continuing progress in CF-related research and care will depend upon multidisciplinary approaches which span the biomedical spectrum and which link biomedicine with psychosocial aspects of treating chronic disease. In this regard, the foundation will continue to stimulate new research approaches to encourage collaborative, multidisciplinary efforts.

27

The Organization of a Cystic Fibrosis Clinic

John D. Lloyd-Still

THE DIRECTORY

The directory published by the CF Foundation[1] lists 128 centers in the United States in 1980. The CF centers provide specialist faciliities for the diagnosis and care of children and adults with CF and other pediatric pulmonary and gastrointestinal diseases. The directory also lists the CF Foundation chapters, the names of the board of trustees, medical advisory council, and headquarters office staff. It is updated at regular intervals, and contains information on the address of the center; phone number for appointments; names of center director, codirector, and other personnel, and the times and days on which the CF clinics are held. This information is of special benefit when families relocate or travel to other parts of the country.

Policies and Rules Governing CF Center Accreditation and CF Center Grants Awarded by the CF Foundation[2]

The Cystic Fibrosis Foundation offers accreditation to institutions for CF center programs which meet criteria established by the foundation. Accreditation is awarded on an annual basis and carries with it assurance that the accredited center program will have access to the resources of the foundation which include the patient registry, meeting announcements, educational materials, eligibility for training grants, eligibility to compete for center financial support, and participation and representation in the various medical and scientific activities of the foundation. All accredited centers will be awarded travel funds for attendance at the foundation's annual center directors meeting and the CF club meetings, and will have their available services, phone numbers, etc, described in the foundation's national directory. In addition, accredited center programs will be represented by the foundation in activities pertaining to legislation and interaction with various government agencies at the national and state level.

FUNDING

Cystic fibrosis center grants are made by the foundation to accredited universities, accredited medical schools, accredited hospitals, or other such institutions in the United States as may be approved by the foundation, as subsidies to help establish and maintain comprehensive, exemplary programs of patient care, teaching and research in cystic fibrosis and related chronic and recurrecent pulmonary and gastrointestinal diseases of children, adolescents and adults.

All CF center programs are categorized and evaluated by the center committee of the foundation. This categorization is according to: (1) what the facility is, ie, care level (level I, II, III), care and teaching center; care, teaching, and resource center; or care and resource center; (2) how good the program is, ie, quality judgment of the activities conducted under the care, teaching, and resource programs; (3) patient load and other factors related to size and scope of the center's operations.

The center committee of the foundation consists of 10 center directors who serve a period on the committee (usually two years) and function by peer review. Each center is visited by a member of the center committee every 3–5 years, and a detailed evaluation is compiled. The report is submitted at the annual meeting of the center committee. The allocation of funds (center grant) for the various CF centers is determined by the recommendations and decisions of the medical advisory committee and the board of trustees of the CF Foundation. The CF Foundation has no direct control over the various CF centers in directing policy, but there are guidelines for the utilization of grant funds.[2]

Cystic fibrosis chapters are usually located in close proximity to many of the larger centers, and a close relationship between the chapters and centers may or may not evolve. The primary aim of the CF chapters is fund raising. The chapters are usually run by a salaried executive director, but some are run by volunteers (see Chapter 26). Since the goal of both chapters and centers is for the betterment of CF patients, mutual collaboration and support are encouraged.

THE PATIENT REGISTRY

The patient registry,[3] in operation since 1966, collects data on each CF patient followed by the care, teaching, and resource centers sponsored by the CF Foundation. At the end of each year the centers submit a report on each patient seen during the year to the patient registry. Initial reports on new patients are prepared by the centers, while reports on current patients are updated on computer-generated forms sent to the centers. The data base contains the following information on each patient: identification number, center number, date of birth, date of diagnosis, sex, race, birth type (single, twin, etc), birth condition (normal, meconium ileus, or intestinal obstruction), current height and weight records, postal code of residence, initials, and status at the end of each report year (alive, transferred, lost to follow-up, dead). If the patient has died during the year, the date and cause of death are also recorded.

The patient registry data base is updated and analyzed annually. Data are also included on patients followed by centers in Canada and other countries. Reports are generated for each center covering the patients reported by that center. The patient registry is designed to provide information about CF as a disease entity, not to provide information about specific patients. Access to individual patient data is not allowed except through the center director or clinician who provided the data. Aggregate data, as for a state or region (but not for a single center), may be made available upon request, when and if facilities allow. A major effort is being made to develop the research potential of the patient registry by increasing its flexibility and by expanding the data base to include more data on each patient.

The minimum criteria established by the CF Foundation for a facility to qualify as a CF care (levels I, II, III), teaching, and resource center are published by the CF Foundation. Although these criteria are the basis on which the site visit evaluation is based, in practice individual CF centers differ markedly in organization, personnel, size, philosophy, and numerous other parameters depending on the demographic, ethnic, economic and other variables in the particular locale. Thus, centers vary from institutions responsible for hundreds of patients with daily clinics, to others that only meet once a month and follow a minimum of 20 patients. Some of the responsibilities and functions of a medium-size CF center caring for between 100–150 patients will be discussed.

FUNCTIONS OF PERSONNEL

Center Director

The center director is considered the key individual responsible for the successful functioning of a center. He or she is usually a board-certified pediatrician or, less often, an internist. Cystic fibrosis is unlikely to be the physician's sole responsibility except in certain large centers. The physician has usually undergone a period of specialized training in CF during postgraduate or fellowship appointments which may have included pulmonary disease, gastroenterology, nutrition, genetics, allergy, or infectious disease. Others have acquired this knowledge by prolonged experience in caring for patients with CF. A center director must be able to fulfill several critical functions.

Leadership and organization The establishment of a "team approach" to CF necessitates an ability to collaborate with and attract other personnel into the clinic. This is required at all levels of care, teaching, and research. Once the clinic assumes a certain size, other back-up physicians are required to help with the "load" of patients and for 24-hr coverage and during periods of absence. The philosophy of individual center directors varies widely from individuals who personally direct all the care of their patients, to others who prefer to delegate responsibility among a number of involved physicians. Likewise, some center directors work very closely with social workers, respiratory therapists, nutritionists, and nursing personnel and encourage a considerable degree of independence and responsibility for the particular area of expertise. However, without strong direction, many ancillary personnel may feel isolated or not functioning to the best of their ability and the spirit of a well-run clinic fails to mature.

Staff relationships Numerous tensions arise in the care of CF patients related to diagnosis, complications of the disease, and various crises, including death. These problems are part of the routine care of CF patients and families, but they also affect the staff of the clinic. Surprisingly, "burnout" in CF clinics is rarely reported, in contrast to intensive care units where the problem is chronic. One of the reasons for its rarity is probably related to the excellent relationships and mutual support system found in so many CF centers.

Patient care This is the primary goal of every physician involved in clinical practice. In a CF clinic the center director has a complicated role related to: (1) the patient's disease status, (2) the family's functioning and capabilities, (3) ancillary support systems, and (4) quality control of laboratory tests (sweat testing).

The treatment of the disease has been extensively covered in the various chapters of this book. Family functioning and the psychological effects on the child or adult with CF have been covered in Chapters 24 and 25. The problems related to quality control of sweat testing are discussed in Chapter 4. The CF center is the referral center for the diagnosis of CF, and it is essential that the sweat test be performed accurately. Ancillary support systems will be detailed.

Teaching Teaching about CF can be performed irrespective of whether or not the director is located in a university environment. Thus, all hospitals have nurses, respiratory therapists, nutritionists, and social workers, as well as students of various disciplines, who can be educated in aspects of CF that involve their particular specialty. The university-based physician has obligations to teach medical students and others about CF. He or she must also educate clinical pathologists from referral hospitals about the correct methodology for performing sweat testing and offer training to laboratory technicians from these institutions if quality control of their sweat testing method is deficient. Education should not be limited to medical personnel, and numerous opportunities exist for participation in chapter activities and cooperation with the press, radio, television, and local organizations that wish to sponsor fund-raising events or educational promotions for the CF Foundation.

Research A major function of the center director is to perform and encourage others to become involved in research into all aspects of CF. This may be either clinical or basic science. The foundation and the National Institutes of Health are especially interested in collaboration with other disciplines and have published detailed guidelines on the areas of special interest.[4]

Lobbying Some physicians feel that lobbying is inappropriate and best left to others. However, the success of lobbying efforts in providing increased appropriations from the federal and state governments for crippled children's services which provide funds for CF patients is impressive. Many of these efforts have been instigated or actively supported by center directors who have provided data to legislators that resulted in major advances for the care of CF patients, such as the Over-21 Program. Details of the state crippled children's services programs for children with CF were surveyed and compiled by the CF Foundation in 1980.[5] The center director should be knowledgeable about these regulations.

Clinic Coordinator

This position in the clinic can be pivotal to the success of the organization. The individual is usually a nurse, the center director's secretary or, in some cases, a dedicated lay person who has become expert in the day-to-day running of the clinic. Responsibilities include the initial contact with the family, usually via the telephone, and the coordinator acts as a triage in arranging the appropriate referral which may be related to consultation, appointments, illness, emergencies, medications, family crises, financial problems, or a specific inquiry about the patient's care. The coordinator is usually present during the clinic and possesses detailed knowledge about the family background.

Continuity of personnel adds greatly to how much these individuals can accomplish. In some clinics the coordinator makes home visits to get to know the family better, and in this way confidence can be established in a more relaxed atmosphere. The coordinator may be involved outside the hospital in local chapter activities or in group sessions for newly diagnosed families or adult patients. The coordinator can also assume a major role in organizing research protocols and encouraging participation of patients and families.

Nursing Personnel

The role of the nurse in the CF clinic would include all the functions of the coordinator if that individual is a registered nurse. Before the clinic takes place, it is advantageous to review the charts of all the patients to be seen. Special functions of the nurse in the clinic include: (1) organization, ie, date of most recent chest radiograph (most clinics take one on an annual basis and at other times when indicated), pulmonary function tests, sputum culture, urine examination, photographs, review of respiratory therapy protocols, social service and nutritional evaluations, immunization status, tuberculin testing and influenza vaccination in the fall; (2) school problems—the nurse may discuss school problems and provide information such as the pamphlet "Teachers Guide to Cystic Fibrosis" on entrance into school, and contact the school nurse if problems arise; (3) education—instruction can be given related to feeding, child-rearing, administration of antibiotics, pancreatic enzymes, and other medications, and older patients may need advice concerning adolescence, sex, and birth control; (4) illness—the nurse is usually the first person to recognize when a patient is sick and can alert other personnel in the clinic; (5) prevention—preventive care can be provided by warning the parents about the dangers of heat prostration in the summer and by organizing the prophylactic influenza immunization program which is recommeded each year in the fall for these patients; (6) crises—the nurse can recognize when families are in need of specialized counseling, or other problems related to finance or nutrition and arrange appropriate referral. When patients are severely ill with cor pulmonale, numerous other functions arise related to difficulties in transportation and oxygen administration.

The nurses in the CF clinic usually develop a close relationship with patients and families and become involved in continuity of care when patients are admitted for hospitalization and in terminal situations.

Respiratory Therapists and Physical Therapists

Physical therapy, including clapping, vibrating, postural drainage, and breathing exercises, is prescribed routinely for all CF patients. Either of the above personnel perform these functions on CF patients in the hospital, and they are responsible for initial education of the parents prior to the home therapy program. Regular revision of postural drainage is advisable and can be performed in the CF clinic. Respiratory therapists also instruct the families in the use of aerosol therapy, and in clinics where mist tents are still used they will be responsible for this therapy.

Social Worker

The role of the social worker in the clinic is essential. Functions are related to (1) diagnosis; (2) preventive counseling, and (3) crisis intervention. When a patient is newly diagnosed, it is beneficial to introduce the social worker to the family to participate in planning the approach to therapy. Assessment of baseline data for family functioning, adaptation, support systems, and financial evaluation will identify areas where difficulties are likely to occur and preventive measures can be instituted. Every clinic has a proportion of problem families, and these will involve an increased amount of the social worker's commitment. At other times crises will develop related to hospitalization, school difficulties, adolescent rebellion, parental problems of separation or lack of support, financial difficulties with loss of job necessitating support from the crippled children's program, and the care of the terminal patient.

We have found it advantageous for the social worker to be familiar with all our families, and in this way when crises arise, the social worker has some relationship that facilitates intervention. Some social workers have organized independent programs for support groups involving newly diagnosed families, group therapy with school-age and young adults, and grief seminars for families who have lost children. The social worker in the CF clinic works very closely with other team members and should always be present for the postclinic conference when the patient evaluation is reviewed and therapeutic decisions are confirmed.

Nutritionist

The contributions of the nutritionist to the care of CF patients are being increasingly appreciated and utilized. Their expertise enables them to accomplish more detailed assessments of dietary intake and identify areas where intervention is indicated. The chapter on growth in CF has stressed the importance of adequate caloric intake for CF patients, especially during periods of acute exacerbation. The nutritionist will have responsibilities to: (1) provide nutritional support to CF patients in an outpatient and inpatient setting; (2) serve as a resource person for patients and staff regarding nutritional composition of food, availability of special formulas, and supplements; (3) interview and counsel families on appropriate diet for age; (4) evaluate dietary intake and, with other pertinent information from the interview, record nutritional assessment in the patient's medical record; (5) check that appropriate vitamin and other supplements are prescribed; (6) participate in the postclinic evaluation conference; and (7) participate in special nutritional projects and resource protocols as needed.

It is useful to evaluate the patient's dietary intake at periodic intervals in the same way that respiratory therapy is reviewed. In some centers, a computer system has been programed to record data on individual patient's dietary intake, and this information can contribute to clinical research studies.

SPECIAL PROBLEMS

The newly diagnosed patient with CF and the adult patient present special problems. These subjects are discussed in Chapter 25.

Genetic Counseling

Until the basic cause of CF is known or a marker becomes available that allows accurate prenatal diagnosis and carrier screening, genetic counseling offers the only contribution to the prevention of CF in families already having an affected child. Limited studies on the usefulness or effectiveness of genetic counseling in CF have been performed, but the problem is complicated because the options available to such couples are limited. It is not known whether this information is best imparted by a genetic counselor or the physician and staff of the CF clinic who are experienced in this field. In most CF clinics the number of children born subsequently to families with a known child with CF has declined in recent years. Whether this reduction is the result of genetic counseling, improved education about the complications of CF, or the fear of ever-increasing financial liabilities is unknown. The physician's responsibilities to the family must involve making them aware of the genetic nature and implications of the disorder. Decisions on future pregnancies, which are the prerogative of the parents, not the staff of the CF clinic, will have to take into account varying religious beliefs, philosophies, and abilities to cope with the possibility of further children with or without CF.

Compliance

Many studies have been made in pediatric practice related to compliance (eg, the prophylaxis of rheumatic fever and the therapy of tuberculosis). Compliance is primarily dependent on three factors: (1) the severity of the disease being treated, (2) the socioeconomic status of the family, and (3) the individual's or family's ability to cope with the implications of the disease. Thus, disorders such as leukemia, hemophilia, and cystic fibrosis tend to have higher rates of compliance than disorders with a less life-threatening prognosis. All CF clinics have a proportion of patients with socioeconomic problems, and they are usually easy to identify. In other situations parents may feel overwhelmed and avoid all contact with the clinic, especially if the child is doing well. These problems are more common in the period after initial diagnosis, and these families are more difficult to identify. Compliance deficiencies will be noted at the postclinic conference and the social worker can be instrumental in helping in these situations.

We have made it policy to telephone families on the day that they have missed an appointment to find the reason for the missed appointment. This contact should be performed in a sensitive and nonpunitive manner expressing concern about their child's health and stressing the importance of regular follow-up. If these families are not identified early, it becomes increasingly difficult to establish regular contact.

Terminally Ill Patient

These patients present a number of different problems that are discussed in Chapter 25.

Community Resources

These may include Medicaid, crippled children's services, vocational rehabilitation, social security, and public welfare. The cooperation of the local CF chapter has been emphasized. In some clinics the United Fund or other voluntary agencies may be actively involved in supporting CF programs. Individual hospitals may provide additional services to help CF patients. The social worker and other administrative personnel can advise patients and families of the availability of these services and direct referral to the appropriate agency. The center director will be available to write letters of support for employment and vocational rehabilitation. Summer camps are organized for CF children in various parts of the country and have specialized medical personnel in attendance for medication, physiotherapy, and nutritional care.

MANAGEMENT OF THE CLINIC

Most clinics use some adaptation of the form reproduced in Figure 27-1, which is taken from the CF Foundation's "Guide to Diagnosis and Management of Cystic Fibrosis."[7] The details of the interval history, date of last visit, height and weight data, medication, and physical examination are included. We would add evaluations of the social worker, nutritionist, and respiratory therapist. Records of immunization schedules, including influenza vaccination, and the family history should be easily available, and we prefer to put these on the face sheet. The results of the chest radiographs, sputum cultures, urine examination, and respiratory function tests should be recorded at each visit. These can be included on a flow sheet for ease of identification and comparison with previous data. Many clinics perform annual photographs, and these can be instructive in following the progress of the disease.

Shwachman Score

This is the standard method of scoring the clinical evaluation for patients with CF and is reproduced (Table 27-1) from the CF publication "Guide to Diagnosis and Management of Cystic Fibrosis."[7] Although other scoring systems have been devised, the Shwachman score is simple to perform, has found widespread acceptance, and is recommended for the majority of clinics. (See Chapter 12 for further detailed discussion of the various scoring systems.)

Sweat Testing

Some centers have found it advantageous to keep a "sweat book" that records several pertinent details such as family history and the reason for referral for the sweat test. It has the advantage that when an abnormal sweat test is found, the referring physician's name can easily be retrieved, and the center director may wish to inform that physician of the diagnosis. This leads to more personal contact with the referring physicians and will usually expedite enrollment in the CF treatment program.

Postclinic Conference

This conference is essential to review the current status of the patient and to collaborate the input of the various members of the team. The postclinic conference also assumes a major role in teaching personnel and students about the disease and its complications. In our experience, the postclinic conference has consistently been evaluated as the most positive learning experience for students and participants. A brief summary

CYSTIC FIBROSIS CLINIC—INTERVAL RECORD

Patients Name ______________
Last Visit ________ Date ________
OPD No. ________ Age ________
Hosp. No. ________ Ht. ______ % ______
Wt. ______ % ______

GENERAL CONDITION: (Same/Better/Worse)

ACTIVITY: (Specify) **EXERCISE TOLERANCE:**

SCHOOL ATTENDANCE: **NEED FOR REST:**

INFECTIONS: (Date/Duration)

RESPIRATORY SYSTEM:

Voice
Wheezing
Dyspnea
Chest Pain

Cough:
Day
Severity
Frequency
Night
Sputum (Amt./Color)
Hemoptysis

Sleeping Respiratory Rate
Clearing Throat Only
Paroxysms
Vomiting

GI: Appetite
Diet
Restrictions
B.M.: Frequency
Consistency
Odor
Volume

Milk: Whole
Skim
Rectal Prolapse:
Flatus:

HOME TREATMENT: (Amount. Duration, Etc.)
Pancreatin
Vitamins
Antibiotics
Other

Aerosol
Postural Drainage
Mist Tent
Other Physical Therapy

UNDUE REACTIONS TO MEDICATION

PARENT'S COMMENT ON PROGRESS:

ADDITIONAL HISTORY: (New sibling, new address, other illnesses, social, economic, toilet training, etc.)

P.E.:
Temp. ______ Pulse ______ Resp. R. ______ B.P. ______
Ht. ______ Percentile ______
Wt. ______ Percentile ______

GENERAL APPEARANCE:
Development
Nutrition
Posture

Skin (Texture)
Muscle Mass
Glands

HEAD:
Mouth/Lips
Teeth
Staining
Tonsils

Nose
Nasal Polyps
Sinuses

Eyes
Ears
Neck
Thyroid

THORAX:
Shape
Symmetry
A-P Diameter
Retraction—Suprasternal
Retraction—Ribs

Circumference: Insp. ____ Exp. ____ Diff. ____
Lat. ______ A-P ______

LUNGS:
Perc.
Aucs.

HEART:

ABDOMEN:
Shape
Liver

Spleen
Masses

Hernia

EXTREMITIES: Clubbing Color

IMPRESSION: General
Specific

TREATMENT PRESCRIBED:
Aerosol
Antibiotic
Other

CURRENT LAB TESTS **PHYSICAL THERAPY:** **NEXT VISIT:**

Clinical Evaluation

Perfect score is 100. Maximum for each item is 25 points.

GENERAL **ACTIVITY** ______ **P.E.** ______ **NUTRITION** ______ **X-RAY** ______ **TOTAL** ______

Figure 27-1 Sample of form used in CF clinics. Reproduced from *Guide to Diagnosis and Management of Cystic Fibrosis,* Cystic Fibrosis Foundation (reference 7), with permission.

Table 27-1
Clinical Evaluation and Grading Criteria for Patients with Cystic Fibrosis*

Points	Case Histories	Pulmonary Physical Findings and Cough	Growth and Nutrition	Chest X-ray
25	Full activity Normal exercise tolerance and endurance Normal motor development Normal personality and disposition Normal school attendance	No cough Normal pulse and respiration No evidence of overinflation Lungs clear to auscultation Good posture No clubbing	Maintains weight and height above twenty-fifth percentile or compatible with familial pattern Good muscle mass and tone Normal subcutaneous fat Normal sexual maturation Good appetite Well-formed almost normal stools	No evidence of overinflation No increase in markings No infiltration or atelectasis
20	Slight limitation of strenuous activity Tires at end of day or after prolonged exertion Less energetic Low normal range of motor development Occasionally irritable or passive Good school attendance	Occasional hacking cough Clearing of throat Resting pulse and respiration normal Mild overinflation Occasional, usually localized harsh breath sounds, rhonchi, or prolonged expiratory phase Good posture Clubbing ± to 1+	Maintains weight and height above 10th percentile or slightly below familial pattern Good muscle mass/tone Slightly decreased subcutaneous fat Slightly retarded sexual maturation Normal appetite Stools more frequent and slightly abnormal	Minimal evidence of overinflation Mild accentuation of bronchovascular markings No infiltration or atelectasis
15	May rest voluntarily Tires after exertion Fair school attendance Moderately inactive Slight motor retardation Lacking spontaneity Passive or irritable	Mild chronic nonrepetitive cough in the morning on arising, after exertion or crying, or occasionally during the day No night cough Respiration and pulse slightly elevated Increased A-P diameter and depressed diaphragms Coarse breath sounds Occasional localized rales, rhonchi, or wheezes Moderate rounding of shoulders 1-2+ clubbing	Maintains weight and height above 3rd percentile or moderately below familial pattern Weight usually deficient for height Fair muscle mass/tone Moderate deficiency of subcutaneous fat Abdomen slightly distended Maturation definitely retarded Fair appetite Stool usually abnormal, large, floating, occasionally foul but formed	Moderate overinflation Increased A-P diameter Lung fields more radiolucent Diaphragms moderately depressed Increased bronchovascular markings Localized or patchy atelectasis Occasional transient infiltration

Table 27-1 continued

10	Limited physical activity and exercise tolerance Dyspneic after exertion Moderate motor retardation Fussy, irritable, sluggish, or listless Poor school attendance, may require home tutor	Chronic cough, frequent, repetitive, productive, and rarely paroxysmal Respiration and pulse moderately elevated Moderate to severe overinflation often with chest deformity Rales, rhonchi, or wheezing usually present and often widespread Rounded shoulders and forward head Clubbing 2-3+ Usually cyanosis	Weight and height below 3rd percentile Weight deficient for height Poor muscle mass/tone Marked deficiency of subcutaneous fat Moderate abdominal distention Failure of sexual maturation and no adolescent growth spurt Poor appetite Stools poorly formed, bulky, fatty and foul smelling	Marked overinflation Marked increase in A-P diameter Diaphragms markedly depressed Narrow cardia silhouette Occasional localized segmental or lobar atelectasis Persistent foci of infiltration Localized cysts Marked increase in markings
5	Severe limitation of activity Dyspnea and orthopnea Inactive or confined to bed or chair Marked motor retardation Apathetic or irritable Cannot attend school	Severe paroxysmal, frequent, productive cough often associated with vomiting or hemoptysis Night cough Tachypnea/tachycardia Barrel chest Generalized fine and coarse rales, rhonchi, musical wheezes Poor posture 3-4+ clubbing Cyanosis	Malnourished and stunted Weak, flabby, small muscles Absence of subcutaneous fat Large, flabby, protuberant abdomen Failure to grow or gain, often with weight loss Bulky, frequent, foul, fatty stools Frequent rectal prolapse	Extensive changes Severe overinflation Lobar or widespread atelectasis and infiltration Widespread cyst formation Bronchiectasis and abscess formation

*This system of clinical evaluation can be used to evaluate patients at each visit or at 6- or 12-month intervals in order to determine the severity the disease and the effect of therapy in any one patient and to compare one patient with the next. The physical findings and chest x-ray are the best indicators of the degree of pulmonary involvement and may be used without the other indicators to simplify and shorten the scoring. References: Shwachman H, Kulczycki LL: *Am J Dis Child* 1958;96:6. Doershuk CF, Matthews LW: *J Pediatr* 1964;65:677. Reproduced from *Guide to Diagnosis and Management of Cystic Fibrosis,* Cystic Fibrosis Foundation (reference 7), with permission.

of the patient's presenting symptoms and previous history is followed by the current findings. The chest radiographs and pulmonary function tests will be reviewed. The nursing staff, social worker, nutritionist, and respiratory therapist may contribute relevant observations and recommendations. The postclinic conference will identify problem areas such as changes in the family situation and deficiencies in care and compliance. Plans to rectify these problems can be devised and decisions made as to the appropriate form of intervention.

SUMMARY

There are scant data elucidating why patients and families select a private physician, specialized CF center, or a combination thereof. The relative efficacy of various facilities in controlling the disease and improving the total well-being of patients and families has not been documented. We are presently unsure whether specialty clinics offer the most effective or economical systems for delivery of care to these patients. (See Chapter 28 for further discussion of this topic.) Retrospective data would indicate that misdiagnosis and delayed diagnosis (commonly present in children with CF) have changed in their spectra and an increasing number of children are now diagnosed at a younger age.[6]

Currently CF centers are highly variable with respect to the composition and expertise of staff, with respect to goals and priorities, and with respect to effectiveness and comprehensiveness of care. Criticisms voiced by consumers at the CF centers relate largely to the lack of facilities for the ever-increasing CF adult population and to criticisms of the quality of care. No matter who delivers it, care must be competently delivered, effective, effcient, personalized, comprehensive, continuous, and compassionate.[4] These directives apply to the physical and psychosocial management of both the patient and the family.

REFERENCES

1. *Directory of Cystic Fibrosis Centers and Cystic Fibrosis Chapters.* Cystic Fibrosis Foundation, 6000 Executive Boulevard, Suite 309, Rockville, Maryland 20852.
2. *Policies and Rules Governing CF Center Accreditation and CF Center Grants Awarded by the CF Foundation.* Cystic Fibrosis Foundation, 6000 Executive Boulevard, Suite 309, Rockville, Maryland 20852.
3. *Cystic Fibrosis Foundation: Report of the Patient Registry,* Vol 1978. Cystic Fibrosis Foundation, 6000 Executive Boulevard, Suite 309, Rockville, Maryland 20852, 1978.
4. *Cystic Fibrosis: A Disease in Search of Ideas. Vol I, Clinical Sciences; Vol 2, Basic Sciences; Vol 3, Model Systems.* Cystic Fibrosis Foundation, 6000 Executive Boulevard, Suite 309, Rockville, Maryland 20852, 1978.
5. *1980 Survey of State Crippled Children's Services Programs for Children with Cystic Fibrosis.* Cystic Fibrosis Foundation, 6000 Executive Boulevard, Suite 309, Rockville, Maryland 20852, 1980.
6. Warwick WJ, Pogue RE: Cystic fibrosis: An expanding challenge for internal medicine. *JAMA* 1977;238:2159–2162.
7. *Guide to Diagnosis and Management of Cystic Fibrosis.* Cystic Fibrosis Foundation, 6000 Executive Boulevard, Suite 309, Rockville, Maryland 20852,1972.

28

The Economics of Cystic Fibrosis

Mark V. Pauly

This chapter will investigate some economic aspects of research and care for persons with cystic fibrosis. The first part will develop some estimates of the gains from reducing the incidence of cystic fibrosis. The most reliable estimates will be those of reductions in the cost of medical care now consumed in treating the disease, but I will also attempt to provide some order-of-magnitude estimates of the value of avoiding lost production and premature death and disability per se. Next, these estimates will be used to comment on the probable net benefits from alternative research and prevention strategies. A final section will deal with the current financing of care for patients with cystic fibrosis.

THE MEDICAL COST

Data on the prevalence, incidence, and medical costs for persons with CF are not very precise. The only real count of persons with CF is provided by the number of such persons under care in CF centers. The total number of patients under care at the end of 1978 was about 11,500, with another 1500 patients seen at some time during the year but who were transferred, lost to follow-up, or died. The number of new CF center patients has been increasing at a rate of 1000–1250 patients per year, suggesting an estimate of about 15,000 at the end of 1980. There is no information on the total number of CF patients outside of centers. There are probably some patients who are receiving care elsewhere, and some with mild symptoms who have not been diagnosed as having CF.

A carrier rate reported in the literature of 1 in 20–22 in the population suggests that there should be 30,000–35,000 patients, considerably in excess of the 15,000 patients in CF centers. However, the deaths reported by CF centers represent about 80% of the total deaths reported by the National Center for Health Statistics, whose information comes from death certificates. Either there are some persons with CF who die without ever being diagnosed, or the appropriate estimate of total patients is at most about 20% more than 15,000, or about 19,000 persons. Figures on the number of newly diagnosed persons seen at CF centers by age indicate that diagnosis beyond the age of 5 is relatively rare. Since one would expect severely ill patients to enter the network eventually, these thoughts suggest that a figure of 19,000 seems to be a reasonable number for the prevalence of the disease.

It is even more difficult to obtain accurate information on the cost of care for CF. A 1977 figure of $10,500 for a patient in "good" health reported by the National Heart, Lung, and Blood Institute appears to have been an educated guess not based on data. The most recent reliable medical expense data is from a 1980 survey of CF adults (over age 18). Average medical expenses from that self-selected sample were $9,532 in 1980, which would have been about $6,200 in 1977 medical prices; median expenses were even lower at $2,640. In addition, there are strong reasons to believe that expenses tend to be higher for adults than for children, because more of the adults are reaching the years preceding death in which expenses are higher. For example, 45% of the sampled adults were hospitalized during 1977, whereas only about 30% of all center patients were hospitalized. In addition, the annual death rate for CF adults is about twice that for children. If we assume that about 25% of the children are hospitalized, that all children have the same mean nonhospital expense as all adults ($4,246), and that the mean hospital costs for hospitalized children are the same as those for adults ($11,745), we get an estimate for the mean cost per child of about $7,200. Since about 14% of CF patients are over 18, the mean expense of all CF patients is estimated to be about $7500 in 1980. This estimate is probably on the high side.* Total medical care costs for all CF patients would therefore be about $150 million, a sizable sum, although one considerably less than that sometimes suggested by the CF Foundation ($450 million). The foundation's projection of 1985 costs (in real terms) of $650 million is probably about three times too high.

OTHER COSTS

For CF, as for many diseases, the direct medical costs probably comprise only a small portion of the total cost of the disease. The total cost is the resources that could be saved if the disease had never happened. These costs would include: (1) the direct money costs to parents of raising a CF child compared to similar costs for raising a non-CF child—extra babysitting, travel, and time costs for seeking medical care would be included; (2) indirect or implicit costs—parents or other family members use what would have been leisure time or work time in caring for CF children; (3) lost earnings (net of schooling costs) associated with premature death or with disability; and (4) willingness of parents and patients to pay to avoid pain, discomfort, and social stigma or to avoid observing such events in one's children. While these costs are obviously difficult to quantify, they do represent real costs in the sense that parents would surely be willing to pay something to avoid the mental anguish and family disruption of caring for a child with a short life span.

---

*In a study of a small sample of Swiss CF patients, mean annual costs was found to be US $4,545 (date not given). Rossi E, Bühlman U, Kraemer R: Social and medical problems of cystic fibrosis in Switzerland. *Monogr Paediatr* 1981;14:192–201.

Another approach to valuing premature death in adults is concerned with the extra wages that have to be paid for riskier jobs. Estimates from such studies suggest that adults are willing to pay up to $500,000 (in 1980 dollars) to avoid one statistical death. It is probable that the analogous figure for children—what parents would be willing to pay to avoid one statistical death for a child—is less. The annual number of CF deaths is estimated to be approximately 500. In any case, despite the imprecision of these estimates, they suggest an order of magnitude estimate of $250 million per year.

The third approach to estimating the cost of illness is to look at earnings lost because of death or disability. We will look at this approach in some detail. The notion is that these earnings represent the additional output that could be made available if a cure for the disease could be implemented. Because people want to avoid disease for additional reasons, this estimate provides a lower bound. For example, a person would value avoiding disability not only because it would allow him to have higher earnings, but also because he would place positive value on reduced pain and discomfort. The foregone-earnings approach does not consider these "non-earnings" gains.

Human Capital Costs of CF

CF causes premature death, and it causes disability during the working years. (Disability among children will not be considered as having consequences for foregone earnings.) Total foregone earnings come from these two causes.

Death We will assume that CF patients would, in the absence of the disease, have had the same life expectancy and labor force participation or housekeeping involvement as people of equivalent age and sex. We also assume that the mean earnings reported by the Bureau of the Census in 1975, updated to 1980 by the rate of growth in nominal earnings, describe the individual's potential earnings. Present value estimates will assume a 1% annual growth in real productivity, and these earnings will be discounted at a real interest rate of 6%. The same procedure is applied to children as to adults. The present discounted value of a child's earnings stream is lower, of course, because more years would have had to elapse before labor force participation and earnings commence.

A recent estimate of the present value of foregone earnings per fatality by age and sex is shown in Table 28-1 (in 1975 dollars).

Table 28-1
Present Value of Average Foregone Earnings per Fatality, by Age and Sex, United States, 1975*

Age Group	Males	Females
0–14	$130,863	$ 92,241
15–24	225,992	156,059
25–34	247,881	153,131
35–44	205,687	126,642

*Source: Hartunian.[2] All figures are discounted at 6%. Household labor was valued at its market value.

The number of deaths in CF centers in 1979, by age and sex, is shown in the first two columns of Table 28-2. Since persons in CF centers represent about 77% of our estimate of all persons with CF, we assume that these deaths represent 77% of all CF deaths. (This probably leads to an overestimate of deaths, because persons outside CF centers are probably less ill.) Making this adjustment, the total value of earnings foregone by the CF deaths that occur in any one year is shown in the third and fourth columns. The total present value of all earnings foregone because of annual CF deaths was therefore about $74 million. As the age composition of CF fatalities changes over time, this estimate will change.

Disability As Hartunian[2] notes, "estimating the present value of foregone earnings for persons experiencing permanent disabilities and a loss of life expectancy is a complex exercise." Here we will try to produce only some order-of-magnitude figures. We will assume that, for children, disability days generate no foregone earnings cost. (There is little evidence that school days lost

Table 28-2
Present Value of Foregone Earnings from CF Fatalities, 1978*

Age Group	Fatalities Total and (in CF centers)		Total Earnings Foregone ($ millions)	
	Male	Female	Male	Female
0–14	90 (69)	129 (99)	14.3	14.4
15–24	92 (71)	78 (60)	20.8	11.4
25–34	23 (18)	26 (20)	6.9	4.8
35–44	6 (5)	0 (0)	1.2	0
All ages			43.2	30.6

*All deaths over age 32 are included in the 35–44 age group. Productivity is assumed to grow at 1% per year, and figures are in 1978 dollars, adjusted by the Consumer Price Index.

due to disability affect eventual performance.) For adults, the CF survey of adults indicates the mean number of work days lost from CF as 26 per person over 18 per year. The number of days lost for other illness, at 13, appears to be about the same as for the general population. For the 59% of CF adults who were employed, we use the Hartunian[2] wage figure of $31 per day (average over males and females in the 25–34 age category). For the 41% of CF adults who were not employed, we assume that the ordinary unemployment rate would have been 6%, and so attribute 35% unemployment to CF. The annual per person cost of that unemployment is then estimated by multiplying $31 per day ($47 in 1980 prices) by 200 working days per year. Table 28-3 shows the estimates of work loss, in 1975 dollars adjusted for productivity gains, for the set of CF patients who were adults in 1980. Total work loss costs amount to $16.2 million per year.

The total foregone-earnings cost from CF deaths was therefore $73.8 million in 1978, and the cost of disability was $16.2 million in 1980. As CF patients live longer and receive better educations, these costs paradoxically will rise, because the death of a young adult "costs" more than the death of a child. I have not tried to project these costs forward to a CF population with a different age composition. Nevertheless, even with the present age composition, foregone-earnings costs amounted to approximately $100 million per year.

Summary All of these figures, it should be emphasized, represent a lower bound for the gain from curing those already born with CF. They indicate the benefits that could be provided if existing cases of CF could be cured. About $150 million now spent on medical care could be made available for other purposes, about $100 million in additional output (and income) could be produced, and perhaps another $100–150 million worth of benefit from avoiding pain and death could be made available. The annual benefits would therefore total about $400–500 million. The present value of the stream of benefits from curing CF would (at 6% interest) therefore be approximately $9.1 billion. To judge whether CF research would then be "worth it" obviously requires more information than this benefit measure, however. It also requires some estimate of how likely it is that a dollar spent in CF research will result in a cure. It also requires some estimate of the cost of implementing whatever cure is discovered.

Research directed at discovering ways of preventing CF births would probably have a lower net benefit (although it may have a higher probability of success). Preventing CF births would avoid the $150 million in medical care costs, but the value of lost productivity and pain avoided would be counted only if the foregone CF births were replaced by other births. If prevention requires married couples to avoid having children when they are identified as carriers, then one should add to the averted medical costs some estimates of the net value to a married couple of avoiding a CF birth but also not being able to have healthy children. Against this benefit one must compare the costs of implementing a screening mechanism, with some adjustment for the possibility that parents may take a chance on having children even if they are identified as carriers. At present, there are no data that would permit even a crude calculation of the costs and benefits from research directed at finding a screening technique (see Chapter 2).

FINANCING CF

Are there better ways to finance care for CF patients than are presently used? At the current time, about $150 million is spent on their medical care. The bulk of this expenditure is associated in some way with the 128 nationwide CF centers, although much of that is incurred in hospitals and is not part of any center's budget. Moreover, it appears that no aggregation of center budgets has been published, so that there is no way of knowing what part of total actually is incurred in centers.

Since the total cost is not known, it should not be surprising that the division of sources of funding is not known. Data from a few centers, and information from the survey of CF adults, suggest that private insurance covers nearly half of CF costs, with the remainder coming from crippled children's, Medicare, Medicaid, or state programs. Even among adults, where insurance coverage should be more difficult to get, 77% were covered by private health insurance. The median percentage of expenses not covered by insurance is 20%, and the median percentage of income paid out of pocket is 10%. For the U.S. population as a whole, about 88% have some insurance coverage, and about 30% of all expenses are not covered by third-party insurance. On the other hand, 21% of CF adults paid more than 30% of income out of pocket for medical expenses, which surely would be regarded as an unacceptably large proportion. In summary, while the typical CF patient has fairly good insurance coverage, there is a nontrivial fraction with poor coverage.

The strikingly large portion of CF costs covered by conventional catastrophic insurance is consistent with the recent results of Zook and Moore[3] in that much catastrophic illness is chronic, and many hospitalizations are repeat admissions for the same disease. One implication of this result is that some out-of-pocket payment, at least over some range of expenses, may serve the useful purpose of limiting use and encouraging economy in the choice of source and method of treatment. In other words, CF costs are not "bolts from the blue," and it may be desirable to give the families of patients some financial incentives to control expenses. Moreover, the gains from these incentives can be shared with the families themselves in the form of lower insurance premiums, at least in a properly designed private insurance arrangement.

While the level of private insurance coverage is quite high, there is also a substantial share of tax-supported finance, support that must be regarded as in jeopardy in the present period of budget cutting. Ultimately, the availability of funds for CF from public sources, as for all such programs, depends on the willingness of the taxpaying public to provide such support. That willingness in turn depends, at least as a first approximation, on taxpayers' generosity as filtered through short-run budgetary considerations. There is no way to argue that more money "ought" to be devoted to CF, at least not without knowing and being able to evaluate the alternative uses to which the

Table 28-3
Annual Foregone Earnings Cost from Disability, Adult CF Patients, 1978–1980

	Percentage of Adults (over 18)	Estimated Number (assuming 3150 patients over 18)	Cost per Patient (1980 dollars)	Total Cost ($ millions)
Employed	55	1733	1692	2.9
Unemployed	45	1417	9400	13.3

funds could be put. The alternative might be national defense (and even here there would be considerable debate on valuation), but it also might be other welfare expenditures, or lower taxes, or care for some other kind of illness.

IMPROVEMENTS IN PRIVATE-SECTOR FINANCING

If one cannot really argue whether more public funds should be devoted to CF care, one can ask about present and alternative private-sector arrangements. To begin this discussion, we first present some stylized facts about the level and distribution of CF medical care costs: (1) The disease is chronic and has an annual average medical cost per patient which is about eight times the average expense per capita. (2) CF can be diagnosed without a great deal of difficulty. (3) The demand for care by individuals with CF varies across individuals. Some will be very severely ill, while others will have only mild symptoms. (4) Care protocols for CF are not standardized; there is considerable variation in the type and cost of care which meets acceptable standards. (5) The bulk of care for CF patients is rendered in (mostly hospital-based) CF centers, coordinated and partly funded by the CF Foundation.

The CF patient can, in principle, be subject to preferred-risk rating and moral hazard. Preferred-risk rating refers to the fact that, unless the insurance market is regulated, persons known to be worse risks will be charged more for health insurance. Moral hazard arises when insurance coverage affects the amount and type of medical care chosen, when people incur larger expenditures because insurance covers the bill. While people with CF cannot choose to avoid medical care entirely, they could potentially have considerable discretion about how much care, where, and at what cost.

To some extent, the social purpose of insurance is to cause moral hazard to occur. One of the reasons why we have an interest in subsidizing insurance coverage for poor people is a desire to encourage them to use more medical care than they would have used without insurance. But once the socially desired level of use is reached, then moral hazard works against efficiency, because it encourages people to use types of care that are not worth their extra cost, because it prevents people from making intelligent and informed choices between cost and quality, and because it offers incentives to overuse in a quantitative or qualitative sense.

Since it is very difficult (and costly in itself) to control use by regulatory measures, economists have favored several ways of encouraging purchasers of medical care to compare costs and benefits, some of which might be suitable for CF. One way is by having the patient pay something out of pocket, so that cost savings for society are matched by cost savings to individuals. Since there is some discretionary care in CF, in style if not in volume, provision of some financial deterrents to overly lavish care would seem to be desirable, at least at the margin for nonpoor families. Bacause the distribution of expenses may be bimodal, with patients either being mildly or severely ill, it might be desirable to combine a small deductible (to discourage marginally useful care in mild cases) with a modest copayment applied to large expenses. In any case, the socially optimal arrangement, for CF as for other illnesses, would probably require an upper limit on total out-of-pocket payments which is positively related to income.

The second way of offering incentives for patients would be to permit the patient to choose between competing health plans (HMOs, health alliances, insurance firms), with each plan providing coverage for a particular style of care (perhaps with closed-panel or exclusive-dealing arrangements), and with less costly plans rewarding their customers with lower premiums. CF centers might consider offering such plans. For example, a CF center might offer a particular regime of care, including hospitalization, in return for a fixed annual payment, and probably with some copayments. It could then "subcontract" hospitalization and other services it did not produce.

While both of these methods begin by operating on demand, by offering incentives to patients, they will also affect incentives to suppliers—doctors and hospitals. When patients pay something out of pocket, they become more conscious of relative costs, and this consciousness serves to discourage the use of care; whatever providers suggest, we know that use falls. There is ample empirical evidence for this proposition for the general public, although it has not been investigated for CF patients or for other chronic illnesses. When a plan must keep its premiums low to remain competitive, it will often choose to offer financial incentives to physicians and hospitals to avoid the care that is costly but only marginally beneficial. These incentives can take the form of capitation, salaries, profit-sharing, or reductions in fees under fee-for-service. Some of the incentives to providers could lead to underprovision of care, but the competition of other plans presumably inhibits such behavior.

In order to bring about this kind of competition, two major alterations in current policy have been discussed. First, current tax incentives to overly lavish insurance coverage should be removed and persons rewarded (perhaps with tax incentives) for choosing lower-cost forms of care. Second, persons should be permitted to make cost-reflecting choices. This could occur if there were several plans in a city offering CF care, and the family could choose which one it preferred. The beneficiary of public funds could be given a government voucher spendable on whatever plan the family selects.

The expectation is that competitive arrangements like these will control costs and improve the efficiency of the health care system. There are two types of questions one may ask about the relationships of competition to the financing of CF: (1) Can competition principles be appropriately applied to financing care for people with CF? (2) Would development of competition in the rest of the health-care system affect the financing of CF? Some concerns about these questions have been raised by the CF Foundation.

COMPETITION IN FINANCING OF CF

At present most CF patients are registered with one of the network of CF centers across the country, accredited by the Cystic Fibrosis Foundation. The centers coordinate care; they are usually affiliated with a hospital that produces inpatient care. To my knowledge, there is no cost information to permit one to judge whether or not these centers are operating efficiently. Cost is not relevant to foundation certification, and no general cost data are available.

While the intent of the CF foundation in establishing these centers seems entirely to have been praiseworthy, and while there is no gross evidence of overly costly practices, this sort of arrangement appears to be extremely questionable on economic grounds. About all one can say is that it would be surprising if the lowest-cost care of acceptable quality were rendered by the centers, since they are nonprofit institutions with considerable de facto monopoly power.

Some investigation of their costliness—even the relative costliness of one center compared to another similar center—might be helpful. In any case, there seem to be few potential benefits, and some costs, from protecting centers from competition. If a center is indeed efficient, it has nothing to fear from competition, and if it is not efficient, it should be subject to competitive pressures. "Efficiency" here is defined in the broad sense to include both low cost for whatever type of care is produced and delivery of the appropriate type of care.

There are two qualifications to this optimistic judgment. The first is that, for competition to work properly, patients have to be able to judge quality. If it is the case for CF (as apparently is true with open-heart surgery) that larger volume leads to higher quality care, and if the CF centers have larger volume, their ability to succeed depends on their ability to convey this message of higher quality. Second, and related, is the point that there may be economies of scale at a given quality. If this is true, the larger CF center will always be able to underprice any competition. Of course, if the CF center must carry some of the overhead cost in a tertiary care facility, then it may not wish to cut its price. However, for efficiency it should do so anyway.

Even if competition among CF providers does not harm and may enhance the care of CF patients, will there not be some adverse consequences from competition in the health care system as a whole? In particular, under competition there will be a reduction in "cross-subsidization"—situations in which revenue from some set of patients or services is less than the cost of services, but the shortfall is made up from the excess of revenue over costs from other products.

How much cross-subsidization there is for CF patients (or even if it is positive) is not presently known, partly because of lack of a clear definition of costs but mostly because of absence of information on costs or revenue. The CF Foundation has apparently accepted the view of the Association of American Medical Colleges that the teaching hospitals, in which most CF centers are located, use revenues from nontertiary patient care to cross-subsidize tertiary care facilities such as the centers.

The fear is that the ending of cross-subsidies would not bring forth direct funding as a replacement. These fears are based on the assumption that additional revenues will not be available for CF, but the reason for this assumption is not clear. Can we assume that present support for CF care, largely private (via insurance or donations) but partly public, represents the maximum that people are willing to pay for care? On the contrary, perhaps private individuals would be willing (indeed eager) to pay more for insurance that covers catastrophic diseases, especially if removal of the cross-subsidy reduces what they have to pay for more routine care.

Other than the general fear of change of established organization, it seems that the worry that funding will not be provided is based on an assessment of "politics," an assessment that support would be politically infeasible. The general theoretical principles of political economy which might be given this matter are clear. In a democratic society, activities of general or public benefit should be decided in a way that permits explicit acknowledgment of the cost and a decision (usually political) on whether benefits exceed that cost. Is replacing the implicit and hidden subsidy by an explicit political choice not desirable? If taxpayers or their representatives would reject a larger subsidy in favor of a smaller one, how can one argue that the larger subsidy is appropriate?

The objectives of the CF Foundation, or of CF patients, do not necessarily coincide with those of the citizenry as a whole; if taxpayers or their representatives are properly informed but are not willing to pay for a high level of care, perhaps there ought not to be a high level of care, despite any inconvenience or reduction in quality imposed on patients. Of course, if it is information that is deficient, then the remedy is obvious. It is just not proper (although it may be politic) to support a self-interested position, to argue against competition on the grounds that it will make apparent a subsidy which was heretofore hidden, and which would be rejected if made a subject of explicit political choice. In short, if reimbursement policies which result from competition would be inadequate to allow higher cost CF institutions to continue to provide their present range of services, then the range of services perhaps ought not to be provided.

The other fear is that, if health maintenance organizations or other closed-panel arrangements dominate a competitive system (and, despite the rhetoric, it is by no means obvious that they will), then those plans may limit the patient's freedom of choice and may restrict their ability to get care from a CF center. Competition does not, however, really limit choice; rather it permits people to choose that combination of (limited) benefits and premium cost that they most prefer. If a family chooses an HMO that provides CF care with its own primary care physicians, because the cost is lower than at a CF center even though the number of services is somewhat limited, the family has chosen this limitation; it has implicitly judged that the extra care it would have gotten at the CF center was not worth the extra cost. All of this assumes, of course, that people will know what they are buying when they pick a plan in a competitive system. Despite positive attempts to foster the flow of information and to simplify choices, some mistakes will occur. If CF centers really do offer a product whose benefits are worth the cost, it will be their job to convince plans and patients of that fact. If what people are willing to pay for such specialized care centers (either directly for care or indirectly through donations) is not sufficient to cover their costs, then their services, even if they are of undoubted value, are not valuable enough.

All of this theoretical discussion assumes that the ability of CF patients to pay for care is adequate, either because of resources they themselves have to draw on or because of public subsidy. "Adequacy" is not an objective concept, but really only reflects a social willingness to devote resources to this purpose. Another possible effect of competition is that, by reducing current subsidies to CF patients, largely hidden in the private sector, the chronically ill will not be able to buy as much health insurance or as much medical care as might be regarded as adequate. "Adverse risk selection" will, it is feared, raise the price of health insurance to chronically ill patients. The concept refers to a situation in which different people have different risks (expected values) of illness and of medical expenses.

There are two conceptually distinct (but often practically combined) aspects of market behavior in this situation. First, and probably most important as far as most people are concerned, if insurers can accurately distinguish high risks from low risks, competition will force them to charge higher premiums per unit coverage to those with higher risks. Second, if insurers cannot accurately distinguish high and low risks, so that premiums do not fully reflect risk differences, then low risks will buy lower levels of insurance coverage and high risks higher levels. Total premiums will be greater for high risks even if they paid the same premium per unit of coverage. (There is also a second-round phenomenon in which insurers may notice that expense per unit of coverage is higher for those with more insurance, and so further raise (experience rate) the premium for comprehensive coverage.) Here, the amount of coverage is used as an (imperfect) signal of the level of risk. The result is that total premiums for the chronically ill will be higher than those of the healthy; it is even possible that the chronically ill will not be willing to purchase coverage at premiums that would satisfy insurers, and will be refused coverage when lower premiums are quoted. The objection then is that, compared to a situation in which total premiums are more uniform, it is "unfair" to charge the ill more for the same nominal benefits (but higher expected payment) than is charged to the well. The problem, for most people, is clearly one of equity, although there are some efficiency aspects as well which seem to be of concern primarily to economists.

Let us consider the first case, partly because it is simpler and partly because it probably approximates the CF case (since an insurer can usually determine at low cost that an applicant has a person with CF in his family). Under competition, such a family would be charged a higher premium for any level of coverage compared to an otherwise similar family. The premium would reflect the differences in expected losses (according to our medical expense data, by about a factor of six to eight for a family with one CF child), plus administrative costs. Actuaries (and economists) would generally regard this situation as "actuarially proper"; after all, the product (insurance) sold to the CF family does cost considerably more, so it should sell for more.

For most of us, however (including most economists), what is proper may not seem fair. It is bad enough that a family should suffer CF; charging more for insurance seems to add insult to gross injury. The critical point, however, is that this unfairness reflects a social judgment about the proper distribution of money income; it is on a par with the judgment that low real income associated with poverty that is not one's fault ought to be offset by taxes and transfers or subsidies. There are two crucial implications: (1) The decision on whether to offset the actuarial difference in premiums, and how much of that difference to offset, ought to be a social decision, made according to the political process we have selected for making such decisions. As argued above, it ought not to be hidden in the complexities of insurance regulation. If we are to have taxation for social goals, it ought not to be concealed as taxation by regulation. (2) The form of taxation used to pay for this social goal ought to be the best one available, judged either by equity or efficiency.

The outcome of all of this would suggest, for the short run at least, that a desirable arrangement would be one involving (1) competition in the market for insurance, along with (2) explicit public transfers (cash payments) to those CF families regarded as deserving, and (3) the transfers financed by explicit (not necessarily earmarked) taxes. Points (2) and (3) could probably be achieved by a system of tax credits (implicit vouchers) along the lines suggested by Enthoven[4] in his competitive strategy, but with the credit substantially increased for families with CF or other chronic diseases.

How would this arrangement compare with the present one? The objection that "adequate" credits would not be politically feasible is not a convincing one, for the same reason as those mentioned above: political acceptability is in itself the touchstone of adequacy. Moreover, compared to community rating, a system of premiums related to risk is superior on three counts: (1) By lowering the premiums to low risks, it encourages them to purchase appropriate insurance. In contrast, under the current arrangement, the implicit excise tax on premiums of low risks discourages coverage, and we know that coverage is lowest among young good risks. Indeed, if premiums were actuarially proper, it is quite possible that low risks would choose high levels of coverage. (2) By raising the premium to high risks, it discourages excessive coverage by them. (3) By using hopefully less distortive taxes to finance transfers to the ill, it avoids both distortions in insurance purchases and the inequity of a poor person who is moderately healthy subsidizing the coverage of a high income family with a chronically ill member.

In the short-run, explicit transfers, and not limits on competition, are the proper way to deal with differentiation of risks. Mandatory community rating and open enrollment, as in the Gephardt-Stockman bill, are an inefficient and duplicitous way of achieving social goals. Such a provision could also make it more difficult for CF patients to obtain coverage, since insurers and health plans would naturally want to avoid offering coverage to CF patients if they could not charge higher premiums. Restriction on premiums is the cause of unavailability of coverage. Having the state provide coverage as insurer of last resort seems desirable, although what the premium should be for such coverage, and how it should be subsidized, should be decided by the principles above. It is undesirable to use a carrier pooling arrangement, since that would continue the implicit excise tax.

One final comment on short-term solutions. I suspect that if tax subsidies to health insurance were eliminated, and health plans were unrestricted in this competition, there would be little more premium differentiation than there is now. In many cases, employers or employees would still choose group purchasing and would cover the CF family at uniform premiums, largely for the "long-run" reasons to be discussed below.

To some extent, these explicit subsidy arrangements are, and will continue to be, imperfect. We know that political choice and taxation are unlikely to achieve perfection. Fortunately, it is possible to think of an alternative arrangement for dealing with CF (or other chronic illness), one with a longer time perspective. The arrangement is based on the idea that the onset of chronic illness, and the higher insurance premiums that would accompany it, is a catastrophic event that people ought to insure against. In particular, it has long been agreed that compulsory coverage of catastrophic illness is in the public interest. Those who favor comprehensive national health insurance, and those who would want to limit its coverage, all agree on the need for protection against catastrophic expense. Even a competitive strategy, as outlined by Enthoven,[4] Feldstein,[5] and others, envisions providing catastrophic coverage to all, although the insurance policy itself could be "produced" in the private sector. What needs to be added is the notion that some, perhaps much, of catastrophic illness is chronic. While such illness may begin as a "bolt from the blue," it often implies high expenses for many years. A catastrophic policy ought, therefore, to include a "guaranteed renewability" feature, which permits the family to continue to purchase coverage at a premium level regardless of whether or not chronic illness strikes. Such a feature would also (ordinarily) specify the amount of coverage that could be purchased at this premium, and the feature would, of course, raise the premium for the catastrophic coverage. Recent economic research strongly suggests that this kind of "multiperiod" policy is likely to be the most efficient way of incorporating experience into insurance premiums. The time to insure against chronic illness is before it strikes. Indeed, such a requirement could also greatly reduce the tendency for high risk people with hidden risk to shop around.

The guaranteed renewability or conversion feature is a part of many health insurance policies currently sold. Moreover, employment-related group health insurance usually contains a kind of implicit guaranteed renewability, in the sense that, despite the onset of chronic illness in the family, coverage will be maintained with no additional premium charge. It is highly desirable that this implicit coverage be made portable and compulsory, at least for that level of coverage and income for which there is social interest.

In summary, adequate provision of insurance for CF patients is part of the general problem of adequate coverage for all kinds of catastrophic illness and should be treated in that context. Competitive arrangements are consistent with adequate coverage, and indeed will help to improve the functioning of markets.

CONCLUSION

Does competitive legislation "rewrite the social contract" to provide access to adequate amounts of medical care? Perhaps not. Competition holds the potential for considerable reductions in cost, for CF patients and for others. It is true that competitive arrangements often will not support cross-subsidies in firms' pricing structures. If a subsidy is desired, it will have to be made explicit, and subjected to explicit political choice. But such an arrangement would seem to be desirable in a democratic society, not objectionable. It is by no means obvious that governmental support will be cut if persons concerned about CF, along with others concerned with other chronic disease, present the facts about needs and costs. There is, after all, no basis in competitive markets for a budget-cutting juggernaut; bureaucrats with a mania for cutting budgets are no more likely to be right or to be invulnerable to criticism than free-spending bureaucrats. The object is to permit people, both as patients and as citizens, to make informed choices about how much medical care they want. If indeed the financing of catastrophic and chronic care makes the medical system only a "little more expensive"—a conjecture that I believe to be true—then the political will to provide the larger personal benefits that come from that small cost should be easy to muster.

REFERENCES

1. Rossi E, Buhlman U, Kraemer R: Social and medical problems of cystic fibrosis in Switzerland. *Monogr Paediatr* 1981;14: 192–201.
2. Hartunian N: *The Incidence and Economic Costs of Major Health Impairments.* Lexington,

Massachusetts, Lexington Books, 1981.
3. Zook C, Moore F: The high cost users of medical care. *N Engl J Med* 1980;302:996–1002.
4. Enthoven A: *Health Plan*. Reading, Massachusetts, Addison Wesley, 1980.
5. Feldstein M: A new approach to national health insurance. *The Public Interest* 1971; 23:93–105.

INDEX